**DeWeese and Saunders'**
# OTOLARYNGOLOGY—HEAD AND NECK SURGERY

*Eighth Edition*

DeWeese and Saunders'
# OTOLARYNGOLOGY–HEAD AND NECK SURGERY

*Eighth Edition*

## DAVID E. SCHULLER, M.D.
*Professor and Chair*
*Department of Otolaryngology*
*Director*
*Comprehensive Cancer Center*
*Arthur G. James Cancer Hospital of Research Institute*
*The Ohio State University*
*Columbus, Ohio*

## ALEXANDER J. SCHLEUNING II, M.D.
*Professor and Chair*
*Department of Otolaryngology–Head and Neck Surgery*
*Oregon Health Sciences University*
*School of Medicine*
*Portland, Oregon*

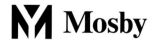
Mosby

St. Louis  Baltimore  Boston  Chicago  London  Madrid  Philadelphia  Sydney  Toronto

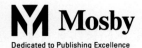

**Dedicated to Publishing Excellence**

Publisher: George Stamathis
Editor: Robert Hurley
Associate Developmental Editor: Lauranne Billus
Assistant Director/Production, Editing, Design: Frances Perveiler
Project Manager: Nancy C. Baker
Proofroom Manager: Barbara M. Kelly
Designer: Nancy C. Baker
Manufacturing Supervisor: Kathy Grone

Printed in the United States of America
Composition by Clarinda
Printing/binding by Maple-Vail

Mosby–Year Book, Inc.
11830 Westline Industrial Drive
St. Louis, Missouri 63146

**Library of Congress Cataloging in Publication Data**
Schuller, David E
    DeWeese and Saunders' otolaryngology—head and neck surgery.—
8th ed. / David E. Schuller, Alexander J. Schleuning.
        p.   cm.
    Rev. ed. of: Otolaryngology—head and neck surgery / David D.
DeWeese . . . [et al.]. 7th ed. 1988.
    Includes bibliographical references and index.
    ISBN 0-8016-6842-5
    1. Otolaryngology.   2. Head—Surgery.   3. Neck—Surgery.
I. Schleuning, Alexander J.   II. DeWeese, David D., (David Downs),
1913-  .   III. Title.   IV. Title: Otolaryngology—head and neck
surgery.
    [DNLM:   1. Otorhinolaryngologic Diseases—diagnosis.
2. Otorhinolaryngologic Diseases—therapy. WV 100 S3845d 1993]
RF46.0753 1993
617.5' 1—dc20
DNLM/DLC
for Library of Congress                                          93-34733
                                                                      CIP

1  2  3  4  5  6  7  8  9  0      98  97  96  95  94

# Contributors

**Thomas F. DeMaria, M.D.**
*Associate Professor*
*Department of Otolaryngology*
*The Ohio State University*
*Columbus, Ohio*

**David D. Hamlar, D.D.S.**
*Resident*
*Department of Otolaryngology*
*The Ohio State University*
*Columbus, Ohio*

**William H. Saunders, M.D.**
*Professor Emeritus*
*Department of Otolaryngology*
*The Ohio State University*
*Columbus, Ohio*

**Alexander J. Schleuning, II, M.D.**
*Professor and Chair*
*Department of Otolaryngology–Head and Neck Surgery*
*Oregon Health Sciences University School of Medicine*
*Portland, Oregon*

**David E. Schuller, M.D.**
*Professor and Chair*
*Department of Otolaryngology*
*Director, Comprehensive Cancer Center*
*Arthur G. James Cancer Hospital and Research Institute*
*The Ohio State University*
*Columbus, Ohio*

**Michael Trudeau, Ph.D.**
*Associate Professor*
*Department of Speech and Hearing Science*
*Department of Otolaryngology*
*The Ohio State University*
*Columbus, Ohio*

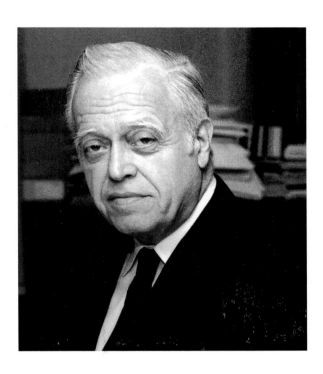

*In memory of*
*David D. DeWeese, M.D.*

*On March 1, 1990, David D. DeWeese passed away at the age of 76. Dr. DeWeese was a major force in the specialty of Otolaryngology–Head and Neck Surgery for over 3 decades and a leader in establishing the resurgence of this discipline. As such, his activities and society honors are too numerous to list, but David DeWeese would be happy to realize that his ultimate, greatest contributions to medicine were his unflagging interest in medical education. Those who knew him realized his greatest pleasure was derived from teaching students and guiding residents in a manner which grasped their attention and interest. David DeWeese's judgments, thoughts, and methods are very important in this textbook and will remain so. We miss his guidance and friendship.*

# Preface

The eighth edition of this textbook marks the first time in its 33-year existence that both of the original authors have not been involved. In order to honor them for their tremendous contributions, we have decided to rename this and all subsequent editions *DeWeese and Saunders' Otolaryngology–Head and Neck Surgery,* so that their names will forever be linked to this textbook. The goals of the eighth edition remain the same as that of all previous editions, and that is to serve as a resource for otolaryngology–head and neck surgeons, primary care physicians, medical students, nurses, dentists, and allied health professionals. The eighth edition is intended to provide a basic foundation for residents in otolaryngology–head and neck surgery as a means of building a comprehensive fund of knowledge with additional study and experience.

We appreciate the evaluations of the seventh edition which were universally positive and supportive of the reorganization of that edition to facilitate easier reference. The eighth edition includes revisions to ensure a contemporary presentation of information in an efficient fashion that did not translate into a notable increase in size of the textbook. We are firmly committed to the concept that the ever-expanding knowledge and technology embraced by contemporary otolaryngology–head and neck surgery can be presented in an introductory fashion in a textbook of this size. Hopefully, the readership recognizes the limitations of in-depth presentations of subject matter accompanied by a textbook of this size.

Once again, our families and staff were fully supportive of the time demands associated with undertaking this revision. We are indebted to them for their help, patience, and understanding. This eighth edition is dedicated not only to the past contributions of Dr. DeWeese, but to Dr. Saunders' continuing input and advice, as well as to the Schuller and Schleuning families and the expert editorial input of Mosby–Year Book.

David E. Schuller, M.D.
Alexander J. Schleuning II, M.D.

# Contents

# PART I
# General Considerations

# 1

# Physical Examination*

## William H. Saunders

Examination of the ears, nose, and throat is basically a study of epithelium. Using brilliant illumination, the physician can inspect directly or indirectly most parts of the upper respiratory passages. A few parts, such as the nasal accessory sinuses and the middle ear, cannot be visualized. Nevertheless, the examiner usually can infer their condition from the appearance of adjacent mucous membranes.

## Lighting

A great many lighting systems are used. Some, such as the flashlight or otoscope, are entirely inadequate when used anywhere except in the ear. Others, such as electric headlights, are of variable worth, depending on their brightness.

The light par excellence is that reflected from the otolaryngologist's head mirror. A clear 150-W light bulb provides the light source and is placed just behind and to the right of the patient.

More and more often, otologists are using the operating microscope for diagnostic examination of the ear (Fig. 1–1) and sometimes for other parts of the otolaryngeal examination. This instrument provides brilliant illumination and also binocular vision and magnification. It may be used with the patient in either the sitting position or the supine position; because of its delicate balance, it is as convenient to use as any other lighting system.

*The text for Chapter 1, with slight modifications, and Figs. 1–4, 1–8, and 1–18 from Saunders WH: Ears, nose, and throat. In Prior JA, Silberstein JS, and Stang J: *Physical diagnosis: the history and examination of the patient,* ed 6, St Louis, 1981, Mosby. Used by permission.

## Adjustment of Head Mirror

To adjust the head mirror, first place it well down over the left eye so that the back of the mirror actually touches the skin or glasses (Fig. 1–2). Then the right eye is closed and the light is focused on the patient's face to a small, brilliant spot. Too often the beginner fails to keep the light bright by neglecting to move his or her head toward or away from the patient. Obviously, since the focal length of the mirror is fixed, the only way the examiner can maintain a sharp focus is by adjusting his or her head position. Once the left eye is focused, the right eye may be opened for binocular vision. After a little experience, focusing becomes automatic and preliminary monocular focusing is not necessary.

If they wish, patients or students can observe part of their own examination.

## Use of Tongue Depressor

The tongue depressor is held in the left hand (Fig. 1–3), so that the right hand is free to hold other instruments or to position the head. Tongue blades may be either wooden or metal. Most examiners prefer the wooden ones.

The blade should be placed on the middle third of the tongue. If placed too far anteriorly, it causes the posterior part of the tongue to mound up, obscuring rather than exposing the pharynx. On the other hand, most patients gag if the blade touches the posterior third of the tongue.

The correct maneuver depresses the tongue and scoops it forward at the same time. The blade is held in the corner of the mouth so that it will not be in the way of the instruments held in the right hand. The examiner should not press the patient's lower lip against the teeth.

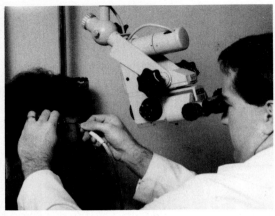

**FIG 1–1.**
Operating microscope used as a diagnostic instrument. Small aural suction tip aspirates serum or pus from the ear canal or middle ear.

The tongue is a strong, muscular organ. One need not (and occasionally cannot) depress the entire tongue at one time. Sometimes, to press more firmly, the examiner may use two tongue blades, one placed on top of the other.

### Warming the Mirror

To prevent fogging, the examiner should use the flame of an alcohol lamp or some other heating device to warm the mirror to be used in exam-

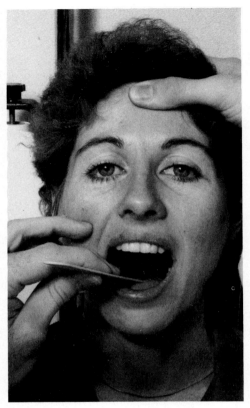

**FIG 1–3.**
Use of the tongue depressor. Note that the left hand is braced on the cheek; the right hand positions the head.

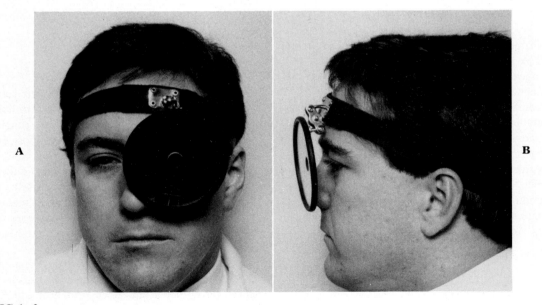

**FIG 1–2.**
**A,** head mirror in position. Note that the mirror is worn *very close to the face*. It is directly in front of the pupil. **B,** lateral view.

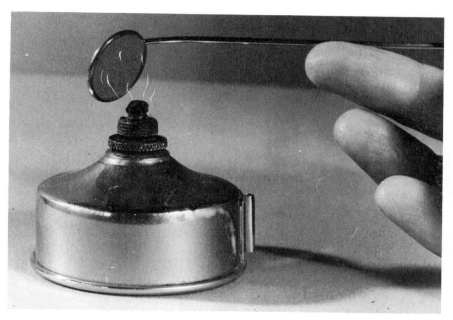

**FIG 1–4**.
Warming the mirror. The glass surface is placed directly over the flame.

ining the nasopharynx or larynx (Fig. 1–4). The glass surface is placed directly into the flame for a few seconds. The back of the mirror is then tested for warmth on the examiner's hand. Because children are sometimes frightened by the open flame, one may simply dip the mirror into a container of warm water before examining a child.

**Patient Position**

The patient's position is very important in otolaryngeal examinations. He or she should sit erect, with knees together and head 10 to 12 inches from the back of the chair (Fig. 1–5). Many patients tend to slump and to slide their hips forward in the chair. The use of a headrest is discouraged because it fixes the head in one position and hinders the adjustments of the head position that are constantly required. The correct position is not restful, but the examination is not so long as to be tiring.

**Cotton Applicator**

The cotton applicator is one of the most useful instruments in otolaryngeal examination. Examiners must learn to prepare their own, because commercial applicators are never satisfactory. A stiff

wire is used, and a small piece of loose cotton is wound around it (Fig. 1–6). The tip of the wire is placed in the center of the cotton, and the cotton is twisted onto the wire, leaving a small tuft at the end. The tuft may be firmed or left loose as the situation demands. Beginners often make their cotton applicators too thick or fail to have a very small tuft at the tip.

**EARS**

**Auricle**

Conditions that affect the auricle are usually obvious and require little explanation. Some patients have congenitally deformed auricles that are too small (microtia) or too large (macrotia). Other ears stand out too prominently from the head (lop ears). Rarely, patients have no auricle at all, or a normal auricle may be associated with an atretric ear canal.

The examiner should inspect and palpate the auricle. Movements of the auricle and tragus are painful in external otitis but not in otitis media. A postauricular scar indicates an old mastoidectomy.

A small dimple just in front of and slightly

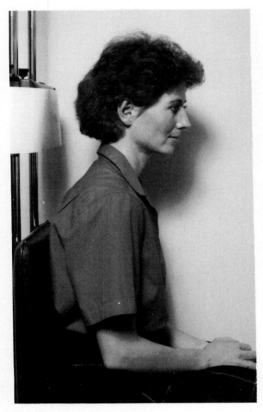

**FIG 1–5.**
Patient position. The head and shoulders are drawn forward, with the hips against the back of the chair. Each patient must be positioned, often several times.

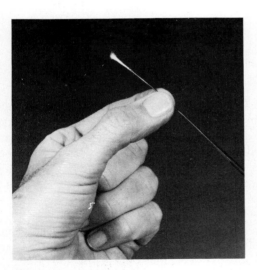

**FIG 1–6.**
Winding a cotton applicator.

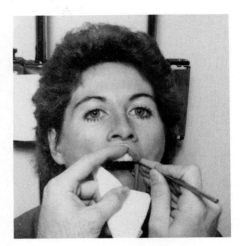

**FIG 1–7.**
Laryngeal examination. See also Fig. 1-22.

above the tragus is a remnant of the first branchial apparatus.

The need for inspection of the external ear is so obvious that it is frequently neglected, although it should require only a few seconds. Occasionally *tophi*, which are small white deposits of uric acid crystals that result from gout, are seen along the margins of the auricle. The gnarled, thickened *cauliflower ear* is the result of repeated trauma to the cartilage. Evidence of injury or congenital malformation is usually obvious.

Next, inspect the external auditory canal and the tympanic membrane. In physical diagnosis, the tympanic membrane, or eardrum, may be regarded as a translucent membrane through which the otologist views normal anatomy and pathologic processes in the middle ear.

### Cleaning the Ear Canal

The most important step in preparing to examine the eardrum is making sure that the ear canal and the surface of the drumhead are clean. Wax, particulate matter, and all pus and secretions must be meticulously removed. This caution seems obvious, but neglect of this preliminary is the rule. Actually, an experienced examiner may take several minutes to remove debris from the ear canal before he or she is ready to study the drumhead.

There are three methods of cleaning the ear canal. Often the simplest way is to remove particulate matter with a cerumen spoon (Fig. 1–8) or

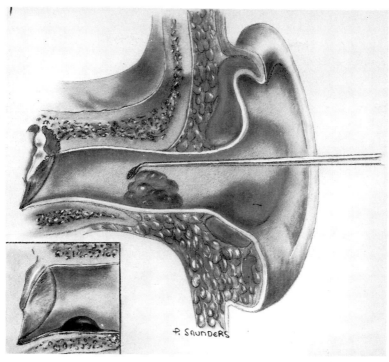

**FIG 1–8**.
Use of the cerumen spoon. *Inset*, hematoma, which is easy to produce unless care is taken.

cotton applicator while working under direct vision through the ear speculum. The cerumen spoon should be inserted above the impacted wax; careful withdrawal of the spoon, which has been engaged in the wax, dislodges the wax. Because the epithelium covering the inner aspect of the ear

canal is exquisitely sensitive, great care must be used in these manipulations to prevent pain and bleeding.

The second method of cleaning the ear canal is by irrigation (Fig. 1–9). Tap water at body temperature is used, because water at any other tem-

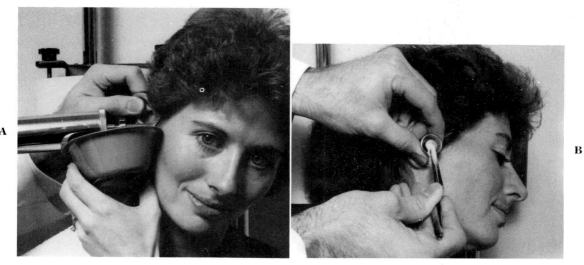

**FIG 1–9**.
**A,** aural irrigation using tap water at body temperature. **B,** drying the ear canal after irrigation.

perature stimulates the inner ear and causes dizziness. If the cerumen to be removed is solidly impacted, and especially if it is dry and hard, irrigation may not be successful unless the patient instills a few drops of mineral oil or so-called sweet oil in the ear for three or four nights before the procedure. This oil softens the cerumen and makes it easy to remove by irrigation. Various proprietary preparations that will soften wax are also available. Most are harmless, although some have been known to cause a local inflammatory response.

The third method involves use of a small, angulated suction tip to aspirate pus or other liquid material from the ear canal (see Fig. 1–1). This method is especially useful when pus coming through a perforated drumhead fills the middle ear as well as the ear canal. Then, by carefully advancing the suction tip, the examiner may clean the ear canal and finally the middle ear space itself of pus so that the ear can be examined.

A good way to begin the examination is to pull the auricle upward and backward and the tragus forward (Fig. 1–10). This maneuver opens the meatus and may even provide a good view of the drumhead. It also lets the examiner select an aural speculum of proper size.

## Examination With Aural Speculum

Most otologists employ a metal ear speculum and a head mirror to examine the drumhead. Generally, other practitioners use an electric otoscope (Fig. 1–11). Whichever instrument is used, the

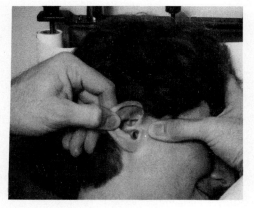

**FIG 1–10.**
Spreading the meatus, a preliminary step.

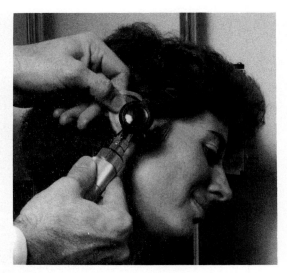

**FIG 1–11.**
Electric otoscope. Traction on the auricle straightens the canal.

principles of examination are the same. *The speculum selected should be the largest that will fit the canal.* The student usually makes the mistake of choosing a small speculum when a large one could be used.

The speculum is inserted to straighten and slightly dilate the cartilaginous ear canal (Fig. 1–12). About halfway to the eardrum the cartilage ends and the supporting wall becomes osseous. Here speculum pressure is painful. The epithelium lining the bony portion of the canal is very thin and exquisitely sensitive. One must be very gentle when cleaning the inner half of the ear canal, even more so than when cleaning the outer surface of the drumhead. In adults the ear canal may be straightened by pulling upward and backward on the auricle; in young children and infants it is straightened by pulling the auricle downward.

The position of the patient's head is important in aural examinations (Fig. 1–13). One might think that with the patient's head perfectly upright the examiner could look directly into the ear canal and see the drumhead. This is a common error. Because of the oblique direction of the ear canal, the patient's head must be tipped sidewise (toward the opposite shoulder) for easy examination of the canal and drumhead. Students who neglect this step find that they are looking at the wall of the ear canal and not at the drumhead. It is usu-

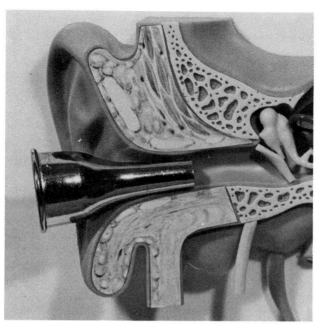

**FIG 1–12**.
Speculum dilates and straightens the cartilaginous portion of the ear canal. If it is pressed against the inner, bony canal, it causes pain.

ally necessary to change the head position several times to visualize all parts of the tympanic membrane.

### Layers of Drumhead

The drumhead has three layers: an outer squamous epithelium, an inner cuboidal epithelium, and a middle fibrous layer. These layers constitute the structure of the pars tensa, which comprises

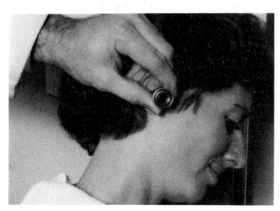

**FIG 1–13**.
Note that the head is tipped to one side. Also, note how one hand holds both the speculum and the auricle.

almost all of the drumhead. In a very small part superiorly, known as the pars flaccida, the middle fibrous layer is absent.

Because perforations in the drumhead heal without formation of a fibrous layer, the area of perforation is often translucent or even transparent. The healing also leaves that portion of the drumhead flaccid and therefore more easily moved by pneumatic pressure (through an otoscope) than the rest of the drumhead.

### Color of Drumhead

The color of the drumhead is important because it is relatively constant in health. The normal drumhead is usually pearly gray. In disease the color may be amber (serum in the middle ear), blue (hemotympanum), dead white (pus in the middle ear), or red or pink (myringitis or infection of the middle ear). Ordinarily the tympanic membrane is quite shiny.

Dense white plaques representing deposits of calcium-like material are seen in some drumheads affected with tympanosclerosis. Other patients with tympanosclerosis have drumheads showing small white flecks scattered throughout the pars tensa. Ordinarily these minor changes merely indicate old, healed disease of the middle ear or tympanic membrane. They do not mean active disease.

**Position of Drumhead**

The position of the drumhead is oblique with respect to the ear canal. The upper posterior part of the drumhead is closer to the examiner's eye than is the lower anterior part. This obliqueness is more pronounced in infants than in adults. Sometimes all of the drumhead cannot be seen because the floor of the ear canal is at a higher level than the lowermost part of the drumhead. Also, the anterior part of the drumhead may be hidden by prominence of the bony wall of the ear canal.

The drumhead is also very slightly conical, with the concavity external. When pus forms in the middle ear because of otitis media, intratympanic pressures are raised and the drumhead actually bulges outward. Sometimes this bulging is in one part of the drumhead only; at other times the entire drumhead bulges so that none of the landmarks are seen.

A "retracted" drumhead occurs when intratympanic pressures are reduced. In such a situation, the entire drumhead is depressed by external atmospheric pressure, the malleus is left in sharp outline, and the malleolar folds are accentuated. This alteration of tympanic pressure is common. It occurs when the eustachian tube is obstructed (because of adenoiditis in children, for example, or as a result of too rapid descent during air travel). Whatever the cause, the tube no longer ventilates the middle ear properly, and oxygen is absorbed from the middle ear and mastoid air cells into the bloodstream. A partial vacuum results. A transudate of blood serum may partially fill the middle ear to relieve the vacuum, and the drumhead appears amber. Also, an air-fluid level may be seen, or bubbles of air may appear in the amber fluid.

**Landmarks**

The landmarks visible in the normal drumhead (Figs. 1–14 and 1–15) vary with differences in its translucency. The *malleus* is the primary landmark. At its upper end the lateral or *short process*

Anatomy to consider

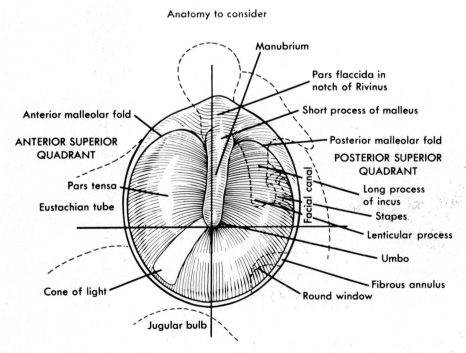

**FIG 1–14.**
Relationships of important middle ear structures. (From Miglets A, Saunders WH, Paparella MM: *Atlas of ear surgery,* ed 4, St Louis, 1986, Mosby. Used by permission.)

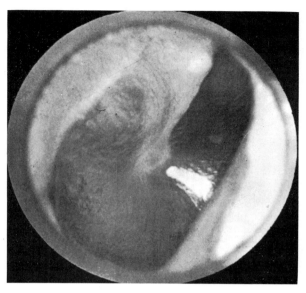

**FIG 1–15.**
Normal tympanic membrane. Note how the anterior wall of the ear canal obscures part of the drumhead. (From Buckingham R: *What's new,* no 193, North Chicago, Ill, 1956, Abbott Laboratories. Used by permission.)

stands out as a tiny knob. The manubrium, or the handle of the malleus, extends downward from the short process to the *umbo*. Both the short process and the manubrium are embedded in the drumhead.

When the drumhead bulges, the manubrium and the short process become less and less well seen until they finally disappear. On the other hand, when the drumhead is retracted, the malleus stands out prominently and the white bone of the short process shines chalky white through the drumhead.

The *anterior* and *posterior malleolar folds* are seen superiorly and enclose between them the *pars flaccida* (Shrapnell's membrane). These folds or epithelium become more prominent when the drumhead is retracted.

The *annulus* is the peripheral fibrous ring of the tympanic membrane that fits in the tympanic sulcus. It looks whiter or denser than the rest of the drumhead. It is complete except superiorly, where it is deficient between the anterior and posterior malleolar folds. The importance of the annulus in aural diagnosis cannot be overstressed. The examiner must follow the annulus completely around. It is at the periphery of the drumhead that important perforations often occur, and they will not be found unless the annulus is systematically examined.

The *light reflex,* or *cone of light,* reflects from the anterior inferior quadrant when the drumhead is in its normal position and its outer epithelium is normal. The light reflex extends inferiorly and anteriorly from the umbo. Sometimes the reflex becomes broken or muddled, and sometimes it is missing altogether. Such changes usually indicate a disease state, but variations of the light reflex alone should not be overemphasized.

The *long process of the incus* is frequently visible posterior to the manubrium of the malleus. Whether or not it can be seen depends on the translucency of the tympanic membrane and the shape of the posterior wall of the bony ear canal. When the incus is seen, the examiner can be fairly certain of a normal middle ear.

Less frequently seen than the incus is the *chorda tympani nerve.* It crosses transversely behind the drumhead at about the level of the short process of the malleus.

### Special Examinations

Special examinations include demonstration of function of the eustachian tube, examination with the pneumatic otoscope, and examination of the temporomandibular joint.

### Demonstration of Function of Eustachian Tube

Function of the eustachian tube may be demonstrated by looking at the drumhead under magnification while the patient holds his or her nose and swallows. This maneuver reinforces the opening of the eustachian tube, which usually occurs during swallowing. At the moment of swallowing, the drumhead can be seen to flick outward and then inward again, a movement indicating patency of the eustachian tube. Also, the patient feels a sensation of pressure in one or both ears at the height of the swallow.

Demonstration of tubal patency is important in some patients who have certain symptoms (deafness, tinnitus, or dizziness) that may be due to occlusion of the tube.

### Examination With Pneumatic Otoscope

The pneumatic otoscope (Fig. 1–16) enables the examiner to compress air in the ear canal. This procedure exerts pressure against the drum-

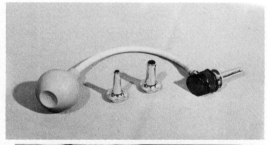

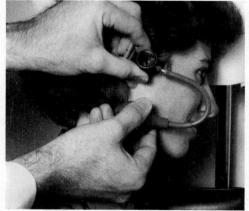

**FIG 1–16.**
**A,** pneumatic otoscope. The speculum that fits this otoscope is attached. The magnifying lens may also be used with the usual type of speculum if magnification only is desired. **B,** pneumatic otoscope in use. Note the lateral tipping of the head, the correct position for all otoscopic examinations.

head, and it moves in and out as a bulb in the examiner's hand is alternately squeezed and released. Pinhole perforations that may not be apparent can be detected as middle ear secretions are drawn through them by suction. Certain drumheads will be found to be more flaccid than normal (usually because of healed perforations), and others will not move at all because they are perforated. Adhesions or fluid in the middle ear may also prevent normal excursions of the drumhead. The pneumatic otoscope can be used to suck down secretions from the epitympanum or mastoid antrum in patients having chronic mastoiditis or to evacuate the middle ear of fluid after myringotomy.

### Examination of Temporomandibular Joint

It is common to see a patient with ear pain that is the result of referred pain from the temporomandibular joint. If the index fingers are pressed into the joint spaces as the patient opens his or her mouth widely, pain may be elicited (often only on one side) when the mouth is closed. This pain is commonly referred to the ear, and the patient complains not of a pain in the jaw joint but of otalgia. A common cause is malocclusion.

## OROPHARYNX

The pharynx is divided into three parts—oropharynx, nasopharynx (epipharynx), and hypopharynx. A patient complaining of sore throat might have a generalized pharyngitis involving all three parts; or only one part might be involved, as in carcinoma of the epiglottis, for example. It is necessary to use *different instruments* to see these three parts; and unless *all* parts of the pharynx are examined, the examiner cannot expect to establish a correct diagnosis for the patient complaining of sore throat.

Before any part of the pharynx is examined, the patient should remove his or her dentures. This is important, not only because the denture itself covers much of the mucosal surface to be examined but also because the lower plate tilts upward, causing gagging, and the upper plate often drops.

### Tongue

The tongue is examined by both inspection and palpation. Palpation is necessary because some diseases of the tongue cause no surface manifestations and otherwise cannot be detected.

### Lingual Papillae
The filiform papillae are the most numerous. Keratinization of these papillae produces the well-known "coated tongue." Fungiform papillae are scattered throughout the filiform papillae and are especially abundant on the sides and apex of the tongue. These papillae look like small red dots because the underlying vascular connective tissue shines through the thin epithelium. The circumvallate papillae are arranged in an inverted V at the posterior part of the tongue. The apex of the V is at the foramen cecum. The circumvallate papillae are best examined with a laryngeal mirror.

### Ventral Surface
The ventral surface of the tongue toward the floor of the mouth is smooth and shows large veins. In older persons these veins may become varicose.

### Frenum
The frenum is found in the midline under the tongue. Rather rarely, this structure is abnormally short and causes so-called tongue-tie. If the patient can protrude his or her tongue between the teeth, there should be no difficulty with speech.

### Glossopalatine Fold
The glossopalatine fold connects the tongue with the palate and is known as the anterior tonsillar pillar.

### Other Structures
Other structures associated with the tongue are the lingual tonsils, the valleculae, and the glossoepiglottic folds. These structures are best seen with the laryngeal mirror and therefore will be described with the laryngeal examination.

## Floor of Mouth

The floor of the mouth is another region where palpation is important. Tissues here are loose, and neoplasms sometimes are detectable only by palpation. The submaxillary salivary ducts may contain calculi that are best felt by palpation. Bimanual examination, using one gloved finger inside the mouth and the other hand outside, is best.

## Submaxillary Salivary Gland

The submaxillary salivary gland empties into the floor of the mouth on either side of the frenum of the tongue. The orifices of the ducts are quite small, but they may be seen as small dark spots from which clear fluid can be expressed by pressure over the submaxillary gland. The orifices of the sublingual glands are not seen.

## Teeth and Gingivae

There are 32 teeth in the full adult dentition. The teeth are inspected for evidence of caries and malocclusion. Sometimes it is worthwhile to percuss a tooth to elicit tenderness in patients suspected of having a dental abscess.

The gums should be inspected and at times palpated. Bleeding from the gums is not unusual and at times is the sole cause of expectorated blood. In adults the gums gradually recede from the teeth and expose a larger and larger amount of tooth root.

## Buccal Mucosa

The parotid duct opens into the buccal mucosa opposite the upper second molar (Fig. 1–17). The orifice is larger than the submaxillary orifices and readily admits a probe. Pressure over the parotid gland produces a clear secretion.

In most adults yellowish glandlike structures may be seen shining through the buccal mucosa. They are sometimes mistaken for an abnormality, but they actually represent sebaceous glands lying directly under the squamous epithelium of the oral cavity.

Frequently a white line of parakeratin in the buccal mucosa is adjacent to the occlusal surfaces

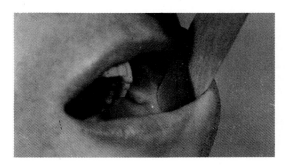

**FIG 1–17.**
Parotid (Stensen's) duct, opposite the second superior molar tooth.

of the molars. This results from invagination of the cheek between the teeth or from sucking on the cheek.

## Palate

There is a distinct difference in color between the hard and soft palates. The soft palate is pink and shows fine vessels under the mucosa. The hard palate is whiter, is more irregular, and has rugae running transversely. Scrutiny shows the orifices of ducts of mucous glands in the posterior part of the hard palate. In heavy smokers the duct orifices look like tiny red dots scattered throughout the hard palate. This is one form of nicotine stomatitis.

## Uvula

The uvula is a muscular organ that varies greatly in length and thickness. It is sometimes bifid. Frequently a small squamous papilloma is attached to the uvula, the free margin of the soft palate, or the anterior tonsillar pillar.

## Tonsils

Normally the palatine or faucial tonsils do not project much beyond the limits of the tonsillar pillars (Fig. 1–18). They are approximately the same color as the rest of the oral mucosa. There are crypts in the tonsils in which squamous epithelium exfoliates. Some patients have deep crypts; in such patients plugs of epithelial debris push toward the surface, where they appear as white spots on the tonsils. In other patients white spots on the tonsils may indicate follicular tonsillitis.

It is sometimes helpful to retract the anterior tonsillar pillar for better visualization of the tonsil. Palpation of the tonsil is important if a neoplasm is suspected.

Tonsillectomy is common. It is usually simple to tell when a patient has had a tonsillectomy because of the changes in the anterior or posterior pillars that occur with healing. Also, lymphoid nodules may remain in the tonsillar fossa and form so-called tonsillar tags.

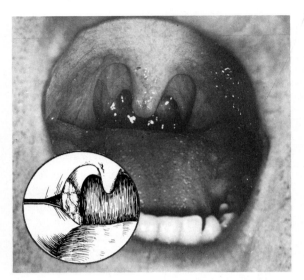

**FIG 1–18**.
Oropharynx. Note the anterior and posterior tonsillar pillars. *Inset,* use of the pillar retractor in withdrawing the anterior pillar.

### Posterior Pharyngeal Wall

The posterior pharyngeal wall is the part of the pharynx that is visible when one uses only a tongue blade. Students are prone to speak of hyperemia or "injection" of the throat when they see any vessels on the posterior pharyngeal wall. Usually these small vessels are normal and do not represent inflammatory changes. The same appearances may be seen on the tonsillar pillars and the soft palate.

Small, irregular spots of lymphoid tissue are common in the mucosa of the posterior pharyngeal wall. They are red or pink. The lateral pharyngeal bands are found behind the posterior pillar, running downward from the nasopharynx toward the base of the tongue. These pink bands are also composed of lymphoid tissue. The lymphoid elements in the pharynx (adenoid, lateral pharyngeal band, faucial tonsil, and lingual tonsil) are commonly known as *Waldeyer's ring*.

## NASOPHARYNX

### Technique of Mirror Examination

The best way to examine the nasopharynx is with the postnasal mirror. A No. 0 mirror is the correct size. Ordinarily, children older than 5 years and most adults can be examined without difficulty. Because of the small size of the mirror, all of the nasopharynx cannot be seen at one time. Instead, the mirror is rotated slightly to bring successive areas into view.

First, after the mirror is warmed, the tongue is depressed to create a large space in which to place the mirror (Fig. 1–19). The light must be focused sharply in the space next to the uvula, where the mirror will be placed. The mirror is placed to one side of the uvula and *almost* touches the posterior pharyngeal wall. It is held in the right hand, and the fingers are braced against the patient's cheek to steady the hand. The left hand holds the tongue blade in the corner of the mouth so that it will not obstruct the examiner's view of the oral cavity.

The patient is instructed to breathe quietly through the nose so as to allow the soft palate to drop away from the posterior pharyngeal wall. Often the patient will protest, "I can't breathe through my nose with my mouth open!" but quiet reassurance and encouragement help to accomplish the desired palatal relaxation.

The beginner is likely to make the following two mistakes:

1. Failing to depress the tongue adequately, so that there is insufficient space in which to place the mirror.
2. Failing to focus the light sharply on the mirror.

## Choana

The choanae are the posterior openings of the nose. Each choana is separated from the other by the posterior end of the vomer. The posterior ends of the turbinates can be seen in each side (Fig. 1–20). The turbinates (especially the inferior turbinate) vary greatly in appearance, even in normal noses. Sometimes they appear engorged with blood and look swollen and bluish. At other times the posterior tips are pale. Such changes may indicate an allergic or vasomotor disorder.

## Posterior End of Vomer

Unlike the anterior part of the nasal septum, the posterior end of the vomer is always in the midline. However, it is not unusual to see a thickening of the vomer caused by hyperplastic mucosa.

## Middle Meatus

The middle meatus is an important space clinically because it is here that pus may be seen running from the maxillary sinus. Pus runs from the ostium (not visible) into the middle meatus and then drips over the posterior end of the inferior turbinate, a pathognomonic sign of maxillary sinusitis. The frontal and anterior ethmoid sinuses also drain into the middle meatus, but they drain

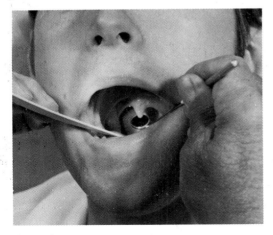

**FIG 1–19.**
Nasopharyngeal mirror in place. The key to this examination is *adequate tongue depression*.

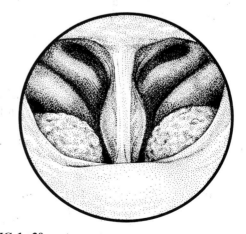

**FIG 1–20.**
Nasopharynx. Superior, middle, and inferior turbinates can be seen. Note hyperplastic mucosa on the septum and inferior turbinates (mulberry turbinates).

higher and more anteriorly, and their drainage is best seen by means of the nasal speculum.

## Inferior Meatus

The inferior meatus is not well seen and has no clinical significance so far as its visualization with the postnasal mirror is concerned.

## Superior Meatus

The superior meatus (above the middle turbinate) blends with the region known clinically as the sphenoethmoid recess and is the site of drainage of the sphenoid sinus and posterior ethmoid cells.

## Eustachian Tubes

The eustachian tubes open laterally into the nasopharynx just under the torus tubarius. Over the torus is the fossa of Rosenmüller. The orifice of the tube usually looks a little pale or yellowish and is about as large as the eraser end of a lead pencil. Normally the tube is closed, but it opens whenever the patient swallows or yawns.

## Adenoid

The adenoid (pharyngeal tonsil) is a collection of lymphoid tissue present in every child and in some adults. It grows from the roof and posterior wall of the nasopharynx, extends into the fossa of Rosenmüller, and blends with that lymphoid tissue known as the lateral pharyngeal band. Sometimes the adenoid, particularly in adults, seems to be only a clump of lymphoid tissue that is centrally located.

In children the adenoid is prone to cause occlusion of the eustachian tube, which interferes with aeration of the middle ear. This causes deafness and predisposes a child to middle ear infection. Large masses of adenoid tissue also produce nasal obstruction and mouth breathing in infants and young children.

## Posterior Aspect of Uvula and Soft Palate

The posterior aspect of the uvula and soft palate and the lateral wall of the pharynx are also visible in the postnasal mirror. Ordinarily no pathologic changes are found here except for nasopharyngitis, causing hyperemia and exudate formation. Many physicians do not locate the site of the patient's sore throat because they fail to examine the nasopharynx. They use only a tongue blade to inspect the oropharynx, but the oropharynx may be normal when the patient has a severe nasopharyngitis.

## Other Methods of Examination

Other methods of examination include palpation and use of the nasal speculum, the nasopharyngoscope, the pharyngoscope, and the palate retractor.

### Use of Nasal Speculum

The nasal speculum may be used to see a small part of the nasopharynx by looking through the anterior nares. Such examination can be done in some patients without previous vasoconstriction, but in most patients a good look depends on careful shrinkage of the inferior turbinate. Anterior rhinoscopy is particularly useful in children who will not permit the use of a nasopharyngeal mirror. In adults it is a convenient route through which to remove tissue from the nasopharynx for biopsy.

### Palpation

The nasopharynx is palpated in some instances, but better and less distressing methods of examination are usually available. If one does use palpation, it is important to place several thicknesses of tongue blades between the patient's molars or to invaginate the patients' cheek between his or her teeth with the right index finger. This is done to prevent the patient from biting the examiner's finger.

### Use of Pharyngoscope

The pharyngoscope (Fig. 1–21), which produces brilliant illumination, is held in the patient's mouth to give a view of the nasopharynx (when the instrument is turned upward) or of the hypopharynx and larynx (when turned downward).

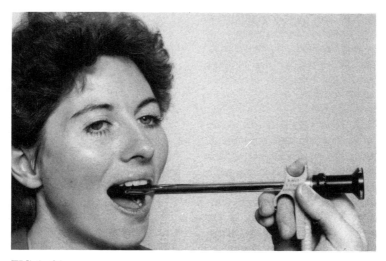

**FIG 1–21.**
Pharyngoscope—shows either the nasopharynx or the larynx.

### Use of Palate Retractor

The self-retaining palate retractor is a useful instrument for the occasional patient in whom there is insufficient space between the soft palate and the posterior pharyngeal wall to afford an adequate view of the nasopharynx. It also is useful when maximum working room is required, for example, during the biopsy procedure.

## HYPOPHARYNX AND LARYNX

The *approach to the patient* is exceedingly important. The examiner must adopt a calm, reassuring attitude and yet conduct the examination with firmness. Admittedly it is difficult to cope with the "gaggy" patient, but annoyance on the examiner's part only worsens the situation.

*Topical anesthesia* such as that provided by 4% cocaine, 2% tetracaine (Pontocaine), or 10% lidocaine (Xylocaine) is permissible but is not often needed by the experienced examiner. One should avoid spraying with compressed-air equipment because too much drug is likely to be administered in this way. Using an atomizer and bulb is safer.

Additional help in visualizing the larynx of a patient who continues to gag even after careful reassurance and application of topical anesthetic can be obtained through the intravenous administration of diazepam (Valium), 5 to 10 mg over 90 seconds. One must be sure to inject the drug into a large vein, since phlebitis may result if a small vein is used. This medication greatly quiets the overactive psyche, which seems responsible for the excessive gagging of certain patients. Its effect lasts about 20 minutes, after which time the patient is ready to leave the office.

The *position* of the patient is paramount in this examination. The patient must not be allowed to slouch or slump in the chair but must sit erect (in military posture). The chin is drawn forward. Both feet are on the floor with the knees together. The head is not placed in a headrest but is left free for adjustment during the examination.

The *tongue* is protruded as far as possible and held firmly by the examiner in a piece of gauze. The gauze is first laid over the tongue and then wrapped under it. This procedure keeps the gauze from wadding up on top of the tongue and obscuring the examiner's vision. It also protects the undersurface of the tongue from the sharp lower incisor teeth. The examiner then holds the tongue between the left thumb and the left middle finger while bracing the index finger against the upper lip or the upper teeth. If the patient cooperates and does not try to retract the protruded tongue, it is not actually necessary to pull on the tongue.

The *mirror* used for adults is a No. 5. The glass surface is warmed over an alcohol lamp, and the mirror back is tested on the examiner's hand for heat. The mirror is held midway along the shaft as a pen is held, not by the handle, and the *fingers are braced* on the patient's cheek.

The mirror is inserted into the mouth so that, as the edge advances, the glass surface is flush with the tongue. Thus the mirror is not introduced in its greatest diameter.

The mirror is placed with its back side against the uvula (Fig. 1–22). The uvula and soft palate are pressed upward in one smooth movement. Once contact is made, the mirror is not shifted about to any extent, although slight changes in its position are necessary for seeing all of the larynx. Touching the uvula and soft palate ordinarily does not cause gagging, but touching the back of the tongue does. In the mirror, anterior and posterior are reversed but right and left remain the same.

The patient is asked to breathe quietly through the mouth and is told that breathing regularly will prevent gagging. Sometimes, gaggy patients do best when they are asked to "pant in and out like a dog." After the examination has been completed during quiet respiration, the patient is asked to sound a highpitched "e-e-e," "a-a-a," or, best of all, "he-e-e." Almost all patients phonate too low and must be told to make a sound high in pitch. Most patients also phonate too briefly. A prolonged singing of "e-e-e" is desired; a short utterance does not give adequate time for examination. The examiner makes the same sound; in effect, the two sing a duet.

Some patients, when asked to phonate, will remain aphonic and shake their heads; others hold their breath. Careful explanation and reassurance do much to obtain cooperation.

The following are the most common mistakes made by the inexperienced examiner:

1. Does not explain what he or she intends to do before doing it.
2. Fails to position the patient properly.
3. Fails to focus light brilliantly on the mirror.
4. Does not elevate the uvula and soft palate with the back of the mirror.
5. Does not insist on a prolonged, highpitched "e-e-e."

## Hypopharynx

The hypopharynx is above the level of the larynx but below the part of the pharynx that can be

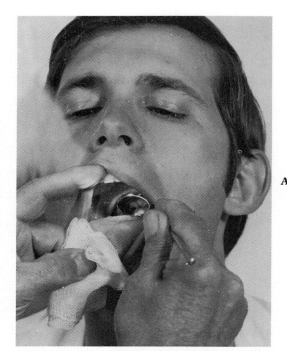

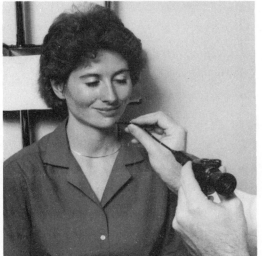

**FIG 1–22.**
**A,** laryngeal mirror in place. Both hands are braced. The instrument is held near the mirror end. One finger retracts the upper lip.

conveniently examined with a tongue blade. The following important structures are seen when one uses a laryngeal mirror.

### Circumvallate Papillae

The circumvallate papillae are arranged in an inverted V, with the apex at the foramen cecum.

The papillae vary considerably in size and prominence, and patients sometimes mistake them for lingual tumors.

### Lingual Tonsils
The lingual tonsils, visible in most adults, lie on either side of the dorsum of the tongue. They vary greatly in size and sometimes are extremely large. In the lingual tonsils one frequently sees small white spots that represent debris in crypts or, if the patient has active lingual tonsillitis, follicular exudate. When the lingual tonsils are enlarged, there is often a deep cleft between them.

### Valleculae
The valleculae are the cup-shaped spaces between the tongue and epiglottis. They are separated from each other by the median glossoepiglottic fold. Large veins are frequently seen in the valleculae, and they are normal. Cysts may form here and are usually thin-walled and yellowish or white. To see the valleculae more distinctly, one asks the patient to phonate.

### Epiglottis
The epiglottis is cartilaginous. Its shape, size, thickness, and color vary from patient to patient. The free edge of the epiglottis is usually thin and slightly curved. Sometimes (always in infants) the entire epiglottis is furled, in which case laryngologists speak of an "omega-shaped" epiglottis. The lateral glossoepiglottic folds and the median glossoepiglottic fold attach the epiglottis to the base of the tongue; the aryepiglottic folds attach it to the arytenoid cartilages.

The epiglottis (especially the tubercle) is usually in the way when the examiner wishes to see the anterior ends of the vocal cords. The patient is asked to phonate in a *high-pitched* "e-e-e" or "he-e-e" to draw the epiglottis out of the line of vision.

Although not a routine part of the examination, palpation of the hypopharynx with a finger is necessary in certain patients, not because visual examination is difficult but because tumors deep in the tongue or beneath the mucosa may not cause visible mucosal alterations.

The lateral and posterior walls of the hypopharynx are inspected along with the rest of the hypopharynx. Ordinarily nothing here confuses the examiner.

### Larynx
In studying the larynx, the beginner too often fixes attention on the true vocal cords alone, because these structures are so striking in their appearance and movement. But inspection of the true vocal cords is only part of the laryngeal examination.

### False Cords
The false cords lie directly above and slightly lateral to the true cords. They are capable of contracting and closing the larynx, but generally they remain quiet during examination. Sometimes, however, the false cords are so active that they preclude a good view of the true cords. Ordinarily the false cords appear dull pink and look thicker than the true cords.

### Laryngeal Ventricle
Directly under the false cords is a space called the laryngeal ventricle. It is not well seen by mirror laryngoscopy, but more of it can be seen by having the patient tilt his or her head sideward (ear toward shoulder).

### True Vocal Cords
The true vocal cords reflect light in such a way as to appear white and sharp edged in the laryngeal mirror. Of course, their color is not really white, and the edges are actually rounded.

Anteriorly the cords meet in the midline, where they are attached to the thyroid cartilage. Posteriorly they are attached to the vocal processes of the arytenoid cartilages. The anterior attachment is fixed, but the posterior attachment is mobile and allows the cords to open and close during respiration and phonation.

### Arytenoid Cartilages
The arytenoid cartilages form the posterior attachments for the true vocal cords. They are mobile and swing in and out with phonation and respiration. Their color is a dull red, and they appear as small mounds at the posterior end of the glottis (the space between the cords). The arytenoids also attach to the epiglottis via the *aryepiglottic folds*. In the aryepiglottic folds are smaller cartilages, the cuneiform and corniculate cartilages. The aryepiglottic folds, the false cords, and the true cords are the sphincters of the larynx. They

protect the lower respiratory passages from foreign bodies and help to build up intrathoracic pressure for coughing and other functions.

From the standpoint of the surgeon, who needs to know as exactly as possible the site of origin of laryngeal tumors, because of different lymphatic distributions, the larynx is divided into (1) a supraglottic area (posterior or laryngeal surface of the epiglottis, ventricular bands or false vocal cords, ventricles, arytenoids, and aryepiglottic folds), (2) a glottic area (true vocal cords), and (3) a subglottic area.

### Pyriform Recesses

The pyriform recesses are situated posterior and lateral to the arytenoids. They will dilate a

little if the patient says "a-a-a" in a low voice. Secretions may gather here, but they should disappear when the patient swallows. If they do not disappear, the patient is said to have a "pooling" sign, which suggests obstruction or paralysis of the upper esophagus.

### Laryngeal Examination

First, the cords are observed during quiet respiration (Fig. 1–23,A). They move only slightly, or not at all, and their color, configuration, and position are noted. The examiner also looks between the cords at the anterior wall of the trachea. In most patients a few tracheal rings can be seen, and sometimes the examiner can see all the way to the carina. He or she can do so best by kneel-

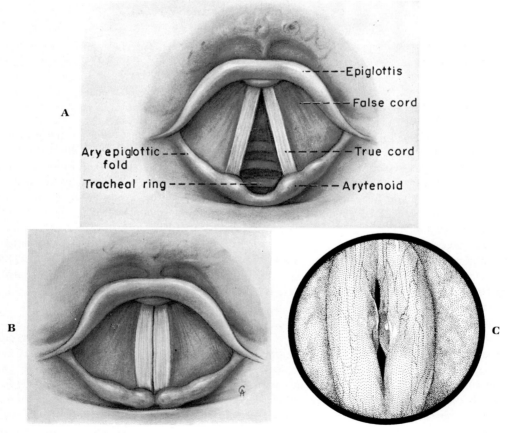

**FIG 1–23.**
**A,** larynx in quiet respiration. **B,** larynx during phonation. The mirror *reverses* anterior and posterior, but right and left remain the same. **C,** bilateral vocal nodules. A common condition to compare with the normal larynx as seen in **A** and **B.**

ing on the floor in front of the patient and looking upward into the laryngeal mirror.

After the larynx has been inspected during quiet respiration, the patient phonates as previously described. Phonation (Fig. 1–23,B) causes adduction of the cords, which can be seen to vibrate as sound is produced. They become more tense and appear elongated. Normally there seems to be perfect approximation of the cords, but in the aged there is a small space that cannot be closed. This space produces the quavering voice of the old man. If one vocal cord is paralyzed, it will lie fixed while the opposite cord moves in and out.

Tumors of the true cords prevent accurate approximation during phonation and therefore cause hoarseness. Malignant tumors of the larynx have a very favorable prognosis if the patient sees a physician as soon as he or she becomes hoarse and *if the physician then examines the larynx.*

The greatest difficulty in examining the larynx is trying to see the anterior commissure, which is often hidden by the tubercle of the epiglottis. Rarely, it is necessary to apply topical anesthesia and to use a retractor to displace the epiglottis. Usually, proper phonation effects adequate retraction.

The attachment of the true vocal cords to the arytenoid process causes a slight, cupshaped depression that is sometimes mistaken for an abnormality. Pellets of mucus resting on the cords may look like small tumors. If the patient coughs, many of these "tumors" will disappear.

The area directly beneath the true vocal cords (conus elasticus) is not entirely visible by mirror (indirect) laryngoscopy. Except for this area and the ventricle of the larynx, all parts of the larynx can be seen well with the laryngeal mirror.

Before the examination is completed, all parts of the larynx should be inspected during quiet respiration and phonation. Sometime during the examination the patient should be asked to turn the head and cough. A sharp cough indicates that the true vocal cords approximate. This functional test helps the examiner to differentiate between so-called hysterical aphonia and other causes of weak voice, or aphonia. Finally, the beginner is again cautioned not to fix attention on the true cords alone.

### External Laryngeal Examination

Complete examination of the larynx calls for palpation of the neck. The shape of the thyroid cartilage is noted, and the space between the thyroid cartilage and the hyoid bone is palpated. This space is a common site for a thyroglossal duct cyst. The space between the thyroid and cricoid cartilages is also palpated. Sometimes a lymph node is felt in patients with carcinoma of the larynx. The cricothyroid space is the site where an emergency tracheotomy may be done with the least bleeding.

Because the cricothyroid muscle is the only laryngeal muscle innervated by the superior laryngeal nerve, the function of that nerve may be tested by having the patient say "e-e-e" in a high pitch. This action causes a contraction of the normal cricothyroid muscle, and the cricoid cartilage is drawn upward. These events fail to happen if the superior laryngeal nerve is not intact.

Laryngeal crepitation is elicited by grasping the larynx (thyroid cartilage) between the thumb and index finger and rocking it vigorously from side to side. This maneuver should cause crepitation that can be felt on either side. If crepitation does not result, a postcricoid neoplasm may be cushioning the movements of the larynx across the vertebral column.

### The Fiberoptic Laryngoscope

The flexible fiberoptic laryngoscope (see Fig. 1–22,B) is the standard of care for the specialist. Rarely is this *not* used if one has difficulty with visualization.

After choosing the roomiest side of the nose, the examiner applies topical anesthesia to the nasal mucosa and also to the pharynx and larynx. Usually this is sprayed first in the nose and then downward into the hypopharynx and the larynx. The scope is passed through the nose until it eventually shows the epiglottis and larynx.

## NOSE AND PARANASAL SINUSES

### Nose

The nasal chambers are examined by inspection. They are inspected anteriorly and posteriorly with the nasal speculum and the postnasal mirror, respectively. A metal applicator wound with cot-

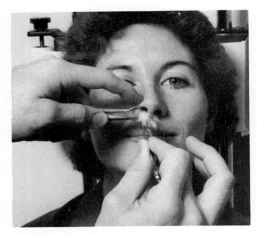

**FIG 1–24.**
Use of a vasoconstrictor. Most shrinkage comes by reducing the inferior turbinate. All intranasal manipulations are done under direct vision.

ton provides a useful instrument for light intranasal palpation.

*Lighting* is the same as already described. The light must be bright and focused to a small spot. Because the nasal chambers are several centimeters long, the position of the examiner's head that allows him or her to focus sharply in the nasal vestibule will not provide a bright spot of light in the posterior area of the nose. Therefore, to maintain adequate lighting, the examiner must constantly alter the relationship between the patient's head and his or her own.

*Vasoconstriction* (Fig. 1–24) is provided by

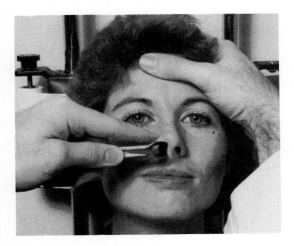

**FIG 1–25.**
Correct way to use a nasal speculum. Note positions of the left *thumb* and *index finger*.

topical application of 3% ephedrine in saline solution. Two percent cocaine has the added advantage of producing topical anesthesia. Shrinking the nasal mucosa (meaning the inferior turbinates in most instances) is necessary in many patients before complete intranasal inspection can be done.

Ephedrine may be sprayed from an atomizer, or it may be applied with wisps of cotton that have been wetted with the drug. The cotton wisps should be introduced along the inferior turbinate and left for several minutes. Sometimes it is important to obtain vasoconstriction in other areas, such as about the middle meatus and middle turbinate.

The *nasal speculum* is held in the left hand whether one is examining the left side or the right side of the nose (Fig. 1–25). The left index finger presses on the ala of the nose to anchor the upper blade of the speculum in place. The blades are inserted about 1 cm into the vestibule. The speculum is opened vertically (not transversely) to avoid painful pressure against the nasal septum.

The *examiner's right hand* is the real key to intranasal inspection, because it positions the head. Except when used for instrumentation, the right hand is placed firmly on the top of the patient's head and is used to change the head position from time to time (Fig. 1–26). Too much emphasis cannot be placed on this point. One must look at small areas successively. For example, with the patient's head erect the examiner can see the floor of the nose and the inferior turbinate but cannot see the septum well unless the head is turned sideways. Similarly, the examiner cannot inspect the middle meatus until the head is tilted backward. Use of a headrest is discouraged because it fixes the patient's head and prevents proper use of the examiner's right hand.

Every beginner makes the following mistakes:

1. Fails to adjust his or her head position to keep light sharply focused.
2. Opens the nasal speculum too little. Actually, unless the speculum is opened as completely as the nose will permit (and often this means as fully as the speculum will open), it is better to use no speculum at all.
3. Fails to tilt and turn the patient's head

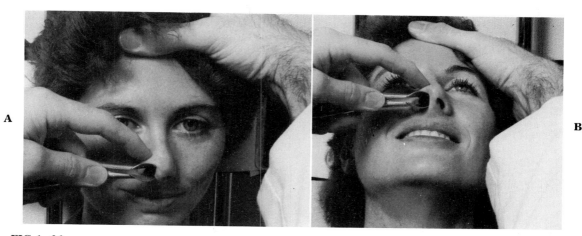

**FIG 1–26.**
**A,** head position necessary to see the floor of the nose, the inferior turbinate, and the septum. Note how *widely* the blades are opened. **B,** head position necessary to see the middle meatus, the middle turbinate, and the superior part of the septum. The *right hand* tips the head backward and thus is the real key to the examination.

with the right hand to see all parts of the nose.

4. Fails to use vasoconstrictors.

### *Examination*

The examination should include the vestibule, the mucosa, the nasal septum, the lateral wall of the nose, and the nasopharynx.

**Vestibule.** The vestibule of the nose is lined with skin and contains the nasal hairs, or vibrissae (Fig. 1–27). Except for folliculitis and fissures, no common diseases involve the nasal vestibule. The vestibule may be examined by tilting the tip

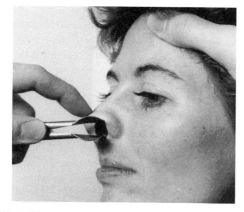

**FIG 1–27.**
Nasal vestibule. This part of the nose is lined with skin.

of the nose upward with the finger. A nasal speculum is also useful.

**Mucosa.** The nose is lined with respiratory mucosa except anteriorly, where there is skin, and far superiorly, where there is olfactory epithelium. The nasal mucosa is redder than the oral mucosa; therefore, students are prone to call normal nasal mucosa "hyperemic" or "injected."

**Nasal Septum.** The nasal septum is composed of both cartilage and bone. In virtually every adult the septum is not straight. Instead it gradually deviates from the midline to a greater or lesser degree, or it has developed a sharp projection (a spur or ridge) or a more rounded projection (a hump). Sometimes the anterior end of the nasal septum is dislocated and projects prominently into one nostril. In any case, such irregularities of the nasal septum ordinarily cause no disturbance unless they are severe enough to obstruct the airway. Sometimes crusting occurs at the site of the nasal septal deviation or spur, and bleeding results.

There is an anterior plexus of blood vessels in the mucosa of the nasal septum, and one can often see small arteries and veins here. This is the most common site for epistaxis (nosebleed).

The posterior end of the septum is formed by the vomer and is best inspected by using a No. 0 nasopharyngeal mirror. Here the septum is normally thin, but sometimes inflammatory tissue

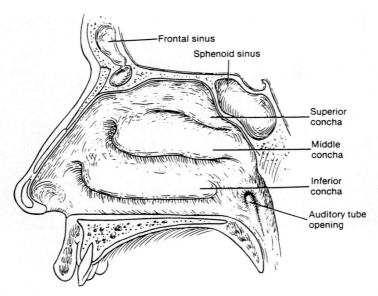

**FIG 1–28**.
Nasal lateral wall. The meati of the sinuses lie under the corresponding turbinate. The nasal orifice of the eustachian tube is located on the same horizontal plane and adjacent to the posterior end of the inferior meatus.

gathered symmetrically on either side gives a plowshare appearance to the vomer.

**Lateral Wall of the Nose.** The important structures of the lateral wall of the nose (Fig. 1–28) are the inferior, middle, and superior turbinates and their respective meatuses.

The *inferior turbinate* is a separate bone; the middle and superior turbinates are parts of the ethmoid bone. The inferior, the largest turbinate, lies like a finger along the lower lateral wall of the nose. It is erectile and swells periodically. This swelling may cause alternating nasal obstruction, which is especially troublesome at night to some patients, who must turn from side to side to relieve the congestion caused by the dependent turbinate.

The two inferior turbinates are not the same size in most patients. When the septum is displaced to one side, the inferior turbinate on the opposite side is prone to swell and fill the concavity. Normally the turbinate is deep pink and similar to the color of the rest of the nasal mucosa, but in allergic states it becomes blue or pale and the tissue becomes boggy and swollen. Inflammation of the nasal mucosa causes redness.

The *inferior meatus* is not seen in its entirety because of the overhanging inferior turbinate. The

nasolacrimal duct, which opens into the anterior part of the inferior meatus, is not seen.

The *middle turbinate* is seen by looking into the nose anteriorly. Sometimes a deflection of the nasal septum partially hides the structure. Occasionally the middle turbinate contains an air cell that enlarges its anterior end. Ordinarily the middle turbinate does not contribute seriously to nasal obstruction.

The *middle meatus* is a very important area; it lies lateral to the middle turbinate. Appearing as a cleftlike space, it often is poorly seen because of encroachment by the adjacent middle turbinate. Vasoconstriction and careful positioning of the head will make the middle meatus visible. Secretions from the frontal, maxillary, and anterior ethmoid sinuses drain here. The ostia of the sinuses are not visible.

**Nasopharynx.** In most patients the examiner can look completely through the nose and inspect part of the nasopharynx. Sometimes this is possible on only one side, because of a deflection of the septum or an unusually prominent inferior turbinate. The use of vasoconstrictors greatly increases the number of patients in whom the nasopharynx can be examined in this manner.

Having the patient say "kick" or "k" causes the

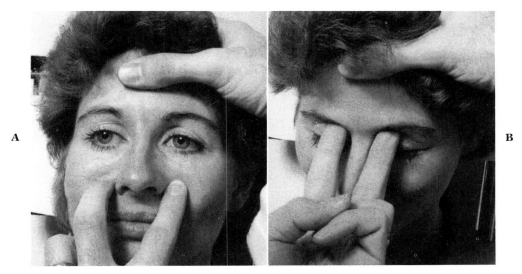

**FIG 1–29.**
**A,** testing the maxillary sinuses for tenderness. **B,** testing the frontal sinuses for tenderness.

soft palate to fly upward. This movement orients the examiner as to how far posteriorly he or she is seeing. It also provides information about the mobility of the palate.

## Paranasal Sinuses

Examination of the paranasal sinuses is done more indirectly than other otolaryngeal procedures. One cannot see into any of the sinuses, and only rarely can one see a sinus ostium. Information about the condition of the sinuses is gained, first, by inspecting and palpating the overlying soft tissues (maxillary and frontal sinuses); second, by noting secretions that may drain from the sinuses; and, third, by transillumination (maxillary and frontal sinuses only).

### Palpation and Percussion

Palpation and percussion may be done over the maxillary and frontal sinuses (Fig. 1–29). Simultaneous finger pressure over both maxillae will demonstrate differences in tenderness (Fig. 1–29,A). Palpation under the upper lip may demonstrate fullness not appreciated by inspection.

The frontal sinuses are palpated by finger pressure directed upward toward the floor of the sinus, where the sinus wall is thin (Fig. 1–29,B). Tenderness may be discovered in this way. Swelling caused by tumors or retained secretions (mu-

cocele) may cause a downward bulge in the floor of the frontal sinus. The ethmoid and sphenoid sinuses cannot be examined except by intranasal inspection.

### Where the Sinuses Drain

It is possible to determine which sinus is infected by discovering where a purulent discharge appears in the nose. It is important to use vasoconstrictors and a sharply focused light if one is to see a small stream of pus in the nose.

**Frontal and Anterior Ethmoid Cells.** The discharge is found well forward in the middle meatus and seems to come from high up.

**Maxillary Sinus.** The ostium is somewhat farther back in the middle meatus, and drainage occurs over the posterior end of the inferior turbinate. Therefore pus from the maxillary sinus often is seen best by using the postnasal mirror.

**Sphenoid and Posterior Ethmoid Cells.** The drainage is far posterior. The examiner sees secretions from the posterior sinuses by using the nasal speculum or the postnasal mirror. The pus runs down between the middle turbinate and the septum.

In addition to the older and more customary methods of examining the nose and nasopharynx, rigid fiberoptic endoscopes are now available. These instruments, which have advantages in certain situations, provide magnification and brilliant illumination and have variously angled lenses. A fiberoptic flexible instrument can be used to inspect the nose and nasopharynx. These are the same instruments used by surgeons and, in general, are better adapted for use in the operating room than in the office.

### What to Look For in Sinus Transillumination

**Frontal Sinuses.** As transillumination is done, the face of each sinus becomes light. Because the frontal sinuses are rarely the same size, the examiner may see a considerable difference in light reflex. Often neither side transilluminates well even in normal patients.

**Maxillary Sinuses.** There are red pupillary reflexes and crescents of light under the eyes, and the faces of the sinuses glow pink.

Although most pathologic changes affecting the ears, nose, and throat are recognized readily after a careful history and a thorough physical examination, some conditions remain obscure and require functional and laboratory tests to establish a diagnosis. The physical examination, therefore, is often supplemented by audiometric examination, vestibular examination, and roentgenography. Cultures and biopsies are also common. Endoscopic examination of the trachea and bronchi and of the esophagus is carried out when necessary.

All these procedures are discussed in detail in the chapters that follow.

# 2

# Basic Principles of Soft Tissue Surgery

All physicians need to understand the basic techniques of suturing, irrespective of their particular disciplines. This matter has particular reference to nonsurgeons. The primary care physician is frequently asked to care for minor lacerations and abrasions. The emergency department physician, family physician, pediatrician, and internist should have the skills needed to provide proper care for these problems. A prerequisite to learning the surgical management of minor soft tissue injuries is a fundamental understanding of the relative anatomy and physiology and an awareness of the pharmacology and toxicity of commonly used local anesthetics. This chapter is intended to provide the basic understanding necessary to allow the medical student and the practicing nonsurgeon to develop the techniques for providing optimal care for these minor injuries. This information will act as a starting point for the medical student with surgical inclinations to develop correct basic surgical skills.

## SKIN ANATOMY

Understanding of the anatomy is important to soft tissue surgery. The epidermis and dermis are the layers of the skin. The epidermis is the outer layer and is stratified squamous keratinizing epithelium. No capillaries go to the epidermis. Its metabolism is supported only by the diffusion from the capillaries in the dermis (Fig. 2–1). The dermis, in contrast to the epidermis, which is derived from ectoderm, originates from mesoderm and is actually a connective tissue. It contains the blood supply that supports the epidermis.

The skin is variable in thickness. Some of the thinnest skin in the body is in the eyelids, while the skin of the back is quite thick. Body skin can vary anywhere from 0.5 mm to 4.0 mm or more in thickness. The epidermis and dermis are anchored to the underlying subcutaneous tissue by bundles of collagen, which extend into the subcutaneous tissue from the dermal layer.

The epidermis, especially those layers which are keratinized, is a barrier to disease organisms. Keratin is somewhat waterproof and acts to protect evaporation of body fluids. This water-containing capability helps regulate body temperature.

The microscopic appearance of skin demonstrates that the epidermis has four or five layers in certain areas. The interface between epidermis and dermis is marked by interdigitating papillae. The dermis is divided into two layers. The papillary layer is thin and adjacent to the overlying epidermis. The deeper reticular layer is thicker. The capillary blood supply is located in the papillary layer of the dermis.

There are numerous skin appendages. Fingernails and toenails are actually a form of keratin. Sweat glands, hair follicles, and sebaceous glands are all skin appendages.

The blood supply of the skin is located within the subcutaneous tissue, which is immediately below the dermis. This subdermal plexus provides the blood supply to the overlying skin. The blood supply to the dermis is not great. Possibly because it consists of connective tissue, the dermis does not have extreme vascular requirements. The actual capillary beds arising from the subdermal plexus are within the connective tissue that is immediately below the epidermis. These capillaries also surround some of the skin appendages.

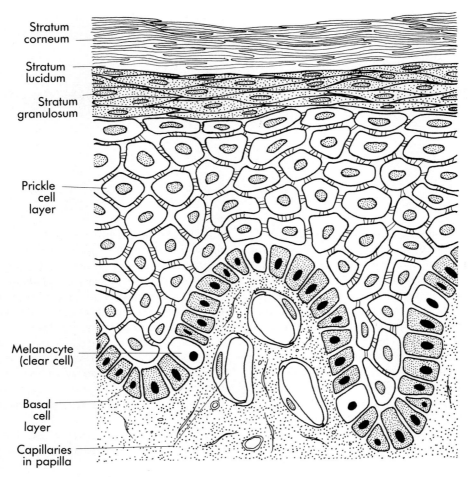

Stratum corneum

Stratum lucidum

Stratum granulosum

Prickle cell layer

Melanocyte (clear cell)

Basal cell layer

Capillaries in papilla

**FIG 2–1.**
The subdermal plexis provides the important blood supply supporting the epidermal and dermal layers of the skin.

There are certain important anatomic factors about the relationship between skin and facial musculature that have clinical relevance. The mimetic muscles actually insert into the undersurface of the dermis. This results in the transmission of mimetic muscular contraction to the facial skin, with the ultimate result being the means of expressing emotion. As the mimetic muscles contract, they cause the overlying skin to fold at right angles to the plane of contraction of the muscle. The fine creases created in the skin from this repetitive folding are referred to as the relaxed skin tension lines (Fig. 2–2). They are excellent locations in which to conceal any incisions on the face or neck. If at all possible, the surgeon should always try to arrange the excision of tissue such that the ultimate skin closure is in a line within or parallel to the relaxed skin tension lines.

It is also interesting to note that facial expression is not as animated in children as it is in adults. The mimetic muscles are not completely developed and active in children. There also is a greater layer of subcutaneous fat between the facial skin and the mimetic muscles that tends to dilute some of the fine, discrete muscular contractions that are transmitted as human emotion.

## WOUND HEALING

The physiology of wound healing is the subject of constant investigation. Certain generalizations can be made about the healing process. It is important for the clinician to understand that more sophisticated explanations and possibly even modifications of general theories continue to oc-

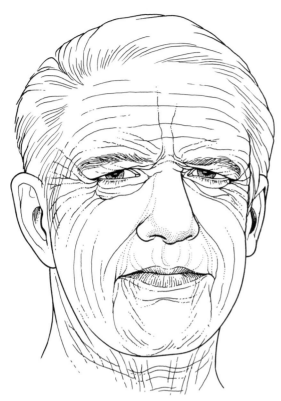

**FIG 2–2.**
The relaxed skin tension lines usually lie at right angles to the long axis to the underlying musculature.

cur. Healing is the series of reparative events following the creation of a wound. Inflammation, fibroblastic activity, and regeneration of vascularity occur during wound healing.

Three general types of healing can occur. Healing by first intention occurs after an incision has been reapproximated. In contrast, second intention healing describes the events occurring when a wound's edges are not reapproximated. Granulation develops between the skin edges, providing the surface for the eventual migration of epithelial cells to complete healing. In third intention healing the skin edges of a wound are left open for a few days and then reapproximated. This type of healing occurs when a contaminated wound is left open for local cleaning and débridement to allow for secondary closure that will minimize the chances for infection.

Healing involves a series of sequential events. The so-called *substrate* phase is the initial occurrence. It is characterized by the thrombosis of cut blood vessels and the movement of plasma and

lymph fluid into the wounded area. Inflammation involves unhealthy tissue that is ultimately removed by macrophages. Mucopolysaccharides are noted within the wound at that time.

The substrate phase is followed by the *proliferative* phase, which is heralded by the appearance of fibroblasts within the wound. The synthesis of collagen begins and actually accelerates. The substrate and proliferative phases tend to overlap somewhat so that collagen lysis is occurring at the same time as collagen synthesis. As the collagen synthesis increases, so does the tensile strength. It has been estimated that the tensile strength of a wound is close to the restraining strength of the sutures by the end of the first week.

The final phase of healing is the *resorptive* stage, at which time collagen is undergoing accelerated lysis. The hyperplastic wounds that are heavily concentrated with capillaries and fibroblasts start to resorb and ultimately assume the appearance of normal tissue. Even during this time, collagen synthesis continues. It has been estimated that collagen synthesis continues for approximately 6 months following the creation of a wound. The tensile strength of well-healed skin is estimated to be 80% of the normal unwounded tissue in a similar region of the body.

In some wounds, tissue has been lost and cannot be primarily approximated. It has been noted that, over a period of time, the area of skin loss decreases; this is referred to as *contraction*. There appears to be a centripedal movement of the surrounding skin so that the defect decreases. It is important to understand that wound contraction is a normal event of healing and is not the same as the exaggeration of this phenomenon, which is referred to as wound *contracture*.

## LOCAL ANESTHETICS

Currently available local anesthetics provide effective and safe anesthesia for the management of minor lacerations and abrasions. These agents generally work by preventing movement of ions across nerve membranes that block impulses. The activity of local anesthetics is definitely affected by the pH of the media. They are inactivated by an acidic environment. An abscess, for example, represents an acidic pH and explains the difficulty that is frequently encountered clinically with the decreased effectiveness of a local anesthetic. Local anesthetics act to block the pain and temperature fibers. It is not unusual for the patient to be aware of the pressure and touch but not to experience any pain with an incision. A variety of local anesthetic agents are currently available. Some are derived from esters of para-aminobenzoic acid (procaine, amethocaine). This group contains effective anesthetics. However, they are rapidly absorbed through the mucous membrane, and toxicity can develop at low dosages.

Amides seem to be preferred because they have a lower incidence of adverse reactions. Lignocaine (Xylocaine, lidocaine) and bupivacaine are two representative amide local anesthetics. Lignocaine is the most commonly used because it has a quick onset of anesthesia.

None of the preceding anesthetics has vasoconstrictive properties. Epinephrine is a commonly used vasoconstrictor that is frequently added to a local anesthetic. It has been experimentally determined that epinephrine in a concentration of 1:200,000 will produce maximal vasoconstriction. However, epinephrine concentrations of 1:100,000 are also commonly used. Maximal vasoconstriction usually occurs approximately 10 to 12 minutes following injection. Cocaine is the only local anesthetic that has both anesthetic and vasoconstrictive properties, but it is used only as a topical agent.

Anyone who uses local anesthetics must have some understanding of toxicities and how to deal with them. The most common toxicity of any of the agents is a change in not only the central nervous system but also the cardiovascular system. Toxicities of the central nervous system are initiated with a stimulatory phase that can involve seizure activity. A depressive stage that can cause respiratory insufficiency follows. The cardiovascular system is affected by myocardial depression. Hypotension occurs as a result of vasomotor depression and prolonged conduction times. Supportive measures for the central nervous and cardiovascular systems are necessary components of the treatment.

## BASIC SURGICAL CONCEPTS

The ideal surgical closure of a wound involves the obliteration of any dead space so that fluid cannot collect, which would predispose to infection. Suture material is used to support the tissues while wound healing occurs. The approximation of tissues is a means of decreasing certain adverse components of wound healing, such as wound contraction and epithelialization. Proper management of a laceration and abrasion requires a minimal number of instruments. A scalpel and scissors are useful to remove any foreign or necrotic material. Toothed forceps used for stabilizing tissues are less traumatic than nontoothed forceps, which can crush the skin. A needle holder is required. Hemostats are sometimes useful to control bleeding that cannot be stopped by direct pressure.

The proper management of an abrasion involves aggressive wound cleansing, followed by the application of a local dressing to promote epithelial migration. Infiltration of a local anesthetic before wound cleansing is helpful because it allows the surgeon to thoroughly clean the wound without discomfort to the patient. The application of a protective dressing to decrease the chance of infection and to keep the wound moist is advisable.

The use of local antibiotic ointments is effective. Neomycin ointment is commonly used. However, it has the highest degree of local sensitivity. Polysporin ointment is particularly useful in the head and neck area. It has the lowest incidence of local sensitivity, and its viscosity is such that the ointment adheres to some of the difficult surfaces of the face and neck. The application of local antibiotic ointment to a dressing impregnated with petroleum jelly provides excellent protection for an abrasion to allow it to heal with minimal scarring.

A laceration is handled in a similar sequence, in that the infiltration of local anesthesia initially allows the surgeon to clean the wound meticulously without creating discomfort to the patient. The abundant vascularity of the head and neck region permits survival of injured tissue that would not be expected to survive in other parts of the body. Therefore the principle of *aggressive cleaning* and *conservative débridement* directly applies to injuries in this area. A wound can be cleaned with scrub brushes if it contains particles of dirt. It is important that all foreign particles, such as gravel or tar, be completely removed from the wound. If the wound is closed with retained foreign particles, traumatic tattooing will occur and become a major challenge to correct later. After the foreign particles have been removed, the wound should be irrigated with copious amounts of saline solution. Following this débridement, the wound can be prepared with some of the usual solutions.

Dead space is eliminated by the suture reapproximation of all tissue layers that have been cut. In a laceration that crosses over or is near critical normal facial landmarks, it is usually best initially to place sutures that preserve or restore the anatomic landmarks in their normal position. If a laceration is long, one can ensure an even approximation of the edges by using a technique referred to as the *principle of halves*. This technique involves placing the initial stitch at one half the distance of the laceration (Fig. 2–3). The subsequent stitches are placed at one half the distance of the new distance created by the end of the laceration with the originally placed suture.

The dermal layer should be closed with stitches whose knot is directed toward the subcu-

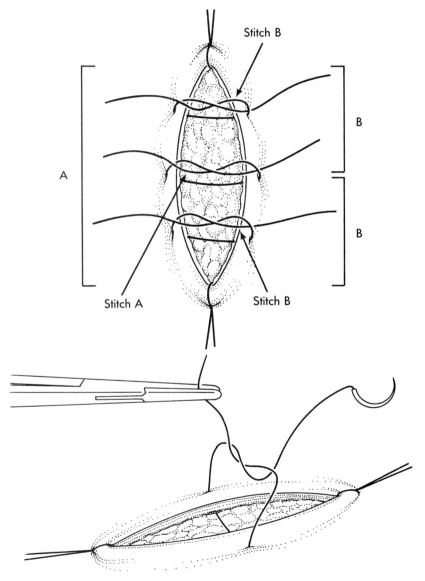

Stitch B

B

A

B

Stitch A          Stitch B

**FIG 2–3**.
The "principle of halves" is a useful technique to ensure an even approximation of skin edges.

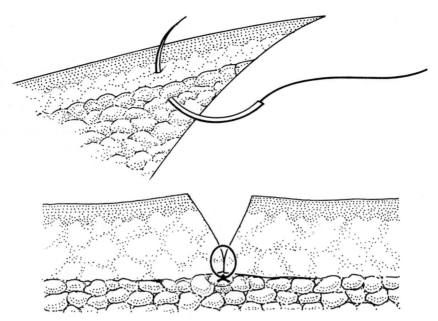

**FIG 2–4.**
Knots of tissues below the skin surface should be directed toward the deep tissues.

taneous tissue rather than toward the skin (Fig. 2–4). Any deep stitches should be closed with absorbable suture material. The clinician's assessment of the required strength of the closure dictates the choice of suture material.

Plain catgut is usually absorbed within 7 days. Chromic catgut is stronger and maintains its strength for a longer period. Some of the newer absorbable sutures can maintain their strength for as long as 90 to 120 days. For the uncomplicated simple laceration of the face or neck that is not under excessive tension with closure, chromic catgut usually provides sufficient strength, and the

more expensive, longer-lasting absorbable sutures are not necessary. The key to the quality of the result rests with the subcutaneous and dermal sutures because they provide strength to the closure and remove any tension on the cutaneous sutures.

Skin sutures should be placed so that the skin edges are slightly everted (Fig. 2–5). This can be facilitated by undermining the skin edges for 1 or 2 mm with a scalpel. This skin eversion allows for the normal wound contraction of healing and

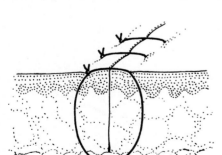

**FIG 2–5.**
Skin edges should be slightly everted after the proper placement of skin sutures.

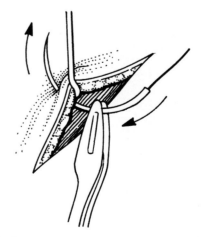

**FIG 2–6.**
Not injuring the blood supply to the skin edges is important in the proper technique of skin handling.

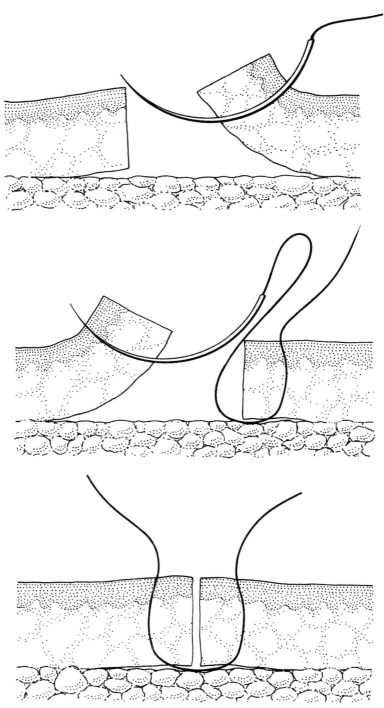

**FIG 2–7.**
The simple stitch.

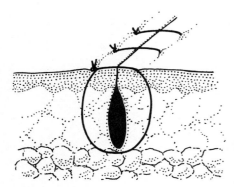

**FIG 2–8.**
Dead space should always be obliterated to avoid accumulation of fluid, which can become infected and impair wound healing.

results in a thin scar. If the skin is not everted, wound contraction will cause spreading and possibly even depression of the final scar.

The proper handling of the skin edges is very important. Either a skin hook or fine-toothed forceps is recommended (Fig. 2–6).

When inserting a needle, the physician should take care to follow the curve of the needle. Instrument ties are recommended because they save time and suture material.

The simple stitch involves placing the needle from outside in on one edge of the laceration, regrabbing it, and bringing it from the inside out on the other side with both entrance and exit sites being equidistant from each skin edge (Fig. 2–7). The author prefers to use a slip knot initially, placing the first two ties in the same direction so that the tension on the closure can be adjusted. The third tie is then placed in the opposite direction to create a square knot and lock the knot at the tension determined by the first two knots. Fig. 2–8 indicates how dead space can be created with the advancement of the needle into the deep tissue when there is insufficient material. If a needle traverses the skin surface at different distances from the edge and incorporates more of the dermis on one side than the other, there is the possibility of asymmetry.

Sometimes a simple stitch is not enough to establish the eversion necessary for optimal healing.

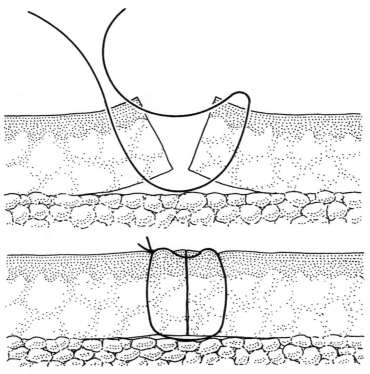

**FIG 2–9.**
Vertical mattress suture.

In that situation, a vertical mattress suture is an alternative. Vertical mattress sutures are not to be used indiscriminately because they compromise the blood supply to the skin edge more than simple stitches.

A vertical mattress suture involves initially tra-versing the skin near the edge and not incorporating a great amount of skin in that passage (Fig. 2–9). It is then passed through the skin a greater distance from the edge to incorporate a greater amount of subcutaneous tissue. The vectors created by this stitch facilitate skin eversion.

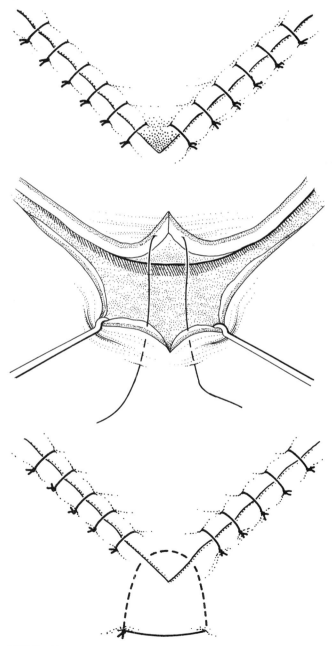

**FIG 2–10.**
Gillies corner stitch.

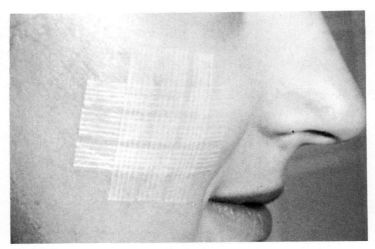

**FIG 2–11.**
Multiple layers of Steri-Strips splint the surrounding tissues and improve wound healing.

Sometimes a laceration will create a pointed flap of skin. In that situation, the placement of simple stitches on either side of this point may compromise the blood supply and result in necrosis of the tip. A Gillies corner stitch is used to decrease the compromise of the blood supply. The needle initially traverses the skin opposite the point and is brought through the dermis at the point (Fig. 2–10). It exits the skin on the other side. This is an effective means of skin approximation that minimizes the stress to the blood supply.

After suturing is completed, the clinician has some options for the care of the wound. To minimize the amount of scarring, a maneuver to decrease the stress to the skin in the area of the laceration is advisable. Multiple layers of Steri-Strips placed at right angles to each other after application of a skin adhesive effectively splint the skin immediately adjacent to the laceration closure (Fig. 2–11). These Steri-Strips are well tolerated by both adults and children. If they can be left in place for an extended period, they will aid wound healing and minimize the amount of scarring. If there is no need for the Steri-Strips, a local antibiotic ointment is applied to decrease crusting, minimize the chance of infection, and keep the wound moist.

Adherence to these basic principles of soft tissue surgery will allow most physicians, both surgeons and nonsurgeons, to obtain excellent results in the care of lacerations and abrasions of the head and neck.

# 3

# Basic Immunology and Immunologic Disorders

Thomas F. DeMaria
David D. Hamlar

## IMMUNOLOGY OVERVIEW

Immunology as a science has developed almost entirely within the past century and has undergone tremendous growth within the last 25 years. Originally the term *immunity* meant "freedom from" or "protection against," but its modern meaning is far broader. For example, it is now recognized that the same mechanisms that protect against infections or noxious agents also produce unwanted or even quite harmful reactions. Allergic rhinitis, transplantation rejection, transfusion reactions, glomerulonephritis, and rheumatic fever are all examples in which the same mechanisms that account for protection against foreign agents turn on their hosts with undesirable results.

Immunologic responses in essence serve three major functions: *defense* or resistance to infection; *homeostasis,* which is the clearance of spent self-produced materials such as red blood cells; and *surveillance,* which involves the detection and elimination of mutant cells that arise spontaneously in the host. Many common clinical problems facing the otolaryngologist involve one or more of these subareas of immunology. Chronic tonsillitis, allergic rhinitis, asthma, nasal polyps, cancer of the head and neck, and middle ear reconstructive surgery all involve immune responses. A broad background in immunology is now a fundamental requisite for the treatment of diseases of the head and neck. This chapter on basic immunology is intended to review only the basics and to alert the student to the need to refer to more advanced texts in the field.

## MAJOR LINES OF IMMUNITY

Immunity may be broadly classified into two areas, innate and acquired. Innate immunity is inherited and cannot be passively transferred from one individual to another. It is nonspecific and relatively constant among all members of a species and results from anatomic and physiologic barriers and activities of the individual. Examples of innate immunity include the skin and epithelia lining internal surfaces, cilia lining the epithelium of the upper respiratory tract, saliva, mucus, and other secretions.

Acquired immunity, on the other hand, is specific and depends on an individual's previous experience with an agent. Not all members of a species have the same level of this form of immunity. Such immunity is not inherited, but a temporary form may be transmitted across the placenta. Acquired immunity can be passively transferred to other individuals, even across species lines. Acquired immunity depends on the development of at least two kinds of substances specifically reactive against the material that stimulated their production: immunoglobulins, or antibodies, and specific lymphocytes. The material that causes production of immunoglobulins and specific lymphocytes is called an antigen. Antigens are generally divided into two classes: those dependent on the presence of functional T-cells and those which can induce an immune response independently of T-cell function. Acquired immunity exists in one of two forms, designated as either humoral or cellular.

Humoral immunity is mediated by lymphoid cells, under maturational control of the bone marrow, called B-cells. B-cells represent between 5% and 15% of circulating lymphoid cells and, unlike T-cells, contain immunoglobulin molecules on their surface that function as receptors for antigen. B-cells possess a series of other surface markers, referred to numerically as CD (cluster designation), that are associated with specific functions or identity. CD19, for example, is a marker present only on B-cells. When stimulated by appropriate materials (antigens), B-cells undergo a maturation and develop into nonreproducing, antibody-forming cells, called plasma cells, and secretory lymphocytes. Their maturation occurs in the presence of T-cells and is induced by a series of T-cell soluble products (lymphokines) referred to as interleukins, which selectively induce B-cells to divide or differentiate. The antibody secretions of B-cells can specifically react with the antigen that stimulated their production, and these reactions between antigen and antibody can occur in the absence of the cells.

Cell-mediated immunity, on the other hand, is not mediated by antibody but by lymphoid cells controlled by another organ system, the thymus; such cells are called T-cells. T-cells represent approximately 20% of the total blood leukocytes in circulation and exist as a heterogeneous population with different subsets and functions. Examples are the T-helper cells designated as CD4$^+$ and the cytotoxic/suppressor T-cells designated as the CD8$^+$ subset. T-cells have on their surface membranes specific receptor sites for antigen, referred to as T-cell recognition molecules. Thus when antigen and effector react, the presence of cells is essential. Antigen reacting with the recognition units on the T-cells causes the release of soluble substances (lymphokines) that initiate other forms of biologic activity comprising the cell-mediated immune response. These will be discussed in greater detail later.

A key component in the development of acquired immunity is the macrophage. The macrophage not only transports antigen (after phagocytosis) to the immune system but also processes the antigen so that it can stimulate production of antibody and immune cells. The macrophage can also ingest and destroy or inactivate antigen.

In reality the immune response is rarely exclusively humoral or cellular but most often includes contributions from both systems. An intricate network of cooperation exists between the various types of immune cells. It is now recognized that T- and B-cells are not homogeneous and that functionally different subpopulations exist.

## CELLULAR BASIS FOR HUMORAL ANTIBODY PRODUCTION

Several kinds of cells participate in antibody production, namely B-cells, macrophages, and T-cells in the case of T-dependent antigens. It is important to realize that the macrophage does not produce antibody, but it does engulf particulate or colloidal antigen, processes it in some way (most likely by forming antigen-RNA templates), and then transmits this information to immunologically competent immature lymphoid B-cells. In the case of T-dependent antigens, the immature B-cells must interact with lymphokines derived from a specific population of T-cells, called T-helper cells, to produce antigen-specific antibody. The lymphokines produced by the T-helper cells are referred to as interleukins. Interleukins exist as a family of proteins, each of which either activates or promotes a specific aspect of differentiation during the B-cell maturation process. Lymphokines are actually a specific lymphocyte-derived subset of approximately 20 soluble mediators referred to as cytokines (soluble products produced by leukocytes in general), which are critical for the immune response. The study of cytokines has taken a giant leap forward over the past decade because of the development of highly purified, recombinant cytokines. Please refer to any of the texts cited at the end of this chapter for a detailed discussion of these mediators.

Once the lymphoid cells are stimulated, two things happen: the lymphoid cell is stimulated to proliferate and differentiate into mature plasma cells, and these cells begin producing antibody. The plasma cell does not itself reproduce but is the product of rapidly dividing precursors. Its sole function seems to be antibody production. Other cells, such as the secretory lymphocytes, may also produce antibody, but the plasma cell seems to be the major antibody producer.

Humoral antibody is closely associated with cells in at least two important ways. (1) The primary function of antibody in vivo is to prepare an antigen for phagocytosis by neutrophils and other phagocytes. The antibody coats the antigen, fixes a group of materials called complement, and stimulates chemotaxis or attraction of phagocytic cells. Such an antibody is called an opsonin. (2) Some antibodies are cytophilic and have a strong attachment to the membrane of macrophages. This association is believed to result in an enhanced ability of the macrophage to capture antigenic material.

The response of the host contacting an antigen for the first time (primary response) differs from that of the host who has had prior exposure to an antigen (secondary response).

In the primary response, introduction of an antigen results in phagocytosis on or near the site of entry and transportation of antigen to the medulla of the regional lymph nodes via the afferent lymphatics. In some cases, the antigen may not be phagocytosed at the site of entry but will be phagocytosed by macrophages in the medulla of the lymph node.

Presumably, antigen is processed and is transferred to plasmacytes (medium to large lymphocytes) in the medulla. The cells undergo proliferation and DNA synthesis and mature into plasma cells and small lymphocytes. The small lymphocytes, derived from the medium to large lymphocytes that occur in the lymph node, are immunologic memory cells. The plasma cells are the primary antibody-producing cells. Most of the antibody is produced initially in the regional lymph nodes. Some antibody-forming cells, however, leave the lymph nodes via the efferent lymphatics and populate other nodes.

In a secondary response, there is a rapid localization of antigen in macrophages at the site of antigen entry and in dendritic macrophages in the cortex of the regional lymph node. The dendritic macrophages have cytophilic antibody on the surface of the dendrites that serves to capture, localize, and concentrate antigen. Memory cells (lymphocytes) contact the antigen bound to the macrophage and transform into antibody-producing plasma cells at a more rapid rate than that of the primary response. The dendritic macrophage and the rapidly proliferating antibody-producing cells then form germinal centers. A germinal center represents an area of intense antibody formation.

When an individual is given an antigen to stimulate his or her own immunocompetent cells to produce antibody, it is called active immunization. Because this process may take some time to produce immunity, depending on the type of antigen or vaccine being used, it is occasionally necessary for medical reasons to establish immunity much more quickly if not immediately. This is done by passive immunization, in which the individual is given antibodies produced elsewhere, for example, in another human (tetanus antitoxin) or in animals (diphtheria antitoxin, rabies antiserum). Passive immunization does not last very long because the individual's immunocompetent cells are not stimulated and the foreign protein will be catabolized without being replaced.

## BIOLOGY OF COMPLEMENT

One of the most important nonspecific humoral factors in immunity is the substance known as complement. It is important to remember that complement is not a product of an immune reaction but is present in all normal sera. Although complement is not a single entity and its nature varies among species, some generalizations can be made. Complement consists of a group of at least 20 plasma proteins that interact much as the elements of the coagulation system do, in that an initial trigger activates a series of cascadelike reactions. The various complement proteins resulting from this activation and cascade function as proteolytic enzymes, inhibitors, positive modulators, or recognition factors, and all promote an amplification of the inflammatory response, an important accessory to the initiation of a humoral immune antibody response. Lytic complement is labile to heat, prolonged storage, shaking, and the addition of certain chemicals, such as acids, alkali, ether, and bile salts. When it is necessary to destroy the complement activity in a serum, heating at 56° C for 30 minutes is sufficient. This process is termed inactivation, and it has no effect on most antibodies. At least one IgM or two IgG molecules reacting with an antigen are required to initiate complement activation. IgA does not activate complement by the classic pathway. Complement combines with an antigen only after that antigen has been sensitized by a specific antibody. This process is known as complement fixation.

The effect of complement activity on the sensitized antigen is usually observed by either lysis or opsonization, depending on the conditions of the system under investigation. If the antigen is cellular, as in the case of erythrocytes, lysis will be the result and is readily observable. If the cellular antigen is bacterial, lysis will also occur; however, it is not readily observable except microscopically. If the antigen is soluble or viral in nature, there is no observable result of antigen-antibody union with complement. Nonetheless, complement is fixed in such systems, and the index of this fixation is cleverly demonstrated in the classic complement fixation tests.

In recent years, the in vivo functions of complement have received greater attention, and it has been found that complement components have many beneficial functions in the normal individual. It is clear that the complement cascade may be activated in different manners and by at least two distinct pathways. The hemolytic reaction that is initiated by antigen-antibody complexes is known as the classic pathway. Additional nonspecific (that is, not requiring specific antibody) means of activating the complement cascade bypass the early components and begin activation with the complement component known as C3. These pathways are collectively referred to as the alternate pathway. Some substances known to activate the alternate pathway are bacterial lipopolysaccharides (endotoxins), aggregated immunoglobulins (need not be specific), inulin, zymosan, plasmin, and antigen-related IgA and IgE.

The complement system makes antibody-reacted antigens more easily phagocytosed and as such is regarded as most important in the body's defenses. This is performed through a mechanism known as immune adherence. After C3 has been mobilized to the complex, it adheres to a platelet or red blood cell. The increase in size of the unit makes it more easily phagocytosed. Other complement components participate in this effort by recruiting phagocytic cells to the area.

More subtle changes may be brought about by still other components, wherein a polypeptide cleavage product called anaphylatoxin is released, stimulating mast cells to secrete histamine. Histamine in turn stimulates smooth muscle contraction, capillary dilatation, and increased vascular permeability, all important functions of the inflammatory response.

Complement activation is thus a very important component in normal inflammation as well as in specific and nonspecific defenses against infectious processes. Furthermore, it is now recognized that the nonspecific activation of complement by means of the alternate pathway is also important in the etiology of certain pathologic processes. Endotoxic shock, tick bite paralysis, hypersensitivity pneumonitis, certain types of urticaria, and trypanosome-induced glomerulonephritis are a few of the diseases that seem to have alternate pathway activation of complement as an important part of their etiology.

Each complement component is antigenic, and serologic methods are available for measuring the levels of each. Knowledge of the levels of certain complement components may be informative clinically. Several examples follow.

### Endotoxin Shock

Because endotoxin is a good activator or substrate for C3 activation, gram-negative infections sometimes result in a systemic activation of C3, causing the release of large amounts of anaphylatoxin. The widespread effect of this substance on vascular permeability contributes greatly to the shock syndrome known to occur in such patients.

### Glomerulonephritis

Complement may become activated in the renal glomeruli through either pathway. The chemotactic and anaphylatoxic properties of the components result in injury to the capillary basement membrane.

### Angioneurotic Edema

With angioneurotic edema, an inhibitor normally present is genetically missing. This allows a runaway, unchecked complement activation owing to normally harmless causes, for example, mild trauma. These patients seem not only to produce excessive complement activation but also to exhibit excessive sensitivity to complement effects in certain tissues, most notably the larynx. The rapid edema of the larynx by this mechanism is an acute situation and can be fatal.

The main purpose of this section has been to emphasize that complement provides the primary nonspecific humoral amplification of an immune reaction, and these reactions may be either harmful or beneficial depending on the circumstances.

A more detailed description of the biologic properties of complement can be found in any of the basic texts cited in the selected readings.

## CELLULAR BASIS FOR CELL-MEDIATED IMMUNITY

Cell-mediated immunity is now viewed in a general sense as any immune response in which cellular elements predominate and antibodies play a lesser role. Examples include delayed hypersensitivity, cytotoxicity, T-cell proliferation, and immune responses to intracellular pathogens. T-cells are the central elements in these immune responses. T-helper cells play a pivotal role in that they act to control and modulate the development of cellular immune reactions through their role as lymphokine secretors. T-cytotoxic cells are effector cells and eliminate virally infected or other foreign cells from the host. Macrophages, under the influence of T-cell derived lymphokines, also play a central role in the elimination of cells infected with intracellular pathogens such as *Mycobacterium tuberculosis.*

Delayed hypersensitivity is classically demonstrated by skin testing with the appropriate antigen, the prototype being the tuberculin reaction. Individuals who have been sensitized to the tubercle bacillus produce specifically sensitized mature T-lymphocytes, which apparently have specific antigen receptor sites on their surfaces. A small amount of tuberculin antigen is injected intradermally, and within 24 to 48 hours an erythema and induration appear at the site of injection in sensitive individuals. This lesion may be severe enough to lead to a necrosis. The time of appearance of the reaction following injection has led to the term *delayed hypersensitivity,* which is synonymous with a cell-mediated immune response.

Whereas delayed hypersensitivity is routinely manifested in response to infectious agents, cell-mediated cytotoxicity is induced on exposure to foreign tissue, such as transplanted organs or certain tumors. T-cell killing is quite efficient, but the exact mechanism remains unknown. Lymphotoxin, discussed later, may play a role.

In both delayed hypersensitivity and cell-mediated cytotoxicity, sensitization may not be passively transferred by means of serum (antibody). It may be transferred only by viable T-lymphoid cells.

When an antigen reacts with specifically sensitized T-lymphocytes, a number of macromolecular, biologically active substances called lymphokines are released. The primary source of lymphokines is the CD4$^+$ T-cell, although all T-cells and even B-cells have been shown to be capable of secreting lymphokines. Examples of lymphokines include the following.

### Interleukins

Interleukins are a family of twelve lymphokines (each numbered sequentially) that promote the growth, differentiation, or expansion of B- or T-cells necessary to amplify the immune response. They are the primary means whereby various lymphocyte populations communicate with one another. Interleukin-2 (IL-2) is an important example of a lymphokine that is primarily a T-cell growth factor but also stimulates B-cell division and monocyte activation.

### Interferon-γ

Interferon-γ has many functions, among which are regulation of expression of the major histocompatibility complex antigens, stimulation of macrophages, activation of cytotoxic T-cells, and promotion of B-cell differentiation.

### MIF

Migration-inhibiting factor (MIF) is demonstrated by inhibitory action against normal macrophage migration. When released in vivo, it promotes defense by causing macrophages to become sluggish and to stick to the capillaries in an area of antigenic invasion, helping to focus defense cells.

### Lymphotoxin

Lymphotoxin kills foreign cells, host cells coated with foreign antigens, and innocent bystander cells. The major beneficial activity of cell-mediated immunity is postulated to be a homeostatic control mechanism that suppresses antigenic mutations of host tissues. This process is also responsible for graft rejections during transplantation. Lymphotoxin production might be involved in this process.

The combined function of all of these lympho-kines is to suppress mutations. Immunologic cells are capable of recognizing "self," but if self is modified either through internal mutations (thus changing the antigens) or by acquisition of a foreign antigen such as tuberculin ("self + X"), the additional antigen to self is not recognized and an immune response is stimulated. Multicellular evolution could not have proceeded unless such a control system had been developed. Day-to-day mutational events are normally controlled by this mechanism, and oncogenic processes develop only in individuals with immunologic abnormalities or those whose immunologic mechanisms have been circumvented.

The cell-mediated immunity that suppresses mutations, rejects grafts, and destroys certain bacterial, mycotic, and viral pathogens may produce such an intense inflammatory response that severe tissue destruction also results. This process of overkill is what differentiates primary from secondary tuberculosis. Secondary tuberculosis is accompanied by a greater amount of tissue destruction, particularly cavitation, as a result of this response. Such severe tissue destruction is undesirable.

It is important to understand what a particular speaker or writer means by "cellular immunity." In addition to that effected by T-lymphocytes, another form, unrelated to antigenicity, may also take place. In tuberculosis, for example, macrophages from unsensitized individuals are killed if allowed to phagocytize virulent tubercle bacilli, whereas macrophages from sensitized individuals are resistant. In fact, such sensitized macrophages exhibit enhanced killing of the tubercle bacilli and are referred to as activated macrophages. Although specifically induced, this type of immunity is nonspecific in execution, since these same tubercle bacilli–sensitized cells also exhibit a greater ability to destroy other intracellular pathogenic bacteria such as *Listeria monocytogenes* and *Brucella abortus*.

## FUNCTIONAL HETEROGENEITY OF T-CELLS

In addition to mediating cell-mediated immune responses, T-cells have several other functions. T-cells consist of a series of distinct subsets. Sev-

eral classification systems have been developed to assist in distinguishing the different regulatory and effector functions mediated by T-cells, based on their phenotypic differences.

Briefly, T-cells can be divided into two major functional categories: effector and regulatory T-lymphocytes. Two distinct populations of effector T-cells have been identified so far: T-cells that are effector cells for delayed sensitivity reactions and effector cells for cell-mediated cytotoxicity. The former play a role in in vivo responses against infectious agents such as the tubercle bacillus in certain viruses; the latter are thought to mediate cell-mediated immunity against foreign tissues such as transplanted organs or certain tumors.

Regulatory subpopulations consist of T-helper cells, which promote antibody production by B-cells against T-cell–dependent antigens, and T-helper cells for promoting cell-mediated toxicity as part of a cell-mediated immune response. At the same time, there are separate and distinct subpopulations that suppress these same responses, and there is even a separate and defined population that induces suppression.

A systemic nomenclature has been developed for cell surface markers present on various leukocytes. The CD system is widely used. $CD4^+$ cells, for example, are T-helper cells. At present over 35 different CD markers are used to identify and designate function for T-cells, B-cells, and other leukocytes.

## NATURE OF ANTIGENS AND IMMUNOGLOBULINS

As discussed, any immune response is induced by the introduction of an antigen into the host. Complete antigens are substances that cause an animal to produce antibodies or stimulate T-cells specifically capable of reacting with that antigen. An epitope or antigenic determinant is an individual site on an antigen stimulating particular clones of lymphocytes. In addition, there are substances called haptens that are antigenic only in the sense that they can react with specific antibodies. By themselves, they are unable to incite antibody production. Haptens must first be linked with a carrier protein molecule to incite antibody production.

As mentioned, antigens can be separated into two types: T-cell–independent antigens and T-cell–dependent antigens. T-cell–independent antigens include substances such as flagellin, ferritin, and polysaccharides, which are all characterized as having many repeating determinants that are identical. These determinants cause cross-binding of receptor sites on B-cells, resulting in transformation of these cells into antibody-producing cells without help from T-cells.

T-cell-dependent antigens require both T-cells and B-cells for antibody production. These antigens lack the linear repeating determinants of the T-cell-independent antigen and must react with T-cells before transformation of the B-cell can occur. The interaction of antigen and T-cell may result in the release of lymphokines that cause transformation of B-cells. Also, interaction of antigen with receptors on the surface of T-cells results in an arrangement of antigenic determinant groups in a linear, repetitive manner (similar to independent antigen). On presentation to the B-cell, these groups result in B-cell proliferation, maturation to plasma cells, and antibody production.

Although it is impossible to predict that a certain substance is antigenic, there are several features that are characteristic of antigens.

## Foreign

In general, substances that are foreign to the species of animal being immunized will be antigenic, although there are important exceptions.

## Molecular Weight

Complete antigens usually have a high molecular weight (on the order of 10,000 or more). There are some important exceptions, for example, insulin (6,000 in the monomeric form) and glucagon (3,600).

## Molecular Complexity

The chemical structure of an antigen must be such that there is a rigid internal configuration as determined, for example, by aromatic groups, disulfide linkages, double bonds, and tertiary configuration. Antigens must also have sufficient number and quality of chemical determinant groups. The type and arrangement of these groups, also known as polar groups, over the surface of the molecule impart specificity to that molecule.

## Ease of Degradation and Elimination

An antigen must be digestible by macrophages but at the same time must not be broken down or excreted too quickly. Its antigenicity depends on its presence in an unaltered state for a certain minimal period of time and its susceptibility to cellular metabolism.

## Particle Size

In addition to molecular weight, larger physical dimensions of antigens seem to increase their effectiveness. Cellular antigens, aggregated proteins, and proteins adsorbed to inert carriers are all more efficient antigens than are the same substances in solutions.

## Competition

Several types of competition among antigens are known. If two antigens are introduced separately into a host within a certain interval, there will be an inhibition of the immune response to the second antigen. Moreover, in mixtures certain antigens are seen to be "stronger" and will mask any response to the "weaker" antigen. Finally, the production of humoral antibody to a given antigen may block the development of cellular responses to that same antigen.

## Whether Living or Dead

In general, living agents are better immunogens than killed organisms. The immunizing agent may be a product of a metabolizing cell. More important, infection by means of a natural route with an attenuated agent might result in a beneficial host tissue modification not possible with a killed agent. Finally, the administration of a living agent permits a continuous dose of antigen, because the organisms are multiplying. A good example of this is the stimulation of the secretory IgA system by the oral polio virus vaccine.

It is important to realize that even the average

antigen defined by these basic criteria will induce a heterogeneous immune response. A variety of antibodies of varying types, and even perhaps a cell-mediated immune response, may be generated by a single simple antigen. We will expand on this in the section on immunoglobulin classes.

## IMMUNOGLOBULIN STRUCTURE

The antibodies produced in response to a particular antigen all have the same basic structure and are referred to as immunoglobulins. Each immunoglobulin molecule consists of at least two kinds of peptide chains: light chains and heavy chains. One class of immunoglobulin, IgA, may have an additional chain or "piece" when that molecule is produced by the secretory system. Finally, any immunoglobulin composed of more than one monomer contains an additional J chain, which serves to bind the monomeric units together into a single unit.

### Light Chains

The light chains have a molecular weight of approximately 20,000 and exists as two types: kappa ($\kappa$) and lambda ($\lambda$). These chains differ chemically, biologically, and serologically. On a given immunoglobulin molecular unit, two light chains are found, and they are of the same type, either kappa or lambda, although any individual will have some molecules with kappa chains (60%) and some with lambda (30%). Single immunoglobulin molecules are not constructed with both types of light chains. In the disease multiple myeloma, light chain dimers are excreted in the urine and are somewhat diagnostic for the disease. These are referred to as Bence Jones proteins.

### Heavy Chains

There are currently five types of heavy chains, and their molecular weights range from 55,000 to 75,000. A single immunoglobulin unit contains a pair of heavy chains, and the type determines the immunoglobulin class, that is, $\gamma$ chains for IgG, $\mu$ for IgM, $\alpha$ for IgA, $\delta$ for IgD, and $\epsilon$ for IgE. These chains are glycoproteins, and they differ according to carbohydrate content. The distinctive

properties of an immunoglobulin class are determined largely by the characteristics of the heavy chains.

### Immunoglobulin Molecules

The specificity of the antigen reactive site resides in the amino terminal end of each chain. The proximity of one of the light chains to the neighboring heavy chain constitutes the reactive site, and because there are at least two places on each molecule where this occurs, immunoglobulins are at least divalent. The amino acid sequence of this amino terminal end is highly variable (V), as one would expect, to account for the diversity among antibody molecules for antigen. This is called the $V_L$ or $V_H$ portion of the light or heavy chain, respectively. The amino acid sequence of the carboxy terminal ends of the chain is much more constant (C) and is referred to as the $C_L$ or $C_H$ portion of the two chains.

The carboxy terminal ends of the heavy chains account for the other diverse properties of immunoglobulin molecules, such as ability to pass the placenta, ability to fix complement, and ability to passively sensitize mast cells.

## IMMUNOGLOBULIN CLASSES

The IgG globulin contains most of the antibacterial and antiviral antibodies that determine immunity against infection. IgG, with a molecular weight of 150,000, passes the placental membranes and is not destroyed by heating at 56° C for 30 minutes, nor is its activity altered by treatment with 2-mercaptoethanol.

Besides the protective antibacterial and antiviral antibodies, the IgG group contains the Arthus reaction antibody, which participates in an allergic-type immune response in immunized animals. The blocking antibody that results from hyposensitization injections in the treatment of allergic patients is also IgG.

The IgG class of immunoglobulins is characteristic of the secondary (anamnestic) immune response and usually possesses a greater antigen-binding affinity than IgM. Human infants do not begin to produce their own IgG in appreciable amounts until about 7 weeks of age, although at birth they possess high amounts of maternal IgG that has been acquired transplacentally. The maternal IgG in the neonate has a half-life of approximately 45 days.

The macroglobulins of IgM have less combining power but greater specificity than those of IgG. They arise first in the course of immunization of an animal and do not respond to reinjection in the anamnestic manner as do IgG globulins. IgM globulins are thought to be composed of five subunits. They do not pass the placenta (molecular weight: 1 million), and their reactivity is destroyed by 2-mercaptoethanol. Most rheumatoid factors, conglutinin, cold-agglutinins, heterophile antibodies, many normal isoagglutinins of human blood groups, complete Rh antibody, leukoagglutinins, some thyroid antibodies, typhoid "O" antibodies, and the Wassermann antibody are all IgMs.

The IgA group contains some antibacterial antibodies. For example, immunity against diphtheria and tetanus may depend on IgA-type antibodies, and patients with deficient IgA are subject to frequent pulmonary infections. A clinical example of this deficiency is seen in patients with ataxia telangiectasia.

Globulins of type IgA do not pass the placenta and do not fix complement; they are heat labile and are denatured by 2-mercaptoethanol. In addition, IgA units frequently exist as dimers or trimers. There are two major types of IgA: a monomeric form in the serum and other internal secretions and a heavier variety, containing a secretory piece, that is associated with saliva, colostrum, mucous membranes, and other external secretions. The heavier secretory IgA is thought to be the body's first line of humoral defense against infection of the respiratory and gastrointestinal tracts. Secretory IgA has an additional chain not possessed by serum IgA that accounts for the difference in molecular weight and serologic specificity.

IgA is not usually detectable at birth, although a free transport piece may be present. Human infants seem to be capable of synthesizing their own IgA at 2 to 3 weeks of age.

A class of human immunoglobulins has been described (IgD) that appears to migrate in the ultracentrifuge with the 7S fraction and is found in the electrophoretic pattern as a fast gamma globulin. IgD is present in human sera only in very small quantities (0.003 mg/100 ml). The precise biological function of IgD is not known but it may play a role in antigen-triggered lymphocyte differentiation. The structure of the molecule is similar to that of IgG.

It has been demonstrated that when IgA, IgG, and IgM are precipitated from sera of patients with allergic disease, the skin-sensitizing antibody activity is still present in the supernatant fluid. Fractions of a microgram of this globulin suffice to initiate the typical tissue reactions seen in such human atopic disease as hay fever, asthma, and urticaria. This IgE antibody can attach itself to skin and other tissue cells much more durably than other antibodies.

As mentioned earlier in this chapter, it is important to realize that when an animal is immunized with even a pure antigen many types of antibody molecules are produced in response to it. A given antigen can summon a response not only from different immunoglobulin classes but also from immunoglobulin subclasses as well (e.g., $IgG_1$, $IgG_2$). Even within an immunoglobulin class, the molecules may be specific for different portions or prosthetic groups on the same antigen molecule. Antibodies with a very close complementary fit for antigen are said to be highly specific, whereas those with a looser fit are less specific. Antibodies produced in response to a single antigen may exhibit a variety of specificities. Finally, each antibody molecule may have a different avidity (strength of association) for the antigen.

Under normal conditions many clones of immunoglobulin-producing B-cells respond to antigen with production of immunoglobulins of several classes and subclasses and with different specificities and avidities.

Under certain conditions, abnormal proliferation of immunoglobulin-producing cells results in excessive production of one or another immunoglobulin. An example of this disease, referred to as a monoclonal gammopathy, is multiple myeloma. A gammopathy is an abnormality of the immune system. The term *monoclonal* refers to a disorder in a single clone of antibody-producing cells. A monoclonal gammopathy refers to an abnormality resulting in production of a single type of immunoglobulin. The monoclonal immunoglobulin is termed *M-component*. In multiple myeloma the abnormal immunoglobulin may be a serum globulin (γG, γA, γD, or γE) or a Bence

Jones protein. Bence Jones proteins are free light chains (kappa or lambda or both), which can be found in urine because of their small size.

Under normal conditions an immune response is composed of a population of antibodies, each different from the next. Such a broad, heterogeneous response is of value to the possessor because it tends to be uniformly effective against minor antigenic differences found in a highly variable pathogen. If the immunoglobulin response were too restrictive, a population of pathogens with sufficient antigenic variations would be selected out and allowed to overcome the host defenses.

## THEORIES AND MECHANISMS OF ANTIBODY PRODUCTION

When an unsensitized individual is injected with an antigen, he or she responds by producing a low level of detectable antibody in 5 to 7 days. The level or titer of this antibody slowly rises, reaching a peak in 3 to 6 weeks, after which time it drops off rather abruptly and reaches a low level again. This general sequence of events is termed the *primary response*. The immunoglobulin produced is primarily IgM. Although the first antibody produced is highly specific, it is regarded as having a low avidity. If at this time more antigen of the same kind is injected into the individual, there will be an immediate but short-lived drop in antibody titer because of neutralization. This is referred to as the immediate antibody decline. This momentary depression will then be quickly followed by a rapid rise in titer. The slope of the curve at this point is steeper than that of the primary curve, the antibody level reaches a higher peak, and a high antibody level is maintained for a longer time. This portion of the generalized sequence of events is called the secondary or anamnestic response.

The primary response is characteristically an IgM one. Toward the end of this response IgG begins to be produced, and when it appears, it acts as a feedback inhibitor for IgM synthesis. The secondary response is characteristically an IgG response only. Occasionally it is helpful to know the class of antibody making up the response, since this tells the individual's state of immunization.

## IMMUNOLOGIC TOLERANCE

Under certain circumstances a host will not respond to a particular antigen. This state of immunologic unresponsiveness to a given antigen is called immunologic tolerance. It is not merely the absence of something, but rather it represents a specific mechanism of inhibiting a response to a specific antigen, not to all antigens in general. Several types of unresponsiveness are known.

### Acquired Immunologic Tolerance

Medawar, Brent, and Billingham shared the Nobel Prize for their work with skin grafts between genetically dissimilar rats. If a skin transplant is made between two such animals, the recipient will reject the donor tissue in about 10 days. These investigators took pregnant rats and injected donor cells directly into the fetuses in utero. After the pups were born and matured, a repeated skin graft was made to these young animals from the original donor. This time the tissue was accepted as self and not rejected. Recognition of self from nonself is one of the cornerstones of understanding the immune mechanism. This form of acquired tolerance may be explained by the clonal selection theory or by the mechanism described subsequently.

### High-Dose Tolerance or Immunologic Paralysis

If too high a dose of purified antigen is given to an animal, it will not respond to that dose or even to a correct dose given some time later. Apparently in such antigen excess the antigen bypasses the macrophages and reacts directly with B-cell receptors. Because the antigen does not have the RNA templates or whatever signal is required from the macrophages, antibody production does not proceed because all available receptor sites are tied up and cannot be stimulated even by antigen that has been processed correctly. Humans do not normally form antibody responses to their own tissue, probably because they are continuously in high-dose excesses of these antigens. This form of tolerance may be broken by immunizing with a slightly altered antigen, and as such the phenomenon of autoimmunity, in which an individual produces antibodies against his or her own tissue, may occur when the body tissues are slightly altered by such events as infection or trauma.

### Low-Dose Tolerance

Low-dose tolerance is a controversial form of tolerance supposedly caused by the administration of exceedingly small doses of antigen. The mechanism for this form, if it exists, is difficult to explain.

Route of administration is believed to contribute to low-dose tolerance. Some materials are antigenic if given intramuscularly but tolerogenic if given intravenously. Of those antigens which are effective intravenously, tolerance can be rendered if the antigen is given through the mesenteric route. In such an instance the antigen is transported first to the liver, where perhaps it undergoes degradation before reaching appropriate lymphoid cells. Thus if the antigen is too quickly degraded, it may not only become nonantigenic, it may even become tolerogenic by being broken down into smaller informational units not large enough to trigger an immune response.

The physical nature of the antigen is another variable that may induce low-dose tolerance. If soluble protein antigens are carefully filtered and centrifuged so that the solution exists only as true aggregate-free monomers, such a preparation is often tolerogenic. Molecules that are of large particle size and aggregated are more apt to be phagocytized, but monomers could react with B-cell receptors without the macrophage informational unit necessary to stimulate antibody synthesis. Further, all reactive cells would be turned off from receiving stimulation from correctly processed antigen at a later date.

### Therapeutic Immunosuppression

At the current state of our knowledge it is difficult, if not impossible, to suppress the secondary immune response. Hence, administering immunosuppressive therapy once sensitization has been achieved is usually fruitless. However, if immunosuppressive agents, either cytotoxic drugs or antilymphocyte globulin, are administered at or near the time of primary antigen contact, specific immune tolerance can be achieved against the antigen. Antigen administered then knocks out the primary immunocompetent cells. These cells are vulnerable to such treatment, but the memory cell appears to be highly refractory to the effect of immunosuppressive agents.

Thus immunosuppression is usually an elective procedure—that is, purposeful steps taken to prevent an immune response from being mounted, as in the case of transplantation surgery. Although immunosuppression has been used to treat some of the autoimmune diseases or diseases with undesirable immunologic counterparts, such treatment has generally not been successful owing to the already established sensitization, which is not amenable to most forms of immunosuppressive therapy. If we define immunosuppression more broadly to include the inhibition of immunologic effectors in addition to the inhibition of specific antibody or cellular response, immunosuppression in this sense becomes useful. A good example would be the administration of disodium cromoglycate, which inhibits the release of substances like histamine from IgE-sensitized tissues following antigen reactivity. Note that the antibody itself is not inhibited or suppressed, only its effectors.

## IMMUNOPATHOLOGY

The same immunologic mechanisms responsible for protection against foreign pathogens and somatic mutations may also produce sufficient inflammation or cytotoxicity to damage the host. Immune and immunelike injuries are the subject of an entire discipline, immunopathology. At the outset, it may be worthwhile to provide an arbitrary classification of the different kinds of *individual* mechanisms that may result in immune injury before discussing them in detail. It should be cautioned, however, that *single* mechanisms do not often occur in a clinical condition, but rather two or more may be operating concurrently.

The most useful system for describing immunologic diseases is the system of Gell and Coombs, in which four types of immunologic injury are noted. To these we have added immunologic deficiencies and diseases of the immunologic system.

## Type I

In type I injury the immune response to an extrinsic antigen is of the IgE class. These molecules have the ability to fix to mast cells and basophils by their Fc fragments. When two or more adjacent IgE molecules are stressed by reacting with antigen, the stress is transmitted to the cell and causes it to secrete various pharmacologically active substances. The effects of these substances account for the symptoms and signs of immediate types of hypersensitivity.

## Type II

Antibodies in type II immune injury are cytotoxic, that is, there is direct injury to the tissue following antigen-antibody reactions. The antigen could be an intrinsic antigen located on the cell or tissue; it could be an extrinsic antigen that has become absorbed to the host tissue; it could be an extrinsic antigen that shares an accidental specificity with host tissue. IgG and IgM immunoglobulins may participate, and complement is usually involved.

## Type III

This form of immune injury is contingent on the ability of antigen and antibody to combine to form soluble complexes in regions of antigen excess. These soluble immune complexes are not phagocytized but are deposited at various anatomic locations such as in renal glomeruli. Here they fix complement and become chemotactic for neutrophils. These cells may release proteolytic enzymes that injure the adjacent tissue.

## Type IV

Unlike the three previous forms of tissue injury, type IV is unrelated to humoral antibody. Instead, this type of immunopathology is caused by specifically sensitized lymphocytes or cell-mediated immunity. Following reaction with antigen, the lymphocytes secrete the various lymphokines that lead to different types of tissue change.

## IMMEDIATE HYPERSENSITIVITY

IgE is the immunoglobulin present in the least amount and apparently is the most specialized immunoglobulin. Although it is found in the serum, it is mainly a product of the gut- and bronchial-associated lymphoid tissue systems. Its unique properties are related to those features of the carboxy terminal portions of the heavy chains which enable the molecule to be attached to specific receptors on basophils or mast cells. IgE is present in very small amounts and only a small amount will have the specificity toward a particular antigen.

The demonstration of IgE antibodies is usually accomplished clinically by one of several methods:

1. Sensitive patients will produce a characteristic wheal-and-flare reaction to intradermally introduced antigen within minutes. The antigen may be injected intradermally in extreme dilutions or merely dropped onto a small area of skin that has been only slightly scratched with a stylet (scratch or prick test).
2. In certain types of sensitivity, especially to insect venoms, the previous method may be dangerous to apply directly to a patient. Instead, serum from the patient is injected intradermally into a nonallergic volunteer. After several hours of incubation to allow the IgE to become appropriately fixed to mast cells or basophils, the same site and additional control sites are injected with antigen. If specific IgE was present in serum, a wheal-and-flare reaction will appear within minutes. This passive test is known as the Prausnitz-Küstner (P-K) test.
3. Histamine release from leukocytes in the presence of antigen.
4. RAST—radioimmunoassay (radioallergosorbent test).

## MEDIATORS OF TYPE I REACTIONS

### Histamine

Histamine is the most widely studied mediator, and it seems to be responsible for most allergic manifestations. Histamine is bound to heparin and other substances within the basophilic granules of mast cells and circulating basophils and is liberated on disruption of the cells. The classic triple response to histamine includes initial erythema at the site of intradermal injection of histamine, then a central wheal and peripheral flare. The most important action of histamine in the pathology of human allergic disease is probably its ability to disrupt the integrity of capillary walls, with resulting edema of mucous membranes or the subepithelial layers of the skin. This partly results in narrowing of bronchial lumen, swelling of nasal turbinates and intestinal wall, and formation of papules or wheals on the skin. The concomitant dilation of capillaries in the area of secretory cells induces the production of large amounts of thin mucus, saliva, and gastric juice. Smooth muscle, including that of the bronchioles, intestines, spleen, and uterus, is contracted.

## Serotonin

5-Hydroxytryptamine is a ubiquitous substance that appears to be liberated together with histamine during anaphylactic reactions. In rodents serotonin is particularly abundant in platelets. Although serotonin can mimic some of the tissue responses that are known to result from histamine effect, the therapeutic use of serotonin antagonists in allergic disorders has only recently become possible.

## Slow-Reacting Substance of Anaphylaxis (SRS-A)

SRS-A is not a single mediator, as previously thought, but a group of sulfidopeptide leukotriene metabolites of arachidonic acid synthesized de novo. SRS-A derives its name from its production of slow and protracted contractions of bronchioles during asthmatic episodes that persist after destruction of all histamines and serotonin.

## Bradykinin

Bradykinin is another slow-reacting substance with powerful constrictor action on certain smooth muscles and a strong vasodilator action with marked capillary hyperpermeability. Like SRS-A, bradykinin does not exist in a preformed stage but is produced de novo. Although it is a functional vasodilator, its role in anaphylactic reaction is uncertain.

## Acetylcholine

Acetylcholine is a physiologic antagonist of epinephrine that is produced at the site of parasympathetic nerve endings and almost immediately inactivated by cholinesterase. Acetylcholine is released during hypersensitivity reactions, but its functional role is not known.

# CLASSES OF TYPE I REACTIONS

## Fungal Spores

Microbial products are often highly allergenic, are small enough to reach the lower airways, and may be produced in large amounts. Their small size also makes them easily airborne, and they remain so for long periods of time without appreciable settling. Some of the most common mold allergens are *Alternaria, Helminthosporium, Aspergillus,* and various mildews.

## Danders and Feathers

Keratinaceous products of animals are potent allergens, particularly those from horses, cats, and birds. Arthropod exoskeleta and egg cases are also extremely powerful allergens and may actually be the component of dander responsible for the allergy.

## House Dust

House dust is a very common source of type I allergy. It follows a seasonal incidence, being most prevalent during hot, humid months and least during the cold, drier months. It does not exist at high elevations or in arid climates. Although mold spores could be the real culprit, the most common offender in house dust appears to be the human dander mite, *Pteryonysinus dermatophagoides.*

## Pollens

Pollen grains that are small enough to remain suspended for long periods of time cause the most trouble. Two pollen seasons exist: one from May to June that is primarily made up of grasses, and one from late August to frost made up of common weeds. Among the most common offenders are orchard grass, fescue, quack grass, red maple, plantain, giant and common ragweed, lamb's-quarters, and thistle.

### Food

A common clinical sign of food allergy is urticaria, although other types, including anaphylaxis, are also known. The most common offenders are tomatoes, strawberries, egg white, flour, milk, and chocolate.

### Miscellaneous Inhalants

More people than is commonly realized are allergic to tobacco smoke. Orrisroot (common ingredient in cosmetics), pyrethrum (common ingredient in insect sprays), and various types of lint from clothing and textiles are common allergens of this type.

### Medicine

Sulfas, penicillin, and horse antisera have caused the most iatrogenic allergies.

## CLINICAL FORMS OF TYPE I DISEASES

### Anaphylaxis

One type of immediate hypersensitivity, anaphylaxis, is a systemic shock reaction resulting from the action of large amounts of mediators affecting smooth muscles and capillaries in many areas of the body simultaneously. Most often such reactions are produced by entry of antigen into circulation through an unnatural route, such as injection of a medication (e.g., penicillin) or the sting of an insect. If an antigenic contact with fixed antibody is made, antigen-antibody complexes are formed on the cells. The resultant stress of these reactions on the tissue cells may then release the mediators that make the response manifest. The symptoms of anaphylaxis vary with the species, but generally there is immediate and violent respiratory distress and circulatory collapse, which is often fatal.

### Atopy

The other major type of immediate hypersensitivity is atopy, a genetically determined abnormal state of hypersensitivity. Atopy in humans assumes a variety of clinical forms (for example, hay fever, asthma, eczema, or hives), but the basic mechanisms are essentially similar to those of anaphylaxis in that the physiologic effects are caused by the hypersensitivity mediators released upon antigen-antibody combination.

1. *Seasonal rhinitis–hay fever* is perhaps the most common type I form of clinical illness. Conjunctivitis, sinusitis, acute nasal congestion, and sneezing are the key signs related to the IgE release of mediators. In general, the particle size of the allergens is large, and they settle out on the upper respiratory tissues.
2. *Bronchial asthma* is essentially an atopic disease of the lower respiratory tract, generally caused by smaller-sized inhalants. Classically it is a recurrent paroxysmal dyspnea with wheezing, characteristically relieved by epinephrine. Environmental conditions (e.g., temperature) and emotional stress may trigger or intensify attacks. Occasionally severe, protracted episodes of dyspnea occur that are not correctable by the usual bronchial dilators (status asthmaticus). Unless this condition is rapidly reversed, it is fatal.
3. *Atopic dermatitis* is an intensely pruritic, erythematous, scaly eruption of the skin, usually chronic in nature. It is often included in the study of allergy, although there is much argument against an immunologic etiology.
4. *Urticaria, or hives,* consists of raised, edematous, erythematous wheals with characteristic areas of blanching surrounded by a red flare or halo. The lesions may be small and discrete or large, confluent plaques. They are intensely pruritic.

### Serum Sickness

Serum sickness is the exception to the rule concerning the short time between challenge and demonstration of symptoms. It has components of both type I and type III mechanisms. This disease occurs when a large amount of antigen, as in the form of therapeutic antitoxic serum, is deposited in the body. After 8 to 10 days the body has built up a certain amount of IgE and precipitins for the antigen that is still present. Fever, lymphadenopathy, generalized urticaria, and painful, swollen joints are the usual result.

## IMMUNOLOGIC THERAPY

Diagnosing the clinical form of an allergic disease like urticaria is not difficult, but determining the etiologic agent may present problems. If the agent is definitely identified, advice or therapy may be given. Sometimes it is a simple matter to avoid the allergen, but when this is not possible or practical, immunologic desensitization may be tried. In this procedure extremely small doses of the offending antigen are given following an empiric schedule for as long as 2 years. One rationale is to stimulate other immunoglobulin classes as a result of artificial immunization to competitively inhibit the IgE globulins with the same specificity. The outcome of IgG reactions with ragweed antigen is inconsequential compared with the same reaction with IgE. In addition to the production of blocking antibody, there is further evidence to suggest that immunotherapy results in an increase of T-suppressor lymphocytes, which suppress the number of IgE-producing B-lymphocytes, resulting in a decrease of circulating IgE. Proof of efficacy of desensitization immunotherapy is obtained from witnessing any clinical improvement following continued exposure to antigen. This tolerance is relatively long lived.

Occasionally, it is necessary to immediately desensitize a patient in order to administer a medication, for example, diphtheria antitoxin to a patient who is allergic to horse serum. The technique of hyposensitization is used in which small doses of antigen are administered while such emergency procedures as administering epinephrine and performing tracheostomy are readily available. After 15 minutes, more antigen is given and so on, until the patient can tolerate the entire dose. It is an empiric procedure taking several hours, but is not long lasting.

## PHARMACOLOGIC THERAPY

Pharmacologic therapy is used to ameliorate symptoms only. It cannot take the place of curing the disease. The attempt is made to counter the effects of the mediators released by IgE-antigen reactions by administering pharmacologic antagonists. Some agents, such as epinephrine, act by exerting an opposite effect on the shock organ. Other agents, such as disodium chromoglycate, act by preventing the release of substances like histamine and SRS-A.

## CYTOTOXIC IMMUNE INJURY

Type II cytotoxic reactions can be broken down into several subcategories for the purpose of explaining mechanisms.

### True Cytotoxic Reactions

True cytotoxic reactions are those in which the cell or tissue is the antigen. The prototype of this is the antiglomerular basement membrane type of glomerulonephritis in which the membrane is the antigen. Goodpasture syndrome is a rare disease affecting both the kidneys and the lungs. It is believed to be the result of an immunologic reaction against an antigen in common with the renal glomeruli and the alveolar capillary membranes. Acute transfusion reactions and erythroblastosis fetalis are isoimmune diseases resulting from cytotoxic antibodies.

### Bystander Reactions

In bystander reactions the antigen is foreign and becomes attached to the cell so that subsequent antibody-antigen reactions destroy the attached cell. The prototype of this form is seen in idiopathic thrombocytopenic purpura, in which platelets may become coated with certain haptens administered as drugs in the treatment of other diseases. Sedormid, digoxin, stibophen, and quinidine are the most well known. If enough of the antibody-antigen reactions occur, a marked decrease in platelets may result.

### Cross Reactions

In cross reactions the body produces an antibody against a foreign antigen that accidentally cross-reacts with normal host tissue. An example is the streptococcal cell membrane antigen that cross-reacts with a myofibrillar antigen in heart muscle. Production of this antibody and subsequent reactivity with the host tissue are thought to be the cause of rheumatic fever. A similar relationship is thought to exist between *Escherichia coli* antigens and colonic mucosa in the disease ulcerative colitis.

### Acellular Antigens

Acellular antigens are not strictly cytotoxic, since the antigens are not cellular, but the materials are involved in certain diseases. Clotting anomalies resulting from antibodies to factor VIII have been described, and some instances of refractoriness to insulin therapy have been traced to anti-insulin antibodies.

## IMMUNE COMPLEX DISEASE

The prototype of immune complex disease is the Arthus reaction. It occurs in individuals who are repeatedly immunized with antigens that preferentially induce a precipitating antibody. As precipitins develop and more antigen is injected, soluble antigen-antibody complexes form because of the antigen excess. These complexes are not large enough to be phagocytized, but they may be deposited at certain anatomic locations such as in a capillary bed or the glomeruli. If they are deposited in a capillary bed, a vascular phenomenon results. This phenomenon is characterized by an inflammatory reaction consisting of edema, hemorrhage, and thrombosis owing to accumulations of complement-attracted phagocytes. The physical effects of the thrombosis, plus the effects of the secreted lysosomal enzymes, damage the tissue severely and necrosis may result. This is most likely to result in a human following insulin injections or after certain immunizations using protein fluids such as any embryonated egg vaccine. It is not a common reaction in humans and is characterized more by pain and swelling than by necrosis. It appears from 4 to 6 hours after injection and is usually gone by 8 hours. It will respond to steroids.

Type III glomerulonephritis, the most common immunologic form, differs from type II reactions in that the antigen is foreign. Under continued antigenic bombardment, as in an untreated streptococcal infection, soluble antigen-antibody complexes are formed and filtered out by the glomerulus. They also fix complement and attract phagocytes, which release proteolytic enzymes that tear holes in the membrane. The complexes that pass through and become lodged either within or on the epithelial side of the membrane appear in an irregular fashion. When viewed by immunofluorescence, the deposits show up as "lumpy bumpy" deposits, as opposed to the continuous pattern of the type II reaction. DNA in lupus erythematosus and certain viruses are also known antigens that can cause type III kidney injury. If the antigenic cause of the disease can be eliminated or controlled, the patient is much more amenable to transplantation therapy. Steroids are helpful in stabilizing the lysosomal membranes from rupture and also interfere with migration of polymorphonuclear neutrophils.

It is more important to bear in mind that clinical disease may be the result of more than one type of immunopathology. Serum sickness has type I and type III components. Hypersensitivity pneumonitis may have types I, III, and IV components, and the clinical course may depend on the relative amount of each component in the mixture. Finally, recent evidence also suggests that there may be type IV mechanisms in glomerulonephritis. Type IV immune injury occurs in two major forms: allergy to infection and contact dermatitis. The former is associated mainly with intracellular bacterial, mycotic, and viral infections. The hypersensitivity to the microbial antigens can be of such an intense nature that tissue is damaged to the point of disadvantage to the host; that is, cavitation, which antibiotics cannot penetrate well, may result within host defenses. These cavities represent a potential source of protected infectious agents that encourages the emergence of drug-resistant strains. It also results in recessive loss of function as a result of devitalized tissue. It should be pointed out that the cell-mediated form of immunity is not wholly undesirable; indeed no animal can live without it. Undesirable activities are noticed only when they occur in excess amounts.

Contact dermatitis results from sensitization to certain environmental haptens that complex with host proteins to become complete antigens. The prototype is poison ivy resin. Certain other materials such as lacquer, nickel, detergents, and inks are other less common contact sensitins. The chemical dinitrochlorobenzene is a universal contact sensitin; that is, everyone exposed to it becomes allergic.

Type IV reactivity may be suppressed or not even appear in patients with T-cell deficiencies, patients under steroid therapy, patients under certain other forms of immunosuppression, and patients with Hodgkin's disease. Known tuberculin reactivity may disappear in the patient who is overwhelmed with infection. This is called the anergic state and is thought to be caused by the saturation with antigen of all lymphocytic receptor sites. It is a poor prognostic sign, but if the tuberculin reactivity reappears, a favorable prognosis is indicated. The tuberculin reaction is also known to be temporarily suppressed in patients with measles, influenza, and certain other viral infections.

Most knowledge of immunopathology was initially obtained from the study of the two immunologic mechanisms involved in the production of glomerulonephritis. As stated, one type, the less common, results from conventional complement-fixing antibodies produced somehow against the glomerular basement membrane. Neutrophils attracted chemotactically to this site release their lysosomal contents and injure the membrane, but the antibody remains fixed to the endothelial side of the membrane, the site of the antigenic groups. The entire membrane is involved and, when viewed with the ultraviolet microscope following reaction with fluorescein-labeled antiglobulin, appears as a thin, membranous, continuous line of fluorescence. Somehow, because of unknown antigens, the body has been tricked into producing an antibody against its own glomerular membranes. Such patients are poor candidates for transplantation therapy, since most destroy the transplanted kidneys by the same immunologic mechanism.

## TUMOR IMMUNOLOGY

The main question of cancer immunology is, why does a tumor that represents essentially new material become established in the presence of a supposedly functioning immune mechanism? There are several plausible explanations:

1. *Antigenic Deletion.* Antigenic deletion is loss of a strong antigen that might stimulate cell-mediated immunity.

2. *Antigenic Modulation.* An antigen may be suppressed when tumor cells are grown in the presence of antibody.

3. *Fetal Reversion.* An antigen that is normally not present in an adult may be found during embryogenesis. During a neoplastic event this "antigen" may become re-expressed, and since it is, no immune response is generated. Carcinoembryonic antigen and $\alpha_1$-fetoprotein are two such antigens, and their sudden production in large amounts correlates well with certain neoplasias.

4. *Immunologic Enhancement by Antibody.* Humoral antibody to a tumor antigen may actually protect it from cell-mediated immunity.

5. *Strong and Weak Antigens.* Strong antigens tend to form antibody, which enhances tumor, and weak antigens tend to form cell-mediated immunity, which is more effective in infiltrating tumors.

The preceding reasons for failure of the immune system to eliminate tumors are related to the expression of antigen, but tumor development may also be related to other predisposing host factors such as:

1. Genetic or familial tendency.
2. Age—As one ages there is not only increased mutability, but also decreased immune function.
3. Immunologic surveillance—The concept that the main function of cell-mediated immunity is to suppress mutations; therefore some consider induction of a neoplasia a failure of the immune response.
4. Tolerance—Little applicability except in newborn animals infected with certain tumor viruses.
5. Immunosuppression—Natural from aging, but environmental and iatrogenic (immunosuppressive therapy) factors are known.
6. Tumor mass—Once established, it could easily exhaust reactivity of competent cells.

Assume a 70 kg patient has a normal blood volume of 5,250 ml and white blood cell count of 15 million ml (15,000 mm). If the patient has a myeloma, 50% of these cells could be plasma cells or $4 \times 10^{10}$ myeloma cells. Considering the average dry weight of a cell and that 90% of a living cell is water, we can readily compute the average weight of a cell ($2 \times 10^{-8}$ g). Using these calculations, we see that a myeloma tumor, although diffuse, weighs 800 g or almost a kilogram! If an anticancer agent with an exceptional killing efficiency of 99.999% is used on a patient, after treatment the patient will still have $4 \times 10^5$ potentially lethal cells!

Immunotherapy for malignant disease is still in the formative stage; however, immunologic tests do provide improved diagnostic and prognostic aids for patients with head and neck cancer. Skin testing, peripheral T-cell counts, lymphocyte reactivity tests, and other tests of cell-mediated immunity appear to be correlated with prognosis in patients with carcinoma of the head and neck, and detection of Epstein-Barr-virus-specific IgA serum antibodies appears to be useful in the diagnosis of nasopharyngeal carcinoma. There is cause to be optimistic about the value of the various immunologic techniques for diagnosis and prognosis, but it is clear that effective immunotherapies will not be available for some time.

## TRANSPLANTATION IMMUNOLOGY

Understanding of the modern aspects of transplantation rests on immunologic and genetic principles. First it is necessary to acquire a familiarity with the terminology in common use. For this discussion we will define the basic types of grafts as follows:

1. Autograft—Self to self.
2. Homograft or allogeneic graft—Between genetically dissimilar members of the same species.
3. Isograft, syngeneic or isogeneic graft— Between genetically similar members of the same species.
4. Heterograft or xenograft—Between members of different species.

## NATURE OF TRANSPLANT REJECTIONS

When full-thickness skin allografts are performed in humans, inflammation and leukocytic infiltrates appear in 4 or 5 days, terminating in necrosis of the grafted tissue by the ninth or tenth day. This reaction is termed *first-set rejection.* Subsequent allografts to the same recipient are rejected more vigorously and quickly (second-set rejection), within 4 to 6 days. A recall flare response is also seen at the site of the first rejection. That this rejection mechanism is cell mediated can be demonstrated by passive transfer experiment. The ability to reject allografts can be conferred on an unsensitized recipient by passive transfer of donor lymphoid tissue, but not by means of donor serum.

Although the rejection of hard tissue grafts cannot be brought about by serum antibodies alone, they do play a part in graft rejection and do cause the fixation of complement. Also, agammaglobulinemic patients reject transplants more slowly than do people with normal immunoglobulin levels. The major component of the graft rejection mechanism is thought to be delayed hypersensitivity. If, after an allograft rejection has taken place, the recipient is intradermally injected with donor lymph node cells, in 24 to 48 hours a typical tuberculin-like skin reaction appears at the injection site. This is thought to be caused by the rapid mobilization of now-sensitized cells of the recipient to act as a host-versus-graft reaction at the injection site. The reverse of this experiment illustrates another aspect of transplantation phenomena. If the same donor is skin tested with lymph node cells from the sensitized recipient, the same reaction is observed. In this case a graft-versus-host reaction has been caused. When lymphoid grafts are made in neonatal animals, there occasionally appears a wasting syndrome of the recipient termed *runt disease.* This is another manifestation of the graft-versus-host phenomenon. It is this same phenomenon that frustrates the use of bone marrow, thymus, and fetal liver transplants in reconstituting immune deficiency syndromes.

## PRIVILEGED SITES AND ACQUIRED TOLERANCE

Not all grafts are rejected similarly. The anterior chamber of the eye, the cornea, the meninges, the hamster cheek pouch, and the placenta are all considered privileged sites in the sense that grafts on these tissues are not always rejected. The tympanic membrane may also be a privileged site. Many such sites are avascular and hence prevent sensitization of the recipient by means of the afferent limb of the immune response. The trophoblast layer of the placenta and a dense layer of connective tissue in the hamster cheek pouch are thought to be nonantigenic and/or to prevent sensitization by exerting a barrier effect. The trophoblast tissue is devoid of H, A, and B isoantigens and is also covered with a nonreactive cellular carbohydrate that masks histocompatibility antigens and repels lymphocytes.

The phenomenon of acquired tolerance was originally demonstrated by experimental allografts in mice. Mouse embryos were sensitized in utero with living spleen cells from an allogeneic donor. When these embryos matured through birth to adulthood, they were found to accept additional grafts from the original donor. These mice were "tricked" into recognizing this foreign tissue as self. This tolerance is specific and may be dose dependent, that is, tolerance remains as long as the original antigen remains. Acquired tolerance can be broken if the original antigen disappears or when a different but closely related antigen is introduced.

## SUPPRESSION OF GRAFT REJECTION

Most immunologists believe that the delayed hypersensitivity mechanism evolved as a means of homeostatic control of somatic mutations (immunologic surveillance). Such mutations, if antigenically distinct, would be quickly removed by this mechanism. This mechanism evolved quite early in vertebrate phylogeny and was probably a key factor that enabled the further evolution and adaptive radiation of the vertebrates to occur. Modern surgical techniques must then employ means of subverting the normal delayed hypersensitivity mechanism for a transplant to be a success. Unfortunately, most means of immunologic suppression are not specific and also suppress the body's ability to cope with ordinary endogenous opportunists as well as the usual pathogens.

Briefly, all of the methods to alter the graft rejection process are aimed at extending the survival time of the graft in an attempt to bring about gradual tolerance or graft acceptance. Some of these methods include:

1. General suppression—This is accomplished by use of either radiomimetic (cyclophosphamide) or antimetabolite drugs (6-mercaptopurine) or else by the use of antilymphocyte globulin.
2. Specific suppression—Because it is very difficult to suppress the secondary immune response or established immunologic memory, transplantation strategy is aimed at timing the administration of the immunosuppressant with the introduction of the primary antigen at the time of transplantation. Such timing effectively inhibits the primary or sensitizing response.
3. Graft adaptation—After the graft has been in place for a period of time, the recipient is gradually withdrawn from the follow-up immunosuppressant (usually a steroid) and monitored carefully for rejection crises. The idea is to present the patient with a high antigen load to establish high-dose acquired tolerance. Possibly humoral, blocking antibody (similar to tumor-enhancing antibody) that blocks the action of cell-mediated immune effectors is produced.

Along with these considerations, proper selection and matching of potential donors with intended recipients with regard to histocompatibility antigens are essential. The closer both parties are with regard to antigenic genotypes, the better the chances of graft acceptance. The line between acceptance and rejection is a thin one and requires diligent attention to detail in postoperative management and follow-up.

## IMMUNOLOGY OF ACQUIRED IMMUNODEFICIENCY SYNDROME (AIDS)

The AIDS epidemic continues to be a major cause of suffering and death in the United States and the rest of the world. No vaccine is available, and despite public education the disease continues to spread. Given the monumental impact of this disease, an understanding of its basic immunopathophysiology and diagnostic and otolaryngologic manifestations is an important requisite for the practicing otolaryngologist. This section briefly summarizes the salient pathophysiologic, diagnostic, and otolaryngologic manifestations of AIDS.

AIDS is caused by the human immunodeficiency virus (HIV), a human retrovirus. By definition, human retroviruses possess RNA as genetic material, a reverse transcriptase, and can cause neurologic or immunologic disease, typically after a long incubation period. Exposure to HIV may not result in disease, and infected persons may remain asymptomatic for years. Some asymptomatic patients develop persistent generalized lymphadenopathy (PGL). Both the asymptomatic and PGL patients may at some point develop what is known as AIDS-related complex (ARC), the hallmark clinical signs of which include chronic fever, weight loss, and persistent diarrhea. Most ARC patients, as well as some asymptomatic patients, and those with PGL can proceed to develop clinical AIDS with one or more severe and often lethal opportunistic infections and/or Kaposi sarcoma. Neurologic disease characterized by encephalopathy, myelopathy, or peripheral neuropathy can also occur as a direct consequence of HIV infection. The mechanisms responsible for the central nervous system (CNS) involvement are not well understood; it is seen most commonly in severely immunocompromised patients.

The primary immune defect in AIDS is a quantitative decrease in T-helper cells(CD4$^+$ T-lymphocytes). The virus selectively infects and kills CD4$^+$ lymphocytes. The virus receptor is the CD4 glycoprotein molecule on the surface of these particular T-cells. Normally these cells play a central role in the immune response by promoting the generation of cytotoxic T-cells and the production of antibody by B-cells. T-helper cells are the source of lymphokines such as IL-2, interferon, macrophage chemotactic factors, hematopoietic growth factors, and various interleukins that serve as differentiation growth factors for B-cells. It is now apparent that the pathogenesis of AIDS is more complex than this and that the depletion of CD4$^+$ T-cells is but one of a myriad of immunologic defects. The CD4 glycoprotein molecule is also present on many other cell types including monocytes, macrophages, Langerhans cells, and follicular dendritic cells. All the afore-

mentioned cells are associated with various immunologic pathways and share a common function as antigen-presenting cells that can support the replication of the HIV.

The immunologic abnormalities associated with AIDS evolve and progress over the duration of the HIV infection. Characteristic immunologic defects induced by infection with HIV include, in addition to the depletion of CD4$^+$ T-cells, a decreased proliferative response to soluble antigens, impaired delayed-type hypersensitivity reactions, decreased antigen-induced interferon production, decreased helper function for B-cell immunoglobulin production, and decreased humoral response to immunization. Other consistently detected abnormalities include lymphopenia, decreased proliferative response to T- and B-cell mitogens, decreased production of IL-2 and other lymphokines, decreased natural killer cell activity, monocyte chemotaxis, and cytotoxicity to virus-infected cells. The eventual net effect of these changes is severe immune dysfunction, opportunistic infections and/or Kaposi sarcoma, and B-cell lymphoma. AIDS has a fatal course at present.

Multiple mechanisms have been postulated for the decline of T4 cells. Infected T4 cells may simply die as a result of prolific viral replication. Additionally, there is direct cell-to-cell spread of virus via fusion of infected with uninfected cells. Fusion of infected cells with formation of syncytia (giant cells) may also be a mechanism of cell death. Fused cells develop "ballooning" and usually die within 48 hours. Concurrently, surface envelope glycoproteins (especially gp 140) shed by the virus may bind to the CD4 receptors on the surface of the T4 cells and induce an autoimmune elimination of T-cells coated with gp140. Finally, HIV infection of the bone marrow decreases production of new T-cells. The number of T-cells infected at any one time is low; most are latently infected, with the viral DNA integrated into the DNA of the T-cell host. The depletion of T-cells takes place over years. Interestingly, mononuclear cells do not die as a result of infection with HIV.

The pathogenesis of the neurologic manifestations of the disease is affected by different mechanisms than those producing disease in the lymphoid system. It has been proposed that infected monocytes may act as a vehicle for entry of HIV into the brain. Once in the brain, the monocytes are somehow activated to release cytokines and other proinflammatory mediators, which recruit other tissue-damaging inflammatory cells. It has also been suggested that the virus can directly infect neural tissue or endothelial cells. HIV has been detected within neurons, oligodendrocytes, and astrocytes.

During the course of HIV disease, antibodies are generated against various viral proteins; however, the HIV-infected host is unable to generate sustained protective immunity. The HIV may escape immune detection by the host by altering its surface-exposed antigens. Additionally, the HIV is constantly undergoing mutation. Several strains may infect a given person, and a recurrent selection process may take place. Finally, HIV may exist predominantly in latent form, integrated in the host cell genome, and thereby be able to "hide" from the host's immunologic surveillance system.

## OTOLARYNGOLOGIC MANIFESTATIONS OF AIDS

The clinical conditions of otitis media, rhinitis, sinusitis, bronchitis, and pneumonia have long been associated with immunosuppressed states such as generalized hypogammaglobulinemia, T-cell defects, combined defects, and selective IgA deficiency. In 1983 seven AIDS patients with head and neck involvement were reported to have died from opportunistic infections. It has been predicted that by 1993 over 350,000 cases of AIDS would be diagnosed in the United States and that 1.5 to 2.0 million Americans would be seropositive.

Human T-cell lymphtrophic virus III (HTLV-III) has been isolated from blood, urine, cerebrospinal fluid, vaginal fluid, tears, and saliva. Its target cells, as the name implies, are T-helper, monocytes, macrophages, certain brain cells, and colorectal epithelial cells. With the risk of HIV infection in heterosexuals ranging from 15% to 20% and increasing, a high index of suspicion and universal precautions are prudent both in treating the patient and protecting the health care team. Public opinion polls show that 86% of respondents want to know their physician's HIV status, and that 65% would change physicians if theirs was found to be positive.

Patients with HIV seropositivity have traditionally been classified as having PGL, ARC, and

AIDS. The Centers for Disease Control have suggested that PGL includes palpable adenopathy greater than 1 cm at two extrainguinal sites. Biopsy is not helpful, especially in absence of constitutional symptoms. ARC is without true symptoms such as associated fever over 37.7° C, weight loss of more than 10%, lymphadenopathy lasting longer than 3 months, diarrhea, fatigue, mental dysfunction, night sweats, decreased T-helper cells, decreased T-helper/T-suppressor ratio, leukopenia, and thrombocytopenia. AIDS has these associated symptoms but in a prolonged or unusual pattern. Arthralgias, sore throat, cervical adenopathy, stiff neck, urticaria, sacral hypesthesia, and abdominal cramps may also be seen.

Forty to sixty percent of HIV-positive patients present with head and neck manifestations. In general these include candidiasis, herpes simplex lesions and stomatitis, chronic cough, rapidly enlarging neck masses, shortness of breath, dysphagia, lymphoproliperative neoplasms, Kaposi sarcoma, hairy leukoplakia, intraoral ulcers, enlarging major salivary glands, and epistaxis.

In 1984 Pass et al. noted the opportunistic organisms most frequently encountered in the head and neck to include *Pneumocystis carinii,* cytomegalovirus (CMV), *Cryptococcus neoformans, Mycobacteria avium* and *intracellarium,* as well as those previously mentioned. By 1984 Patow et al. had described pharyngeal Kaposi sarcoma.

In 1986 Alshari et al. reported squamous cell carcinoma associated with HIV. That same year, Penn discussed cofactors of neoplastic disease, with a high percentage of lymphomas, squamous cell carcinomas, and Kaposi sarcoma seen in these patients.

In 1987 Williams described pediatric AIDS patients with manifestations including candidiasis, cervical adenopathy, parotid enlargement, and microsomia. From a historical context, Phelan described xerostomia, exfoliative cheilitis, patchy tongue, gingival bleeding, perioral *Molluscum contagiosum,* and brown hairy tongue in 1987. In the same year, Roberts added acute necrotizing gingivitis, periodontal disease, and aphthous ulcers to the findings.

The culmination of these findings suggests the following approach: (1) correct the underlying cause, (2) maintain a high index of suspicion, (3) culture suspected areas, (4) consider antibiotic prophylaxis, (5) biopsy and re-examine available areas, (6) use computed tomography and/or magnetic resonance imaging for detection and staging, and (7) be acutely aware of airway management.

**Initial History and Physical Examination**

All prior medical, surgical, and psychiatric hospitalizations should be explored and chronic medical conditions should be described in detail. Of particular concern is any history of hepatic and renal disease. A full obstetric history should be elicited. Any parenteral drug use or infectious diseases, especially sexually transmitted and tuberculosis, require investigation. Specific information concerning an AIDS-related infection or tumor can help to confirm suspected head and neck manifestations.

Any examination should be carried out using universal precautions. This includes eyewear, masks, and latex gloves. A cursory whole body examination follows, including a thorough head and neck examination. Dermatologic changes include folliculitis, herpes zoster and simplex, *Molluscum contagiosum* infection, seborrheic dermatitis, psoriasis, and Kaposi sarcoma. Retinitis is usually accompanied by visual complaints. Pathologic murmurs are suggestive of endocarditis. Hepatosplenomegaly may be associated with

HIV-related conditions such as immune thrombocytopenic purpura, disseminated mycobacterial infection, or lymphoma.

**Testing and Laboratory Data**

HTLV-III antibodies can be detected using enzyme-linked immunosorbent assay (ELISA), immunofluorescent assays (IFAs), and radioimmunopreciptation tests (RIP), all of which have known false-positive and false-negative results. Western blot is usually the confirmatory test. Quantitative abnormalities in circulatory cell populations are seen, including decreased T-cell populations, leukopenia, thrombocytopenia, and anemia.

**Clinical Manifestations**

In 71% of reported cases, AIDS manifests itself in anatomic regions treated by the otolaryngologist–head and neck surgeon.

***Oral and Oropharyngeal***
The mouth serves as the "window to the soul" of HIV infection. Dry mucous membranes generally reflect volume depletion. Angular stomatitis

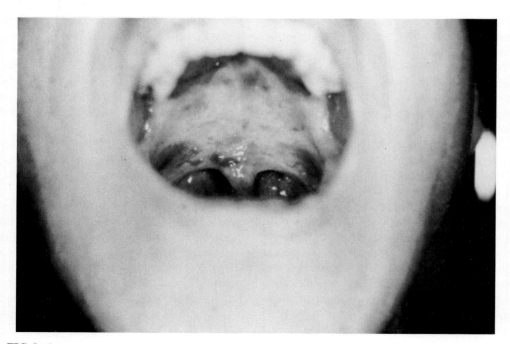

**FIG 3–1.**
Kaposi's sarcoma of hard and soft palate.

or cheilitis may be associated with candidiasis. Periodontal disease can be very aggressive in patients with HIV. Opportunistic infections are frequent, including those previously mentioned, as well as herpetic stomatitis; "hairy" leukoplakia; aphthous stomatitis; and fungal, streptococcal, or gonococcal pharyngitis. Oncologic manifestations include Kaposi sarcoma, lymphoma, and squamous cell carcinoma. Kaposi sarcoma appears as an atypical elevated purplish blue lesion, most commonly on the hard palate (Fig. 3–1). The other lesions can present as ulcerations, plaques, exudates, diffuse inflammation, or nodules.

Candidiasis usually responds to nystatin solution, while symptomatic care and antibiotic or antiviral therapy are used for the other lesions. Kaposi sarcoma is amenable to carbon dioxide laser therapy in localized areas. Biopsy of nonhealing lesions confirms their diagnosis.

### Sinus and Nasal

Rhinosinusitis is most commonly caused by *Haemophilus influenzae* and *Streptococcus pneumoniae* bacteria, with *Pseudollescheria boydii* being the most common fungi. Treatment is usually conservative, with appropriate antibiotics and early sinus irrigation.

Granular, erythematous nasal mucosa is indicative of invasive vascular endothelial cells and squamous metaplasia of cytomegalovirus. Treatment is with ganciclovir.

*Acanthamoeba castellani,* a free-living amoeba, may cause swelling of the turbinates, opacification of the ethmoids, antral mucosa hypertrophy on computed tomography. Treatment is with rifampin or ketoconazole.

*Alternaria alternata* causes a clear rhinorrhea with black necrotic lesions on the septum. Treatment is with a Caldwell-Luc operation and amphotericin B, repeated if necessary.

*Cryptococcal* infection requires endoscopic sinus surgery, in addition to amphotericin B and fluorocytosine.

*Pneumocystis carinii* is associated with septal abscesses. Treatment is with pentamidine, cephalexin, or trimethoprim/sulfamethoxazole (Bactrim).

Benign nasopharyngeal masses are seen in patients with PGL and those at risk for HIV with no significant cervical adenopathy. One study reported seven patients whose chief complaints consisted of nasal congestion and hearing loss. In such cases, physical examination reveals otitis media with effusion and type B tympanograms. Biopsy via curettage is important to rule out lymphoma. Histologic study shows benign lymphoid hypertrophy dispersed with giant cells in granulomatous formations. The mass is described as glistening homogeneous tissue. HIV testing with consent is necessary. Bilateral myringotomies and/or tubal insertion can accompany the biopsy.

Seventy-three percent of patients at high risk for AIDS presented with herpes simplex in one study. In some cases giant herpetic nasal ulcers, up to 3 cm, extend to the septum or face. Acyclovir is currently therapeutic.

Seborrheic dermatitis has a prevalence of 22% to 83%, involving the facial skin, extremities, and chest; it can also involve the nares. Treatment is with steroids but is not always successful.

Candidiasis most commonly is seen in a pseudomembranous form with cheesy white patches. Scraping reveals an erythematous base. Diagnosis is via a potassium hydroxide preparation; treatment is as described previously or with oral ketoconazole.

Non-Hodgkin's lymphoma can present with a foul-smelling nasal discharge. CT shows soft tissue density without bone destruction. Biopsy most commonly shows high-grade, undifferentiated tumor. Radiation and chemotherapy are recommended.

Kaposi sarcoma is seen in 47% of AIDS patients. Involvement of the nasal skin, vestibule, nasal cavity, and septum have all been reported. Clinically, nasal obstruction, epistaxis, and rhinorrhea are the result of the violaceous, nodular tumor. Treatment includes radiation and/or chemotherapy.

### Salivary Glands

Multiocular cysts of the parotid gland, as well as mycobacterial sialadenitis of the submandibular gland, have been noted in patients with AIDS. Treatment is expectant.

### Upper Airway Involvement

Epiglottitis is rare in adults. A series of 5 patients is presented to illustrate this manifestation. Ages ranged from 29 to 46, and all were HIV positive. All presented with tachypnea, one with stridor. Flexible nasopharyngoscopy revealed edematous supraglottic structures and a pale, large epiglottis. Temperatures ranged from 102° to 105° F, bilateral upper jugular lymphadenopathy was present, and medical management failed. All patients were intubated and decanulated 48 to 72 hours later. Cultures obtained grew *S. pneumoniae* and *Staphylococcus aureus*. Treatment was continued with cefuroxime or ampicillin and chloramphenicol. Other studies have shown that AIDS alters the rapid progression of the disease, precluding conservative management.

A case report illustrates tracheal-laryngeal involvement of Kaposi sarcoma, which is found in approximately 20% of AIDS patients. The patient presented with dysphagia and hoarseness which required an emergent tracheotomy. Subsequent direct laryngoscopy revealed a mass between the cords with a 5 to 7 mm opening. Biopsy caused uncontrolled hemorrhage that resulted in respiratory arrest. This has been documented in one other case as well. Intubation is the preferred management scheme. Chemotherapy will decrease the size of the tumor if time is available—60% in 2 to 3 days. Laser therapy and radiation may be used. In one case, autopsy revealed Kaposi sarcoma of the larynx, pharynx, esophagus, and lungs.

CMV laryngitis presents with odynophagia, hoarseness, and weight loss. Computed tomography findings are consistent with endoscopy, with supraglottic involvement that shows no involvement of the true vocal cords but possible esophageal ulcers. A greenish exudate was seen in one case, and biopsy was positive for CMV. Histologic findings for this patient included large cells with homogeneous eosinophilic nuclear inclusions and granular cytoplasm (Figs. 3–2 and 3–3). Another patient showed a true vocal cord lesion that was positive for CMV on rapid immunofluorescence assay. Treatment is with ganciclovir.

Laryngeal lymphoma has been reported. It appears to be more aggressive in unusual sites. Airway obstruction is a concern with either of the above.

### Lymph Nodes

Generalized lymphadenopathy is an early consequence of HIV infection. Most HIV-infected patients have palpable lymph nodes. Any of the following characteristics should prompt immediate evaluation to exclude regional or systemic opportunistic infection: size greater than 1.5 cm or rapid change in size; asymmetry; pain, tenderness, or fluctuance; hard or fixed nodes; cutane-

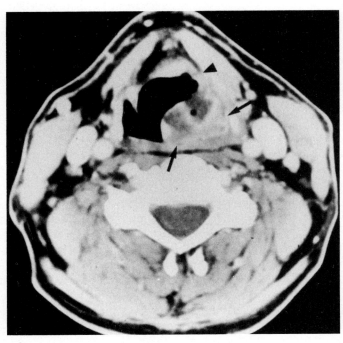

**FIG 3–2.**
Cytomegalovirus of left pyriform sinus. (From *Arch Pathol Lab Med* 116:540, 1992. Used by permission.)

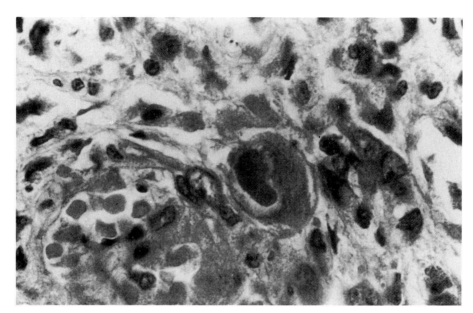

**FIG 3–3.**
Cytomegalovirus of larynx. (From *Arch Pathol Lab Med* 116:540, 1992. Used by permission.)

ous discoloration above, or purulence; and unexplained constitutional symptoms in conjunction with new or diffuse lymphadenopathy. Initial antibiotic therapy is warranted but prolonged resolution demands further workup, including HIV testing, and not to exclude carcinoma. Fine needle aspirates are usually nonproductive, and biopsy may lead to difficulty with wound healing. Treatment is for the underlying cause.

### Ear

Reports by Real (1987) and others have suggested direct involvement of HIV with auditory function. Potential causes that must be eliminated include CMV, hepatitis B virus, herpes simplex virus, syphilis, herpes zoster-varicella, toxoplasmosis, ototoxic medications, encephalitis, meningitis, and hemorrhage with neuropathy resulting from lymphoma or mononeuritis multiplex. Neuropathologic studies suggest some subcortical changes including the brainstem that may predict CNS degeneration.

Review of the literature reveals that AIDS patients may present with both sensorineural and conductive hearing loss; accelerated otosyphilis; *Pneumocystis carinii* involvement; peripheral cranial nerve VII paralysis with hearing loss; with otalgia, tinnitus, and vertigo presenting separately. HIV does not seem to affect the cochlear

end-organs as other viruses do. Chandrasekhar et al. noted endosteal membrane elevation, subepithelial damage with buckling of the otoconial membrane, and inflammatory precipitate in the semicircular canals. All of these findings lend credence to the suggestion that HIV directly involves the auditory system.

Ho et al. (1985) found HTLV-III to be neurotropic, with resultant meningitis, dementia, and encephalopathy. However, they could not isolate the virus from the spiral ganglion or the eighth cranial nerve.

### Sudden Hearing Loss

Viral agents cause up to one-third of cases of sudden sensorineural hearing loss. The fourth most common agent to affect AIDS patients is *Cryptococcus neoformans*. This class of fungi has a 27% incidence of sensorineural hearing loss through invasion of the cochlear and vestibular nerves to the organ of Corti. Retrocochlear loss is seen with positive short increment sensitivity index (SISI) scores but without recruitment (see Fig. ). A case report demonstrated clinical loss of hearing, frequent headaches, and difficulty walking. Tympanometry was normal, along with acoustic reflex, but there was poor progression on ABR. Computed tomography was normal. Diagnosis was made at surgery when the patient's con-

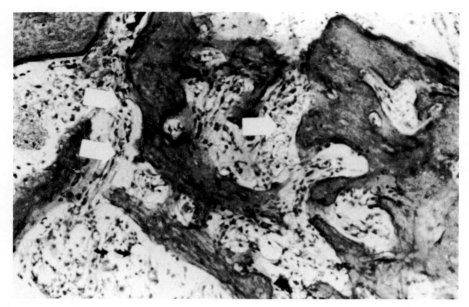

**FIG 3–4.**
Cryptococcal invasion of Scarpa's ganglion.

dition worsened. He was treated unsuccessfully with amphotericin B and 5-fluorocytosine for his meningitis. At autopsy, *Cryptococcal* organisms were noted to have invaded the bilateral internal auditory canals with extension and necrosis of the cochlear and vestibular nerves to the geniculate ganglion. Scarpa's ganglion was involved, but the facial nerve was free of disease (Figs. 3–4 and 3–5).

More commonly seen is a conductive or mixed hearing loss as a result of opportunistic infections of the external ear canal. These include *Aspergillus* and *Pneumocystis carinii*. One-third of HIV-infected individuals have extrapulmonary *Pneu-*

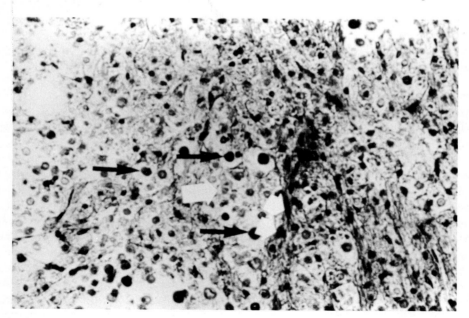

**FIG 3–5.**
Cryptococcal invasion of the spiral ganglion.

*mocystis* involvement. In the external ear it causes a polypoid lesion that can extend to the middle ear and mastoid. Clinically, this results in unilateral hearing loss and a foul discharge. At surgery a tympanic membrane perforation is noted with erosion of the ossicles. On histologic examination, cysts are seen with silver stain. Treatment is with trimethoprim/sulfamethoxazole and dapsone. The pathogenesis is unknown, though carriage in the nasopharynx is common and the infection is disseminated hematogenously.

Otosyphilis remains a clinical diagnosis requiring a high index of suspicion. The patient experiences unilateral or bilateral sudden sensorineural hearing loss, tinnitus, and fullness. A low-frequency hearing loss is most frequently noted. A flourescent trepenemal antibody absorption (FTA) is the best test and is positive in 65% of patients testing positive for HIV. Treatment is with penicillin combined with steroids, but further immunosuppression is of concern. Response rate ranges from 15% to 58%. Patients are usually followed with audiograms.

Lymphoma and Kaposi sarcoma have been reported to affect the external ear, canal, and tympanic membrane. Treatment includes argon and carbon dioxide laser.

### Neurologic

Ten percent of AIDS patients present with neurologic problems. Eight-eight percent have evidence of CNS involvement on autopsy. This may result from infection, tumors, or primary neuropathology; the AIDS-associated pathogenesis is unknown.

Mycotic and bacterial infections contribute to intracranial hemorrhages in immunocompromised patients. The pathogenesis involves the formation of aneurysms along major and small cerebral vessels. The incidence is less than 4% for bacterial and even lower for fungal infections.

*Toxoplasma gondii* causes focal or diffuse seizures, mental status changes, or focal neurologic deficits resembling strokes. Serologic testing is nonspecific, making brain biopsy necessary.

Patients with Cryptococcal meningitis present with fever, severe headaches, and mental status changes. Diagnosis is based on positive Cryptococcal antigen response or culture. Therapy is as noted previously with amphotericin B, with or without 5-fluorocytosine.

Oncologic CNS involvement includes lym-

phoma and Kaposi sarcoma. Patients with dementia should be managed with a high index of suspicion.

### Associated Neoplasia

Kaposi sarcoma may affect as many as 80% of HIV-infected individuals, though recent data suggest the incidence is declining. One study placed it as low as 14%. Originally described by Moritz Kaposi in 1872, the epidemic Kaposi sarcoma seen in AIDS is aggressive, with cutaneous visceral or nodal involvement. Histologic study shows spindle-shaped cells with cleft formation. The tumor is highly resistant to treatment, though traditional radiation and carbon dioxide laser treatment have been palliative. Further investigation has found partial success with cryotherapy, and with chemotherapy via intralesional injection and α-interferon.

Nearly one-half of AIDS patients present with a malignant diagnosis at some time. The incidence of extranodal lymphomas ranges from 4% to 10%, with no site predilection. Patients with lymphoma rarely manifest Kaposi sarcoma. Seventy percent of the non-Hodgkin's lymphomas are found to be high grade, while 30% are intermediate. Case reports demonstrate clinical fevers, anorexia, night sweats, and generalized adenopathy, with lesions found on the hard palate, postauricular area, external ear canal, intranasal area, and pyriform sinus. Diagnostic workup includes computed tomography, chest x-ray, and peripheral blood smear as well as bone marrow examination and lumbar puncture. Direct laryngoscopy with guided biopsies is beneficial. Response rate to chemotherapy varies from 33% to 57%, to the most effective regimen being methotrexate, bleomycin, cytosine arabinonide, cyclophosphamide, vincristine, and doxorubicin.

High-grade non-Hodgkin's lymphoma is described histologically as small non-cleaved cell or immunoblastic lymphoma. It has been associated with Burkitt's lymphoma or Burkitt's-like findings. Ziegler et al. noted that patients with non-Hodgkin's lymphoma were younger with unusual presentations in nontraditional sites. They had a 53% remission with chemotherapy and additional radiation and bleomycin, but a 59% relapse rate. Overall mortality rate was 73%, 90% from CNS involvement. Lymphoma should therefore be considered an immediate life-threatening condition.

Five percent of other associated neoplasms include Hodgkin's lymphoma and squamous cell cancer. Stage 3 and 4 Hodgkin's lymphoma is seen most commonly with T-cell dysfunction and AIDS. Squamous cell carcinoma has thus far only been documented with venereal contact and not in the head and neck.

### Pediatric Infection With HIV

Many children with congenital HIV infection show signs and symptoms of disease in their first year of life. These may include diarrhea, fever, recurrent night sweats, generalized lymphadenopathy, unexplained enlarged parotid glands, and hepatosplenomegaly. A dysmorphic syndrome with microcephaly, flat nasal bridge, patulous lips, short nose with a flattened columella, obliquity of the eyes, hypertelorism, and a boxlike appearance of the forehead has been described. Opportunistic infections, most notably viral, are common in the first year. Chemoprophylaxis against specific organisms can be instituted. Immunization schedules should be modified because of the child's immunosuppressed condition. Ultimately, antiviral agents are therapeutic for children as well as adults.

### Treatment of AIDS

Initial success with azidothymidine through inhibiting HTLV-III reverse transcriptase lengthens patient survival and prevents development of recurrent opportunistic infections. Recombinant interferon-2 has a positive response in vitro. Interferon-2 and IL-2 are currently being investigated. The remainder of therapy is directed, supportive, or symptomatic.

### Management of HIV Infection in the Health Care Setting

To date 82 health care workers have acquired HTLV-III, with no documented cases being otolaryngologist–head and neck surgeons. The seroconversion rate after needlesticks is 0.2% to 0.3%; after splashes, it is 0% to 0.1%.

### Prevention

Guidelines set by the Occupational Safety and Health Administration specify that there should be no direct contact between patients' blood, secretions, and excretions and employees' skin or mucous membranes. This includes the handling of examination instruments and disposable waste.

After possible exposure to HTLV-III, prompt cleaning is recommended; back bleeding with expression of blood at the puncture site and disinfection with alcohol or iodine are beneficial. Immediate arrangements should be made for HTLV-III antibody testing and hepatitis screening. If the patient's status is unknown, consent should be obtained for testing. If the employee is seronegative, testing should be repeated at 6 weeks, then at 3, 6, and 12 months. Counseling should be arranged, and azidothymidine should be offered to the employee if the patient is HIV positive.

This chapter was designed as a basic review of major concepts of modern immunology. The general principles outlined are only guidelines, and the student should consult standard texts on immunology for a more comprehensive review. Many excellent books are available that focus on the specific nuances of the immunobiology of the head and neck.

## SELECTED READINGS

Bernstein JM, Ogra PL, eds: *Immunology of the ear*, New York: 1987, Raven.

Rose NR, Friedman H, Fahey JL, eds: *Manual of clinical laboratory immunology*, ed 3, Washington, DC, 1986, American Society for Microbiology.

Poliquin JF, Ryan AF, Harris JP, eds: *Immunobiology of the head and neck*, San Diego, 1984, College-Hill.

Roitt IM, Brostoff J, Male DK, eds: *Immunology*, ed 2, London, 1989, Gower.

# PART II
# Nose and Paranasal Sinuses

# 4

# Anatomy and Physiology

## ANATOMY

### External Nose

Terms commonly used to describe the external nose (Fig. 4–1) are the *tip* or *apex*, the *base* (which includes the nares), the *root* (where the nasal bones join the skull above), the *dorsum* (between the root and the tip), and the *bridge* (the upper part of the dorsum).

The two nasal *bones* vary in size and sometimes are even absent. They join each other in the midline and articulate above with the frontal bone and laterally with the frontonasal processes of the maxillary bones.

Only the upper third of the external nose is bony. The lower two thirds are cartilaginous. Variations in the size and shape of the nose result in large part from differences in the cartilages. The *lower lateral (major alar) cartilages* form the rim and the flaring curve of the ala. There is a lateral crus and a medial crus. The major alar cartilages form most of the tip of the nose. The *upper lateral (lateral nasal) cartilages* lie in the middle third of the nose, between the nasal bones above and the lower lateral cartilages below. These cartilages account for the shape of the middle third of the nose. There are several *sesamoid* and *minor alar cartilages* lateral to the two large cartilages of the external nose. Also contributing to the shape of the ala and middle third of the nose is fibroadipose tissue.

The *nasal septum,* discussed in detail in the section on the internal nose, forms part of the dorsum as it extends upward between the two upper lateral cartilages and between the medial crura of the lower lateral cartilages.

Muscles of the external nose are rather rudimentary in humans. The *procerus muscle* extends between the nasal bones and the frontalis muscle; the *depressor septi muscle* and certain fibers that cause dilatation of the nasal alae are also recognized.

### Internal Nose

On each side of the nose are anterior and posterior openings called the nares. The posterior nares are also called the *choanae.* The *vestibule* is the anterior, skin-lined part of the nasal cavity that contains the vibrissae, or nasal hairs, the follicles of which often become infected. A *recess* of the vestibule reaches upward into the tip. The junction of the skin and nasal mucous membranes occurs at a variable distance inside the nose. Usually the junction is clearly defined because of the difference in color between skin and mucosa.

The *nasal septum* (Fig. 4–2) divides the nose into the two nasal fossae. It is cartilaginous in front and bony behind. The septum is straight at birth and in early life but becomes deviated or deformed in almost every adult. Only the posterior end, separating the posterior nares, remains constantly in the midline. Anteriorly, the *quadrilateral,* or *septal, cartilage* is frequently dislocated into one nasal vestibule. Posteriorly the septal cartilage joins the perpendicular plate of the ethmoid above and the vomer below. The other bony parts of the septum (palate bone, crest of the maxilla, and rostrum of the sphenoid) are small.

The lateral wall of the nose (Fig. 4–3) is a complicated area anatomically and a very important area clinically. There are four nasal turbinates, or conchae. Named from below upward, they are the inferior, middle, superior, and supreme turbinates. The *supreme turbinate* is very small and is not seen during clinical examination;

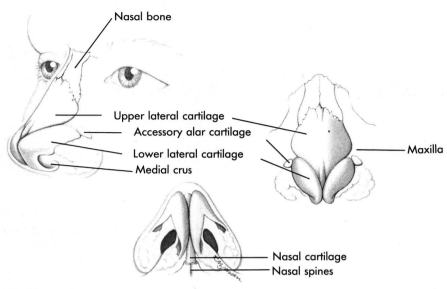

**FIG 4–1.**
Anatomy of external nose.

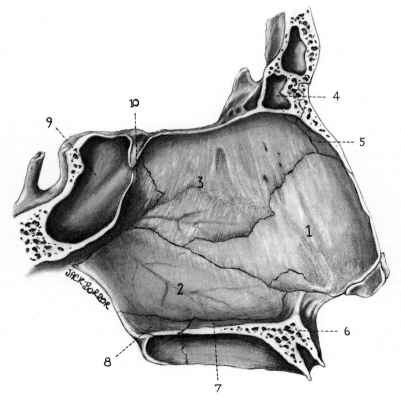

**FIG 4–2.**
Nasal septum. *1*, septal cartilage. *2*, vomer. *3*, perpendicular plate. *4*, frontal sinus. *5*, nasal bone. *6*, maxilla. *7*, maxillary crest. *8*, palatine bone. *9*, sphenoid sinus. *10*, rostrum of the sphenoid.

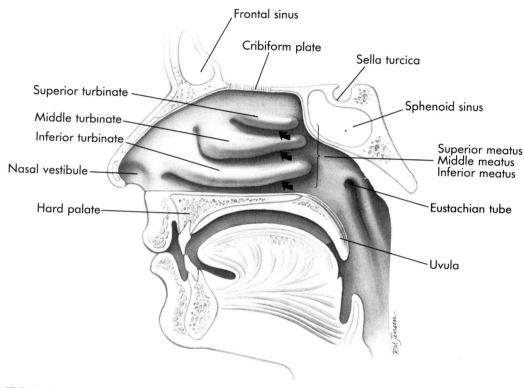

**FIG 4–3.**
Lateral wall of nose.

the *superior turbinate* is so placed that usually it can be seen only with a postnasal mirror.

The *inferior turbinate* is a separate bone, whereas the other turbinates are part of the ethmoid bone. The mucous membrane of the inferior turbinate is very rich in blood vessels and is semierectile. Vasoconstrictors affect this structure the most. Sometimes the bony part of the inferior turbinate lies close to the lateral nasal wall, but at other times it juts out prominently into the airway and causes nasal obstruction. Often the mucosa of the inferior turbinate touches the septum.

The *middle turbinate* is somewhat smaller than the inferior turbinate because it is shorter. It often contains an air cell, which sometimes dilates the turbinate enough to produce nasal obstruction.

The several nasal meatuses are named according to the turbinates that overlie them. Thus, the inferior meatus lies under the inferior turbinate, and the middle meatus under the middle turbinate. Above the superior and supreme turbinates is the *sphenoethmoid recess,* into which the sphenoid sinus opens.

The *inferior meatus* may be large or small, depending on the position of the inferior turbinate and its state of vascular engorgement. The only channel opening into the inferior meatus is the *nasolacrimal duct,* which opens toward its anterior end. Posteriorly there are large blood vessels (sphenopalatine branches) under the mucosa of the lateral wall of the inferior meatus, which may be a site of bleeding.

The *middle meatus* contains the drainage sites of the maxillary, frontal, and anterior ethmoid sinuses. About midway along the meatus, the ethmoid bulla (an air cell) bulges from the lateral wall of the nose into the meatus. Just anterior to the bulla is a groove, the *infundibulum,* which curves from above downward and then posteriorly around the bulla. This area is very important clinically because it is into the upper end of the infundibulum that the *nasofrontal duct* drains, whereas the maxillary sinus drains into the posterior and lower part of the infundibulum. The anterior ethmoid cells drain, along with the frontal sinus, anteriorly and superiorly. By knowing the general sites of sinus drainage, the clinician, looking at a stream of pus, is better able to differentiate between maxillary and frontal (or anterior ethmoid) sinusitis. The actual ostia of the sinuses, except rarely the sphenoid, are not seen during clinical examination.

The posterior ethmoid cells drain into the *superior meatus.* Pus from the sphenoethmoid recess and the superior meatus is usually best seen with the postnasal mirror. As seen anteriorly (with the nasal speculum), pus from the frontal, anterior ethmoid, and maxillary sinuses drains under the middle turbinate (into the middle meatus), but pus from the posterior sinuses drains medial to the middle turbinate (between it and the septum).

The *olfactory* area is a 2.5 cm area located high in the nose in a narrow niche formed by the superior turbinate, the upper septum, and the cribriform plate. The olfactory epithelium consists of three types of cells: receptor, supporting, and basal cells. The supporting cells serve secretory and nutritional functions and provide firm attachment between cells. The unmyelinated axons of the receptor cells ascend through the cribriform plate and eventually reach the rhinencephalon, the uncus, the hippocampus, the mamillary bodies, and the amygdaloid nucleus. Unlike other senses, olfaction is not relayed through the thalamus.

## Blood Supply of the Nose

Both the *external* and the *internal carotid systems* provide a blood supply to the nose (Figs. 4–4 and 4–5). The external carotid does so chiefly through one of its terminal divisions, the internal maxillary artery, and to a limited extent through nasal branches of the facial artery. The internal maxillary artery, and more particularly its terminal branch, the sphenopalatine, has been called the rhinologist's artery because it supplies so much of the nose. The sphenopalatine artery supplies most of the posterior part of the nasal septum and most of the lateral wall of the nose, especially posteriorly.

The *anterior* and *posterior ethmoidal arteries,* branches of the ophthalmic artery, derive their blood from the internal carotid system. The anterior ethmoidal artery is the second largest vessel supplying the internal nose. It gives blood to both the anterosuperior part of the septum and the lateral wall of the nose.

The *external nose* receives blood from approximately the same arteries as does the internal nose. The venous drainage is important because part of it, through the angular vein, leads to the inferior ophthalmic vein and eventually to the cavernous sinus. Most of the venous drainage, however, is downward through the anterior facial vein.

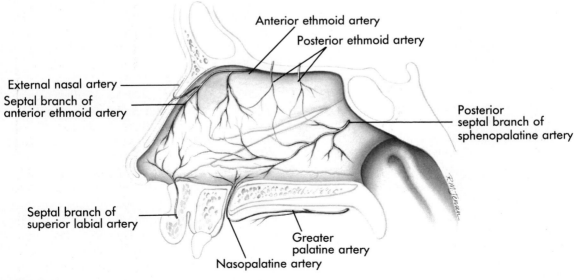

**FIG 4–4.**
Blood supply to the nasal septum.

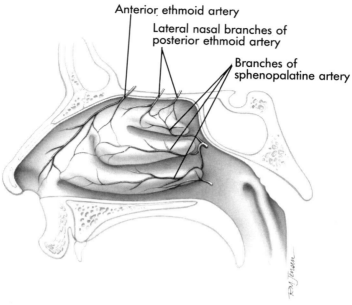

**FIG 4–5.**
Blood supply of lateral wall of nose.

## Lymphatics of the Nose

Lymphatic drainage of the nose is extensive and parallels the venous drainage. Lymphatics along the anterior facial vein terminate in submaxillary lymph nodes.

## Nerve Supply of the Nose

The muscles of the *external nose* are supplied by the seventh cranial nerve; the skin receives its sensory supply from the first and second divisions of the fifth nerve (Figs. 4–6 and 4–7).

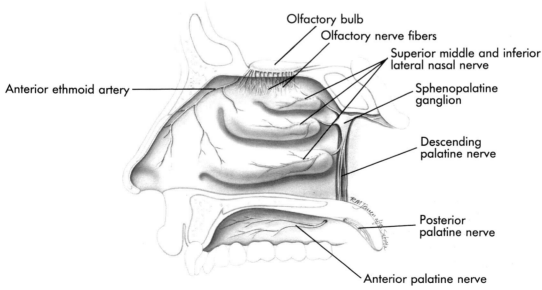

**FIG 4–6.**
Nerve supply to lateral wall of nose.

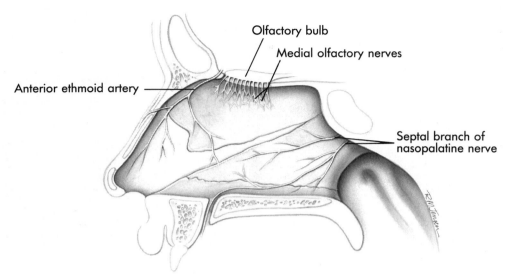

**FIG 4–7.**
Nerve supply to lateral nasal septum.

The *internal nose* has a more complicated nerve supply. The olfactory nerves have been mentioned. Their cell bodies (in the mucous membrane) send fibers upward through the cribriform plate. These fibers enter the olfactory bulb. Olfaction is disturbed or lost when there is enough nasal obstruction to keep air currents from the olfactory mucosa (as in nasal polyposis). Anosmia also results from fractures through the cribriform plate, tumors of the frontal lobe or meninges, and some viral infections.

The general sensory nerve supply to the internal nose comes from the first and second divisions of the fifth cranial nerve. The *nasociliary,* or *anterior ethmoidal, nerve* is a branch of the ophthalmic (first) division and supplies some of the superior and anterior parts of the septum and lateral nasal wall. Sphenopalatine branches of the maxillary division supply most of the posterior part of the nose.

*Parasympathetic fibers* with cell bodies in the sphenopalatine ganglion are distributed to the nasal mucosa. *Sympathetic fibers* that reach the nose come from fibers around the carotid plexus. These carotid fibers join and form the deep petrosal nerve, which joins the greater superficial petrosal nerve (branch of the facial nerve) to form the vidian nerve. The vidian nerve thus carries preganglionic parasympathetic fibers and postganglionic sympathetic fibers to the sphenopalatine ganglion. Here the parasympathetic fibers synapse.

It is sometimes thought that the general sensory nerve supply of the nose is from branches of the sphenopalatine ganglion, but actually the ganglion is parasympathetic; the maxillary fibers merely branch off at this level. Other *parasympathetic* ganglia of the head are the *otic,* associated with the parotid gland; the *submaxillary,* associated with the tongue and submandibular salivary gland; and the *ciliary,* associated with the eye. Besides supplying the nose, the *sphenopalatine ganglion* supplies the lacrimal gland and palate.

The *mucous membrane* of the nose is described in detail in the discussion of the physiology of the nose.

**Paranasal Sinuses**

There are four paranasal sinuses (air-filled spaces lined by mucous membrane) on each side of the head (Fig. 4–8). The *ethmoid sinus* is often called the ethmoid labyrinth because of its many cellular divisions. The others are the *maxillary,* the *frontal* (Fig. 4–9), and the *sphenoid sinuses.* The sinuses develop as outpocketings of nasal mucous membrane. At birth only the maxillary and ethmoid sinuses are present. The frontal sinus develops from one of the anterior ethmoid cells but does not start to pneumatize the frontal bone until the first or second year of life. It is not significant until about the age of 9. Similarly, the sphenoid sinus begins to invade bone in about the

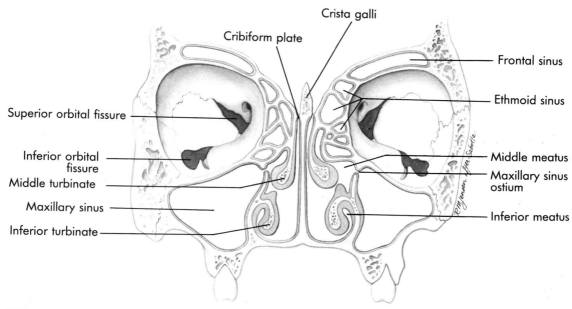

**FIG 4–8.**
Frontal section of paranasal sinuses.

third year of life but is not clinically significant until 10 to 12 years of age.

**Practical Considerations**

There are fewer glands in the mucosa of the nasal sinuses than in the mucosa of the nose. Most nasal discharge of a mucoid type is pro-duced by nasal glands and does not come from the sinuses. The walls of the sinuses are less sensitive to pain than are their ostia or most parts of the nasal mucosa. *A great deal of the head pain and mucoid nasal discharge ordinarily attributed to chronic sinusitis is in reality caused by other disease.*

Sometimes one frontal sinus is missing; at

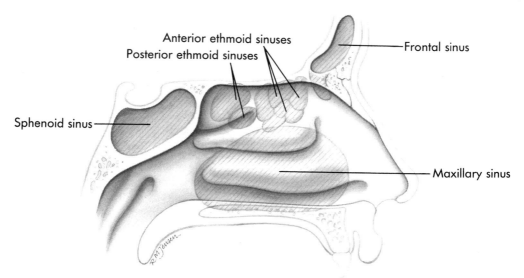

**FIG 4–9.**
Lateral wall of nose with location of paranasal sinuses.

other times there are more than two frontal sinuses, each with a separate drainage canal into
the nose. When disease of the frontal sinus occurs, complications are most likely to occur in the
orbit and the anterior cranial fossa.

The relationship of the maxillary sinus to the
upper teeth is important because of the frequency
with which pain from dental abscess is confused
with pain from sinusitis and because tooth extraction may result in loss of a root tip (or even a
whole tooth) into the maxillary sinus.

The ethmoid air cells pneumatize not only the
ethmoid bone but also parts of adjacent bones.
The lamina papyracea is a thin plate of bone separating the ethmoid labyrinth from the orbit. This
"paper plate," often incomplete, is a common
place for infection from the sinuses to enter the
orbit.

The sphenoid is the most deeply placed of the
sinuses. The two sphenoids are seldom the same
size and are sometimes very small. Directly above
the sphenoid sinus is the sella turcica. From there,
pituitary tumors may erode downward and fill the
sphenoid. Lateral to the sphenoid sinus is the cavernous sinus, with the third, fourth, fifth, and
sixth cranial nerves. The brainstem is located posteriorly.

## PHYSIOLOGY

### Functions of the Nose

Because the nose is exposed to constant differences in temperature and relative humidity, as
well as to particles present in the atmosphere, it
must be able to perform a variety of functions
(see box). These functions are aided by the turbinates. Projecting into the nasal cavity, the turbinates produce a broad surface covered by mucosa
that supports a specialized epithelium.

Nasal obstruction, produced by a variety of
conditions, usually seems worse to a patient when
he or she is lying down. This is because tissue

```
FUNCTIONS OF NOSE
Olfaction
Humidification
Temperature control
Cleansing
Antibacterial/antiviral activity
```

fluids and blood tend to pool in the head more
when the patient is recumbent. This phenomenon
is analogous to the swelling of the feet and lower
extremities that some patients notice toward the
end of a long day of standing and the relief that
follows when they are able to elevate the lower
extremities. Patients also commonly complain
that at night, when they lie on one side, the dependent side of the nose becomes obstructed and
they find it necessary to roll over in bed to
breathe better. Subsequently, the other side becomes obstructed, and they turn over again.

### Olfaction

The olfactory area is located high in the nasal
vault above the superior turbinate. Sensory hairs
extend from the surface of the olfactory area to
the cells that lie deep in the mucosa. The central
axons of the cells penetrate the cribriform plate
and travel to the olfactory area of the cortex
through the first cranial nerves. These nerves lie
under the frontal lobes of the brain and on top of
the cribriform plate.

In human beings, the sense of smell is much
less important than it is in other mammals. A
wild animal may depend on the sense of smell to
warn him of an impending attack or to locate a
source of food. Humans' use of the olfactory
sense is primarily for pleasure. With training, the
sense of smell can be developed to a high degree
of sensitivity, as in persons engaged in the testing
of wine, cheese, or perfumes.

Under ordinary conditions the human being is
aware only of odors that are pleasant or unpleasant. When the sense of smell is poor or absent,
the only immediate discomfort is a change in
taste. The taste of food is recognized and enjoyed
through simultaneous stimulation of the taste buds
of the tongue and the olfactory cells of the nose.
When odors cannot reach the olfactory area or
when the sense of smell is absent (anosmia), food
tastes flat and unpalatable. Alteration of the taste
of food is a common complaint of the patient with
a blocked nose caused by acute infection or, more
often, by nasal allergy associated with nasal polyps. When the sense of smell is absent for a long
time, the sensitivity of the taste buds apparently
increases.

**Anosmia.**   Anosmia may be the result of
simple nasal obstruction—for example, nasal

polyposis—that prevents air currents from reaching the olfactory area high in the nose. Some patients with anosmia, however, have no nasal obstruction whatsoever but rather a neural defect. The onset of anosmia is often sudden. A patient may have a normal sense of smell one day but will not be able to smell anything the next. He or she may remember a severe upper respiratory infection, or may have had perfect health before losing the sense of smell.

A multitude of conditions, including drug toxicity, skull fracture, tumor, congenital defects, and viral infections, can be responsible for anosmia in patients in whom intranasal appearances are normal.

Inflammation and edema, as seen in acute rhinitis, sinusitis, allergic rhinitis, nasal polyps, or atrophic rhinitis, may be accompanied by anosmia. This type of anosmia is usually transient, with the sense of smell almost always returning as the tissues heal.

Trauma to the head, with injury to the olfactory nerves as they pass through the cribiform plate, may cause anosmia. Anosmia may occur in 2% to as many as 20% of such cases, depending on the severity of the injury. If the sense of smell is going to be recovered, return of function should be expected in the first few weeks following the injury.

Patients in whom the larynx has been removed (usually from cancer) have anosmia. The most obvious explanation is the lack of airflow through the nose, since they must breathe through a tracheostomy. There is evidence of probable neural feedback between the vagus nerve and the olfactory system, which may be the true mechanism of this type of anosmia.

Intracranial tumors, most commonly olfactory meningiomas, may cause anosmia. Frontal lobe tumors may create a syndrome of anosmia, ipsilateral optic atrophy, and contralateral papilledema (Foster Kennedy syndrome).

Agenesis of the olfactory bulb, an X-linked recessive combination of anosmia and hypogonadism (Kallmann syndrome), is seen rarely.

Viral infections, often unsuspected, are the *most common* cause of anosmia. In addition to the loss of the sense of smell, symptoms include dryness of the nose and decreased quality and quantity of nasal discharge. Examination reveals only that less than normal moisture is present in the nose. Viral hepatitis may also include anosmia or hyposmia as an associated complaint.

Treatment of anosmia has been unsatisfactory. Vitamin A, given orally or by injection, has been used with partial success in some patients.

**Testing.** Testing of olfactory function may be done in several ways. Various familiar odors, such as those of coffee, chocolate, tobacco, and perfume, may be used to test each side of the nose separately, with the eyes closed. Water and mineral oil, which have no odor, can be used as controls. A method of testing for malingering is to use coffee and ammonia. The anosmic patient will not recognize the coffee but will react to the ammonia, since it will stimulate the trigeminal nerve rather than the olfactory nerves. The malingerer will deny smelling either one. Other, more exact and quantitative tests may be used. Most of them require closely controlled laboratory conditions.

**Parosmia.** *Parosmia* is an alteration of the sense of smell in which a person may smell odors that do not exist or may interpret existing odors incorrectly. Such persons often complain of smelling disgusting odors such as burning chicken feathers or decaying garbage, and they are likely to be more annoyed by their symptoms than are persons with complete anosmia. The explanation for parosmia is not clear, but the disorder often occurs after a preliminary period of anosmia. It may be that after destruction by a viral infection, for example, regenerating nerve fibers find their way along unaccustomed pathways. An analogous situation is thought to be present in some patients who recover from Bell's palsy. In them, regenerating fibers of the facial nerve apparently do not reach the same muscles that they originally reached, resulting in uncontrolled "mass motion" of the face. Nasal or intracranial tumor must be excluded in patients with parosmia.

### Air Conditioning

The primary function of the nose is to condition the inspired air for its entrance into the trachea, bronchi, and lungs. The atmosphere varies in temperature, relative humidity, and cleanliness. Whether the outside air is 100 degrees in the shade or 40 degrees below zero, the temperature of the inspired air is changed to approximate body temperature during its brief passage through the nose.

The relative humidity of atmospheric air may vary from less than 1% to more than 90%. The nose can add moisture to or remove moisture from the inspired air so that the air that reaches the pharynx is of almost constant relative humidity.

The air around us is never gaseous alone. At all times it contains particles of smoke, dust, pollens, and bacteria, as well as products of combustion. The nose attempts to remove these particles before the air reaches the pharynx and the lungs.

When the nose is functioning normally, it accomplishes these tasks efficiently.

**Temperature Control.** Air entering the nose travels primarily through the space between the turbinates and the nasal septum. It also passes over the broad surface of the turbinates. Numerous capillaries make the blood supply of the turbinate tissue as rich as that in any other area of the body. These capillaries are associated with erectile tissue that contains large spaces filled with rapidly circulating blood. The erectile tissue enables the blood spaces to enlarge or contract rapidly, as is necessary for temperature alteration. Because of this ability to change size, the blood spaces have been called swell spaces.

Cold air causes blood to fill the swell spaces. This induces swelling of the turbinates. Their resultant enlarged surface area allows greater transfer of heat from the blood to the incoming air. The process is reversed when air that is warmer than the body temperature enters the nose.

Air reaches the nasopharynx approximately one-quarter second after it enters the nose. During this time the air is warmed or cooled to the proper temperature, regardless of its temperature before entering the nose. The nasopharyngeal temperature ranges from 96.8° to 98.6° F.

**Humidity Control.** The surface of the nasal mucosa is covered with a blanket of mucus. This is supplied by the mucous and serous glands of the respiratory mucosa of the nose (Fig. 4–10). Air reaching the nasopharynx has a constant relative humidity of 75% to 80%. When the outside air is cold and dry, large amounts of water must be transferred to the inspired air during its passage through the nose. When relative humidity is high, little, if any, fluid is lost from the mucous membrane.

It is estimated that as much as 1,000 ml of moisture can be evaporated from the nose during normal breathing in a 24-hour period. The actual amount of fluid lost varies with the relative humidity of the inspired air. As the air absorbs water from the mucosa, the submucosal glands replenish the supply. Unless the epithelium of the nose is damaged, the mucosal surface rarely becomes dry.

Extensive surgical removal of intranasal tissue may produce a nasal cavity in which the air space is large and the moist surface small. Atrophy of the nasal mucosa and turbinates may so alter the normal surface that dryness and crusting develop and become distressing symptoms.

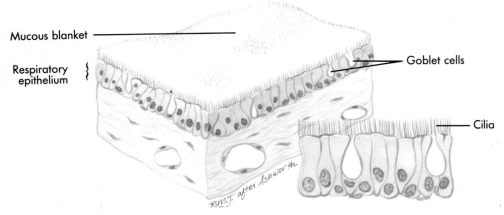

Mucous blanket

Respiratory epithelium

Goblet cells

Cilia

**FIG 4–10.**
Respiratory mucosa.

**Particle Control (Cleaning).** The entire lining of the nose is covered with a thin blanket of moisture. This is known as the mucous blanket of the nose. A similar blanket of moisture covers the mucosa of the sinuses, the eustachian tube, the trachea, the bronchi, and the bronchioles.

The mucous blanket rests on top of the cilia of the respiratory epithelium. On this blanket are deposited bacteria and other particles present in the inspired air. Constant ciliary action carries these particles to the nasopharynx and pharynx, after which they are swallowed. The nose empties itself and replaces the mucous blanket by a continuous process simulating a moving belt.

**Respiratory Epithelium and the Mucous Blanket.** The respiratory tract, with the exception of the pharynx, is lined by specialized respiratory epithelium. This epithelium is pseudostratified columnar in type and is ciliated. Beneath the surface cells three or four layers of replacement cells lie on a submucosa that is thickest in the most exposed areas of the nose and thin in the paranasal sinuses. The same epithelium lines the paranasal sinuses and the eustachian tube. In the anterior third of the nose the cell type differs; the epithelium is squamous in character and has no cilia. The epithelial cells are less columnar, and the entire epithelium is thinner inside the sinuses.

Beneath the submucosa are found both tubular and racemose glands that supply both serous and mucous secretions. Goblet cells, intermixed with the columnar epithelial cells, are numerous and add to the secretion of the respiratory epithelium.

*Cilia and Ciliary Movement*

Each surface cell of respiratory epithelium has 25 to 30 cilia. The cilia are 5 to 7 $\mu$ in length. The cilia seem to work automatically, and contractions continue in a rhythmic manner even after a cell has been artificially broken into small pieces. The cilia beat in such a way that anything carried on their surface is propelled in the direction of the ciliary motion. This is accomplished by a rapid beat in the direction of the flow and a slower recovery phase in the opposite direction. During the recovery phase the cilia are bent and the motion is slower than during the active phase, when the cilia are straight. In humans, the cilia beat approximately 250 times per minute.

*Mucous Blanket*

The submucosal gland and the goblet cells of the respiratory epithelium supply a continuous flow of secretion that forms a viscid blanket. This mucous blanket is continuous throughout the nose, the sinuses, the pharynx, and the tracheobronchial tree. Its surface promptly collects any particle that comes into contact with it. Dust, bacteria, pollens, and other airborne particles cling to it on contact.

The pH of the secretion remains fairly constant near 7. The secretion contains lysozyme and enzyme that destroys most bacteria. Lysozyme effectively causes disintegration of bacteria on contact. Ciliary action and lysozyme activity are most effective at pH 7. Serious alteration of the pH of the nasal secretion, whether by disease or medication instilled into the nose, can slow or stop ciliary action and inhibit the action of lysozyme.

Secretion is continuously produced from the epithelium of the sinuses, the nose, and the tracheobronchial tree. Ciliary action carries the blanket with its contained particles toward the pharynx, where it is swallowed. In the stomach the gastric juice and hydrochloric acid destroy residual bacteria. The mucous blanket in the nose travels approximately 5 to 10 mm per minute. It is somewhat faster near the ostia of the paranasal sinuses. The secretion is replaced about every 20 minutes. Its volume approximates 600 to 700 ml every 24 hours.

The protective action of the mucous blanket is obvious. When this action is altered by trauma, drying, irritating chemicals, or any other factor, the nose, sinuses, and lower respiratory tract become more susceptible to infection.

# 5

# Special Diagnostic Studies of the Nose and Sinus

There is no place in the head and neck where radiographic examination is more critical or more frequently used than in the nose and sinus. Though computed tomography has replaced standard films of the sinuses in many areas, high-quality sinus x-rays can be useful and diagnostic.

## SINUS RADIOGRAPHS

Four standard radiographs are taken as part of a sinus evaluation: the Waters view, Caldwell view, lateral view, and submental view.

The Waters view is a projection in which the patient's nose tip and chin are against the film surface. This projects the petrous ridge below the level of the maxillary sinus. The Waters view is the best view for the maxillary sinus and intranasal structures. With the mouth open, the sphenoid sinus can often be visualized through the sinus. The Waters view is also the best view for determining fractures of the floor of the orbit (Fig. 5–1).

The Caldwell view is obtained by positioning the patient so that the forehead and the tip of the nose are in contact with the film. In the Caldwell view the frontoethmoid sinuses are best visualized. Because of superimposition of other bony structures, the maxillary sinus is not well visualized. This view is generally best for the posterior medial and inferior portion of the maxillary sinus. It is generally a good view demonstrating the floor and rim of the orbit and the infraorbital canal (Fig. 5–2).

The lateral view of the sinuses is generally taken to visualize the sphenoid sinus, which is seen to best advantage with this view. This view is also useful in determining the integrity of the posterior wall of the maxillary and frontal sinuses (Fig. 5–3).

The submental vertical view, or base view, is obtained by passing the x-rays at right angles through the base of the skull. In this view, the sphenoid sinuses are shown to excellent advantage, as are the posterior maxillary wall, posterolateral wall of orbit, and zygomatic arch. Posterior ethmoid cells are often well seen on this exposure (Fig. 5–4).

Not all views are necessary in follow-up of patients with chronic sinus disease; however, initially, all four views are advisable.

## COMPUTED TOMOGRAPHY (CT)

The CT scan has provided a major advance in radiography of the paranasal sinuses. As each new generation of system has been developed, the quality of CT scan visualization of the paranasal sinuses has improved markedly. Computed tomography is now the procedure of choice to determine bony or tumor erosion of the ethmoid, sphenoid, or maxillary sinuses and to visualize the region of the cribriform plate. Visualization of certain cellular regions of the ethmoid involved

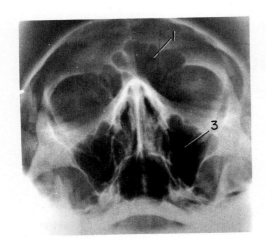

**FIG 5–1.**
Waters view. The orbits and frontal *(1)* and maxillary *(3)* sinus can be seen clearly.

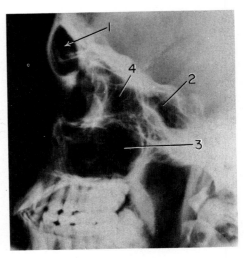

**FIG 5–3.**
Lateral view. This view is particularly valuable for demonstrating the sphenoid sinus *(2)* and the posterior wall of the frontal sinus *(1)*. The ethmoid sinus *(4)* and the maxillary sinus *(3)* are seen.

by infection, for example, is much better with the CT scan than with x-ray films, which superimpose normal and abnormal sinuses on one another (Fig. 5–5). One additional advantage of CT has been the ability to reproduce by computer various projections of anatomic areas that are difficult to demonstrate on standard CT views (Figs. 5–6 and 5–7).

Because of the high quality and decreasing

cost of CT studies, they will eventually replace conventional x-ray studies.

## MAGNETIC RESONANCE IMAGING

Magnetic resonance imaging has less value than CT in the study of paranasal sinuses because

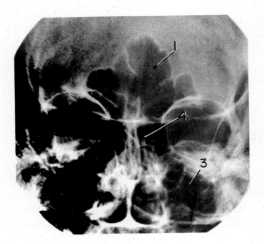

**FIG 5–2.**
Caldwell view. The frontal sinus *(1)* can be seen clearly. Ethmoid cells *(4)* lie between each orbit in the nasal septum. The maxillary sinus *(3)* is partially obscured by the petrous ridge.

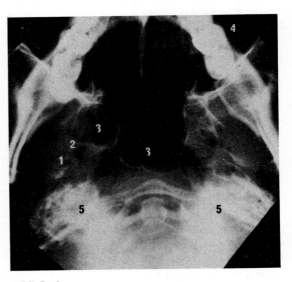

**FIG 5–4.**
Submental vertical view. Visualized are the foramen spinosum *(1)*, foramen ovale *(2)*, sphenoid sinus *(3)*, maxillary sinus *(4)*, and petrous bone *(5)*.

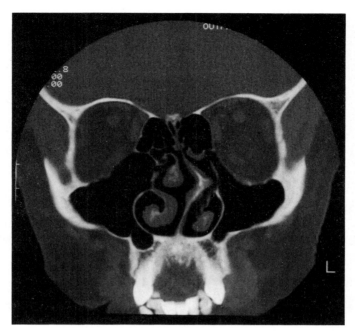

**FIG 5–5.**
CT scan of maxillary and ethmoid sinuses. Note septal deviation, maxillary sinus ostia, turbinates, and ocular muscles.

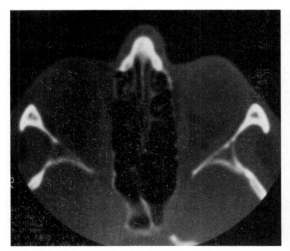

**FIG 5–6.**
CT scan demonstrating the ethmoid cell complex. The thin bony wall separating the medial orbit from the ethmoids is defined. Posterior cells represent the sphenoid sinus.

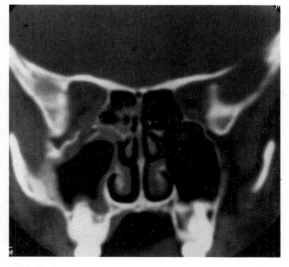

**FIG 5–7.**
Coronal view of the maxillary sinus. The maxillary sinus is well defined along with the inferior and medial turbinates. The ethmoid air cells on the right may have some very slight mucosal thickening.

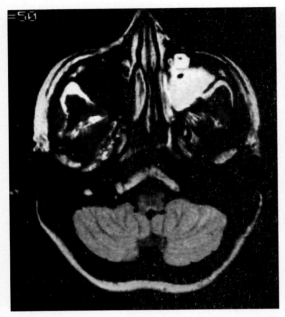

**FIG 5–8.**
MRI study of the maxillary sinus. The right maxillary sinus is occluded either with a mass or fluid. The one on the left is clear. The bony structures and air-containing spaces appear as lucencies while the opaque areas represent soft tissue. The septum and portion of the inferior turbinate are visualized.

it does not define the bony structures, which are so important in determining abnormalities of the sinuses. Further refinement of this technique may, however, present a noninvasive means of visualizing the sinuses (Fig. 5–8).

# ANGIOGRAPHY

Angiography still has significant use, particularly in the diagnosis of tumors of the nose and paranasal sinuses, and can be used to demonstrate blood flow, from either the external or internal carotid system. With the use of subtraction techniques in which superimposed bony structures are removed (subtracted) from the film exposure, excellent visualization of tumor extension and vascular involvement can be demonstrated. Angiography maintains an important place in the management of uncontrollable epistaxis or traumatic injuries of the head and neck with significant bleeding (Fig. 5–9).

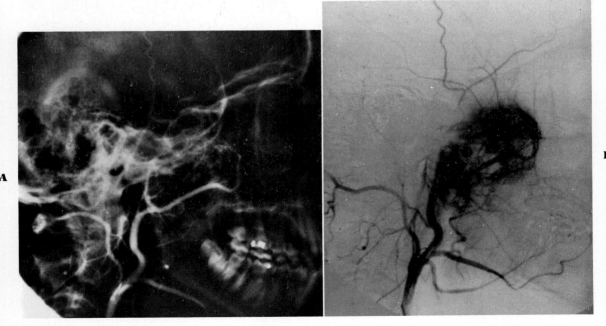

**FIG 5–9.**
**A,** angiogram of the external carotid demonstrating blush in posterior nose and nasopharynx (angiofibroma). **B,** subtraction film (same patient) more clearly demonstrating vascular source of tumor.

# 6

# Embryology and Congenital Disorders of the Nose

## EMBRYOLOGY

At about the third to fourth week of gestation, development of a nasal placode of ectodermal origin appears between the eyes. By the following week, the placodes become depressed below the surface and appear as invaginated pits (Fig. 6–1). The nasal pit extends backward toward the oral cavity but remains separated from it by the bucconasal membrane. Failure or rupture of this bucconasal membrane is the primary cause of choanal atresia. The membrane generally ruptures at about the eighth week. Olfactory epithelia develop in the upper portion of the nasal cavities bilaterally. At the same time the lateral nasal processes fuse with the medial nasal processes and the maxillary process, creating anterior nares. The frontal nasal process, which lies between the medial nasal processes, extends inferiorly as the nasal septum and also forms the primitive palate. Palatal shelves of the maxilla grow medially around the tenth week, fusing with each other and the septum to form a posterior secondary palate at about the twelfth week. Failure of fusion of these elements creates a variety of clefts and defects manifested as congenital abnormalities (Figs. 6–2 and 6–3). As the nose develops during embryologic life, the lateral wall of the internal nose develops several folds. Eventually, at about the third month, the maxillary sinus arises as a prolongation of the ethmoid infundibulum. By birth, it is approximately the size of a pea, about 1 cm. The ethmoid sinus arises from evagination of the nasal mucosa into the lateral ethmoid mass at about the sixth fetal

month and is present as a small series of air cells at birth. The frontal sinus and sphenoid sinus develop after birth. The maxillary sinus generally continues to grow during childhood, achieving maximum size around the age of 15. The ethmoid sinus becomes fully pneumatized around 7 years of age and reaches full size about puberty. The frontal sinus develops as an outpouching of the middle meatus, and ethmoid air cells superiorly become pneumatized after the age of 2 and do not achieve full size until early adulthood (Fig. 6–4). Although it may be present as a very tiny invagination at birth, the sphenoid sinus generally starts developing at about that time, achieving full size about puberty. It is not uncommon to have only one maxillary sinus develop or to have total agenesis of the maxillary sinus.

## DISORDERS RESULTING FROM CONGENITAL ABNORMALITIES

### Choanal Atresia

Choanal atresia is caused by failure of the bucconasal membrane to rupture at around the second month of embryonic life. There tends to be a familial tendency (Fig. 6–5). Though usually unilateral, it may be bilateral. When the atresia is bilateral, symptoms of choking, inability to nurse, and bouts of cyanosis usually lead to an early diagnosis. When the atresia is unilateral, the infant may nurse and breathe normally but may have a unilateral nasal discharge. The discharge is thick

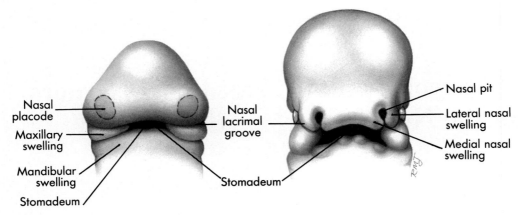

**FIG 6–1.**
Embryos at the fourth and sixth weeks of development.

and viscous but rarely infected. To make the diagnosis, the physician should attempt to pass a small rubber catheter through the nose into the pharynx. Normally such a catheter can be passed without difficulty, but in an infant with choanal atresia, it fails to enter the pharynx when inserted through the obstructed side of the nose. X-ray films taken after installation of Lipiodol will demonstrate a posterior blockage. Atresia is bony in about 90% of cases. In the remainder of cases, it is membranous.

At birth the infant with bilateral choanal atresia presents as a respiratory emergency. The diagnosis calls for immediate insertion of an oral airway with a variety of devices specially formed for feeding and breathing. It must be remembered

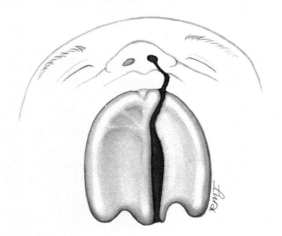

**FIG 6–2.**
Developmental anomaly in cleft lip and palate resulting from embryonic failure of fusion of the palatal process and medial and lateral nasal process.

that a newborn infant is an obligate nasal breather. However, by 2 to 3 weeks of age the child may learn to mouth breathe. Therefore a tracheotomy generally is not necessary.

A variety of approaches have been used to correct choanal atresia. These have included transnasal puncture of the occluding membranes with a hemostat or blunt instrument followed by placement of a rubber or Silastic tube. Another procedure to open the stenosis, usually done under magnification, involves a cruciate incision made over the nasal mucosa under direct vision. This is followed by either laser or microdrill removal of the obstructing bone and enlargement of the nasal cavity. The nasal mucosa is preserved. A nasal tube is then placed and held in position for 2 months.

Another popular technique for repair of unilateral atresia is a transpalatal approach. This procedure is performed by a palatal incision and removal of the obstructing portion of nasal bone under direct vision through the oral pharynx.

Cleft lip and cleft palate create a variety of defects about the nose. Generally, the lip is repaired at about 3 months of age, and the palatal defect is repaired at 12 to 18 months of age. Even after repair of the defect, growth will be altered and repeat surgery and extensive orthodontic procedures may be required.

## Nasal Glioma

Three developmental abnormalities of the nose that are frequently confused are nasal glioma, encephaloceles, and nasal dermoids. *Nasal gliomas*

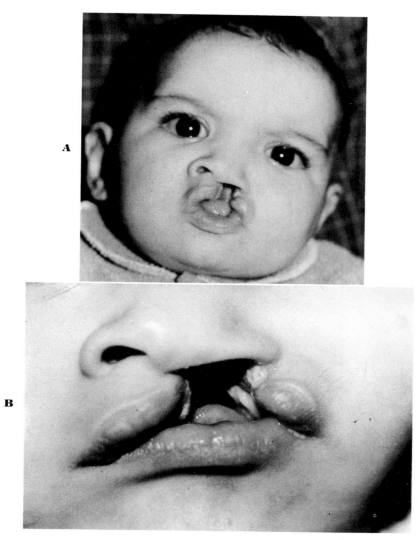

**FIG 6–3.**
Cleft lip and palate demonstrates the lack of migration and fusion of tissue from the palatal and lateral nasal process toward the midline.

are deposits of glial tissue in an extradural site. Encephaloceles are similar to gliomas but maintain connection to the central nervous system and contain cerebrospinal fluid or brain tissue. Gliomas can occur extranasally or intranasally. Extranasal gliomas are smooth, firm, and noncompressible masses. They usually occur along the glabella or the lateral wall of the nose off midline. Intranasal gliomas may manifest as a cyst or mass within the nose, are polypoid in appearance, do not distend with bending over or with crying, and appear quite firm. *Encephaloceles,* when extranasal, are generally soft and compressible and

always associated with a bony defect. This is in contrast to gliomas, which are not compressible. Intranasal encephaloceles are soft and cystic lesions that can be compressed and enlarge with crying or bending over. These lesions generally are pulsatile. Encephaloceles usually require intracranial repair followed by intranasal or extranasal removal of the tumor. When problems arise, they are usually a result of biopsy of this lesion within the nose under the mistaken belief that it is a nasal polyp.

*Dermoid cysts* are formed by trapped dermal elements external to or between the nasal bones

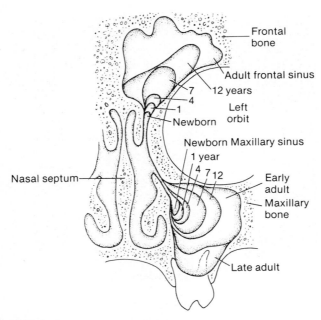

**FIG 6–4.**
Developmental stages of maxillary and frontal sinuses.

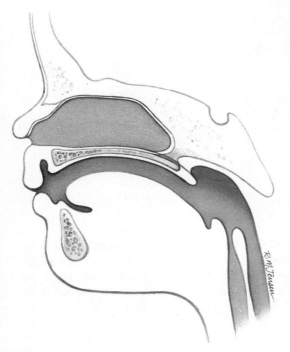

**FIG 6–5.**
Choanal atresia.

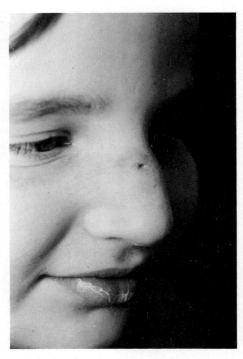

**FIG 6–6.**
Nasal dermoid of the bone.

(Fig. 6–6). They are painless swellings found generally in the midline in the nose, often with a small pitlike opening into the skin. Dermoid cysts can be found almost anywhere along the midline of the face but are most commonly found about the bridge of the nose. The cysts may extend superiorly with sinuses through defects in the frontal bones superiorly or nasal bones inferiorly. Therefore, they must be handled carefully surgically and followed to the source of their origin.

# 7

# Clinical Problems

## ACUTE AND CHRONIC DISEASES OF THE NOSE

Inflammation of the tissues of the nose can be localized or diffuse. Inflammation involving the vestibule is localized and does not ordinarily extend to the mucosa of the nasal cavity. Inflammation of the mucous membranes of the nose is usually diffuse, but it does not produce concomitant infection of the skin of the vestibule.

When the nose is partially or completely blocked, even for a short time, most people complain. Obstruction to the normal free passage of air through the nose creates a sensation of fullness in the face, shortness of breath, and often headache. Nasal obstruction can be temporary or fixed. It is caused by changes in the tissue of the nasal cavity, septum, or turbinates; disease of the nasal vestibule; or tumors of the nasal cavity. Most conditions that cause nasal obstruction can be treated successfully.

## DISEASES OF THE NASAL VESTIBULE

### Vestibulitis (Folliculitis)

The vestibule of the nose contains numerous hair follicles, which can become infected. The typical complaint is recurrent crusting inside the vestibule and recurrent tenderness of the nasal tip or ala. The symptoms vary in severity and seem to disappear after several days, only to recur a few weeks or months later. Examination shows a mild inflammation at the base of one or several hair follicles. The infection spreads from one group of hair follicles to another.

Unless treated, this mild but annoying infection

sometimes lasts indefinitely. The usual treatment consists of applying ointment to the skin of the nasal vestibule two to three times daily. Ointments containing antibiotics, with or without cortisone, are frequently used and are effective. Ointments containing bacitracin or neomycin are most effective. Ammoniated mercury ointment (5%) is also useful in recurrent staphylococcal infections that are resistant to other treatment. Treatment should be continued for 2 to 3 weeks after symptoms disappear. If it is discontinued as soon as the tenderness and crusting have stopped, recurrences are more frequent. Bactroban (Mupirocir ointment 2%) is another topical agent frequently useful for recurrent vestibular irritation.

Ammoniated mercury ointment should not be used continuously. Indiscriminate use over long periods (months) can lead to chronic mercury poisoning.

### Furunculosis

Furunculosis of the nasal vestibule is common (Fig. 7–1). Usually trauma from picking or vigorously blowing the nose causes a break in the skin, which allows staphylococcal or streptococcal organisms to enter the subcutaneous tissue. The nose becomes tender as the infection develops, and the entire tip of the nose, the ala, and the upper lip may become swollen and red. There is mild fever. Often signs of systemic toxicity appear. After 2 to 3 days, the furuncle localizes and can be seen inside the nasal vestibule.

Sometimes the infection becomes diffuse, and cellulitis spreads as a result of attempts to squeeze the furuncle or to incise it before pus has localized. This area, as well as the upper lip, has direct venous drainage through the angular vein to

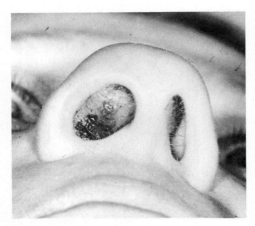

**FIG 7–1.**
Furuncle inside the right nasal vestibule.

the cavernous sinus. Attempts to express pus from a furuncle or to incise it in an area where there is cellulitis may cause the infection to spread to the cavernous sinus. The triangle formed by lines drawn from the corners of the mouth upward to the glabella is referred to as the danger triangle. Infections of the skin in this area (including the vestibule of the nose) should be treated without mechanical manipulation to avoid the possible complications of cavernous sinus thrombosis, which still carries a high mortality.

Treatment consists of adequate doses of appropriate antibiotics, hot wet packs, and analgesics or narcotics to relieve pain. Until cultures are obtained, antistaphylococcal agents are the antibiotics of choice. Antistaphylococcal penicillins (dicloxacillin, cloxacillin) are the primary drugs of choice; cephalosporin, clindamycin, and erythromycin are alternatives for penicillin-resistant individuals. There should be a "hands-off" policy regarding any surgical treatment until the surrounding inflammation has subsided and the furuncle has localized. Then, with sterile technique, it can be incised safely.

## Fissures

Small breaks in the skin of the vestibule often occur at the junction of the skin and mucous membrane. A crust forms that the patient removes from time to time. Under the crust is a painful fissure. Fissures are not dangerous and rarely become infected. Superficial cautery of the fissure with silver nitrate, followed by application of an-

tibiotic ointment, such as bacitracin or Neosporin, is usually satisfactory treatment.

## Squamous Papilloma

Small wartlike growths may develop on the squamous epithelium of the vestibule (Fig. 7–2). The cause of these papillomas is unknown, although a virus is implicated. Malignant degeneration of this type of papilloma has not been reported. These benign papillomas usually occur singly, and some of them regress spontaneously. However, because patients tend to pick at them, spontaneous regression is often prevented, and excision is required. Simple excision along the base of the lesion will not prevent recurrence. Effective removal of the lesion requires a small incision. Some of the surrounding normal tissue should be included in the excised tissue.

## DISEASES OF THE NASAL CAVITY

### Acute Rhinitis (Common Cold)

The most common cause of acute rhinitis is the common cold. The symptoms are familiar to both physician and patient. The common cold is caused by filterable virus and can be transmitted after as many as 80 transfer subcultures. It is probably the most common infectious disease in humans. Children less than 5 years of age are the most susceptible. Susceptibility is progressively

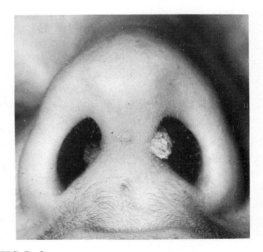

**FIG 7–2.**
Squamous papilloma of the columella of the left nasal vestibule.

less from the age of 5 years to 18 or 20 years. Thereafter it remains constant. On the average a child or an adolescent may have three to five colds a year, depending on contacts and certain environmental factors.

The disease is spread by droplet contact from sneezing. Chilling of the body, fatigue, crowded living quarters, and poor hygiene are predisposing factors. The immunity lasts approximately 1 month. So far no vaccines to increase the length of immunity have been developed.

The typical symptoms are well known. The onset is usually manifested by a feeling of irritation and a burning sensation in the nasopharynx. Sneezing and copious nasal discharge soon follow. Mild fever and malaise are usually present. As the disease progresses, the nose becomes more obstructed and the discharge becomes purulent. Headache is a common symptom during the first 2 days. Sore throat is not a characteristic complaint of the patient with a common cold. Any significant pain should make the physician wary of a complication. When uncomplicated, the common cold is self-limited, and most symptoms subside in 4 to 5 days. The nose returns to normal in 6 to 7 days. However, when the condition is complicated by a secondary invasion of virulent bacteria, the symptoms persist and worsen. Then there may be symptoms and signs of sinusitis, otitis media, bronchitis, tonsillitis, or pneumonia.

Treatment of the common cold is symptomatic. Rest, adequate fluids, and a regular diet are as effective as any known medication. Overheating and chilling should be avoided. Aspirin or other general analgesics may help the general feeling of malaise. On occasion the use of antihistamines during the first day of the disease will alleviate some of the symptoms, but antihistamine decongestants are not curative. There is no indication for the use of antibiotics during an uncomplicated cold. Nose drops may be prescribed for nasal obstruction but should be used infrequently and only to allay prolonged nasal obstruction. There is a great tendency for some patients to continue the use of nose drops longer than necessary and thereby to addict the nasal mucosa to their use (rhinitis medicamentosa). Some investigators believe that closure of the nose during the acute symptoms may be a protective mechanism and that use of nose drops may cause infection to spread. This is not proved, however. Drops or sprays, when given, should be used for only 4 days (Table 7–1).

When possible, isolation of the patient is advisable. Usually the symptoms are not so severe that the patient will stop work during the contagious first 2 or 3 days of the disease. If isolation could be accomplished, the incidence of the common cold in the general population might be lowered appreciably.

## Allergic Rhinitis

Often called hay fever, allergic rhinitis may be acute and seasonal or chronic and perennial. The usual symptoms are obstruction of the nose, sneezing, and recurrent thin nasal discharge. Itching of the nose and eyes, tearing, and frontal headache are common.

Not infrequently the patient with perennial allergic rhinitis will complain of frequent colds. However, a careful history will reveal that the patient has symptoms of allergic rhinitis rather than the acute symptoms of the common cold. The final diagnosis may depend on examination of the nose during an attack and microscopic study of the nasal secretions. The discharge from the nose in allergic rhinitis usually contains large numbers

**TABLE 7–1.**

Nasal Sprays, Drops, Mists, Inhalants

| Generic Name | Trade Name |
| --- | --- |
| *Vasoconstrictors* | |
| Ephedrine | |
| Epinephrine | Adrenalin |
| Naphazoline | Privine |
| Oxymetazoline | Afrin |
| | Dristan |
| | Neo-Synephrine 12-hour |
| Phenylephrine | Alcon Efrin |
| | Coricidin Nasal Mist |
| | Neo-Synephrine |
| Propylhexedrine | Benzedrex |
| Xylometazoline | Neo-Synephrine II |
| | Otrivin |
| | |
| *Prevention of histamine release* | |
| Cromolyn | Nasalcrom |
| | |
| *Topical corticosteroids* | |
| Dexamethasone | |
| Beclomethasone | Beconase |
| | Vancenase |
| Flunisolide | Nasalide |

of eosinophils, whereas that in the common cold contains desquamated cells, lymphocytes, and large numbers of polymorphonuclear leukocytes.

Seasonal allergic rhinitis is usually caused by pollens from trees, grasses, or flowers. It lasts several weeks, disappears, and recurs the following year. Perennial allergic rhinitis may occur intermittently for years with no pattern, or it may be present constantly. This more constant type of allergic rhinitis is usually caused by sensitivity to house dust (house dust mite), newspaper, wool, feathers, foods, tobacco, or other contacts always present in the environment. The symptoms of perennial allergic rhinitis are usually less severe than those of acute hay fever, but they present a greater problem in therapy because identification of the offending allergen is difficult. Perennial allergic rhinitis is often associated with allergic sinusitis.

Treatment in all forms requires identification of the allergen and its avoidance if possible. In mild forms antihistamines are effective for most individuals (Table 7–2). In more severe episodes (which may often include asthma) systemic steroids are effective. For many years a single injection of long-lasting steroid (e.g., methylprednisolone acetate susp.) has been used for seasonal (grass or tree pollen) symptoms.

More recently topical steroid sprays have been effective in about 70% of patients with seasonal allergic rhinitis. These sprays do not appear to cause adrenal suppression or elevated steroid levels. Through the years identification of the allergen by means of skin test, intradermal injection, or scratch test has been advocated. More recently, diagnostic measurement of allergen-specific IgE in serum has been used.

Allergen immunotherapy has been widely advocated through the years. Three methods are presently used: (1) the traditional method of starting with an arbitrary safe dose of allergen in high dilution, with gradual increasing of strength over weeks and months; (2) skin endpoint titration methods involving large doses of antigen, ten times the volume required to cause a positive skin reaction, with increasing doses; and (3) the radioallergosorbent test method, based on the amount of serum allergen-specific IgE. The latter two techniques more rapidly reach therapeutic maintenance levels of immunization.

**TABLE 7–2.**

Antihistamines

| Generic Name | Trade Name |
|---|---|
| Butyrophenone | |
|   Terfenadine | Seldane |
| Ethanolamine | |
|   Carbinoxamine | Clistin |
|   Clemastine | Tavist |
|   Dimenhydrinate | Dramamine |
|   Diphenhydramine | Benadryl |
|   Doxylamine | Decapryn |
| Ethylenediamine | |
|   Pyrilamine | |
|   Tripelennamine | PBZ |
| Piperidine | |
|   Azatadine | Optimine |
|   Cyproheptadine | Periactin |
|   Diphenylpyraline | Hispril |
|   Phenindamine | |
| Piperazine | |
|   Hydroxyzine | Atarax |
| Alkylamine | |
|   Brompheniramine | Dimetane, |
|   Chlorpheniramine | Chlor-Trimeton, Histaspan, Teldrin |
|   Dexchlorpheniramine | Polaramine |
|   Triprolidine | Actidil |
| Miscellaneous | |
|   Astemizole | Hismanal |
| Phenothiazine | |
|   Promethazine | Phenergan |
|   Methdilazine | Tacaryl |
|   Trimeprazine | Temaril |

## Vasomotor Rhinitis

Many patients complain of chronic, intermittent nasal obstruction or nasal stuffiness. The obstruction may be accompanied by increased nasal discharge, either thin or viscid. These symptoms are often considered by the patient (and sometimes by the physician) to be allergic, even when there is no good proof of nasal allergy.

Sometimes nervous, tense persons complain about normal postnasal discharge. The 500 to 700 ml of nasal mucus that normally must be swallowed daily is distasteful to some patients. Reassurance and careful explanation of nasal physiology will satisfy some of these patients. Treatment with nose drops or other medication is rarely helpful and should be avoided.

Nasal stuffiness may also result from certain endocrine disturbances that cause the turbinates to become boggy and edematous. The most important of these is hypothyroidism. When no obvious cause can be found for a chronic nasal obstruction, hypothyroidism must be considered. In many patients, thyroid hormone replacement will alleviate the condition. Most of these patients do not have typical myxedema but are regarded as having a subclinical hypothyroidism. In patients with true myxedema, a pale, boggy mucosa and chronic nasal obstruction are characteristic.

Recently, allergic and immunologic studies have indicted aspirin as the sensitizing substance in some patients who have a history of intermittent asthmatic attacks and progressive, bilateral nasal obstruction with recurrent, multiple nasal polyps.

Occasionally, severe nasal obstruction develops during pregnancy. The complaint usually begins near the end of the first trimester. The mucosa is pale, and the turbinates are swollen. They press against the nasal septum and completely obstruct the nose. Treatment is generally ineffective. The nose resumes its normal appearance and function shortly after delivery.

Some patients react to any stress with the development of nasal symptoms. Emotional, sexual, and financial problems may cause stuffiness or dryness of the nose or increased nasal discharge. These patients are often diagnostic enigmas and may require psychiatric consultation.

A very common cause of nasal obstruction is deviation of the nasal septum. If symptoms are mild and intermittent, treatment may not be necessary. However, if the obstruction is constant, whether unilateral or bilateral, septoplasty or submucous resection is indicated.

*Rhinitis medicamentosa* is an important cause of nasal obstruction because it is so common. This condition develops in patients who are habitual users of nose drops or sprays, and the nasal mucosa often becomes fiery red. They can breathe for an hour or two after using nose drops, after which the nose becomes obstructed again. Because the state of engorgement of the turbinates is controlled by the autonomic nervous system and because vasoconstrictors stimulate the sympathetic nerves, there tends to be a compensatory relaxation of the turbinal vessels after the effect of the nose drops has stopped. Thus, after temporary relief, the nose becomes more stuffy than it was originally. This cycle of medication and obstruc-

tion may continue for months or even years. *Any patient who complains of nasal obstruction and in whom there is no obvious cause for the obstruction should be asked if he or she is a longtime user of nose drops.* The treatment is to have the patient throw away all intranasal vasoconstrictors. After 2 or 3 weeks, the normal reflexes return, and the nose may function properly again. Systemic or topical steroids along with oral decongestants are helpful in easing the patient's complaints during the transition when nasal stuffiness may be severe.

## Hypertrophied Turbinates

The combination of long-standing allergic rhinitis and low-grade inflammation may produce permanent enlargement of the turbinates, particularly the inferior turbinate. When this occurs, the turbinate loses most of its normal ability to expand and to shrink. The result is continuous nasal obstruction (Fig. 7–3). Nose drops, antihistamines, and allergic desensitization do not relieve the obstruction.

In some instances injection of a sclerosing solution beneath the mucosa of the turbinate will reduce its size. In others careful submucosal electrocoagulation gives similar results. In still other cases successful treatment is possible only by submucous resection of the turbinate itself.

*Submucous resection* is performed with the patient under local anesthesia. The mucosa and submucosa along the free margin of the turbinate are incised. Some or all of the bones of the inferior turbinate are removed, and the mucosa is reapproximated. Packs are left in the nose longer than

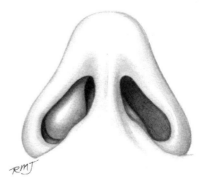

**FIG 7–3.**
Hypertrophic turbinate.

they are after the routine submucous resection operation (nasal septum) because of a tendency toward postoperative bleeding. After healing, the turbinate is smaller, but the functioning mucosa remains.

### Nasal Polyps

Nasal polyps are most often seen in patients with allergic rhinitis (Figs. 7–4 and 7–5). A nasal polyp forms gradually from recurrent localized swelling of the sinus mucosa or from the nasal mucosa. At first the polyp is small. With each succeeding increase in submucosal edema, it becomes larger until, when fully developed, it appears as a smooth, pale tumor. The base is pedunculated but is not seen. In most instances nasal polyps are multiple. They can be moved back and forth. Turbinates, with which nasal polyps are often confused, cannot move freely, and they are tender when probed. Polyps cause symptoms because they protrude into the airway. They may be large or numerous enough to occlude the nose completely. If untreated for years, they can cause gradual spreading of the nasal bones and widening of the nasal bridge.

Sometimes cortisone, given systemically or injected locally, will cause nasal polyps to disappear. However, when the cortisone is discontinued, the polyps usually reappear. Steroid sprays have been particularly useful for polypoid disease and in many cases will cause significant resolu-

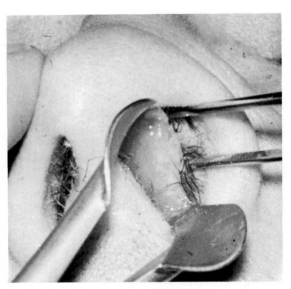

**FIG 7–5.**
Typical nasal polyp—soft, pale gray, nontender, and mobile.

tion of the polyps. For the most part, nasal polyps require surgical removal. This is performed with the patient under local anesthesia. Two cotton applicators, moistened with 5% cocaine, are used. One is placed between the posterior end of the middle turbinate and the septum (sphenopalatine block), and the other is placed high in the anterior part of the nose to block the anterior ethmoidal nerve (Fig. 7–6). A maximum of 200 mg of co-

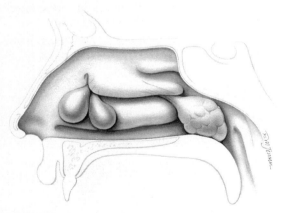

**FIG 7–4.**
Nasal polyps. A choanal polyp is usually single, originating in the maxillary sinus and extending into the nasal pharynx through the maxillary sinus ostia. Most other polyps are found in the middle meatus.

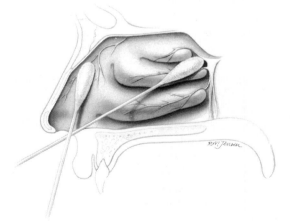

**FIG 7–6.**
Local anesthesia inside the nose. Applicator No. 1 is placed between the posterior end of the middle turbinate and the nasal septum. Applicator No. 2 is placed opposite the junction of the nasal bone and the cartilage high in the nasal vault.

caine can be safely used. Each polyp is avulsed with a wire snare. Often, because the underlying allergy cannot be well controlled, the polyps tend to recur.

Many nasal polyps actually arise from the paranasal sinuses, and one should not be surprised to see changes on x-ray films. Intranasal polypectomy may have to be repeated at intervals of months or years. In patients in whom the condition is severe, a more extensive operation, such as intranasal ethmoidectomy and sphenoidectomy and the Caldwell-Luc procedure, is needed to prevent recurrence.

In an asthmatic patient the presence of nasal polyps suggests aspirin hypersensitivity. Although authorities tend to disagree on the subject, many surgeons believe that polypectomy in such a patient may precipitate a severe asthmatic attack, even though the patient is not given aspirin.

### Atrophic Rhinitis

The cause of atrophic rhinitis is unknown. Fortunately it seems to be a disappearing disease. Symptoms begin near the age of puberty, and women are affected more often than men. When the atrophy is well established, the nose is dry and often filled with crusts. Paradoxically, even though the nasal airway is more open than it is normally, the patient with atrophic rhinitis complains of nasal stuffiness. The condition is painless. Often a foul or fetid odor called ozena accompanies the crusting of the nose and may be the most disturbing symptom.

Examination reveals yellow or green crusts associated with some surface purulent exudate. After removal of the crusts, the nose is wide open and the nasopharynx can usually be clearly seen. The turbinates are thin and atrophic. These changes are usually present on both sides of the nose. Atrophic rhinitis is rarely unilateral. The nasopharynx and pharynx frequently appear smooth, dry, and shiny rather than pink and moist, as they do normally.

Atrophic rhinitis is resistant to most forms of treatment. In the past, nasal sprays of oily solutions containing estrogens were used. Cortisone has been tried in recent years. All antibiotics have been used. None appears to be effective. In most instances gentle, daily irrigation of the nose with

isotonic saline solution provides as much symptomatic relief as any known medical treatment.

Some patients have subjective improvement when ordinary confectioner's (powdered) sugar is blown into the nose with a powder blower once or twice daily. In these patients the appearance of the nasal mucosa may also improve.

Surgical procedures designed to narrow the airway have been effective in some patients. Bone chips from the crest of the ilium can be implanted in a subperiosteal pocket in the lateral wall of the nose. This procedure narrows the airway and may end odor and crusting.

## UNILATERAL NASAL DISCHARGE

As mentioned, choanal atresia, when it involves only one side, will cause a unilateral, generally mucoid discharge. Often the diagnosis is not made for many years, and the child is treated for such conditions as allergies and infection.

### Foreign Bodies

Children often put foreign bodies into the nose, just as they do in the ear. Rubber erasers, paper wads, pebbles, beads, and beans are the most common objects (Fig. 7–7). The cardinal symptom is unilateral purulent nasal discharge. Usually there is no pain or other symptoms. The parents usually have no knowledge of the foreign body. It is easy to make an erroneous diagnosis of sinusitis if the nose is not carefully cleaned of secretions before it is examined.

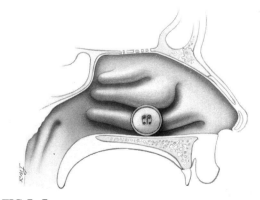

**FIG 7–7.**
Foreign bodies in the nose usually lodge in the anterior or middle third of the nose and rest on its floor.

In removing the foreign body, one must have good visualization of the object and the proper instruments. Often the child must be restrained. General anesthesia may be necessary at times. After shrinking the nose with a vasoconstrictor, the physician removes the foreign body with grasping forceps.

Rarely, a foreign body will remain in the nose for many years, and calcium will become deposited around it. After the surrounding purulent secretion has been removed, a chalky white foreign body called a rhinolith is found.

### Malignancies

Unilateral bloody discharge from the nose should always make the physician think of a neoplasm of the nose or sinuses. This type of discharge tends to be scanty and intermittently blood tinged. Sometimes, chronic sinusitis with granulation tissue can also cause a bloody nasal discharge. This type of bleeding should not be confused with the fresh, brisk bleeding of ordinary epistaxis.

### Cerebrospinal Rhinorrhea

Occasionally, unilateral nasal discharge will be sparkling clear. Such discharge may occur spontaneously, or it may follow a head injury or tumor. When clear fluid flows from one side of the nose in any significant amount, and particularly when the symptom recurs, cerebrospinal rhinorrhea should be suspected. Lowering the head or compressing the jugular veins may increase the flow. The mucosa of the nose looks normal. When cerebrospinal rhinorrhea is suspected, a sample of the discharge should be collected. A simple test for the presence of glucose will confirm the diagnosis.

Treatment requires surgical closure of the defect, usually near the cribriform plate. The operation is performed by an otolaryngologist or a neurosurgeon or both.

## ACUTE AND CHRONIC SINUSITIS

For many years nonmalignant disease of the paranasal sinuses has been poorly understood by the medical student, the general physician, and the laity. Too often the paranasal sinuses have been indicated as the underlying cause of nasal obstruction, headaches, fever of unknown origin, chronic sore throat, chronic fatigue, recurrent cough, chronic dyspepsia, and almost any symptom of the upper respiratory or upper gastrointestinal tract.

The misconceptions regarding sinusitis are common among lay persons, and they are unwittingly fostered by the physician. The laity use the term *sinus* rather than *sinusitis,* and the physician may speak of "sinus trouble." Such thinking has become so common that many headaches and most nasal symptoms are referred to as sinus trouble. Frequently the lay person thinks that a simple intranasal operation for relief of nasal obstruction is a sinus operation. Acute hay fever and chronic allergic rhinitis are erroneously called sinus infection. The normal postnasal discharge resulting from the physiologic cleansing function of the mucous blanket has been improperly blamed for the ill effects of tobacco, alcohol, and drugs. The student will benefit from a review of the causes of nasal obstruction and vasomotor rhinitis, as well as of headache, before studying sinusitis.

As the suffix *-itis* indicates, sinusitis means an inflammatory change in the mucosa of a sinus. When such a pathologic change occurs, definite signs and symptoms are produced. Most of the signs can be seen on physical examination of the nose or can be demonstrated by x-ray films or other special diagnostic procedures. If the symptoms and signs are not present, many other local or systemic conditions may need to be investigated to discover the cause of the nasal symptoms. Of every 100 patients who consult an otolaryngologist because of "sinus trouble," fewer than 10 have sinusitis. Sinusitis may be conveniently classified as acute, subacute, and chronic suppurative sinusitis; allergic sinusitis; and hyperplastic sinusitis.

### Acute Suppurative Sinusitis

Acute suppurative sinusitis most often accompanies or follows the common cold. It sometimes occurs endemically from a specific organism when there has been a sudden drop in temperature. It may also occur when infected water is forced into the nose when the patient is swimming or diving.

The bacteria most often responsible for acute suppurative sinusitis are *Streptococcus pneumoniae,* beta-hemolytic *Streptococcus, Haemophilus influenzae,* coagulase-positive *Staphylococcus aureus,* and *Klebsiella pneumoniae.* By far the most frequent are *S. pneumoniae* and *H. influenzae,* which account for more than 50% of maxillary sinus infections. Anaerobic bacteria may be present in as many as 30% of infections. Very often they are of dental origin. Cultures often do not provide specific information because they generally reflect multiple organisms.

The onset of acute sinusitis is not abrupt except when it occurs after swimming or diving. The first symptom is usually a stuffy feeling in the nose, followed by a slowly developing pressure over the involved sinus. There is mild general malaise and toxicity, and headache may be present. The temperature is only slightly elevated

(99° to 99.5° F.) or may be normal throughout the course of the disease. The white blood cell count remains normal in most patients. If the temperature is high and the blood cell count is elevated, complications should be considered.

Symptoms progress over 48 to 72 hours until there is severe localized pain and tenderness over the involved sinus. In maxillary sinusitis the pain is over the cheek and the upper teeth (Fig. 7–8). The patient frequently attributes the pain to an infected tooth. The pain may involve all or several teeth in the upper alveolus rather than a single tooth. In ethmoid sinusitis, the pain is usually medial and deep to the eye (Fig. 7–9). There may be mild discomfort with eye motion. In frontal sinusitis, the pain is in the forehead, above the eyebrow. In infection of the sphenoid sinus, the pain is deep behind the eye, over the occiput, or sometimes is referred to the vertex of the skull. In acute frontal and maxillary sinusitis, pain is typically not present in the early morning after a night

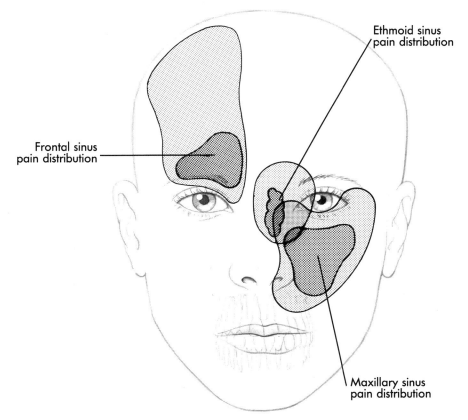

**FIG 7–8**.
Sinus pain—area of local tenderness and pain referral. Maxillary sinus pain frequently refers to teeth. Frontal pain is generally localized to supraorbital area. Ethmoid pain is generally deep to eye.

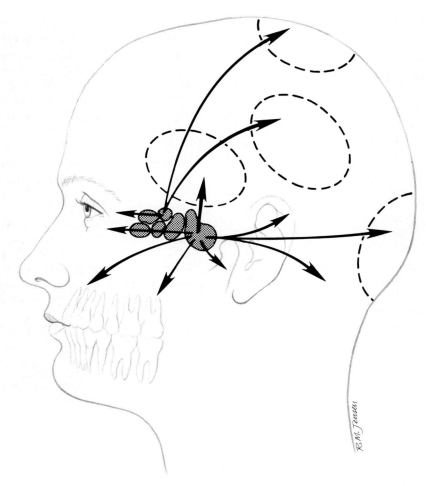

**FIG 7–9.**
Pain from anterior ethmoid deep to eye. Pain from postethmoid cells and sphenoid is referred to the eyes, teeth, the ears, or the temporal area of the occiput.

of rest. It usually appears 1 or 2 hours after waking, increases for 3 or 4 hours, and becomes less severe in the late afternoon and evening. This is particularly true of frontal sinusitis, hence the term for the daytime pain is *union headache.*

Discharge from the nose may be bloody or blood-tinged in the first 24 to 48 hours of the disease. It rapidly becomes purulent and copious. The nose becomes more blocked, and the throat may become inflamed and sore on one side as a result of the purulent discharge.

The nasal mucosa on the involved side is hyperemic and edematous, and the turbinates are enlarged. They fill the air space of the nose and usually press against the nasal septum. In most patients purulent discharge is visible in the nose. When only swelling and redness are seen, pus can

be demonstrated after a vasoconstrictor is applied to shrink the turbinates and afford visualization of the posterior middle meatus. Ciliary action directs the pus toward the nasopharynx in the middle or superior meatus or in both. Localized tenderness over the involved sinus is a constant finding. The tenderness is easily demonstrated and is sharply localized to the anatomic boundaries of the involved sinus (Fig. 7–10). X-ray films or computed tomography show the involved sinus to be cloudy, and sometimes a fluid level is visible. However, these studies are usually not necessary to establish the diagnosis. If the history is one of multiple or recurrent episodes of acute sinusitis, a CT scan is indicated to rule out underlying disease (Fig. 7–11).

Treatment of acute suppurative sinusitis is

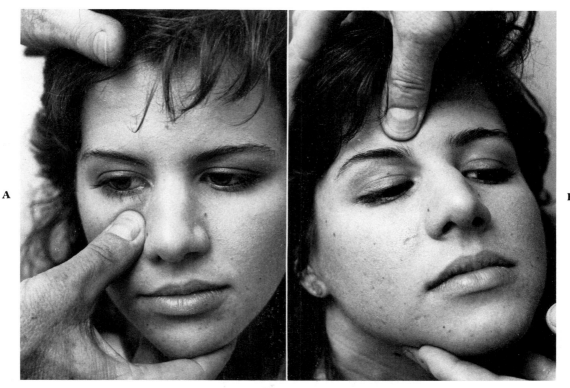

**FIG 7–10**.
Pressure over the maxillary sinus, **A,** or over the frontal sinus, **B,** elicits pain or tenderness in acute sinusitis.

medical, not surgical. The only exception to this rule is when the natural ostium of the sinus is completely blocked, resulting in an empyema. In that circumstance, pain becomes unbearable, and extension of the infection outside the walls of the sinus may occur.

Treatment is directed at relief of pain, shrinkage of the nasal mucosa, and control of infection. Codeine, meperidine (Demerol), or other narcotic analgesics are often required to control the pain. It may be necessary for the patient to take narcotic preparations for several days. The application of heat affords symptomatic relief. Wet heat often gives more relief than dry heat. Hot wet packs applied to the face or over the involved sinus either continuously or for 1 to 2 hours at a time, four times a day, will hasten resolution of the inflammation and may open the nasal passages.

The nose should be kept open as well as possible. This can be accomplished by the use of nose drops or a nasal spray containing vasoconstrictors such as 2% ephedrine, 0.25% phenyleph-rine (Neo-Synephrine), or other, longer-acting nasal mucosal shrinking solutions (Afrin) (see Table 7–1). Solutions containing antibiotics or corticosteroids neither hasten the resolution of the infection nor make the patient more comfortable. Antihistamine decongestant combinations may be of benefit, particularly in providing symptomatic relief (Table 7–3).

Although most patients with sinusitis would clear their infection satisfactorily without antibiotics, antibiotics are the treatment of choice in acute sinusitis. The antibiotics most effective in alleviating sinus infections are penicillin, ampicillin, amoxicillin, trimethoprim-sulfamethoxazole, and cefaclor. Ampicillin or amoxicillin is effective in most adults and in those patients in whom the sinusitis develops as a result of dental extraction. In children and adults the use of amoxicillin or ampicillin is indicated because of the high incidence of *H. influenzae*. The cephalosporins and the sulfas are satisfactory medications in individuals who are sensitive to penicillin. *Staphylococcus* organisms are unusual in acute sinusitis, and

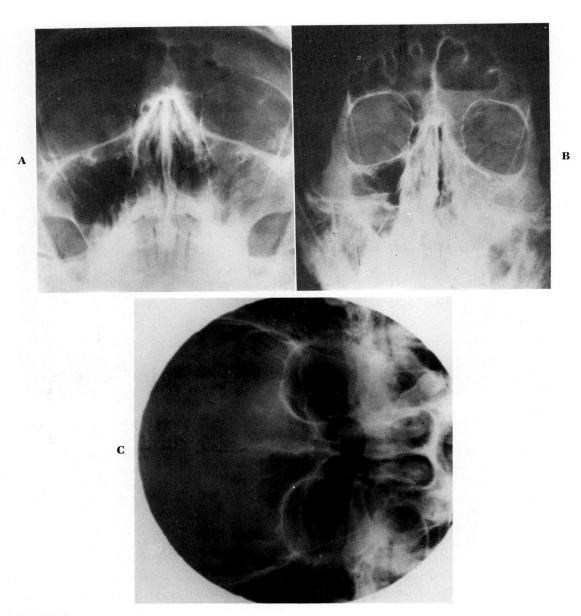

**FIG 7–11.**
**A,** Waters view showing clouding of left maxillary sinus. **B,** Caldwell view showing clouding of left maxillary sinus and a fluid level in the left frontal sinus. **C,** Caldwell view demonstrating left acute frontal sinusitis as well as ethmoid and maxillary clouding.

generally antistaphylococcal agents are not necessary.

ganisms are unusual in acute sinusitis, and generally antistaphylococcal agents are not necessary.

In some patients the natural ostium of the involved sinus is completely occluded by edema or the viscosity of the purulent discharge. The frontal sinus is the most common site of obstruction, but the maxillary sinus may become occluded as

well. In the presence of virulent infection, blocking of the ostium of the frontal sinus may lead to an early spread of infection through the posterior wall of the sinus. The immediate threat is meningitis, epidural abscess, or frontal lobe abscess.

When pain is out of proportion to the usual picture, and when pus fails to drain into the nose after the usual treatment (local application of heat and nasal decongestion), drainage of the involved

**TABLE 7–3.**

Oral Decongestants and Combinations (Tablets, Capsules, and Liquids)

|  | Alone | Combination | Plus |
|---|---|---|---|
| Pseudoephedrine | Novafed | Actifed | Triprolidine |
|  | Sudafed | Co-Tylenol | Chlorpheniramine |
|  |  | Sinutab | Acetaminophen |
|  | Afrinol | Deconamine | Chlorpheniramine |
|  |  | Novafed A |  |
|  |  | Histalet DM |  |
|  |  | Isoclor |  |
|  |  | Sudafed Plus |  |
|  |  | Drixoral | Dexbrompheniramine |
|  |  | Phenergan compound | Promethazine |
|  |  |  | Aspirin |
|  |  | Phenergan D | Promethazine |
|  |  | Rondec | Carbinoxamine |
|  |  |  | Azatadine |
|  |  | Benadryl decongestant | Diphenhydramine |
|  |  | Dimetane DX | Brompheniramine |
| Phenylpropanolamine |  | Allerest | Chlorpheniramine |
|  |  | Novahistine |  |
|  |  | Contac |  |
|  |  | Dehist |  |
|  |  | Ornade |  |
|  |  | Sinutab | Phenyltoxamine |
|  |  |  | Acetaminophen |
|  |  | Triaminic | Pheniramine |
|  |  |  | Pyrilamine |
|  |  | Coricidin D | Chlorpheniramine |
|  |  |  | Aspirin |
|  |  | Dimetapp | Brompheniramine |
|  |  | Nolamine | Chlorpheniramine |
|  |  |  | Phenindamine |
|  |  | Tavist-D | Clemastine |
| Phenylephrine | None | Comhist | Phenyltoloxamine |
|  |  | Comhist LA | Chlorpheniramine |
|  |  | Dristan | Chlorpheniramine |
|  |  | Novahistine |  |
|  |  |  | Chlorpheniramine |
|  |  |  | Pyrilamine |
|  |  | Dristan-AF | Chlorpheniramine |
|  |  | Dimetane | Acetaminophen |
|  |  | Demazin | Brompheniramine |
|  |  | ENTEX | Chlorpheniramine |
|  |  | Naldecon | Guaifenesin |
|  |  |  | Phenyltoloxamine |
|  |  |  | Chlorpheniramine |
| Ephedrine | Generic |  |  |

sinus may be necessary. The operative procedure can be performed with local or general anesthesia. For the frontal sinus, a small incision is made just under the eyebrow. The periosteum is retracted, a small opening is made into the floor of the frontal sinus with a trephine, and a drain is placed into the cavity of the sinus. Occasionally it is necessary to puncture the medial wall of the maxillary sinus when drainage cannot be established by conservative means (see discussion of antral puncture in section on subacute suppurative sinusitis). Both of these procedures are reserved for unusual situations. Ordinarily any surgical procedure involving the bony walls of the sinus is contraindicated during the acute phase of sinusitis. Osteomyelitis of the facial bones or of the skull may occur as the result of ill-advised puncture during acute sinusitis.

A single episode of acute sinusitis does not necessarily predispose the patient to chronic sinusitis. It can do so, however, if the acute sinusitis is neglected or complicated by another disturbance of nasal physiology, such as allergy.

### Subacute Suppurative Sinusitis

More than 90% of patients with acute suppurative sinusitis are cured by conservative treatment. Many patients may not have had any treatment. In the remaining 10% the condition persists as a subacute infection. During the subacute stage of infection, persistent purulent nasal discharge is the only constant symptom. The nose may remain stuffy or obstructed. Although localized tenderness is no longer present, there may be vague intermittent discomfort over the involved sinus or face. There may be a feeling of fatigue or of tiring more easily than usual. A nonproductive cough may become annoying. The chief physical sign is persistence of pus in the nose.

Computed tomography sinus studies are indicated during the subacute phase of the infection to determine whether more than one sinus is involved (Figs. 7–12 and 7–13). A culture of the nasal discharge should be made. Because it is uncommon for the disease to persist, the causative organism may be an unusual one. One should also keep in mind that, because many instances of sinusitis are caused by anaerobes, special culture techniques may be needed to demonstrate the organisms. Antibiotic sensitivities are important. The most common organisms isolated are *H. influenzae, Haemophilus pneumococcus,* and *Branhamella catarrhalis* (a common pathogen of the upper respiratory tract that may cause a low-grade continuing nasal discharge for weeks when the maxillary or ethmoid sinuses are involved). A culture revealing this organism *(B. catarrhalis)* should not be disregarded. Treatment requires systemic sulfonamide therapy, or erythromycin with a sulfonamide, since the bacterium is not sensitive to penicillin or amoxacillin (the antibiotics of choice for *H. influenzae* and *S. pneumoniae*).

The possibility that the patient has an underlying allergy should be considered because patients with allergic symptoms often have persistent sinus infections.

During the subacute stage, treatment can be more vigorous than during the acute phase without the danger of spreading the infection. No medication is necessary to relieve pain. Nasal vasoconstriction should be part of the treatment. Heat may be beneficial, and irrigation of the involved sinus may afford some relief. In some patients the frontal sinus can be irrigated through the natural ostium by means of specially designed cannulas; however, if irrigation cannot be accomplished easily, it should not be performed. Trauma to the natural ostium may produce adhesions and narrowing. Obstruction to normal sinus drainage hinders successful treatment and may lead to future difficulties.

The maxillary sinus (antrum) can be irrigated through the thin bone of the medial wall of the sinus under the inferior turbinate or through the face of the maxilla. Otolaryngologists–head and neck surgeons use either approach, according to their preference. Trauma to the natural ostium should be avoided.

Antral puncture is not a difficult, painful, or dangerous procedure. It is probably the most beneficial method of treatment in subacute and early chronic suppurative sinusitis. It can be repeated many times without permanent damage to the nose or the maxillary sinus.

The puncture is performed using the following procedure. A cotton-tipped applicator, moistened in 5% cocaine solution, is placed high under the inferior turbinate against the lateral wall of the nose. The applicator should be placed immediately under the attachment of the inferior turbinate. A small second applicator can be placed under the middle turbinate. After 5 to 10 minutes a large needle (16- to 18-gauge) is inserted under the turbinate, and firm, controlled pressure is applied until the needle pierces the medial wall of the antrum and enters the cavity of the sinus (Fig. 7–14). A syringe is then attached to the needle either directly or with a plastic tube. Suction brings purulent material or air into the syringe to prove its presence in the sinus. This is an essential part of the procedure. Culture should be obtained at this time. No solution should be irrigated through the needle until the open tip of the needle is clearly in the cavity of the sinus. Injection of

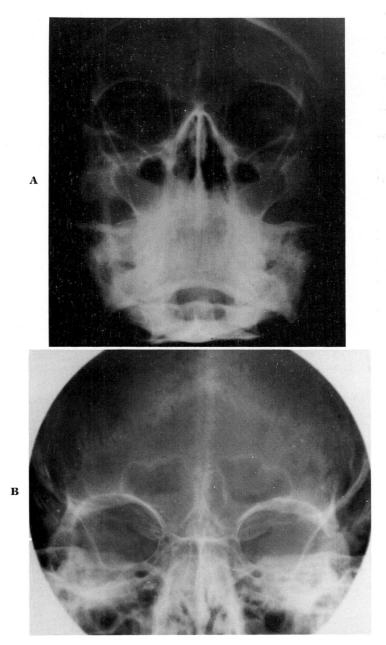

**FIG 7–12.**
**A,** Waters view revealing bilateral maxillary sinus clouding with fluid and membrane thickening. Note small under-developed frontal sinuses. **B,** Caldwell view of frontal sinuses showing bilateral fluid level and cloudy ethmoid si-nuses.

air or solution into any surrounding soft tissue may spread infection or produce an air embolism. When proper placement of the needle is proved, the sinus is washed with saline solution. As saline solution enters the sinus through the needle, it flows out into the nose through the natural ostium of the antrum. The patient is instructed to lean over a basin, into which the fluid and purulent matter drain (Fig. 7–15).

The second method of antral irrigation, which

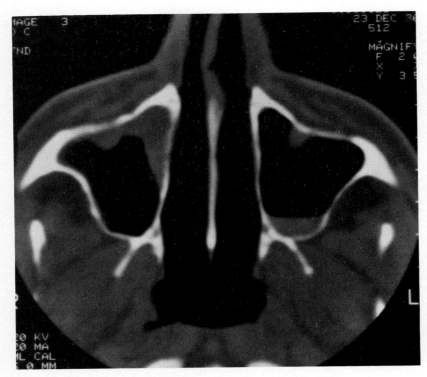

**FIG 7–13**.
CT scan revealing fluid left maxillary sinus and membrane thickening, notable on right.

is increasingly preferred, is to puncture the anterior wall of the maxillary sinus. An injection of 2 to 3 ml of 1% lidocaine (Xylocaine) with 1:100,000 epinephrine is made under the upper lip, and then a 16-gauge needle (with stylet in place) is tapped or preferably rotated through the soft tissue and bone (Figs. 7–16 and 7–17). This approach has the advantage of being the most direct.

Many solutions, including antibiotics, have

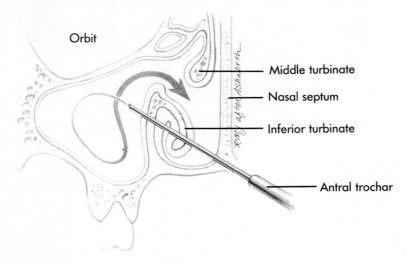

**FIG 7–14**.
Trocar inserted under the inferior turbinate (through the medial wall of the antrum). Contents of the sinus are washed into the nose through the natural ostium.

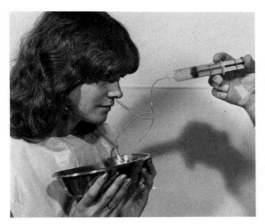

**FIG 7–15.**
Irrigation of the maxillary sinus. With the head tipped forward, solution returns via the natural ostium and out the anterior nose for examination and/or culture.

been used to irrigate the maxillary sinus for treatment of subacute or chronic infection. However, the mechanical cleansing of the sinus is more important than the solution used. Normal ciliary activity can return within a few hours after irriga-

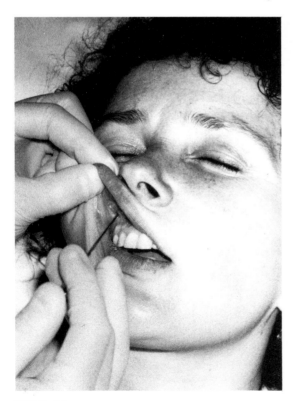

**FIG 7–16.**
Placement of 18-gauge needle with stylet after local injection.

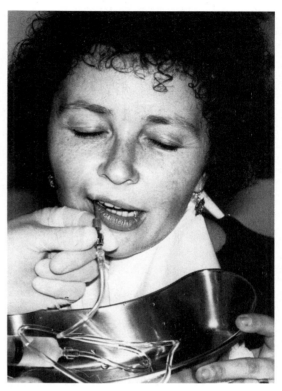

**FIG 7–17.**
After penetration of needle into maxilla, irrigation of sinus with saline. Care must be taken not to penetrate floor of orbit.

tion, after which further clearing of the purulent material may occur spontaneously. During the subacute stage of infection, one irrigation will often suffice. More than two or three irrigations are required only rarely.

Antral puncture can be used for diagnosis as well as for treatment. Puncture and washing of the antrum will demonstrate whether active infection is present or absent.

Whereas the maxillary sinuses can be easily irrigated, it is not possible to irrigate the ethmoid sinuses directly. Infection of the sphenoid sinus is usually associated with infection of the posterior ethmoid cells or of all the ethmoid cells. Isolated sphenoid sinusitis rarely occurs. Although almost all cases of subacute sinusitis and ethmoiditis are controlled by antibiotics, it may be necessary to remove retained purulent material from the ethmoid and sphenoid sinuses through the Proetz displacement method. Now used much less frequently than in the preantibiotic era, this method is most effective when disease is present in the

the small and inaccessible ethmoid air cells.

The systemic antibiotics used for subacute sinusitis are generally the same as those used for acute sinusitis. It is more likely that the organism represents a less sensitive organism and the use of the antibiotics should be continued for 10 to 14 days. Anaerobic organisms must be considered. The systemic administration of corticosteroids for short intervals (3 to 5 days) may be helpful in patients with severe symptoms and boggy inflammatory changes within the nose. This is most useful in patients with allergy.

Proper treatment of subacute sinusitis is the best means of preventing chronic purulent sinusitis.

## Chronic Suppurative Sinusitis

When suppurative sinusitis is neglected during the attack or subacute phase, or when recurrent attacks damage the mucosa, permanent change may occur. It has been proved conclusively that bacteria can invade the tissue of the sinuses, become walled off, and produce chronic inflammation. At some time during any prolonged infection of soft tissue, pathologic change may become irreversible. The term *chronic suppurative sinusitis* indicates that the physician believes irreversible tissue changes have occurred in the lining membrane of one or more of the paranasal sinuses.

Symptoms of uncomplicated chronic suppurative sinusitis are similar to those of the subacute process. Purulent nasal discharge is the most common and often the only symptom. Contrary to popular belief, chronic infection of the paranasal sinuses is not a common cause of recurrent headache. Although low-grade headache can be a symptom, it rarely results from sinus infection. A more common cause of headache in the frontal region or between the eyes is allergic rhinitis. Swelling of the nasal mucosa can create increased intranasal pressure and thus headache. The mere presence of pus in a sinus, without accompanying positive or negative pressure, does not usually produce pain. When persistent pain occurs in a patient with known chronic sinus infection, the physician should be alert to the probability of an impeding complication or of the presence of unsuspected neoplasm. Symptoms of allergy are common in patients who have chronic sinusitis.

Because purulent nasal discharge is the one common sign of chronic suppurative sinus disease, proof of the presence or absence of pus in a sinus is essential to diagnosis. Visible pus in the nose in the absence of acute respiratory disease should be considered to come from one of the sinuses until proved otherwise. If pus cannot be seen in the nose but a purulent nasal discharge is suspected because of the history, further examination should be performed to prove or disprove the presence of pus in a sinus. X-ray films, CT scan, antral puncture, and displacement should be used to establish the diagnosis or refute the suspicion of chronic suppurative sinusitis (Fig. 7–18).

There is not always a good correlation between the information obtained from sinus x-ray films and irrigation or displacement. Sinuses either clouded or clear on the x-ray film may contain pus or have no active infections. It is here that the CT scan is most helpful. Therefore all methods must be used at times to confirm the diagnosis. Antral puncture and displacement are the most distinctive, and it is on the results of these procedures that a final opinion on treatment must be based.

Treatment of chronic suppurative sinusitis is primarily surgical. In a small percentage of patients, repeated irrigation or displacement, antihistamines, and antibiotics may cure the disease. In most patients, however, an operation is necessary.

The physician must remember to investigate general systemic conditions that adversely affect the body's ability to overcome infection. Allergy has been mentioned. Hypometabolism, anemia, malnutrition, immunodeficiency, and neoplasm are others. These conditions may require treatment before either medical or surgical treatment of chronic inflammatory disease will be successful.

## Surgery

Sound operative treatment of chronic suppurative sinusitis requires removal of all diseased soft tissue and bone, adequate postoperative drainage, and obliteration of the preexisting sinus cavity where possible. A specific technique is used for each sinus. The aim of each operation is to eradicate the infection but to leave contiguous struc-

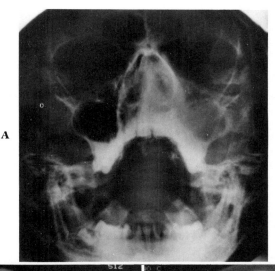

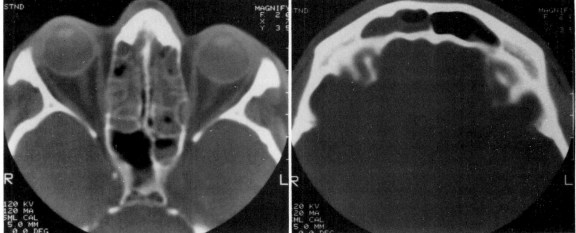

**FIG 7–18.**
**A,** Waters view showing chronic maxillary-frontal sinus, maxillary-frontal sinusitis. **B,** CT scan of ethmoids demonstrating clouding and membrane thickening. **C,** CT scan of frontal sinus demonstrating clouding of right frontal with membrane thickening.

tures normal. Partial removal of involved inflammatory tissue is generally successful.

When subacute infection of the maxillary sinus will not respond to systemic treatment, nasal shrinkage, and antral washing, drainage is necessary. This can be accomplished by making a window, called the antral window, through the lateral wall of the nose under the inferior turbinate. The operation is performed through the nose by fracturing the inferior turbinate medially or by removing a portion of its anterior end. The bony wall between the nose and antrum is removed widely, producing a permanent window. This window allows retained pus to drain into the nose by gravity and may cure the sinusitis. In some patients, multiple recurrent acute maxillary sinusitis can be treated in this manner. Most chronic suppuration requires a more radical operation.

The Caldwell-Luc operation, named after two surgeons, is the most generally accepted operative procedure for chronic maxillary sinusitis. It is also referred to as a radical antrum operation. Either local or general anesthesia can be used.

The maxillary sinus is entered through an incision under the upper lip and above the level of the roots of the maxillary teeth. Part of the anterior

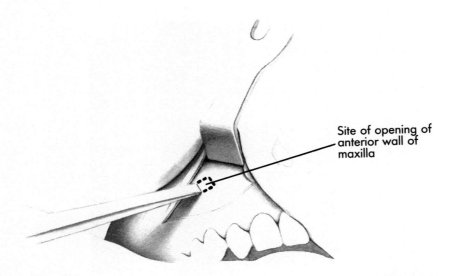

Site of opening of
anterior wall of
maxilla

**FIG 7–19.**
Incision for Caldwell left procedure with exposure of the face of the maxilla. Window is then made into the maxillary sinus.

bony wall of the antrum is removed. Through this window in the bone all of the diseased mucosa and periosteum is removed. The bone of the lateral wall of the nose in the inferior meatus, which divides the nose from the antrum, is removed. The mucous membrane and periosteum of the lateral wall of the nose are preserved, fashioned into a hinged flap with the base down and turned from

the nasal cavity into the floor of the antrum. The incision over the upper alveolus is then closed (Figs. 7–19, 7–20, and 7–21).

The antrum may be packed to control bleeding. However, bleeding from the exposed bone is often so slight that packing is not required. Twenty-four to 48 hours after the operation the packing should be removed through the nose and

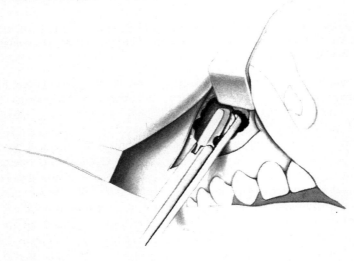

**FIG 7–20.**
With biting forceps and rongeur the anterior face of the maxilla is opened, exposing the maxillary sinus pathology.

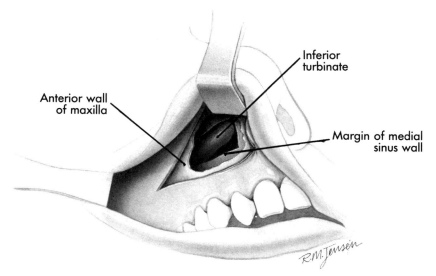

Anterior wall
of maxilla

Inferior
turbinate

Margin of medial
sinus wall

R.M.Jensen

**FIG 7–21.**
After removal of the sinus mucosa or polypoid tissue, a window is made into the nose along its floor, allowing dependent drainage from the maxillary sinus. Incision is closed with absorbable sutures.

the nasoantral window that has been created. During the postoperative period the maxillary sinus heals and the exposed bone is covered by mucosa.

Total exenteration of the ethmoid air cells can be accomplished by an operation (ethmoidectomy) through the nose or through an incision around the inner canthus of the eye. The external approach is recommended by some because it affords greater visibility, making possible a more thorough removal of tissue. The incision heals well and does not result in any cosmetic deformity.

Intranasal ethmoidectomy can be performed with local or general anesthesia. The middle turbinate is fractured medially toward the nasal septum and may be partially removed to gain access to the ethmoid sinuses. The ethmoid air cells and all infected tissue are removed to the medial wall of the orbit, and the nose is packed. If the nasofrontal duct is involved by infection or obstructed, the floor of the frontal sinus is removed to provide an adequate opening into the nose for future normal discharge of mucus from the frontal sinus. The sphenoid sinus, when involved, can be widely opened from this approach.

### Endoscopic Sinus Surgery

A new surgical procedure called functional endoscopic sinus surgery has increased in popularity and is a substitute for some of the more extensive sinus procedures. Like other surgical procedures on the sinuses, it is reserved for patients who fail traditional noninvasive therapy. The underlying principle in endoscopic sinus surgery is to focus the procedure on the actual site of pathology and thus perform a more limited operation. These procedures endeavor to open normal sinus ostia more widely and to ensure adequate drainage from the sinuses and thus alleviate recurrent infection. Thus under direct vision the maxillary sinus ostia can be enlarged, specific ethmoid cells opened and drained, or the sphenoid sinus widely exteriorized. The development of advanced optical and endoscopic instruments allows excellent visualization of the nose and the sinus ostia. These procedures are replacing many of the standard surgical approaches previously used.

External ethmoidectomy can be performed using either local or general anesthesia. After the skin, subcutaneous tissue, and periosteum have been incised with a curved incision around the inner canthus, soft tissue is dissected subperiosteally to expose the lateral bony wall of the ethmoid area. This is the common bony wall separating the ethmoid sinuses from the periorbital fascia, which encloses the eye and eye muscles. The ethmoid air cells, all infected tissue, and the lateral wall of the nose medial to the ethmoid bones are removed (Figs. 7–22, 7–23, and 7–24). If the

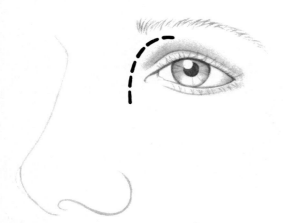

**FIG 7–22.**
Medial canthal incision for external ethmoidectomy.

sphenoid sinus is involved, its anterior face and lining mucous membrane are removed. The operative area is packed, and one end of the packing is brought into the nose. The skin and soft tissues are closed with sutures. The packing is removed through the nose during the postoperative period.

The floor and anterior wall of the frontal sinus can be exposed by extending the incision used for external ethmoidectomy into the eyebrow and carrying it toward the lateral limit of the eyebrow (frontoethmoidectomy). The floor of the frontal sinus, or its anterior wall above the supraorbital

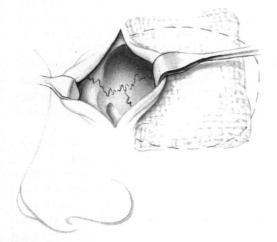

**FIG 7–23.**
Orbit contents retracted gently laterally, demonstrating lateral wall of ethmoid sinuses, e.g., ethmoid/sphenoid bone. Note frontal ethmoid suture line, which demonstrates the level of the cribriform plate, an important landmark.

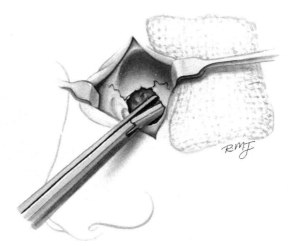

**FIG 7–24.**
Entry into the ethmoid sinus with removal of inner sinus walls and opening into the nose with biting forceps.

ridge, can be removed in order to remove all the lining mucosa of the frontal sinus. The extent of bony removal necessary depends on the size of the frontal sinus and the accessibility of its lateral and superior extent through the incision into the eyebrow. Ethmoid cells are always removed when the frontal sinus is exenterated by this approach to provide adequate drainage into the nose during healing. The cavity created during the operation is packed. The packing is brought into the nose and later removed through the nose. The external soft tissues are closed. When possible, it is advantageous to create a superiorly based hinged flap from the mucosa of the lateral wall of the nose. Such a flap can be turned up into the cavity and used to line the medial wall of the frontal sinus. It will prevent obstruction from scarring.

When infection is present in both frontal sinuses, or when a frontal sinus is pneumatized high into the frontal bone (approaching the hairline), an osteoplastic frontal sinus approach is used. This approach provides excellent direct access to the frontal sinuses. Though ethmoid cells can be removed by this approach, exposure is often incomplete and requires a separate approach for ethmoid disease. In this procedure, an incision is made through the skin and subcutaneous tissue of the scalp either in the eyebrow region or above the hairline (coronal incision) (Fig. 7–25). After elevation of skin and soft tissue down to the brow, a vibrating bone saw is used to cut into the

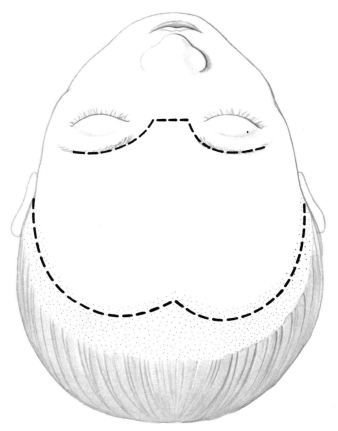

**FIG 7–25.**
Incisions for frontal sinus exploration. The coronal incision should be placed above the hairline while the brow incision should be placed just adjacent to the superior edge of the eyebrow. The brow incision may be unilateral if only one frontal sinus is to be exposed.

frontal sinus. With the lower or eyebrow margin left uncut, the anterior sinus wall is fractured from above downward so as to leave a hinged attachment (to periosteum) inferiorly (Fig. 7–26). This opens the sinus widely and permits removal of all mucosa. Drilling of the bony walls themselves will doubly ensure that all mucous membrane is removed. Fat taken from the abdominal wall is placed in the sinus cavity, and the osteoplastic flap (anterior wall of the frontal sinus) is replaced in its former position. The periosteum, subcutaneous tissue, and skin are then carefully closed. With no mucous membrane to regenerate, there is little likelihood that a mucocele—one of the complications after frontal sinus operations—will form postoperatively. This direct approach to the frontal sinus is used when there is osteomyelitis of the frontal bone, a rare but serious complication.

## COMPLICATIONS OF SINUSITIS

As long as infection remains within the paranasal sinuses, the symptoms remain localized. However, when it extends beyond the limits of the sinuses, usually new symptoms and signs appear that are no longer localized to the anatomic region of the involved sinus. Many of these symptoms and signs indicate spread of the infection to vital structures. Infection of the ethmoid and frontal sinuses is particularly dangerous because these sinuses are intimately associated with the orbit, the optic nerve, and the dura covering the frontal lobe of the brain. Complications of maxillary sinusitis are less common, and except for osteomyelitis of the superior maxilla, they are not considered dangerous.

Complications of sinusitis usually follow the acute stage of the disease or occur during an acute

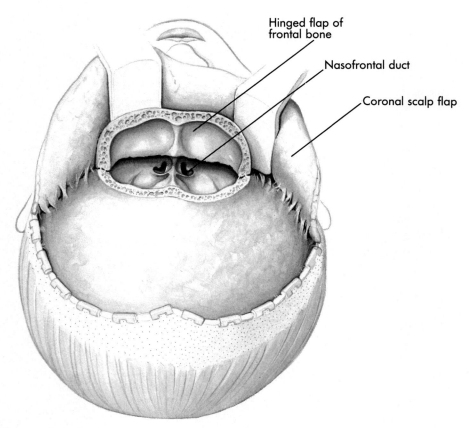

Hinged flap of
frontal bone

Nasofrontal duct

Coronal scalp flap

**FIG 7–26.**
After osteotomy the anterior table of the frontal bone is fractured over the superior orbital rim and tipped down, exposing the entire frontal sinus and nasofrontal duct.

exacerbation of a chronic infection. They are most frequently caused by inadequate therapy during the acute stage or by a delay in treatment. If antibiotics are indicated, they should be continued until the infection has subsided for no less than 10 days.

**Signs of Complications**

Certain signs occurring with, or shortly after, apparent subsidence of acute sinusitis are danger signals. The following symptoms should alert the physician to the possibility that infection may have spread from the involved sinus and is threatening important structures:

1. Generalized persistent headache
2. Vomiting
3. Convulsions
4. Chills or high fever
5. Edema or increasing swelling of the forehead or eyelids
6. Blurring of vision, diplopia, or persistent retroocular pain
7. Signs of increased intracranial pressure
8. Personality changes or dulling of the sensorium
9. Any combination of signs and symptoms in which the patient appears to be more ill than he or she should be with uncomplicated sinusitis (includes any sudden increase in white cell count above 20,000)

When any of these symptoms or signs are present, complications must be suspected and every effort made to find the probable site of origin. Thus, in addition to the careful evaluation of the condition of the sinuses, a general survey must be made to rule out other acute infections that may be the cause of the generalized symptoms.

## Orbital Complications

In 75% of patients orbital infections are caused by extension from paranasal sinusitis. The ethmoid sinuses are most frequently involved. The orbital complications of sinusitis include:

1. Inflammatory edema
2. Orbital cellulitis
3. Subperiosteal abscess
4. Orbital abscess
5. Cavernous sinous thrombosis

### Inflammatory Edema

Patients with inflammatory edema present with soft tissue swelling of either the upper or lower eyelids. There is no limitation of motion or loss of visual acuity and generally no evidence of chemosis. This is the earliest stage of spread of infection, and although it may occur from many other causes, the sinuses must always be considered. Treatment is appropriate antibiotics for the sinusitis. These patients can be followed on an outpatient basis but must be closely managed until all signs of infection subside.

### Orbital Cellulitis

When the infection spreads from the ethmoid sinuses through the lateral ethmoid wall, it may cause a diffuse cellulitis in the periorbital tissue. Typically a chill accompanies the initial invasion. The temperature is elevated, and there is a dull pain deep in the involved eye. Edema and inflammation of the eyelids in the region of the inner canthus often occur early (Figs. 7–27 and 7–28). As the process develops, the eyeball may protrude, usually in a straightforward direction. Eye movements become painful, but the eyeball can be moved until the inflammation is far advanced and the proptosis pronounced. Later, the conjunctiva becomes red, edematous, and thickened (chemosis) and the patient becomes acutely ill. Still later the eyeball may become completely fixed, the lid swollen and red, and the conjunctiva so edematous that the lids do not close. Patients with any significant degree of orbital cellulitis must be treated aggressively with intravenous antibiotics such as penicillinase-resistant penicillins and/or cephalosporins in large doses. Frequently a combination of two or more antibiotics may be necessary to resolve the infection. Early recognition

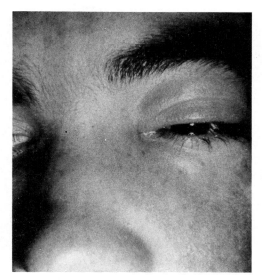

**FIG 7–27.**
Early orbital cellulitis.

and prompt, adequate treatment will prevent serious late sequelae. Patients (especially children) with orbital cellulitis should be hospitalized.

### Subperiosteal Abscess

When the infection extends through the lateral ethmoid plate but does not penetrate the perior-

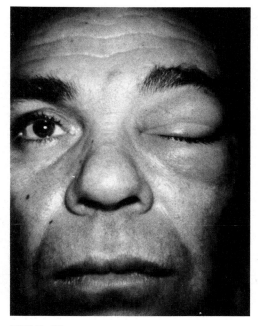

**FIG 7–28.**
Extensive orbital cellulitis.

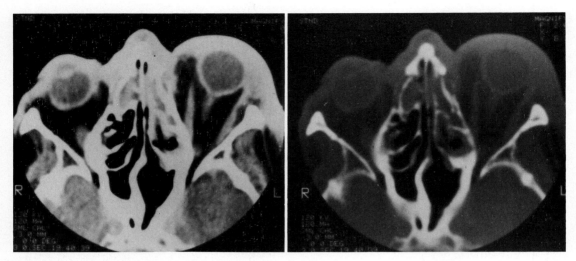

**FIG 7–29**.
CT scan with evidence of ethmoiditis, periorbital edema, and proptosis on the left. The medial rectus is displaced laterally, suggesting abscess formation.

bita, pus collects between the bone and the periorbita, producing a periorbital abscess. The general symptoms are not as severe as those caused by orbital cellulitis. However, the patient is often toxic. There is an increase in fever, some pain during motion of the eye, and edema in the region of the inner canthus. The eye may be slowly forced slightly outward and downward. There is little or no chemosis, but there may be extensive proptosis and limitation of extraocular mobility. Pressure over the inner canthus will cause pain. If unrecognized or neglected, the abscess may later break into the cone of the eye muscles and produce an orbital cellulitis. The diagnosis of subperiosteal abscess is generally made on the basis of the history and physical findings and clinched by classic appearance on CT scan, which shows a mass along the medial aspect of the orbit (Figs. 7–29 and 7–30).

Periorbital abscesses must be drained to prevent spread to the eye or the dura. An incision around the inner canthus of the eye and subperiosteal separation of the periorbita from the ethmoid wall will allow drainage. After drainage in-

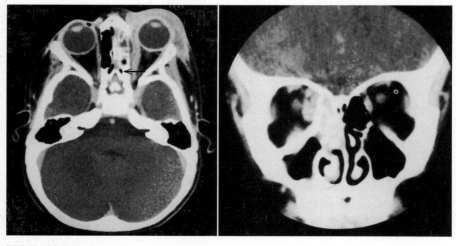

**FIG 7–30**.
**A,** CT scan demonstrating periorbital abscess. **B,** coronal view of periorbital abscess.

tranasally and externally and the use of adequate intravenous antibiotic therapy, recovery is almost always certain.

### Orbital Abscess

Patients with a collection of pus that has either ruptured from a subperiosteal abscess or formed within the orbit have severe proptosis, chemosis, ophthalmoplegia, and loss of vision. If inadequate primary treatment and prompt treatment are not instituted, the loss of vision is often irreversible.

### Cavernous Sinus Thrombosis

Cavernous sinus thrombosis occurs when there is an extension of infection through the venous pathways (usually the angular vein) to the cavernous sinus (Fig. 7–31). A septic thrombus forms. The symptoms occur abruptly and are severe. Chills and a rise in temperature to as high as 106° F are the rule. Pain deep behind the eyes is present. The patient rapidly becomes toxic and may become semicomatose. The third, fourth, and sixth cranial nerves are closely associated with cavernous sinus and are involved. Initially there is selective ocular palsy, which helps to differentiate the condition from orbital cellulitis, in which complete ophthalmoplegia is the rule. Eventually the infection affects both eyes with complete fixation, lid edema, and chemosis. If cavernous thrombosis is unrecognized or inadequately treated, death may occur in 48 to 72 hours. Despite adequate management, more than 25% of patients who develop cavernous sinus thrombosis will die. Primary treatment consists of intravenous antibiotics. The administration of heparin and steroids may improve the prognosis.

The bacteriology of orbital complications of sinusitis confirms the presence of *H. influenzae* as the most common organism cultured, since the majority of these episodes occur in children.

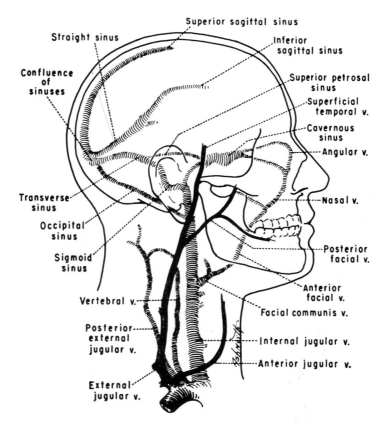

**FIG 7–31.**
Venous drainage of the brain. Note the continuity of the nasal vein, angular vein, and cavernous sinus. Note also the transverse sinus, sigmoid sinus, and internal jugular veins.

When abscesses have occurred, *S. aureus* and *Streptococcus* organisms are commonly found. Approximately one third to one half of cultures are negative in cases of orbital complications because of either the use of antibiotics or the presence of anaerobes that are not discovered.

Fungal infections are now more frequently being diagnosed as a complication of sinusitis. A particularly virulent fungal infection that causes nasal and orbital complications of sinusitis is mucormycosis. This is caused by a fungus of the family Mucoraceae. Infection generally starts in the nose and rapidly spreads into the sinuses, orbit, and cranial structures through the walls of vessels. The disorder is almost always seen in patients who have severe acidosis or are immunologically suppressed. Patients with uncontrolled diabetes are particularly prone to this type of infection, which occurs in both young and old. Characteristic signs are vascular thrombosis, including black nasal turbinates; a brownish watery discharge, which may actually be bloody; and thrombosis involving the palate or maxilla (Fig. 7–32). Ocular signs are common with involvement of the third, fourth, and sixth cranial nerves. Diagnosis is made on the basis of history and physical findings, awareness of the disorder, and appearance of nonseptate hyphae readily demonstrated in the tissue culture. X-ray films generally show cloudiness of the sinus. Because of the ful-

minant nature of the disorder, no significant bony changes are noted. Untreated, mucormycosis is fatal within a few days, but with treatment survival is possible. Treatment includes administration of amphotericin B, local drainage, resection of infected or necrotic tissue, and control of acidosis and systemic disease.

The ravages of human immunodeficiency virus have greatly increased the number of complications from sinus disease. The patient with acquired immunodeficiency syndrome will often present with sinusitis, usually caused by a variety of opportunistic organisms. It is in this population that tissue specimens and culture are most important. If appropriately treated early, the secondary sinus disease and/or complications can be alleviated. (See Chapter 3, section on Sinus and Nasal.)

## Intracranial Complications
### Meningitis

Infection from the frontal, ethmoid, or sphenoid sinuses may spread through the inner table of bone to the meninges or the frontal lobe of the brain. Extension of an infection occurs most often as a result of septic thrombophlebitis. Veins within the submucosa of the sinuses pierce the skull and join with dural vessels. Sterile thrombosis of these veins is the normal protective mechanism by which the body prevents such extension.

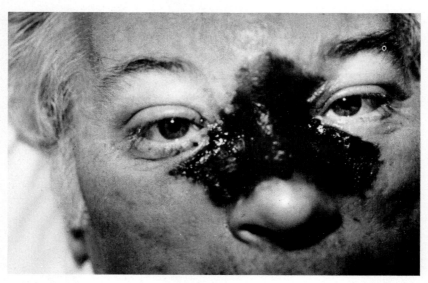

**FIG 7–32.**
Extensive mucormycosis with a vascular necrosis of anterior face.

However, in some abrupt infections, particularly those which occur as a result of swimming and diving, bacterial invasion may be so rapid that sterile thrombi may not have time to form. A chill usually marks this invasive stage, but several days may elapse after the chill before the symptoms of intracranial disease occur. Purulent invasion may also occur as a result of long-standing and neglected chronic sinusitis in which the bone of the inner table has eroded. However, this is much less common than meningitis secondary to acute infection.

The symptoms of meningitis following sinusitis are the same as those of meningitis from any cause—stiff neck, chills, variable sensorium changes resulting in coma, focalized convulsions, headache, and vomiting. Spinal fluid must be examined and cultured early to find the causative organism. General supportive measures, fluids, and massive doses of intravenous antibiotics such as penicillinase-resistant penicillins, cephalosporins, and/or chloromycetin are required. The prognosis is excellent if treatment is started promptly.

### Epidural Abscess

An epidural abscess is more difficult to diagnose than meningitis. After an initial invasive stage (usually a chill), symptoms and signs are minimal. The white blood count may be only slightly elevated. There is often a predominance of lymphocytes in the differential white blood count. Dull, persistent headache is common. There may be tenderness to percussion of the skull over the involved dura. Late in the course of the disease there may be erosion of the inner table of the skull over the abscess. When the headache persists and the patient's general condition does not suggest a subsiding sinusitis, daily evaluation of the patient's condition, including consultation with a neurosurgeon, is necessary. The symptoms of epidural abscess are often vague and confusing, and unless the patient is followed closely, they will not be recognized before they spread to the brain or rupture into the subarachnoid space to produce meningitis. Treatment consists of draining the abscess and administering intravenous antibiotics. Recovery is the rule.

### Subdural Abscess

Occasionally a subdural abscess occurs and even more rarely, epidural hemorrhage. Both re-quire daily evaluation of symptoms and signs by the otolaryngologist and the neurosurgeon (Fig. 7–33).

### Brain Abscess

Abscesses of the frontal lobe of the brain are often difficult to recognize. The frontal lobe is frequently called a "silent" area of the brain because disease here must be extensive to produce any obvious neurologic signs. A brain abscess must be suspected when a patient with sinusitis appears to be responding well to treatment and yet continues to have signs of retained pus. Slight personality and mood changes may occur. Facial muscles on the side opposite the involved lobe may show slight weakness. Signs of increased intracranial pressure occur late in the disease process. Careful daily observation of the ocular fundi may reveal early papilledema, which does not occur in epidural abscess. Ultimately the diagnosis is made when confirmatory signs appear. The CT scan and, more recently, magnetic resonance imaging have proved excellent aids in the diagnosis of these lesions and should be obtained if there is

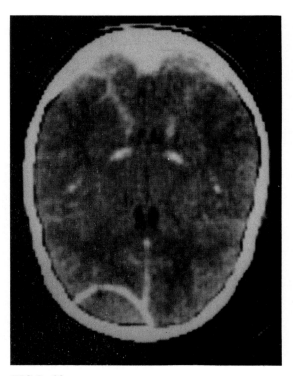

**FIG 7–33.**
CT scan demonstrating subdural abscess secondary to frontal sinusitis.

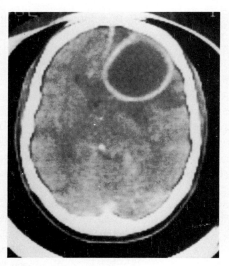

**FIG 7–34.**
Axial brain CT scan with large left frontal abscess secondary to underlying left frontal sinus infection.

any suspicion of abscess (Fig. 7–34). Drainage or aspiration of the abscess is required as well as control of the offending primary sinus infection. Cooperation with the neurosurgeon is important.

In general, the intracranial complications must be recognized and managed before any operative approach to the sinus infection is attempted. If any infection remains in the sinuses after the complication is controlled or drainage has been established, definitive surgery on the involved sinus should be performed to prevent further recurrence of the intracranial infection.

## Osteomyelitis of the Skull

Since antibiotics and chemotherapeutic drugs have been available, the incidence of osteomyelitis of the skull has diminished steadily. It still occurs in untreated or neglected patients. The primary signs of this complication are continuation of low-grade fever, dull headache, and slow development of doughy, tender thickening of the periosteum over the infected bone. Edema of the upper lids is common when the frontal sinus is involved (Fig. 7–35). The patient does not have overwhelming symptoms but rather appears chronically ill. X-ray films of the skull may show localized decalcification or destruction of bone. This may also be clearly visible on CT scan. Bone scan may be of diagnostic value in questionable diagnoses. Etiologic factors include trauma, frontal sinus surgery, or hematogenous spread. *Staphylococcus* is the most common organism, although *Streptococcus* and pneumococcus are frequently found. Formerly, treatment demanded an extensive excision of skull and removal of bone. More recently, antibiotics with high bone penetration—for example, clindamycin (Cleocin)—have been used in early cases of osteomyelitis with success and without the requirement for surgery. Generally, however, in extensive osteomyelitis, wide exposure of the frontal bone with surgical removal of the diseased bone is required. If bony removal is extensive, an alloplastic plate may be placed to protect the underlying brain from external injury, as both the

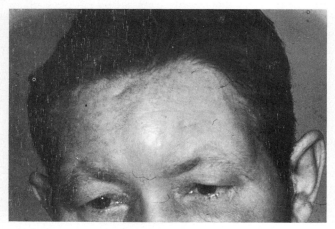

**FIG 7–35.**
Doughy swelling over the left frontal sinus, typical of osteomyelitis—often called Pott's puffy tumor.

inner and outer cortical plates have been removed.

## Osteomyelitis of the Superior Maxilla

Osteomyelitis of the superior maxilla is rare. It may occur spontaneously in infants and young children as a result of sinusitis or serious dental infection. In adults it is almost always caused by unnecessary intranasal procedures performed while a patient is suffering from acute maxillary sinusitis. It can also result from trauma in the face of an infection. Removal of polyps, fracture of turbinates, and puncture of the antrum should always be avoided during the acute stage of maxillary sinusitis prior to antibiotic treatment.

When osteomyelitis occurs, the soft tissue over the maxillary sinus becomes red, swollen, and tender. There are signs of spreading infection with sepsis. Purulent matter fills the nose. If treatment is neglected, osteomyelitis rapidly spreads to involve the entire maxilla, orbit, and lateral wall of the nose. Subperiosteal abscesses, slough of necrotic bone, and spreading cellulitis of the face may occur. Septicemia or extension into the cavernous sinus may complicate the condition in untreated patients. Prolonged treatment is required and may involve excision of sequestra or portions of the maxilla.

## Mucocele and Pyocele

When there is complete blockage of the nasofrontal duct or of the ducts of one or more of the ethmoid sinuses, no mucus can drain from the sinus into the nose. Because the mucosal lining of the sinus continues to produce mucus, the result is a slowly developing swelling above and medial to the eye. This is caused by erosion of the floor of the frontal sinus or the lateral wall of the ethmoid labyrinth as a result of pressure from the retained mucus. Such swelling occurs slowly and may take years to become evident. The eye is slowly pushed downward and outward, eventually causing diplopia (Fig. 7–36). There is no redness, inflammation, or pain. Except for diplopia, there are no visual changes.

Examination of the nose usually shows no abnormality. Sometimes evidence of a past intranasal operation can be seen. The cardinal sign is a rubbery mass under the inner third of the supraor-

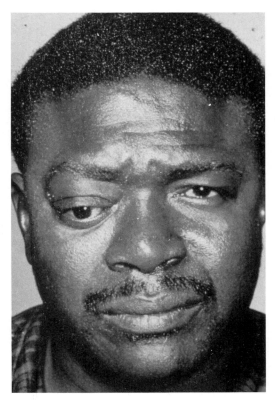

**FIG 7–36.**
Frontoethmoid mucocele with eye pushed outward and downward.

bital ridge. The mass is smooth and partially compressible. Often a firm edge can be felt where the mucocele joins the remaining uneroded bone. The eye can be moved in all directions, but there is restriction of motion upward and inward. When the swelling is severe, the eyeball is forced partially out of the orbit, giving a downward and outward proptosis. X-ray films show a loss of continuity of the bony suborbital ridge or displacement of the bony floor of the frontal sinus (Fig. 7–37). The CT scan will similarly demonstrate a mass involving the superior ethmoids or frontal sinus with displacement of the orbital contents (Fig. 7–38).

Chronic dacryocystitis may cause swelling at the inner canthus of the eye, but such swelling is usually below the medial canthal ligament. The swelling of a mucocele is above and medial to the eyeball (Fig. 7–39).

If a mucocele becomes infected, it is called a pyocele. Pyoceles tend to flare intermittently, with pain developing and the size of the mass

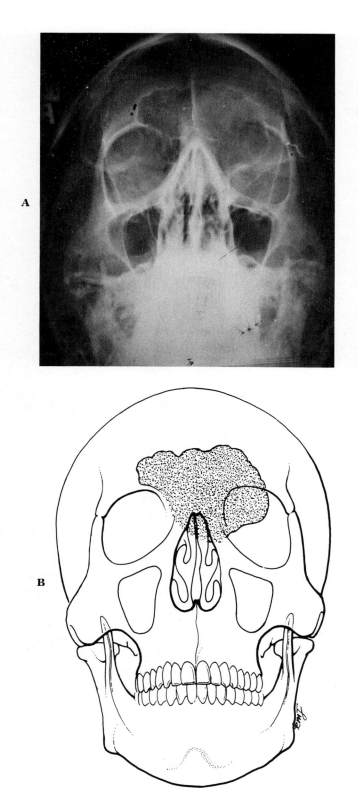

**FIG 7–37.**
**A,** x-ray film (Waters view) of a mucocele in the left frontal sinus. Note that the floor of the sinus is depressed into the orbit to cause proptosis. **B,** represents line drawing of **A.**

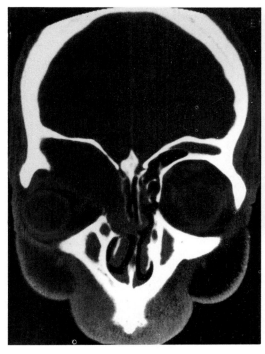

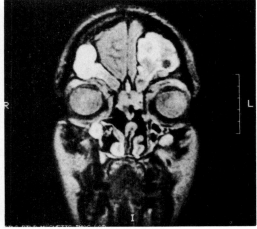

**FIG 7–38.**
**A,** CT scan demonstrating left frontal sinus mucocele.
**B,** MRI study showing bilateral frontal sinus mucocele
with compression of frontal lobe.

fluctuating. Treatment is directed toward the infection and must include surgery.

In most instances, a careful history reveals that some intranasal manipulation or surgery was performed many years previously. The possibilities of facial trauma must not be disregarded. Attempted cannulation of the nasofrontal duct or removal of the turbinates may have caused formation of scar tissue that blocks the normal ostia, or displacement of bone as a result of trauma may have occluded the normal openings of the sinus. In any event, the block or obstruction generally occurs years before visible signs of the mucocele appear. Mucoceles can also occur within the maxillary sinus, although they are generally less common and are usually discovered inadvertently on routine x-ray studies. Treatment is operative. The area is opened in the same manner as for a radical frontal ethmoid operation. The usual finding is a large cavity filled with thick, tenacious mucus and lined with a thin, secreting membrane. The entire membrane is removed, along with any remaining ethmoid air cells. A new opening is made into the nose and is kept open during the postoperative period by means of a mucosal flap or nonreactive plastic tubing. Total cure is the rule. The eye will assume its natural position as soon as the postoperative tissue reaction has subsided.

The differential diagnosis of the complications of sinusitis frequently involves both the possibility of tumor, which must never be excluded, and the possibility of unusual or secondary infections of immunologic basis. One disorder that deserves additional discussion is malignant exophthalmos. This is not a complication of sinusitis, but it does produce signs and symptoms similar to those of the complications of sinusitis. Because treatment involves the sinuses, the condition is discussed with sinusitis. The exophthalmos is a result of an endocrine disturbance of the pituitary-thyroid relationship. It most often occurs in a person who has had hyperthyroidism and who, a short time before the exophthalmos, had a thyroidectomy. This is not always the case, however, and the underlying pathologic condition is a large increase of orbital fat (Fig. 7–40). This may occur slowly or rapidly. The eye may be forced out by the pressure of the fat in the muscle conus behind the eyeball. The pressure may progress to the point where the lids cannot close over the globe, and edema, chemosis, and inflammation of the conjunctiva may occur. Vision may be threatened by stretching of the optic nerve. In early stages of the disease, treatment of the underlying endocrine disturbance may arrest the further development of proptosis. However, in later stages surgery is al-

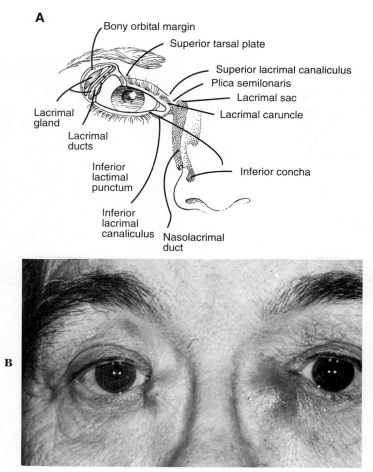

**FIG 7–39.**
**A,** relationship of the eyelids and eye to the lacrimal apparatus and the nose. (Modified from Jacob SW, Francone CA: *Structure and function in man,* ed 5, Philadelphia, 1982, WB Saunders. Used by permission.) **B,** chronic dacryocystitis. Note that the swelling is *below* the inner canthus.

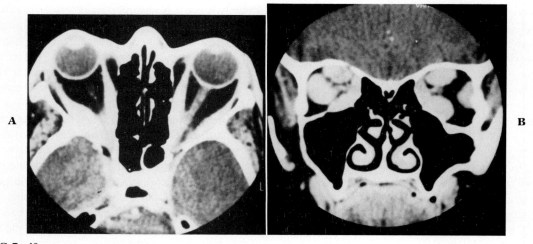

**FIG 7–40.**
**A,** axial CT scan showing malignant exophthalmus on left. **B,** coronal CT scan of same patient showing muscle edema on left.

most always necessary. The operative procedures include (1) decompression of the orbit through a modification of ethmoidectomy, removal of ethmoid cells, and opening of the frontal sinus; (2) removal of a portion of the floor of the orbit, allowing the fat to herniate into the maxillary sinus; or, (3) the release of orbital fat by removing the lateral wall of the orbit.

## DISORDERS OF THE NASAL SEPTUM AND NOSE

### Deviated Septum

At birth the nasal septum normally is straight, and it remains straight and thin throughout infancy and early childhood. However, as a person ages, there is a tendency for the septum to become deviated to one side or the other, or for an irregular projection to develop (called a septal spur, shelf, or hump, depending on the shape) (Fig. 7–41). Often, there is no history of injury to account for the irregular septum. In some persons the nasal septum seems to lose its midline position during the growth process rather than as a result of injury. Few adults have a septum that is altogether in the midline.

Sometimes the septum is bent as a result of birth trauma, and the infant's nose appears twisted. Usually there is no bleeding. Often the nose will right itself after a few days (greenstick injury), but sometimes the deformity persists. It is

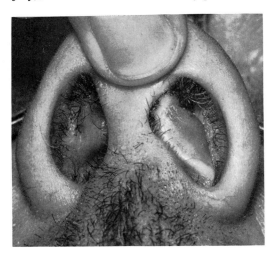

**FIG 7–41.**
Dislocation of the columellar end of the septal cartilage.

worthwhile to reduce the deformity when the patient is first seen. Correction is usually simple and can be made by applying light pressure of the thumb on the convex side of the nose or by twisting the tip between the thumb and index finger to pull the septum back to midline. No packing or splint is required.

When trauma causes a septal injury during childhood or adulthood, similar maneuvers may suffice to correct the deformity. However, more forceful manipulation with the patient under local or general anesthesia may be necessary.

Physicians do not always agree on the symptoms that may be caused by deviated septum, but one symptom, nasal obstruction, is recognized by patients and physicians alike. However, there are many other causes of nasal obstruction, and a deviated septum may be the least important of them. A septum that appears severely obstructed may not, in fact, cause the patient any discomfort at all. In a group of patients with the same apparent degree of obstruction, some will have no complaint, whereas others will be in distress. Except for nasal obstruction, other symptoms resulting from septal malformations are not well defined. Headache is frequently attributed to a septal spur impinging on the inferior or middle turbinate or to a septal deviation when it causes nasal obstruction, yet many patients seen with these conditions have no headache. The possibility of coincidence in patients who have both head pain and septal deformity is great. Great care must be taken before a causal relationship is suggested.

Sinusitis may be influenced by a deviated septum that occludes a sinus ostium, but this is rare. The physician should be careful not to promise that a septal operation will cure sinusitis. The reputation of nasal surgery suffers when a patient fails to obtain relief after an operation. The patient blames the operation, whereas the fault was in the diagnosis. Sometimes nosebleeds are produced as a result of air currents drying the mucosa that covers the deflected septum. As the mucosa is traumatized, crusts form and bleeding results when they are picked off or come loose. Such trauma is confined to the anterior part of the nose. Occasionally a patient may feel irregularity just inside the nasal vestibule and be inclined to pick at it.

On inspection, the deviated septum is seen to be inclined or bent to one side (sometimes an S-curve blocks both sides) and the airway is greatly reduced. The obstruction may be anterior (cartilaginous) or posterior (bony). Sometimes the anterior (caudal) end of the septal cartilage is dislocated into one nasal vestibule. In such conditions, an operation called a nasal septal reconstruction or a submucous resection is performed to relieve the nasal obstruction. It is dangerous, however, to suggest to the patient who has a deviated septum that an operation to straighten the septum will do anything more than improve the nasal septum. The operation is not ordinarily intended to correct headache (unless there is specific coincidence to conclude nasal turbinate compression causes the symptoms) or reduce nasal mucous discharge (postnasal drip).

### Nasal Septal Reconstruction

Many procedures are used to straighten and thin the septum. In the most common procedure an incision is made through the mucosa and perichondrium (on one side) just behind the mucocutaneous junction. The mucoperichondrium and the mucoperiosteum are elevated on that side. The cartilage is then cut through at the site of the original incision. (Great care must be taken not to cut through the opposite mucoperichondrium.)

Similar mucoperichondrial and periosteal flaps are elevated on the opposite side until the septal cartilage and bones are freed of all soft tissue attachments. The obstructing pieces of cartilage or bone or both are removed or placed in better position (Figs. 7–42 and 7–43).

In one technique (submucous resection), almost all the framework of the septum, except a strut at the top and in the front, is removed. In other techniques, an effort is made to excise as little cartilage and bone as possible. The obstruction is corrected by shaving off the thickened cartilage and breaking its spring, leaving the septum thinned and straightened. In another approach, an incision cuts through the entire membranous columella just in front of the cartilage, affording an end-on view of the free edge of the cartilage. This approach is especially useful when the inferior edge of the cartilage is dislocated and appears in one vestibule rather than in the midline.

Great care must be taken to avoid two opposing incisions (or tears) in the mucoperichondrial flaps. If this occurs, perforation of the septum may result. Also, care should be taken to leave sufficient support for the nose so that the nasal dorsum does not fall down or become pulled down by scar contracture (saddle deformity).

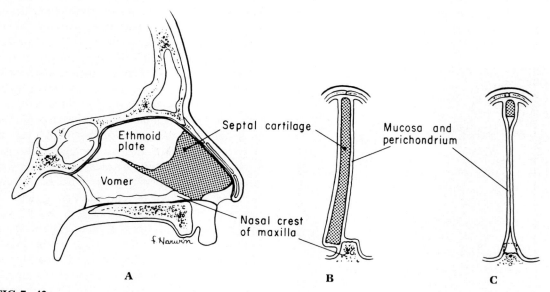

Ethmoid plate

Septal cartilage

Mucosa and perichondrium

Vomer

Nasal crest of maxilla

f Narwin

**A**    **B**    **C**

**FIG 7–42.**
**A,** chief components of the septum. **B,** septum with a deviated cartilage and spur at the junction of the nasal crest and septal cartilage. **C,** part of the cartilage and bone have been resected, allowing the mucoperichondrium of the two sides to grow together in the midline.

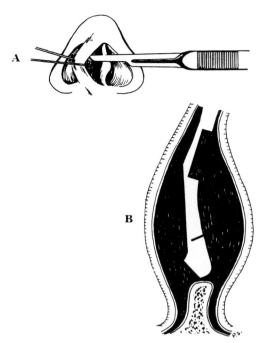

**FIG 7–43.**
Another type of septal operation. **A,** complete transfixation of the membranous portion of the columella just in front of the septal cartilage. **B,** the cartilage is shaved down, and cuts are made to break the spring, but very little is resected.

## Rhinoplasty

Rhinoplasty is discussed in the chapter on facial plastic surgery; however, rhinoplasty is often a concomitant procedure following nasal trauma. In this procedure, the entire structure of the nose is mobilized and repositioned in straight or normal position.

## Septal Perforation

The most common cause of nasal septal perforations is chronic infection initiated by repeated trauma (nose picking), operative procedure, or cocaine addiction. Perforations resulting from syphilis and tuberculosis, once quite common, are now seldom seen. Carcinoma may also cause septal perforations, but rarely. Other causes of septal perforation are Wegener's granulomatosis, lethal midline granuloma, and chronic inhalation of acid fumes. Septal perforations do not always cause symptoms. When they do, recurrent nosebleeds and nasal crusting are common symptoms. Small perforations may produce a whistle when the patient breathes (Fig. 7–44).

A septal perforation is usually obvious but may be overlooked when the septum is crusted. There is a tendency to look through a large septal perforation and see the normal mucosa of the opposite side of the nose without realizing which mucosal surface is being seen. Perforations are usually in the cartilaginous septum anteriorly but may also involve the bony septum.

Surgical closure of septal perforations is possible, but operations are not always successful. In general, discomfort can be kept at a minimum if the patient avoids picking the nose, uses bland ointment such as vaseline to control crusting, and treats symptoms as they occur. Bleeding from the margins of the perforation may require packing or cautery.

## Septal Abscess

Although unusual, a septal abscess is important because it is painful and serious consequences may result. The septum balloons out on both sides and becomes red (Fig. 7–45). The widening begins just behind the columella and extends a variable distance posteriorly. Pressure with a probe or bayonet forceps causes pitting of the swollen area and increases pain. Incision releases the collection of pus. Purulent matter between the cartilage and its perichondrium affects the blood supply to the cartilage. Necrosis of the cartilage may result, and after the infection resolves, the dorsum of the nose may depress (Fig. 7–46). Thrombosis of the cavernous sinus may occur as infections about the nose drain through

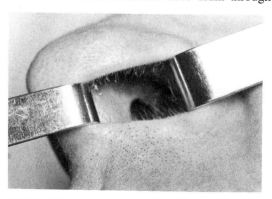

**FIG 7–44.**
Septal perforation.

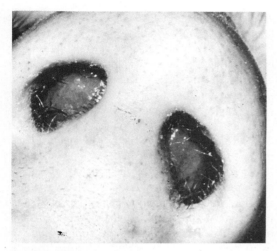

**FIG 7–45.**
Septal abscess.

the angular vein, to the inferior ophthalmic vein, and thus to the cavernous sinus.

A septal abscess should be incised and drained, but bilateral drainage is contraindicated because septal perforation may result. Systemic antibiotics (antistaphylococcal) are prescribed in full dosage.

**Septal Hematoma**

After facial trauma, or sometimes after a nasal operation, a hematoma may develop in the sep-

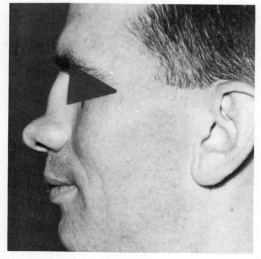

**FIG 7–46.**
Saddle deformity of the nose caused by loss of support of the septal cartilage secondary to abscess.

tum. The intranasal appearance may be similar to that of a septal abscess, but instead of pus, there is blood between the cartilage and perichondrium. The proper treatment is incision and drainage, although often the incision heals so quickly that blood reaccumulates. Packing the nose helps prevent additional bleeding. Treatment with antibiotics is customary to prevent a septal abscess, even if no active infection is present.

## TUMORS OF THE NOSE AND SINUS

### External Nose

Any variety of benign lesion that can be found on the face can be found on the nose, including solar keratoses, sebaceous cysts, and nevi. One more common dramatic tumor specific to the nose is *rhinophyma* (Fig. 7–47), a benign tumor caused by an overgrowth of sebaceous glands of the tip of the nose. Sometimes the condition is marked and will produce lobulated tumors so that the patient is said to have a "potato nose." Treatment is simple and effective. The excess tissue is shaved off until the nose has a normal configuration. Various means of reshaping the nose include the use of the "hot knife" surgical excision, electrocautery, or the carbon dioxide laser. The area is allowed to reepithelialize, generally without the need for a skin graft.

Both squamous cell carcinoma and basal cell carcinoma involve the external nose (Figs. 7–48 and 7–49). The squamous cell lesions usually grow faster and may metastasize to the neck at any stage. Basal cell lesions often remain very small for a long period and then gradually spread locally. They do not generally metastasize. However, in advanced stages, basal cell carcinoma may erode the entire nose and adjacent cheek and cause death. These lesions are particularly aggressive when they involve the mucous membrane on the portion of the internal nose. Treatment of either type of carcinoma in early stages should be very successful. Wide local excision is generally proposed, although small squamous cell lesions can be treated with radiotherapy or curettage. It is particularly difficult to determine margins for basal cell carcinomas, and frozen-section evaluation of margins of the excision is critical at the time of the initial surgery. Recently a surgical technique (Mohs technique) has been used for le-

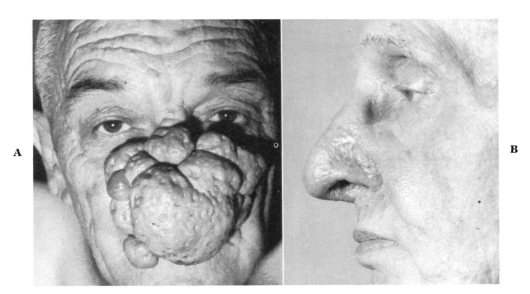

**FIG 7–47.**
**A,** large rhinophyma. **B,** appearance of the nose in another patient after removal of a rhinophyma without a graft. (**A** Courtesy of Dr. James A. Harrill, Winston-Salem, NC)

sions of the skin. The lesion is excised and serial pathologic sections are taken of margins at the time of surgery. This is done in an attempt to more closely define the total extent of tumor and any extension. It has been a useful technique preserving as much normal tissue as possible about the face and nose, as well as more accurately defining the tumor.

**Internal Nose**

Squamous papillomas occur in the nasal vestibule. They generally cause local irritation and are easily removed by excision and diathermy. Nasal polyps, the most common tumors of the nose, arise from the sinuses, sinus ostia, or turbinates

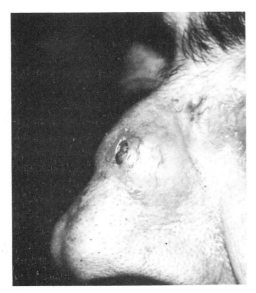

**FIG 7–48.**
Basal cell carcinoma. Note how the tumor undermines the skin.

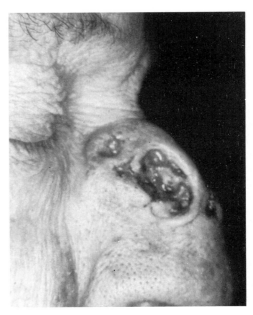

**FIG 7–49.**
Squamous cell carcinoma.

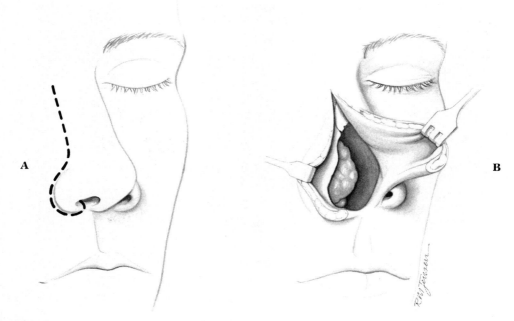

**FIG 7–50.**
**A,** incision for lateral rhinotomy. **B,** exposure of nasal tumor via lateral rhinotomy. Additional exposure can be obtained by removal of the adjacent maxillary and nasal bone.

and then project down into the nose. Nasal polyps were discussed earlier.

Inverting papilloma of the nose and sinus is a rather unusual tumor that, although histologically benign, clinically tends to act malignant, since it may by continuity involve adjacent structures beyond the interior of the nose. Furthermore, there is a strong tendency toward recurrence if the lesion is not completely excised. Inverting papilloma usually arises from the lateral wall of the nose and presents as a fleshy polyp. Characteristically, it demonstrates microscopic invagination of surface epithelium into the stroma of the polyp. Treatment is wide local surgical excision, often requiring a lateral rhinotomy (Fig. 7–50). Irradiation is contraindicated. About 10% of inverting papillomas undergo malignant degeneration.

Less common benign tumors include adenomas, lymphangiomas, and hemangiomas. Angiofibromas, which are generally more frequently found in the nasopharynx, are discussed in the chapter on the nasopharynx.

## Sinuses

### Benign Tumors

Benign tumors of the sinuses include chiefly osteoma and chondroma. Osteoma is a true bone tumor, most commonly found in the frontal sinus (Fig. 7–51). It is occasionally seen in the ethmoid and the maxilla. These tumors enlarge very slowly. Symptoms result from pressure or obstruction of the drainage of the sinuses. Osteomas are generally easily removed through external op-

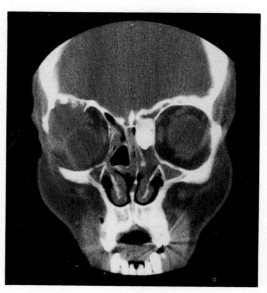

**FIG 7–51.**
CT scan showing frontal ethmoid osteoma.

erations on the sinus. Small exostoses found on the frontal sinus are different from osteomas in that they do not enlarge and generally tend to be stable. Chondromas are rare tumors of the nose and are generally found on the septum. Mucoceles, which may easily be confused with neoplasms, appear as smooth, rounded lesions, generally within the maxillary sinus, although they are often found within the frontal and ethmoid sinuses. They enlarge slowly and are generally asymptomatic.

Polyps in the sinuses, particularly the maxillary sinuses, are often reported by the radiologist as tumors. These tend to be multiple, often arising from the roof and lateral walls of the sinus. They generally cause no symptoms. The polyps are noted on x-ray film as a smooth, rounded mass without bone destruction. Treatment is generally unnecessary, but occasionally polyps that grow may require investigation.

### Fibrous Dysplasia

Fibrous dysplasia (of bone) is a benign growth in which the bone is soft and is replaced by relatively avascular, abnormal fibrous tissue. This occurs primarily in the maxillary but also in the ethmoid and frontal sinuses. It is a relatively rare condition that causes deformity and obstruction of the sinus ostia, displacement of the eye, nasal obstruction, and erosion of the skull (Figs. 7–52 and 7–53). Generally, when it develops in the maxilla, it is noted as an enlargement and asymmetry of the face over the maxilla. The treatment is surgical, with resculpturing, but generally not radical excision of the tumor, and with preservation of all other bony and soft tissue structures. It is found in young individuals and tends to stop growing after adolescence.

### Nasal Cysts

A variety of other cysts may occur about the sinuses and develop on the floor of the maxillary sinus or nose. These include radicular cysts, globulomaxillary cysts, and nasoalveolar cysts. The more common nasoalveolar cyst is a developmental cyst located in the soft tissues of the junction of the premaxilla and alveolar process of the maxilla. It presents as a cystic lesion growing into the floor of the nose.

### Squamous Cell Carcinoma

Squamous cell carcinoma is the most common malignant neoplasm occurring in the nasal cavities and paranasal sinuses. Squamous cell carcinomas arise more frequently in the maxillary sinus than in any other sinuses. Unfortunately, carci-

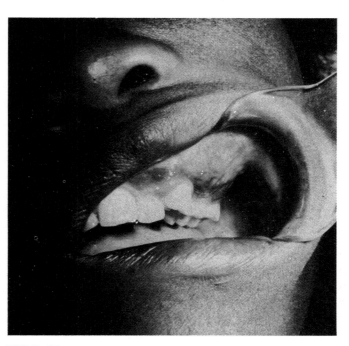

**FIG 7–52.**
Fibrous dysplasia of the maxilla.

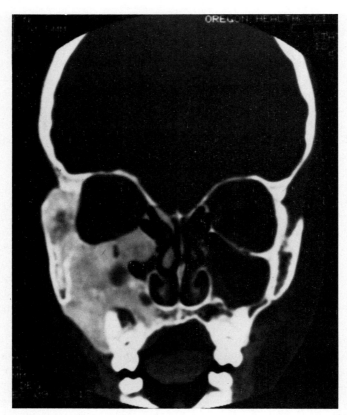

**FIG 7–53.**
CT scan demonstrating fibrous dysplasia of maxilla.

noma of the maxillary sinus causes no early symptoms to warn the patient. When the tumor is large, it erodes into the nose and causes nasal obstruction or bloody discharge. If it erodes into the periosteum of the posterior or lateral wall of the antrum, persistent pain in the face develops. The pain may follow the distribution of the second division of the fifth cranial nerve. If there is erosion of the superior wall of the antrum, the orbital contents may be displaced upward and produce proptosis and double vision. If the superior alveolar ridge is invaded, the maxillary teeth may become loosened.

The diagnosis is generally confirmed by biopsy and x-ray evaluation. X-ray films generally demonstrate erosion or destruction of bone (Fig. 7–54). The CT scan is particularly useful in differentiating between benign lesions and malignant lesions and extension of tumor, particularly posteriorly (Fig. 7–55). In most instances the specimen for biopsy can be obtained from the nose. When the tumor has not involved the nose, it may

be necessary to open the maxillary antrum through a sublabial incision to obtain a biopsy specimen.

Treatment usually consists of irradiation followed by complete surgical excision of the maxilla. Radiation therapy alone for carcinoma of the antrum is usually palliative. The combination of irradiation and maxillectomy is more effective than either procedure alone. The timing of irradiation remains controversial, however. Some physicians prefer to use the tumor dose of x-ray therapy 8 to 10 weeks before maxillectomy. Others favor similar irradiation following surgery. The use of chemotherapeutic drugs in conjunction with irradiation or surgery may improve long-term survival, especially in large tumors.

Whether or not irradiation or chemotherapy is used, successful treatment generally is based on complete surgical excision of the maxilla. The surgery is performed through an incision that begins along the lateral border of the nose, is extended through the upper lip to the midline, and is

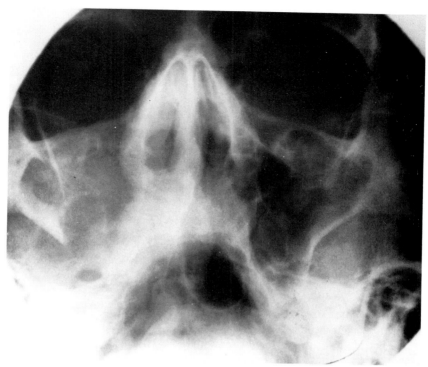

**FIG 7–54.**
Demonstration of bony erosion from squamous cell carcinoma of the maxillary sinus (Waters view).

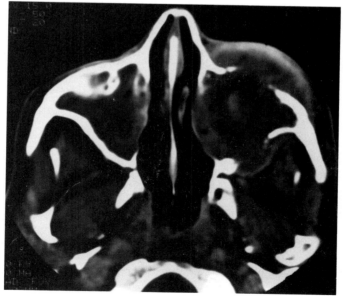

**FIG 7–55.**
CT scan demonstrating tumor involving the maxillary sinus. Note erosion into pterygopalatine fossa posteriorly, nose medially, and face anteriorly.

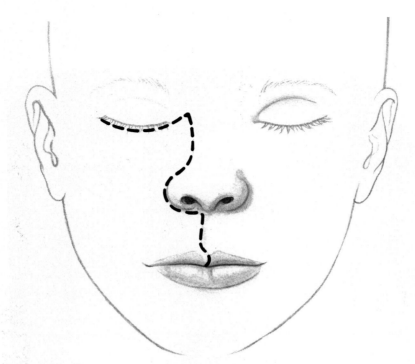

**FIG 7–56.**
Weber-Fergussonn incision for maxillectomy.

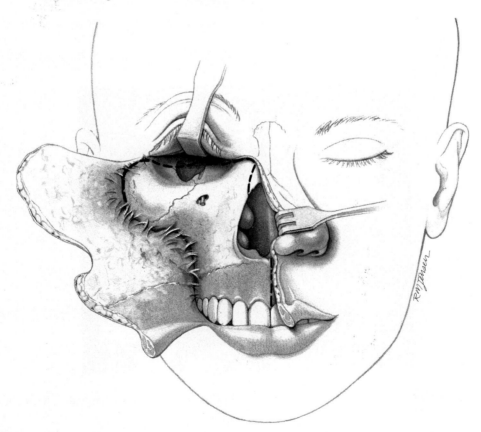

**FIG 7–57.**
Demonstration of exposure and block removal of maxilla with eye preservation. If the tumor extends through the floor of the orbit, the eye must be removed with the maxilla.

continued laterally along the upper alveolus (Weber-Fergusson incision) (Fig. 7–56). All the soft tissue of the maxillary region of the face is reflected laterally. The entire maxilla is then resected in block manner (Fig. 7–57). In addition, it may also be necessary to resect the contents of the orbit if the superior wall of the maxilla (the floor of the orbit) has been invaded. The resulting oral defect is grafted with split-thickness skin. After healing, a dental prosthesis replaces the resected hard palate and floor of the nose. This allows nearly normal speech, swallowing, and appearance.

Just as with any other malignant lesion, early diagnosis greatly improves the surgical result. To that end, the use of diagnostic antrotomy through a sublabial excision is a relatively benign procedure advocated by many when there seems to be a possibility of antral carcinoma or when the course of unilateral sinusitis is prolonged and different from what is expected. Also, some clinics incorporate a screening x-ray film (Waters view) in multiphasic screening programs for patients over the age of 40.

Malignancy of the frontal sinus is much more unusual than that of the maxillary sinus. Often there are no early symptoms. Nasal bleeding, pain, or even proptosis may be the first symptom. Treatment is usually a combination of surgery and irradiation, and the prognosis is poor. Carcinomas are more common in the ethmoid sinus and nose than in the frontal sinus. In these cases the nose is filled with tumor. The eye is pushed outward, and shortly thereafter the skin near the inner canthus breaks down. It is difficult to localize the extent of these tumors, and CT scan is imperative. Irradiation and extensive external ethmoidectomy with en bloc excision, often incorporating removal of the cribriform plate and the floor of the frontal fossa with the aid of neurosurgeons, is indicated.

Malignancies of the sphenoid sinus are rare. Occasionally other types of tumors are found within the nose and sinuses, including melanomas. Patients with melanoma, which arises in the mucous membranes, are generally treated with a combination of chemotherapeutic drugs and radiation therapy. Neural tumors of the nose are not uncommon, and neuroblastoma is perhaps the most common. This is an extremely slow-growing tumor that arises generally high on the vault of the lateral wall of the nose or septum. It rarely metastasizes but continues to enlarge. Total excision is the treatment of choice but is often impossible because of the location. Surgical incision in conjunction with neurosurgical support is indicated.

# 8

# Epistaxis

## CAUSES

The most common cause of nosebleed is trauma. In some instances the type of trauma may be quite obvious, as when a crust has been picked off the nasal septum or when there is excessive drying of the nasal mucosa. In other instances the cause may be less obvious—for example, when there is a defect intrinsic in the blood vessel. Nosebleeds are more common in patients who have hypertension or sclerotic blood vessels.

Patients receiving chemotherapy or suffering from leukemia or thrombocytopenia may have nosebleeds. These patients represent only a small number of patients suffering from nosebleeds. Even in such patients, trauma may be the precipitating cause.

Often the cause of epistaxis may be obscure. The patient's nose simply starts to bleed spontaneously. Dry air causes the nasal septum to crust, and as the crusts are removed by blowing or picking, the mucosa is torn and small vessels are opened.

Bleeding from the posterior half of the nose is unlikely to be caused by external trauma. Instead, it results from splitting of a sclerotic blood vessel. The defect is intrinsic to the vessel and is worsened if the patient is hypertensive.

Certain conditions commonly thought to cause nosebleeds have been overemphasized. For example, a disturbance in the blood-clotting mechanism is often considered a common cause of nosebleed. However, alterations in the vitamin C or K level, changes in the prothrombin time, or changes in bleeding and clotting are not commonly associated with epistaxis. If these conditions were the cause of epistaxis, the patient would bleed from other mucous membranes and into the skin and viscera rather than only from the nose. A patient who is not bleeding from any other part of the body rarely has nosebleed resulting from a hematologic disorder.

The distinction between nosebleed caused by trauma and nosebleed resulting from a generalized systemic disorder is important in treatment. If a patient's nose is not packed accurately, the bleeding continues. Then, instead of replacing the packing, the physician ascribes the bleeding to a hematologic disorder and prescribes various medications designed to promote coagulation. The rent in the vessel wall remains, however, and the patient continues to bleed. The proper management of nosebleeds depends on the physician's ability to look into the nose and discover the exact site of bleeding.

### Sites of Bleeding

#### Anterior Part of the Nose

Most nosebleeds in the anterior part of the nose start from the vascular network in the anterior part of the nasal septum (Kiesselbach plexus, Fig. 8–1). Occasionally, bleeding occurs from the anterior end of the inferior turbinate. Most of the blood that supplies the anterior part of the nasal septum comes from the external carotid system.

#### Posterior Part of the Nose

In the posterior part of the nose the bleeding vessels may be derived from either the external or internal carotid system. They are large vessels, and bleeding is usually severe. A very common site of hemorrhage from the posterior part of the nose is under the posterior half of the inferior turbinate (in the inferior meatus).

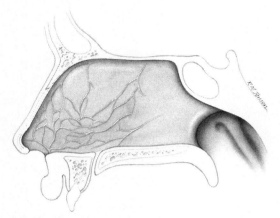

**FIG 8–1.**
Kiesselbach plexus.

Vessels in this area are branches of the internal maxillary artery (external carotid). The anterior ethmoid artery, a branch of the ophthalmic artery (internal carotid system), supplies the upper portion of the posterior part of the nose. Bleeding from this artery usually is seen high in the nose between the nasal septum and the middle turbinate.

### Other Sites

Sometimes blood oozes from the anterior end of the middle or inferior turbinate. Blood may come from the paranasal sinuses following severe head injury or in the presence of a neoplasm. When a patient has hereditary hemorrhagic telangiectasia or a blood dyscrasia, virtually all of the nasal mucosa may bleed. However, patients with blood dyscrasias do not bleed only from the nose; they also have skin petechiae, ecchymoses, hematuria, or other manifestations of a generalized hematologic disturbance.

The nose is expected to bleed from only one place at a time. Frequently, when bleeding is serious, blood passes behind the nasal septum and appears in the unaffected, as well as the affected, side of the nose. This seems to represent an instance of bilateral nosebleed. (Actually, bilateral nosebleed is uncommon except in nasal fractures or after instrumentation in the nonbleeding side.) Except for these special situations, bleeding is expected to be from one side only and then usually from only one spot. The history of the side of onset is critical.

### Diagnosis of the Site of Bleeding

Before treatment is instituted, the exact site of bleeding must be determined. Obviously, effective treatment for bleeding from the Kiesselbach plexus will not control bleeding from the posterior part of the nose. A satisfactory approach for determining the site of bleeding is as follows:

1. The patient and the examiner are gowned.
2. The patient is seated in a chair. The patient should not be examined in the recumbent position unless he or she is weak or in shock.
3. Any blood clots are sucked from the nose with an angulated sucker and a strong suction pump. If suction apparatus is unavailable, the patient is instructed to blow his or her nose to clear it of blood clots.
4. With a bright light (either a head mirror or head lamp), the physician inspects the anterior part of the nose. If a bleeding spot is seen on the nasal septum, the search has ended.
5. If the blood does not seem to come from the anterior part of the nasal septum and the patient continues to swallow blood as it trickles down the back part of the throat, it may reasonably be assumed that the bleeding is from the posterior part of the nose. It may be from a vessel in the inferior meatus or from the ethmoid artery.

It is not uncommon to see a patient bleeding from the Kiesselbach plexus whose nose has been packed with yards of petroleum gauze pushed back so far that the bleeding vessel is not compressed. Conversely, it is not uncommon to see a patient bleeding from the posterior part of the nose whose nose is packed anteriorly only. In both situations the packing merely acts as a wick for the blood and the patient continues to bleed.

## Treatment

### Nosebleeds From the Anterior Part of the Nose

The easiest nosebleeds to treat are those from the Kiesselbach plexus. Epistaxis is easy to control because the anterior part of the nasal septum is readily accessible and the bleeding vessels are

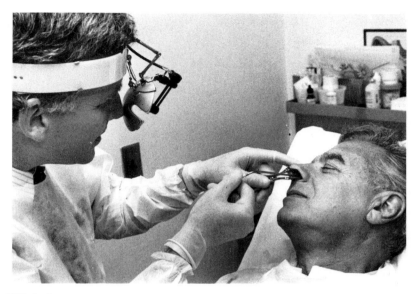

**FIG 8–2**.
Removal of clots and blood from the nose and direct inspection of the bleeding site.

relatively small. After the exact site of the nose-bleed has been determined, the following procedure will usually stop the bleeding:

1. With the use of suction, blood clots and fresh blood are aspirated from the nose (Fig. 8–2).

2. Topical epinephrine, 1:1000, is applied to a cotton ball, which is placed into the bleeding nostril over the bleeding site (Fig. 8–3).

3. After pressure is applied, the cotton ball is removed and the bleeding point cauterized with a silver nitrate stick (Fig. 8–4), tri-

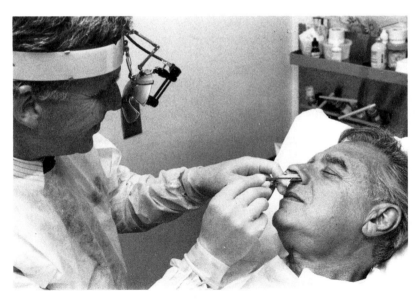

**FIG 8–3**.
Placement of a cotton wick soaked with epinephrine 1:1,000 into the bleeding nostril over the bleeding site. Note gowns on both the patient and physician.

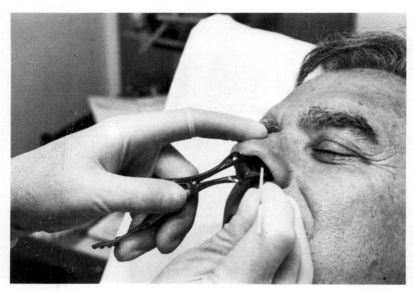

**FIG 8–4.**
Cautery of the bleeding vessel with a silver nitrate stick.

chloroacetic acid, or suction cautery (Fig. 8–5). The septum should be dried after chemical cautery so that the medication does not spread over the mucous membrane excessively. Five percent cocaine, 2% tetracaine, or 4% xylocaine provides sufficient anesthesia for intranasal cautery. In adults, chemical cautery may be done without anesthesia. Children who will not voluntarily submit to nasal cautery and who have recurrent, severe nosebleeds may have to be given a general anesthetic.

After the bleeding has been controlled, patients are warned not to pick or blow their noses. After a week it may be desirable to prescribe petrolatum or mineral oil to be applied to the nasal septum. It should not be necessary to pack the nose after the bleeding point has been adequately cauterized.

### Intractable Nose Picking
Some patients who will not stop picking their noses may actually cause septal ulceration or even septal perforation. Nose picking may be a habit, or it may be done of necessity to remove crusts from around an ulceration or a perforation that was already present. In either case, healing of the mucous membrane can be accomplished, if usual

methods fail, by prolonged packing of both sides of the nose with cotton greased with either Neosporin or oxytetracycline (Terramycin) antibiotic ointment. The cotton balls or gauze used as packing are left in place 7 to 10 days, with the nose carefully taped shut (Fig. 8–6). Although this treatment annoys patients because it forces them to breathe through their mouths, it is effective both in healing the mucosa and in discouraging nose picking.

If packing is needed in the anterior or upper parts of the nose, special nasal packs of folded petrolatum gauze; antibiotic-coated continuous quarter-inch gauze; or a long, continuous strip of half-inch gauze coated with an antibiotic ointment can be used. The usual antibiotic ointments used are bacitracin or Neosporin. The packing must be placed under direct vision, assisted by use of a nasal speculum and bright light reflected from a head mirror or head lamp. It should be placed in layers, one over the other, somewhat like the folds of an accordion, until all available space adjacent to the bleeding site of the nose is packed.

The use of gauze impregnated with antibiotic ointments such as Neosporin, Terramycin, or bacitracin will prevent odor. A preliminary spraying of the nose with 5% cocaine solution, 1% tetracaine, or 4% lidocaine makes the procedure less unpleasant.

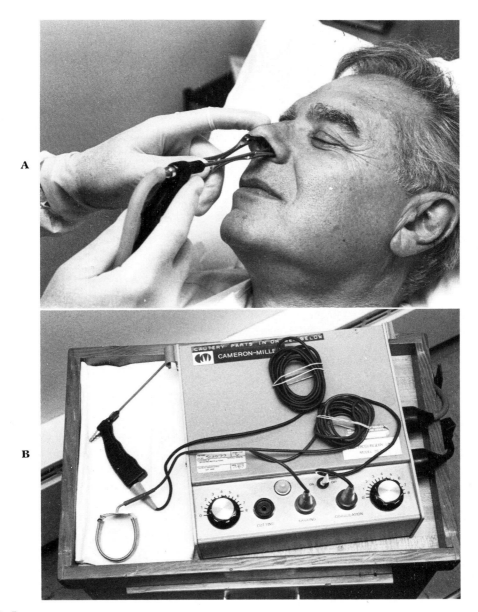

**FIG 8–5**.
**A,** Cautery of the bleeding site using the suction cautery with the bipolar cautery touching the bleeding vessel. **B,** Suction bipolar cautery unit. This equipment is extremely useful in nosebleeds.

Complete packing of this type may be done in conjunction with a postnasal pack. It is also used in some patients who bleed from the ethmoidal artery. In such cases, however, a small piece of greased packing should be wedged tightly into the space between the septum and the middle turbinate to obtain more discrete pressure at the bleeding site.

### Nosebleeds From the Posterior Part of the Nose

Epistaxis from vessels in the posterior part of the nose is often profuse. Because of the bleeding and because the posterior part of the nose is difficult to see, treatment is complicated. If it were technically possible, the same principles of treatment that apply to nosebleed of the anterior part

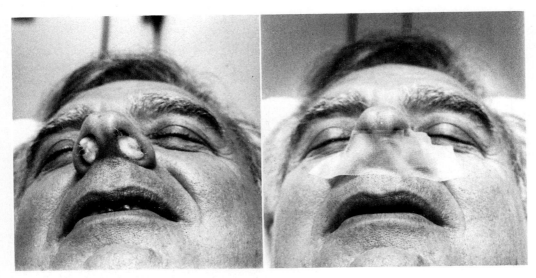

**FIG 8–6.**
Treatment for intractable nose picking. Cotton impregnated with antibiotic ointment is placed in the anterior nose and the nose taped shut. Risks of nasal occlusion must be considered before placement of obstructive packing in the nose of the elderly, and occasionally tubes are brought out inferiorly to the packing to allow a nasal airway.

of the nose would apply to bleeding from the posterior part—namely, excellent illumination, accurate suction, and point cautery. Practically, however, it is often impossible to see the exact bleeding site in the posterior part of the nose.

To aid in finding the site, the patient should be seated rather than supine, because lying on the back causes blood to run down the throat, choking the patient. By using suction and clearing blood as the suction tip advances, the physician eventually reaches the spot at which the nose fills with blood when the suction tip is passed farther. This is the site of the bleeding, although usually the bleeding vessel itself cannot be seen. It may be well back in the inferior meatus (under cover of the inferior turbinate) or high above the middle turbinate. The nose fills with blood rapidly even when strong suction is used.

The use of cautery in the most posterior part of the inferior meatus is impractical because of the difficulty in reaching the bleeding spot and the quantity of blood. Suction cautery can be used in some widely open noses.

### Methods of Postnasal Packing

Because cauterization usually cannot be done effectively in the posterior part of the nose, bleeding must be controlled by compression of the bleeding vessel. Packing must be positioned so

that it will remain in place and provide enough pressure to stop the bleeding.

**Local Packing.** Otolaryngologists sometimes use a small piece of gauze or a small cotton ball soaked in epinephrine and wedged firmly into the inferior meatus at the approximate bleeding point (Fig. 8–7). This localized pack is placed with a bayonet forceps. The pack should be left in place 1 or 2 days and then removed with forceps. In localizing and treating the bleeding point, the physician may find it helpful to fracture the inferior turbinate medially (toward the nasal septum) to

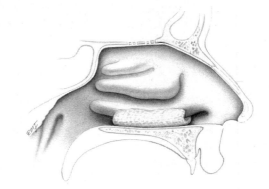

**FIG 8–7.**
Local packing under the inferior turbinate for control of hemorrhage from the posterior part of the nose.

gain a better view of the inferior meatus. In comparison with a postnasal pack that obstructs the nose completely on one or both sides, the great advantage of a local pack is the comfort to the patient. The disadvantage of local packing of this sort is that it may slip and not maintain proper pressure, necessitating a conventional postnasal pack. As the physician's skills increase, most posterior nasal bleeding can be stopped by a well-placed anterior pack.

**Postnasal Pack.** Treatment of postnasal hemorrhage may require the use of a postnasal pack. A postnasal pack is made of gauze in which stout silk sutures or umbilical tape is sewn to give it shape and to provide a means of traction (Fig. 8–8). It is then impregnated with an antibiotic ointment. A pack can easily be constructed by cutting a large vaginal tampon in half, adjusting the tampon so that the two strings are in the center, and sewing a third string to the opposite end (to be used in withdrawing the pack). A variety of balloons have also been devised for control of epistaxis, but do not appear to be as effective in controlling hemorrhage, although they are more comfortable.

Postnasal packs are often constructed too large so that they occlude both choanae. Then the patient has no nasal airway. Preferably, bilateral posterior nasal packs should be avoided, particularly in the elderly. Significant problems are described with obstruction of nasal airway, including depressed $Po_2$ and elevated $Pco_2$ levels with resultant secondary respiratory and cardiac complications. If posterior packs are placed bilaterally in elderly individuals, these patients should be hospitalized and closely monitored. Large packs also may compress the eustachian tube and cause ear symptoms. The physician should look at the patient's eardrum every day to see if the pack is causing otitis media or hemotympanum. Postnasal packs are unpleasant to the patient at the time they are placed and for as long as they are in place. The pack is removed in 48 to 96 hours. If the patient bleeds seriously after it is removed, the pack should be replaced.

For placement of a postnasal pack (Fig. 8–9), a catheter is passed through the bleeding side of the nose and pulled out through the mouth with a hemostat. The doubled strings are then tied to the catheter, which is then pulled back out the nose. This maneuver pulls the postnasal pack into the mouth and up behind the soft palate into the nasopharynx. A finger inserted above the soft palate helps to seat the pack. After the postnasal pack is in place, the anterior part of the nose (on one side only) is packed with a long strip of treated gauze (Fig. 8–10). Finally, the two strings brought out on the same side of the nose are tied tightly around the gauze.

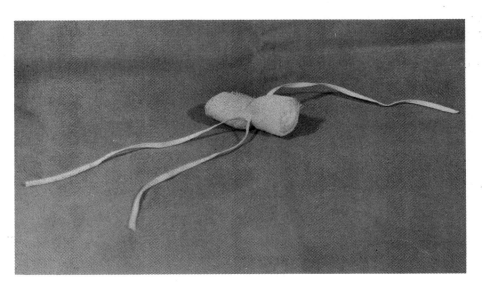

**FIG 8–8.**
Postnasal pack made from fine mesh gauze and umbilical tape. Note that two tape ends come through the nose and the third hangs down in the nasopharynx to assist in later removal of the pack.

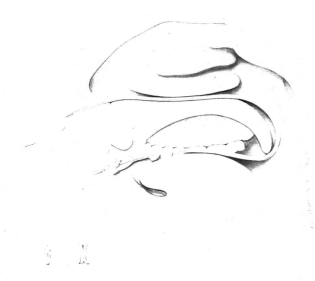

**FIG 8–9.**
Nasal packing. A pack consisting of lamb's wool or gauze is attached to a catheter placed through the nose and brought out the mouth. Placement of the pack is facilitated by pulling the catheter pack into position behind the palate.

Another popular type of postnasal pack can be devised using a Foley catheter with the balloon blown up in the nasopharynx. Although this device does not in itself create pressure against the bleeding site, which is not usually in the nasopharynx but in the nose, it does provide a posterior buttress against which additional anterior packing can be placed. It also has the advantage of easier availability and probably is easier for the inexperienced physician to place.

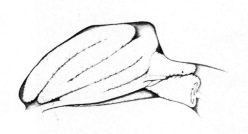

**FIG 8–10.**
A posterior pack is in place with anterior packing layered firmly against it and the nasal walls. The tag attached to the postnasal pack extends behind the palate and allows for removal.

**Patient's Position.** Bleeding tends to be less if the patient is kept in a sitting position. Also, in this position blood does not drip into his throat and gag the patient. Many times, merely elevating the head of the bed eliminates oozing of blood in the packed nose. Paradoxically, removing the nasal packing may also stop the bleeding. It occasionally does so in the patient with oozing blood around nasal packing that has been in place for several days.

*Arterial Ligation*

Many reports in the literature concern treatment of epistaxis by ligation of either the external carotid artery or the anterior ethmoidal artery (blood derived from the internal carotid artery). Arterial ligation is occasionally required, but in most patients more efficient packing would probably serve better. When a serious nosebleed is uncontrolled even after proper packing, arterial ligation is necessary. Some authorities believe that the discomfort to the patient is much less with ligation than with prolonged packing, and they begin with ligation rather than packing.

A common error is to assume, without a careful search, that the source of bleeding is the external carotid system. Most of the blood supply to the nose is from this system, but when bleeding is from high in the nose posteriorly, the bleeding is from the internal carotid system via the anterior ethmoidal artery. It is safe to ligate the anterior ethmoidal artery. With the patient under local anesthesia, an incision made along the side of the nose near the inner canthus of the eye can be used to expose the artery. The periosteum (periorbita) is elevated carefully, and the artery is identified as it crosses from the orbit to the interior of the nose. A silver clip makes a convenient ligator.

The surgeon who decides to ligate the external carotid artery must bear in mind the only certain way to distinguish the external carotid from the internal carotid: the external carotid has branches; the internal carotid has no branches in the neck. To make certain, the surgeon should identify two branches before ligating. An alternative to ligating the external carotid artery in the neck is ligation of one of its terminal branches, the internal maxillary artery. Because this artery supplies so much blood to the nose, it has been called the "rhinologist's artery." The approach to the internal maxillary artery is by way of an incision made under the upper lip, as for the Caldwell-Luc operation (Fig. 8–11). After an opening has been made through the anterior wall of the normal maxillary sinus, the operating microscope is used and the posterior wall of the maxillary sinus is removed. It is then that the internal maxillary artery can be isolated and ligated. Proponents of early ligation of the internal maxillary artery say that patients find this procedure less uncomfortable than suffering with the postnasal pack for several days.

### Other Means of Control

Another method of controlling epistaxis from the internal maxillary artery is by transpalatal injection of saline solution into the greater palatine foramen. When this simple measure works, it is an easy one, but often the control of epistaxis is only temporary.

When a patient has bled enough to be in shock, immediate transfusion is required. However, this situation is unusual. Because hematocrit determinations made immediately after a nosebleed may not represent the patient's true condition as a result of hemoconcentration, the hemoglobin/hematocrit values should be rechecked when fluid balance has been restored.

Patients with epistaxis often become pale and

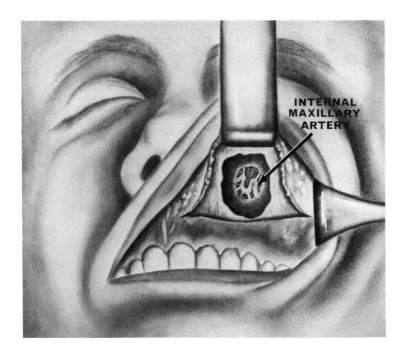

**FIG 8–11.**
Caldwell-Luc approach to the maxillary sinus and removal of the posterior bony wall of the sinus to expose the internal maxillary artery. One or more clips on this vessel will be used to control posterior epistaxis. (From Chandler JR, Serrins AI: *Laryngoscope* 75:1151, 1965. Used by permission.)

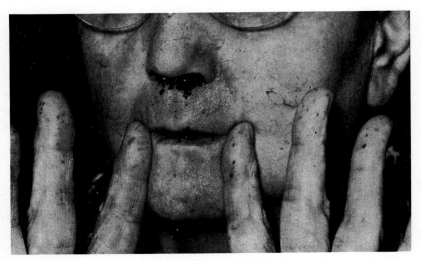

**FIG 8–12.**
Severe nasal crusting is common in patients with hereditary hemorrhagic telangiectasia. Note also telangiectases on the lips, fingertips, and face—all common sites. (From Saunders WH: *Arch Otolaryngol* 76:245, 1962. Used by permission.)

may be in shock but rarely die. (Some authorities state that death may occur from coronary insufficiency resulting from severe nosebleed, but such instances must be extremely unusual.) When a patient bleeds enough to go into shock, the blood pressure falls and bleeding almost always stops. Thus, there tends to be a check on the amount of

blood a patient can lose from epistaxis at any one time.

Hemorrhagic hereditary telangiectasia, also known as Rendu-Osler-Weber disease, is an unusual cause of recurrent and severe nosebleeds (Fig. 8–12). The disorder affects most organs and epithelial surfaces, but usually the patient

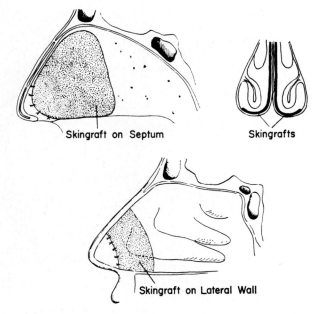

Skingraft on Septum

Skingrafts

Skingraft on Lateral Wall

**FIG 8–13.**
Septal dermoplasty operation. The skin grafts can be considered posterior extensions of the normal vestibular skin. (From Saunders WH: *Arch Otolaryngol* 76:245, 1962. Used by permission.)

bleeds only from the nose or gastrointestinal tract.

Septal dermoplasty is an operation used for this disorder, with varied results. The principle of this operation is that although these patients have telangiectases on the skin and oral mucosa, lesions covered by squamous epithelium rarely bleed because squamous epithelium is tough and resists trauma. Nasal mucosa, on the other hand, is exceptionally fragile.

A graft of split-thickness skin from the thigh is placed in the nose to cover the anterior parts of the septum and the floor and lateral walls of the nose anteriorly. A raw surface for grafting is created by scraping the mucous membrane but not the perichondrium (Fig. 8–13). The grafts are held in place 5 days by appropriate nasal packing. Usually there is great reduction in the severity and frequency of epistaxis after septal dermoplasty. Some patients never bleed again.

### Other Operative Procedures

Sometimes, when projecting parts of the septum are traumatized by the drying effect of inspired air, the occluding nasal septum is resected. Usually, however, operative procedures on the nasal septum are not required for the control of nosebleeds. In many instances, the use of a lubricant such as petrolatum or mineral oil permits healing, making an operation unnecessary.

# 9

# Trauma—Maxillary Fractures

Patients with maxillofacial trauma usually have associated injuries. Therefore, it is imperative that the physician have a standardized approach to evaluating the patient. Initial evaluation should include three basic considerations: airway, control of bleeding, and evaluation for cervical or cranial injury.

## AIRWAY

In the initial assessment, attention must be directed at the airway and the establishment of adequate airway exchange. *In complex injuries it is very important to note any blunt trauma to the larynx because laryngeal fracture or tear can cause rapid development of total obstruction.* The physician must sweep his or her fingers through the mouth to rule out any dentures, blood, or foreign bodies obstructing the upper airway. An endotracheal tube must be passed or tracheotomy performed immediately if necessary.

## CONTROL OF BLEEDING

Usually, bleeding from the head and neck can be controlled by pressure or packing. However, in multiple injuries one must look for other areas of hemorrhage, particularly in the thorax and abdomen. Blood and fluid volume must be replaced before any further evaluation of the facial injury can be completed.

## CERVICAL INJURY

After head and neck trauma, great attention must be given to the possibility of cervical frac-

ture. If such fracture is present, manipulation of the head, as occurs during movement of the patient for x-ray studies and laryngoscopy, could easily cause an injury to the cervical spinal cord that will result in tragic neurologic consequences. Therefore, in any severe head injury, x-ray views of the cervical spine and anterior-posterior-lateral projections are required. Extreme caution must be used in positioning and manipulating these patients.

Depending on the nature of the associated injuries, management of intrathoracic, cervical, and abdominal injuries takes precedence over the maxillofacial injury.

The level of consciousness, amnesia, or the development of progressive neurologic distortion must be evaluated. X-ray films of the skull may show fractures, and CT examination may detect early intracranial bleeding. In these cases, neurosurgical consult is required.

The thoracic and abdominal injuries must be looked for. Fractured ribs, penetrating wounds, and splenic or hepatic rupture must be excluded. Blood in the urine or the rectum demands full work-up. A serial hematocrit study will assist in the discovery of continuous bleeding.

Facial trauma among adults is primarily related to motor vehicle accidents. Domestic violence also accounts for some injuries, and its frequency shows geographic variation. The major urban centers have a greater occurrence of facial trauma related to domestic violence than do other regions. Decreased speed limits in the United States seem to have resulted in an apparent decrease in facial trauma related to motor vehicle accidents. Most victims of automobile accidents suffer injuries to facial structures. The face is the most commonly injured anatomic region, with the lower extremi-

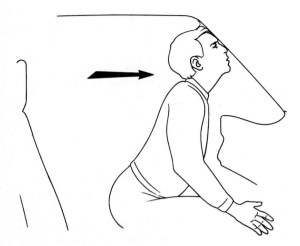

**FIG 9–1.**
The face can be struck against a windshield in a deceleration accident.

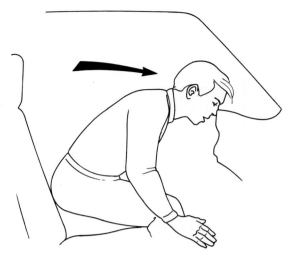

**FIG 9–2.**
The face can also make contact with the dashboard in an automobile accident.

ties being the second most involved area. Soft tissue facial injuries occur more frequently than bony injuries.

A person has a greater chance of sustaining facial trauma in a motor vehicle accident if he or she is sitting on the front seat. The passenger seat tends to entail the greatest frequency of injury. Many of these front-seat car injuries are avoidable with the use of seat-shoulder straps. It will be interesting in the future to compare the frequency of facial injuries in states with mandatory seat-belt laws with that of those states with no such legislation.

Accidents may involve the person being thrust through the windshield in a deceleration event (Fig. 9-1) or making direct contact with the dashboard (Fig. 9-2). Windshield accidents usually produce lacerations of the head and neck, and dashboard accidents generate injuries consistent with rapid compression of the tissues, with shearing and crushing. The steering wheel can protect the person in the driver's seat from hitting either the windshield or the dashboard. However, it is not uncommon for direct facial trauma to result from hitting the steering wheel (Fig. 9-3).

Trauma to the facial bones in children is uncommon. The resilience of the facial bones and the decreased inertia from the low body weight usually act as protective mechanisms. The mandible serves as a protective hood against direct impact to the larynx because of the more superior position of the larynx in the child's neck. Excluding nasal fractures, mandibular fractures are the most common in children.

Invariably children sustain facial trauma as a result of motor vehicle accidents as a passenger or pedestrian or as a result of child abuse. Child abuse is disturbingly becoming more frequent.

The nature and chronology of the injury must be understood to fully evaluate and manage the trauma patient. This is particularly important in dealing with facial nerve injury. The clinician must seek information from those who are in-

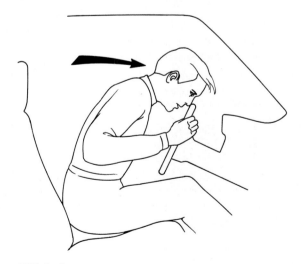

**FIG 9–3.**
The steering wheel is another source of blunt trauma to the facial soft tissue and bones.

volved with the initial management of the patient to determine whether or not facial paralysis was present immediately or developed gradually after the injury. If the paralysis was present immediately it is likely that the nerve has been transected. However, if the paralysis occurred several hours after the injury, it is probable that the nerve is not transected but is compressed by edema or some other mechanism. This determination has therapeutic implications. Immediate paralysis is usually surgically explored, and delayed paralysis is observed. The true sequence of facial paralysis is often overlooked by those who are initially involved with the evaluation of the patient because they tend to become preoccupied with other matters and forget to assess facial nerve function.

Similarly important is the cause of the trauma: e.g., car accident, fall, gun shot, or fight, because each creates a specific type of injury.

The examination must be systematized. The general inspection is an important component of the examination. This is sometimes made more difficult with the rapid onset of soft tissue edema which obscures and alters any facial prominences or depression that may have been created by an underlying displaced fracture. One also must not overlook soft tissue injuries. Cranial nerve evaluation is critical, with particular reference to anesthesia of any portion of the face. The loss of facial motion also must be similarly observed by looking for movement in closing of the eyes, wrinkling of the forehead and nose, and smiling. Injuries of the carotid or salivary duct often occur in severe lacerations to the lateral aspect of the face and must be identified. In the process of evaluating the possibility of fractures, examining from a superior to an inferior direction is one means of ensuring a complete examination.

Palpation is a means of identifying any areas of local tenderness or underlying boney displacement. The scalp can be initially palpated. The orbital rims are circumferentially palpated followed by the zygomatic arches, the maxillae, and the mandible. The patient is asked to open the mouth while pressure is placed on the temporomandibular joints. Eliciting localized pain with any of this movement should arouse suspicion of a fracture at the site of the pain. It is important to ask the patient to bite down on a group of tongue blades on

one side of the mandible in order to create stress on the mandible as a means of potentiating any pain. Often the palpation of the mandible will illicit local tenderness over the fracture site.

The orbits should be examined by doing a gross check of visual acuity using both monocular and binocular vision. If there is an alteration in monocular visual acuity it may indicate an intraocular injury which should be followed promptly with an evaluation by an ophthalmologist. Extraocular muscle function should also be noted. The eye is located in a boney socket surrounded by subcutaneous fat and any direct pressure to the globe causes transmission of that pressure in the boney socket. The weakest points of the socket are the orbital floor and medial wall. Fractures of the orbital floor or medial wall are referred to as "blowout fractures."

Following orbital examination one should examine the mid-facial boney structure. If the patient has teeth, the dental relationships provide useful information. Often the palpation of the infraorbital rim will reveal step-offs which indicate a displaced maxillary fracture. Nasal deviation or tenderness should be noted. In addition, the patient who has sustained facial trauma may have trismus. This condition is usually related to injury of the mandible. However, it can also be a result of a medially displaced zygomatic arch, which impinges on the temporalis muscle (Fig. 9-4).

Facial fractures often cannot be detected on the basis of radiographs of the skull. CT (preferred) or x-ray films of the nasal bones, sinuses, floor of the orbit, zygoma, and mandible are required. In mandibular fractures, panorex views are particularly helpful. Older x-ray procedures such as polytomography may still be useful for fractures along the floor of the orbit, but CT has generally replaced all these studies in fractures of the face.

Facial lacerations do not require immediate management; therefore, a delay of up to 24 hours can be allowed to establish diagnosis and patient stability. If wounds are kept covered and clean, there is no increased incidence of infection by delay.

Several rules apply to the closure of facial wounds:

1. All bony and cartilaginous supporting structure must be replaced as close as pos-

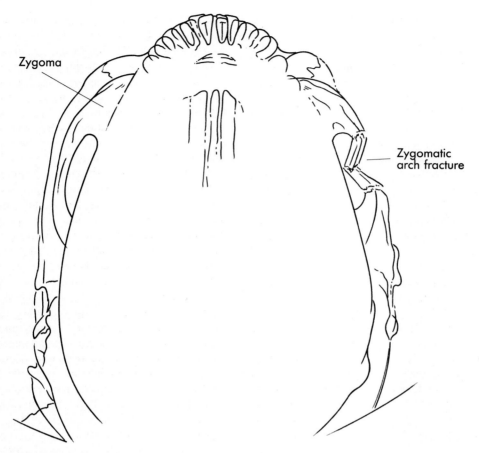

**FIG 9–4.**
A medially displaced zygomatic arch, which impinges on the temporalis muscle.

sible onto the original site, no matter how torn or comminuted. This tissue may be indispensable in secondary cosmetic repair of extensive lacerations or bony loss.

2. If one is not willing to spend a significant number of hours in the closure of small lacerations, the physician should not be doing the procedure. Closure of facial lacerations requires meticulous layered closure of muscles, subcutaneous tissue, and skin with fine sutures under atraumatic conditions to obtain the best result. Many serious lacerations can be repaired cosmetically with the initial closure.

3. The physician must be cognizant of injuries to the seventh nerve, the parotid duct, lacrimal apparatus, and other areas prior to the closure of facial wounds.

## NASAL FRACTURES

Nasal fractures are the most common fractures of the maxillofacial complex. Occasionally, during birth the nose is fractured in the birth canal. Such fractures are usually of the greenstick type, and the nose inclines a little to one side. The treatment of these fractures is extremely simple. The nose can be straightened by merely grasping its tip and pulling it toward the midline or pushing slightly on the convex side.

In adult life, nasal fractures commonly result from a "right cross" that smashes both nasal bones to one side; a frontal blow that depresses the nasal bones; or various other injuries that cause misalignment of the septum, with or without nasal bone fracture. Nasal fractures are usually associated with fractures of the ascending process of the maxilla or the nasal process of the frontal bone. Other facial fractures, particularly of the inferior orbital rim, or zygoma, may be associated with severe nasal trauma. If the external nose is lacerated, a compound fracture may exist. Usually, however, nasal fractures are simple, or comminuted, rather than compound. Frequently, the mucosa of the internal nose is torn, which results in bleeding. If the cartilage of the septum is injured, but not the nasal bones, the tip of the nose may deviate to one side and the upper bony part of the nose remains straight. The opposite may also occur, or both the septum and the nasal bones may be twisted (Fig. 9-5). Occasionally, the tip is injured independently of the rest of the nose, in which case there is usually a hematoma of the upper lateral cartilage and the swelling pushes one side of the nasal tip outward.

The diagnosis of nasal fractures is often complicated by ecchymosis and swelling. However, palpation of the nose may reveal crepitus or deformity. Previous photographs are particularly

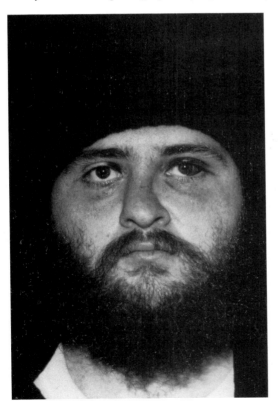

**FIG 9–5.**
Acute nasal fracture.

valuable in determining whether a fracture is recent or old. Although x-ray films are taken of nasal fractures, they generally provide very little additional information. However, when nasal fractures are associated with other facial injuries, radiographs of the paranasal sinuses are important.

Treatment of most fractured noses is not difficult. The aims of reduction are to obtain a satisfactory airway and to restore the original appearance of the nose.

In the lateral type of fracture in which one nasal bone is smashed inward and the other outward, simple thumb pressure on the convex side is often enough to push the nasal bones back into position. The nasal septum may also be displaced, but it returns to normal position when the nasal bones are repositioned. It is important to be certain that the nasal septum rests within the maxillary crest. The lateral type of fracture is the most common. Depressed fractures are more difficult to reduce than fractures of the lateral type. Reduction must be done with the patient under either local or general anesthesia. Children always require general anesthesia.

When a local anesthetic is to be used, the patient can be given preliminary medication for sedation. These may include barbiturates, analgesics (e.g., meperidine [Demerol]), hypnotics such as diazepam (Valium), hydroxyzine (Vistaril), or promethazine (Phenergan). These medications should be given 30 to 45 minutes before the procedure. Either cocaine 5%, or lidocaine 4% (Xylocaine) can be used to induce local anesthesia. It is initially sprayed into the nose.

The nose is gently packed with cotton that is moistened with the same solution. Another sedative hypnotic such as propofol (Diprivan) can be utilized during the course of the procedure. Local anesthesia can also be induced by placing two applicators soaked in either 5% cocaine or 4% xylocaine in each side of the nose. One is placed high in the nose adjacent to the septum to block the anterior ethmoidal nerve and the other far back at the end of the middle turbinate blocking the sphenopalatine ganglion (Fig. 9-6). The maximal tolerable dose of topical medication must be kept in mind (e.g., cocaine, 200 mg), because topical medications are rapidly absorbed in the nose.

Additional anesthetic for the external nose can be obtained by injection of 2% lidocaine (Xylo-

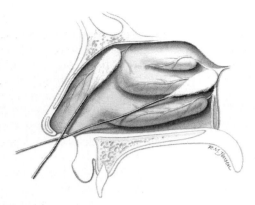

**FIG 9–6.**
Placement of local anesthetic in the nose blocking the anterior ethmoidal nerve superiorly and the sphenapalatine ganglion at the posterior end of the middle turbinate.

caine) near the infratrochlear and infraorbital nerves. Usually about 5 mL should suffice for both sides (Fig. 9-7). A nasal elevator, large forceps, or a hemostat covered with thin rubber tubing is used to elevate the nasal bones (Fig. 9-8).

In the occasional difficult case, wiring, packing, or splinting is required. In most instances, however, the replaced bones stay in position without packing or splinting, though a small degree of packing may be necessary for hemostasis (Fig. 9-9). A new injury will disturb the fragments, but with reasonable care the patient will not dislocate the nose.

Nasal fractures may be associated with septal fractures and septal hematomas, which are discussed separately.

**Common Errors**

Following are some common errors associated with treatment of nasal fractures:

1. The physician attempts to set a nose that was fractured many years previously. In such instances, the patient becomes aware of the deformity only when new trauma calls attention to the nose.
2. X-ray films or a CT scan may reveal no fracture, when there actually is one present. In general, x-rays are of little practical value in the management of nasal fractures. The clinical judgment is much more important; however, CT of the adjacent structures are of great value in the management of associated fractures, especially those of the zygoma and infraorbital rim.
3. The physician regards an easy-to-reduce fracture too seriously (gives general anesthesia) or a severe fracture too lightly

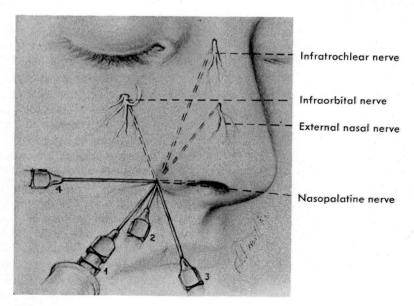

Infratrochlear nerve

Infraorbital nerve

External nasal nerve

Nasopalatine nerve

**FIG 9–7.**
Anesthesia of the external nose. (Courtesy of Dr. Lewis Jordan, Portland, Oregon.)

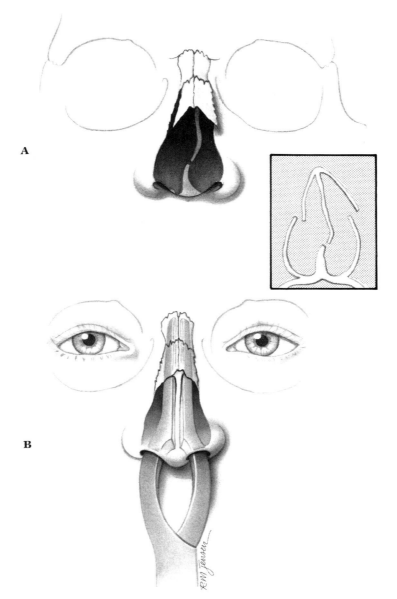

**FIG 9–8.**
**A,** nasal fracture with displacement of nasal bones to the left. Note fracture and displacement of septum, a common occurrence in displaced nasal fractures. **B,** elevation of nasal fracture with commonly used Ash-Walsham elevator.

(treats it in the office rather than in the hospital).

4. The physician waits too long to reduce the fracture. If treated within 5 or 6 days after injury, a nasal fracture can be reduced easily. Thereafter, reduction may be difficult.
5. Secondary injuries to the septum, for example, septal hematoma or hematoma of the upper lateral cartilage, may be overlooked.

## ZYGOMATIC FRACTURES

The zygoma (malar bone), frequently injured when the maxilla is fractured, may be fractured independently of the maxilla. The zygomatic arch, composed of the malar and temporal bones, is usually depressed, so that its normal convexity is lost (Fig. 9-10). An x-ray film made in the submentovertical dimension shows this deformity best (Fig. 9-11). In arch fractures, one

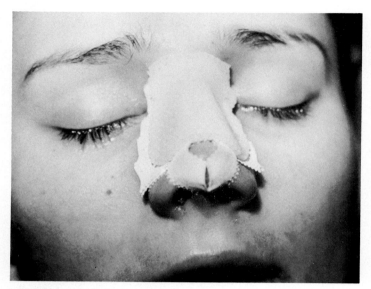

**FIG 9–9.**
Typical nasal splint for fracture.

must rule out coexistent fractures of the maxilla. Physical examination usually demonstrates depression of the lateral aspect of the cheek along the zygomatic arch (Fig. 9-12). Occasionally, patients will have trismus (inability to open their mouths) because the fragment compresses the temporalis muscle.

In reducing fractures of the zygomatic arch, the physician can use numerous techniques to elevate the depressed bone. One good technique (Gillis) is to make a small incision above the fracture (and above the hairline) to insert an elevator under the temporalis fascia and pry the depressed fragment upward. This can also be done by a lateral orbital approach (Fig. 9-13). Sometimes one can use a towel clip (less aesthetic but equally satisfactory) to grasp the depressed bone through the skin and pull it forward and outward. Third, an intraoral (Keene) incision can be made and the zygomatic arch elevated inferiorly through the

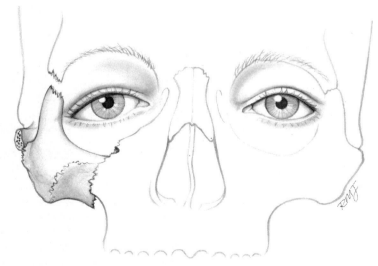

**FIG 9–10**.
Zygomatic fracture with distraction of bony fragments. Note inferior displacement of lateral canthus.

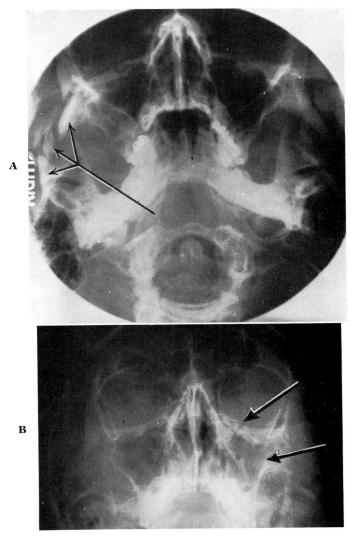

**FIG 9–11.**
**A,** comminuted zygomatic fracture. **B,** palpable steplike fracture of the infraorbital rim. Note clouding of the maxillary sinus caused by blood.

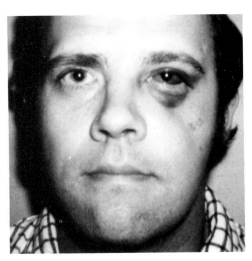

**FIG 9–12.**
Flattening of malar eminence, secondary to depressed zygoma.

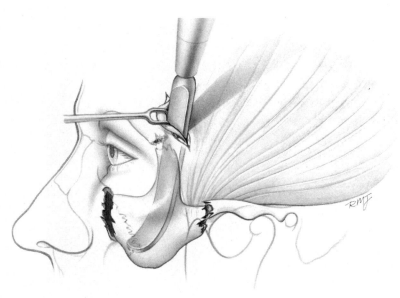

**FIG 9–13.**
Elevation of zygomatic maxillary complex fracture through lateral rim incision. Incision is deep to temporalis fascia with insertion under the zygoma. Unstable fractures may require wire fixation of the lateral orbit and rim fracture.

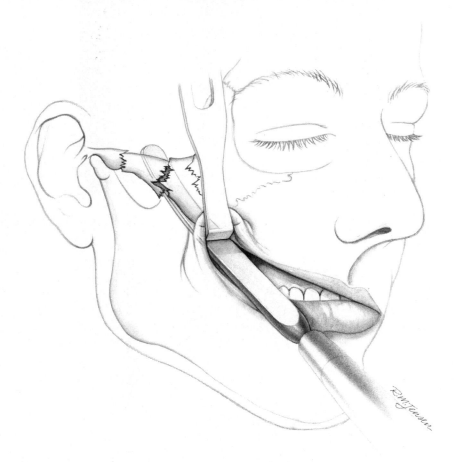

**FIG 9–14.**
Intraoral approach with an elevation of zygomatic arch fracture.

mouth (Fig. 9-14). Zygomatic arch fractures often snap into position, and only infrequently is packing necessary to hold the fragments laterally. Some pitfalls in management of zygomatic fractures are (1) failure to diagnose because of ecchymosis and edema, and (2) failure to appreciate fractures of the maxilla or floor of the orbit.

## MAXILLARY FRACTURES

Fractures of the maxilla usually result from severe, direct trauma such as a blow with the fist, a fall, or an automobile accident. The history of the injury and direction of the blow are helpful in evaluation. The maxilla tends to fracture in certain ways, which have been classified as Le Fort I, II, and III injuries (Fig. 9-15). The Le Fort I fracture is a transverse fracture above the level of the apexes of the teeth (alveolar fracture). A Le Fort II fracture is a triangular fracture that includes the nasal bone but excludes the zygoma. A Le Fort III (cranial-facial dysfunction) includes the separation of the maxilla, nasal bones, and zygoma from the cranium. However, only rarely will there be the classical Le Fort fracture. Automobile accidents often produce a type of Le Fort III injury, in which both maxillae are fractured in several places and the entire middle third of the face, including the nose, is driven backward. The resulting deformity is a very flat face, with the mandibular teeth protruding beyond the maxillary teeth so that normal occlusion is impossible. The entire maxilla can be rocked back and forth when the examiner holds the upper teeth and palate and moves them. This "middle third fracture" usually occurs when an automobile is stopped suddenly and the passenger in the right front seat is thrown forward, his or her face striking the hard dashboard. The driver is usually protected by the wheel and steering column and seldom experiences this injury.

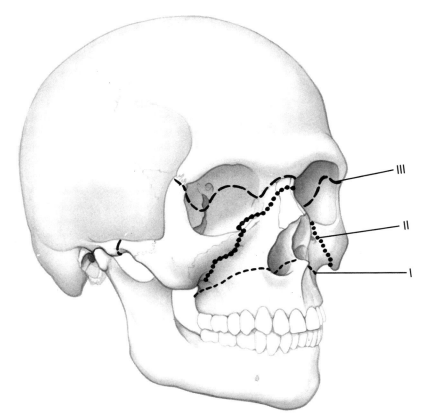

**FIG 9–15**.
Representation of midfacial fracture classification. Le Fort I: aveolar fracture. Le Fort II: zygomatical maxillary complex fracture. Le Fort III: cranial facial dysostosis with separation of midface from the skull.

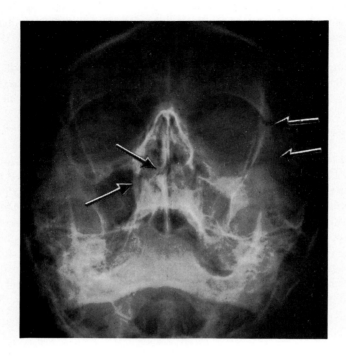

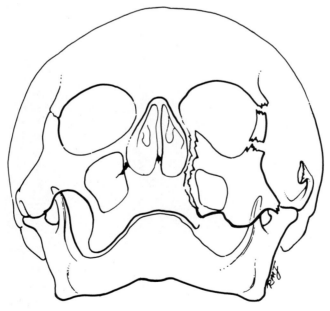

**FIG 9–16.**
Severe zygomatic and maxillary fracture. Note depression of the infraorbital plate and rotation of the zygoma into the maxillary sinus. Note on-line drawing the placement of the fractured fragments.

The diagnosis of the Le Fort fractures may be difficult. Edema rapidly obscures all visual landmarks, the face may be elongated, and occlusion may be disrupted by the trauma. There is often extensive ecchymosis about the eyes. The physical examination, though difficult, is critical. Palpation along the superior rim of the maxilla (the infraorbital area) may reveal a steplike segment where a piece of orbital rim is displaced downward into the maxillary sinus. In the patient with severe middle third fracture, the entire upper jaw will be loose to palpation and the examiner can move it in and out readily. The teeth ordinarily should occlude properly. If they do not, either the maxilla is pushed posteriorly or the mandible is fractured. X-ray films are indispensable in diag-

nosis. Several views should be taken, including standard sinus films (the Waters, Caldwell, lateral, and submental vertex views (Fig. 9-16). Because maxillary fractures are sometimes associated with unrecognized mandibular fractures, x-ray films of the mandible should be taken if there is any doubt. The zygomatic arches should be observed on the submental vertex view.

## Treatment

After stabilization of the patient (who generally with the more extensive Le Fort fractures has multiple injuries or some compromise of upper airway), one may consider surgical repair. In the Le Fort I fracture (upper alveolar fracture), the al-

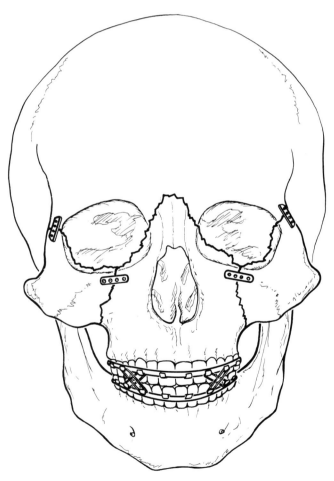

**FIG 9–17.**
Demonstration of repair of a Le Fort III fracture with plate fixation of the frontal zygomatic suture and maxillary fracture. Frequently suspension wires from zygomatic process of the frontal bone are necessary to hold the fracture in position (not illustrated here). Interdental fixation further supports the maxilla.

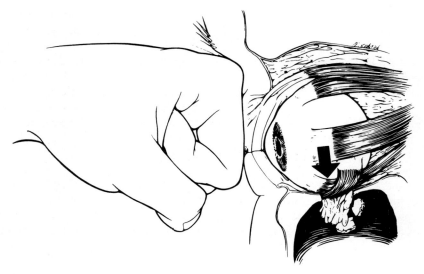

**FIG 9–18.**
Gravitational forces acting on the thin floor of orbit increase likelihood of fracture caused by blunt trauma to orbit. (From Holt JE, Holt GR: *Ocular and orbital trauma,* Washington, DC, 1983, American Academy of Otolaryngology-Head and Neck Surgery Foundation, Inc. Used by permission.)

veolus must be reattached to the fixed facial structures superiorly. This may be accomplished by internal wiring, dentures, or plating. In Le Forte II fractures in which nasal bones and infraorbital rims are fractured, wiring or plating of the infraorbital rim, stabilization of the nose, and interdental fixation to stabilize the maxilla are required. In the absence of dentures, dental splints may be used. With the more extensive Le Fort III fractures, the zygoma must be suspended from the frontal bones by wiring or plating into position, and the alveolar segment supported by fixation to the cranium by suspension wires or plates (Fig. 9-17). Recently the use of mini plates has frequently replaced suspension devices. These plates tend to solidify the maxillary fracture segments and obviate the need for suspension. Temporary dentures attached to the palate or mandible can often be wired to one another to maintain reduction.

Small local fractures of the orbital rim may be reduced by elevation through a Caldwell Luc antrotomy and packing, or by direct incision over the fracture with wiring or plating the loose fragments. Even when multiple fragments are present, fixation plates are possible.

Fractures of the nasal bones are often associated with more severe facial injuries. The tendency is not so much to overlook fractures of the

nasal bones in the presence of known maxillary fractures, as is the reverse.

In all cases of severe facial injury, it is important to determine whether there has been any intracranial or cervical damage before correcting major facial fracture. Immediate reduction of any of the facial bones is not imperative. Satisfactory results can be obtained 2 to 6 days later. An important fact to remember in fractures of the maxilla is the importance of reestablishment of good occlusion, and maintenance of the orbital structures in the normal position (for example, the medial canthus and floor of orbit).

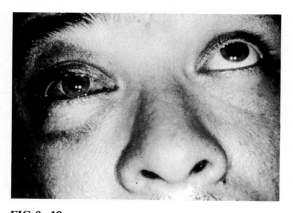

**FIG 9–19.**
Restriction of upward gaze in right orbital blow-out fracture.

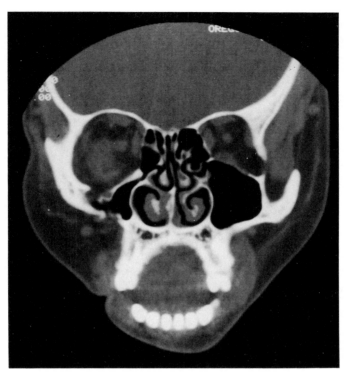

**FIG 9–20.**
Coronal CT demonstrating right orbital blow-out fracture with displacement of orbital contents.

## BLOW-OUT FRACTURES

Blow-out fractures result when blunt trauma to the orbit suddenly raises intraorbital pressure and drives orbital fat and muscles through the fracture in the bony floor of the orbit (Figs. 9-18 and 9-19). This results in the orbital contents hanging into the maxillary sinus. The orbital rim is intact, even when there is a significant depression of the bony floor. Double vision (diplopia) may result from incarceration of intraocular musculature (inferior rectus) in the fracture line (Fig. 9-20). Surgical exploration using either an orbital or a transantral approach, or both, is required if the posttraumatic symptom of diplopia and enophthalmus is to be avoided. This type of floor fracture can frequently occur in association with fractures of the maxilla.

The diagnosis of blow-out fracture is generally established by signs of diplopia, inability to move the eyeball on upward gaze, and enophthalmos, with drooping of the upper lid. In addition, there may be bleeding from the nose.

# PART III

# Oral Cavity, Oropharynx, and Nasopharynx

# 10

# Anatomy and Physiology

The area of the mouth that extends from the lips to the anterior tonsillar pillar is defined as the oral cavity. It contains the lips, gums, tongue, inner lining of the cheeks (buccal area), and tissue underneath the tongue between the point of attachment of the tongue and the mandible (floor of mouth) (Fig. 10–1). The pharynx is the area of the throat that extends from the tonsillar pillar to the posterior pharyngeal wall. The oropharynx extends superiorly from the horizontal plane of the free edge of the palate to the tip of the epiglottis (Fig. 10–2). That portion of the pharynx extending from the oropharynx to the skull base is the nasopharynx, and extending below it to the esophageal inlet is the hypopharynx.

The mucosal lining of the oral cavity and pharynx is lubricated by the salivary glands. The parotid duct orifice opens opposite the maxillary second molar on either side, and the orifices of the submandibular duct open on either side of the midline of the floor of the mouth anteriorly. Just deep to the mucosa of the floor of the mouth are the sublingual salivary glands, each of which has multiple ducts draining into the oral cavity.

The musculature of the floor of the mouth and tongue has a considerable number of loose fascial planes that permit the quick development of interstitial edema fluid in response to inflammation and infection (Fig. 10–3). The fascial planes also permit easy submucosal extension of malignancies beyond the point of being grossly detectable. The tongue, innervated by the hypoglossal nerves bilaterally, is quite mobile, and its movement is critical.

The contraction of the soft palate musculature causes a "knuckle" configuration of the palate, which touches the posterior pharyngeal wall to seal the nasopharyngeal inlet. The motor innervation of the palate is primarily from the vagus nerve (cranial nerve X), with some contribution from the third division of the trigeminal nerve (cranial nerve V) to the tensor veli palatini muscle. Any anatomic or neurologic dysfunction of the palate impeding this contact can cause alterations in deglutition and speech.

Deep to the mucosa of the pharynx are the constrictor muscles, which come to join in the midline raphe posteriorly. The motor innervation to the pharyngeal constrictor is by means of the vagus nerve. The primary sensory innervation of this area is the glossopharyngeal nerve (cranial nerve IX). There is some contribution to the sensation of the palate from the trigeminal nerve and also a slight component from the facial nerve (cranial nerve VII).

The nasopharynx contains the adenoid tissue in its central compartment. In each lateral recess of the nasopharynx is the eustachian tube orifice. It remains closed unless the palatal musculature (tensor veli palatini and levator veli palatini) is functioning properly. These muscles act to open the eustachian tube orifice, which permits equalization of pressure within the middle ear. The mucosa of the oral cavity, oropharynx, and nasopharynx contain thousands of minor salivary glands that contribute to total salivary outflow.

The physiology of this area is primarily concerned with mastication, deglutition, and phonation. The process of mastication involves biting, chewing, and the preparation of a bolus of food. The act of biting is actually first developed at approximately 7 months of age. Chewing does not develop until the infant is somewhat older, about 10 to 12 months of age. Biting and chewing are

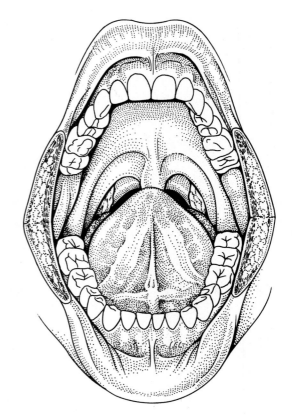

**FIG 10–1.**
The oral cavity extends from the lips to the anterior tonsillar pillar. (Redrawn after Hollinshead W: *Anatomy for surgeons*. vol 1, ed 3, Philadelphia, 1982, Lippincott. Used by permission.)

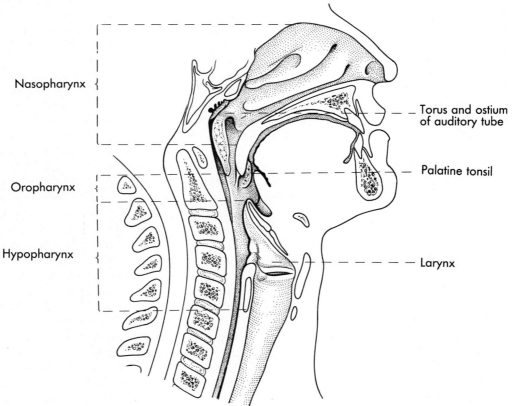

**FIG 10–2**.
The oropharynx is that portion of the throat which can be seen readily on inspection with a tongue blade. (Redrawn after Hollinshead W: *Anatomy for surgeons,* vol 1, ed 3, Philadelphia, 1982, Lippincott. Used by permission.)

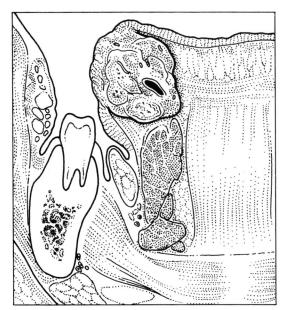

**FIG 10–3.**
The loose submucosal tissue contains numerous avenues for collection of fluids and extension of infection. (Redrawn after Lore J: *An atlas of head and neck surgery,* Philadelphia, 1973, WB Saunders. Used by permission.)

functions of the proprioceptive nerve endings from the muscles of mastication, mandibular movement, and the oral sensory receptors of the trigeminal nuclei. Chewing is a series of forward, backward, and/or lateral rhythmic motions of the mandible. The strength of closing the mandible with biting can be rather substantial, being measured at more than 200 pounds per square inch. During the chewing phase of mastication, the tongue and cheek muscles keep the food between the biting surfaces of the teeth. The sensory innervation of the oral cavity is critical to all of this, and it has been determined that the touch functions of the oral mucosa exceed those of the skin in sensitivity and in discrimination. The mixture of the particles of food with the oral mucus and saliva and the manipulation with the tongue and the oral musculature result in the formation of a food bolus.

Deglutition is considered the most elementary component of feeding. It is elicited by the stimulation of either the superior laryngeal (cranial nerve X) or glossopharyngeal nerves. Touching the tonsillar pillars or adjacent areas of the soft palate, pharynx wall, and tongue in the human will initiate the act of swallowing. Swallowing in

the human can be initiated voluntarily, but it is necessary to have the capacity to develop a bolus. Voluntary "dry swallows" cannot be performed in succession in the human. After deglutition is initiated, it becomes a reflex-elicited event that cannot be modified by any sensory input. Swallowing occupies a dominant position over respiration in the arrangement of pharyngeal function in the brainstem so that the initiation of the swallowing act results in an inhibition of respiration.

With the initiation of swallowing, the pharyngoesophageal segment of the hypopharynx relaxes, permitting entrance of the descending bolus. The act of swallowing is a coordinated event in which one activity is a function of the other. In fact, the swallow can actually be stopped at this pharyngeal segment if the next step, which is elevation of the larynx, is prevented by the examiner's finger restricting elevation. The bolus is formed between the tongue and the palate near the junction of the hard and soft palates (Fig. 10–4). The onset of deglutition begins with the tongue posteriorly displacing the bolus along the palate to the relaxed pharynx (Fig. 10–5). It then enters either pyriform sinus and begins its descent into the cervical esophagus. The cricopharyngeal sphincter relaxes to allow the bolus to enter the

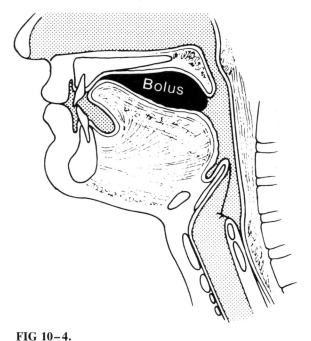

**FIG 10–4.**
The tongue initially forms the food bolus with compression against the hard palate.

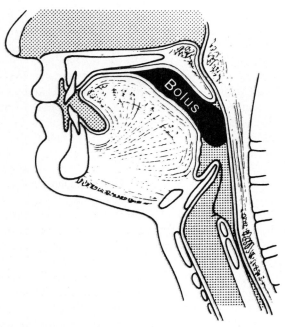

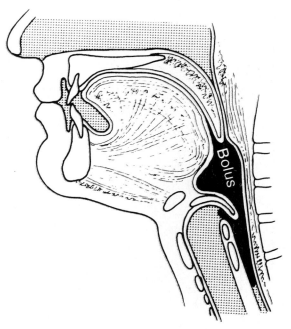

**FIG 10–5.**
Displacement of the bolus into the pharynx by the tongue initiates deglutition.

**FIG 10–6.**
Relaxation of the cricopharyngeal sphincter permits access of the bolus into the cervical esophagus.

cervical esophagus (Fig. 10–6) and move inferiorly into the stomach.

The oral cavity and pharynx are critical to phonatory activity. It is necessary for the nasal cavity to be relatively sealed from the oropharynx and oral cavity. This is accomplished by the contraction of a palatal musculature so that the "knuckle" of the palate approximates the posterior pharyngeal wall. It is important to understand that it is not the free edge of the palate that opposes the posterior pharyngeal wall. It is not possible to determine whether there is velopharyngeal competence by merely looking into a patient's mouth.

Some type of radiographic study, such as a speech ciné study, is useful to examine this relationship. Flexible fiberoptic nasopharyngoscopy is another means of evaluating velopharyngeal closure. Misarticulations can occur when there is neurologic injury to either the hypoglossal (cranial nerve XII), trigeminal, or facial (cranial nerve VII) nerves. The presence and position of a patient's dentition will also affect phonation. The presence of large palatine tonsils or other mass effects in the oropharynx or oral cavity also can alter the resonating features of the oral cavity and oropharynx.

# 11

# Special Diagnostic Procedures

Disorders involving the oral cavity, oropharynx, and nasopharynx frequently can be diagnosed solely on the basis of the presenting symptoms and physical findings. However, at times certain diagnostic procedures provide useful additional information that is not readily available otherwise. Physical examination, for example, often will not provide adequate information about the amount of adenoid tissue in the nasopharynx. In this situation, a lateral soft tissue radiograph of the nasopharynx allows assessment of not only the amount of adenoid tissue but also its relationship to the superior surface of the palate. This radiograph also indicates the length of the palate.

In the patient sustaining maxillofacial trauma, routine radiographs provide some information about the extent of injury, but these can be difficult to interpret because of the overlapping bones.

Computed tomography (CT) is invaluable in the evaluation of the patient with facial trauma. It reveals precise detail about both the soft tissue and bony alterations of the trauma patient (Fig. 11–1). It is especially useful in evaluating the extent of any neoplasms because of its high degree of resolution. The CT scan can detect subtle differences in tissue density that help define the relationship of tumors (Fig. 11–2) to the normal structures.

Ultrasonography is a means of assessing the characteristics of a particular lesion. Its main use is in distinguishing solid from cystic tumors. This technique is most commonly used in the evaluation of neck and thyroid masses.

Magnetic resonance imaging is a diagnostic technique that has numerous possibilities for evaluating tissue (Fig. 11–3). Its primary advantage over other currently available imaging studies is that it uses no ionizing radiation, so there is no risk to the patient. Dramatic advances in magnetic resonance imaging are occurring, and it is currently considered one of the most precise means of analyzing soft tissue detail.

Angiography is a widely used examination in which radiopaque dye is injected into vessels by means of transcutaneous catheter insertion. It visualizes the internal wall and caliber of the vessel lumen, as well as the position of the vessel, which is useful in the evaluation of certain parapharyngeal masses. It is difficult to assess the position and extent of a tumor in the parapharyngeal space with only physical examination. Although CT is helpful in defining anatomic relationships, surgical resection demands information about the position of the carotid artery. Arteriography provides that capability (Fig. 11–4). When the results of arteriography are combined with those of CT, surgical resection (Fig. 11–5) can be done more safely than was previously possible.

Tissue diagnoses for any neoplasms are often made during endoscopic evaluation in the operating room. However, biopsies of certain neoplasms of the oral cavity and oropharynx can be done using fine-needle aspiration, and the histologic identity of the tumor can be determined before hospitalization. This helps the patient's psychological adjustment to the diagnosis before treatment is instituted.

The special diagnostic evaluations required for patients with sleep disorders involve a battery of measurements recorded continuously over an extended sleeping period. These techniques are discussed in more detail in Chapter 13 under the discussion of sleep disorders.

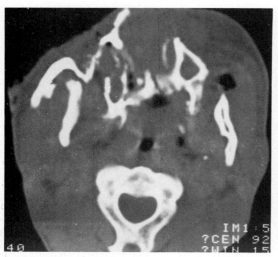

**FIG 11–1.**
CT scan showing extensive comminution of midfacial bones with posterior displacement of the facial soft tissues in a patient with a head crush injury.

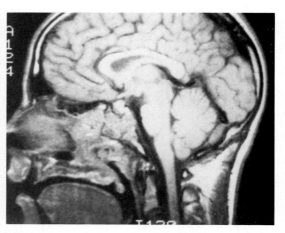

**FIG 11–3.**
Magnetic resonance image of large recurrent nasopharyngeal angiofibroma that has eroded the clivus.

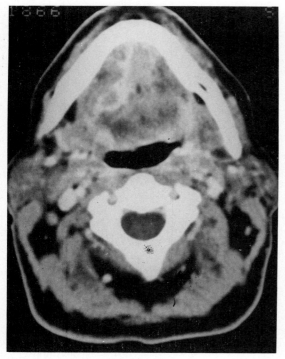

**FIG 11–2.**
CT scan defining the extent of a large tongue cancer.

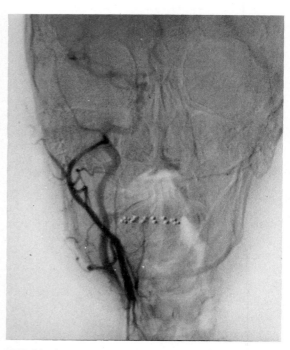

**FIG 11–4.**
Posterolateral displacement of carotid artery by large parapharyngeal tumor.

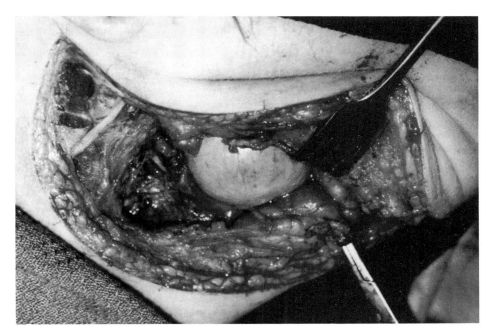

**FIG 11-5.**
The combination of CT and arteriography allowed accurate tumor localization and identification of the position of critical structures to facilitate resection of a parapharyngeal benign mixed tumor of the deep lobe of the parotid gland.

# 12

# Embryology and Congenital Disorders

It is important for the clinician to have some basic understanding of developmental anatomy because this core of knowledge facilitates comprehension of the pathophysiology of the oral cavity, oropharynx, and nasopharynx.

The digestive canal is composed essentially of entoderm. In fact, the entire digestive system is derived of epithelium from the entoderm. The primitive gut is in the form of a tubule. This primitive tubular system ultimately differentiates into the mouth, the pharynx, and the rest of the intestinal tract. The foregut ultimately forms the mouth and all of the pharynx (Fig. 12–1). The differentiation occurs when the pharynx is undergoing changes from the stage of the branchial arch when the breathing of air is evolving. The branchial arch and pouches are profoundly altered during this course of embryologic development.

The blind cranial extremity of the foregut ultimately forms the buccopharyngeal membrane that separates the foregut from the stomodeum. The stomodeum is actually a shallow ectodermal depression. Superiorly is the forebrain, and laterally are the maxillary processes. The mandibular processes develop caudal to this area. The branchial arches are five or six bars on each side of the foregut (Fig. 12–2). The pharyngeal grooves develop into pouches and ultimately come in contact with the more shallow ectodermal grooves. The first and second arches meet their opposite members in the midline, and the medial portions of the first arch develop into a small pair of swellings. A small eminence, the tuberculum impar, eventually appears. Another median prominence located more caudally is the hypobranchial eminence. It prevents the third and fourth arches from reaching the midline. These arches and grooves continue their development (Fig. 12–3) and result in the formation of the pharynx and the structures of the oral cavity.

Many congenital disorders of this area are related to the cleft deformity, which is discussed in a later chapter.

*Median rhomboid glossitis* (Fig. 12–4) represents persistence of the tuberculum impar in the middle third of the tongue. It separates the lateral halves of the tongue, and this depapillated area persists as a shiny area. It gives that portion of the tongue a reddish appearance. It is not a pathologic abnormality, and no treatment is necessary. Many other congenital anomalies are associated with the cleft deformity, such as a double lip, as are numerous dental anomalies. Extra or missing teeth is a common congenital dental disorder seen in children with a cleft lip or palate.

Sometimes the lateral portions of the tongue fail to fuse, and a child is born with a so-called cleft tongue. This is a defect of the first branchial arch. Some believe that macroglossia, fissured tongues, and geographic tongues all represent congenital anomalies. The *Melkersson-Rosenthal syndrome* is another congenital disorder and is characterized by facial swelling, fissured tongue, and facial nerve paralysis.

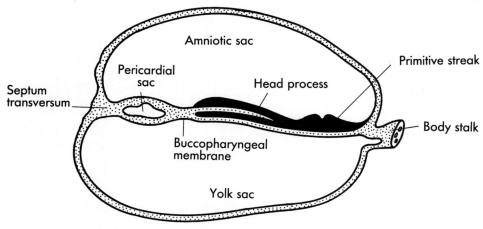

**FIG 12–1.**
The foregut eventually differentiates into the mouth and pharynx. (From Paparella M, Shumrick D: *Otolaryngology—basic sciences and related disciplines,* vol 1, Philadelphia, 1973, WB Saunders. Used by permission.)

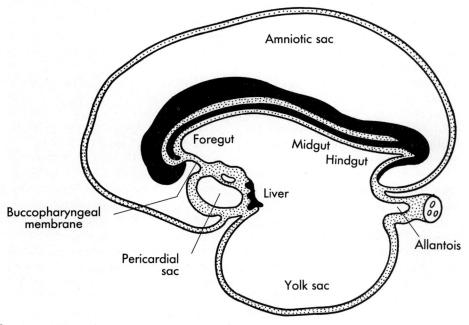

**FIG 12–2.**
Branchial arches are bars flanking the foregut. (From Paparella M, Shumrick D: *Otolaryngology—basic sciences and related disciplines,* vol 1, Philadelphia, 1973, WB Saunders. Used by permission.)

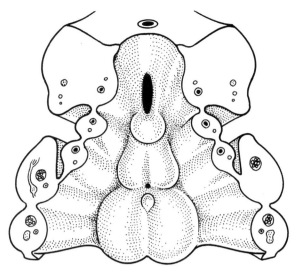

**FIG 12–3.**
Important structures in the pharynx and the oral cavity are derived from the arches and grooves. (From Paparella M, Shumrick D: *Otolaryngology—basic sciences and related disciplines,* vol 1, Philadelphia, 1973, WB Saunders. Used by permission.)

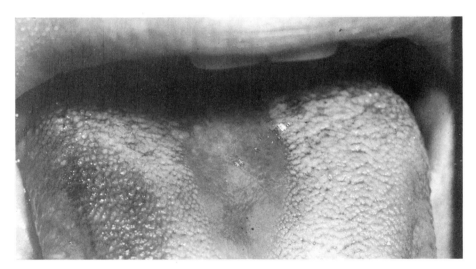

**FIG 12–4.**
Median rhomboid glossitis. The central area is slick and red because it has no papillae.

# 13

# Clinical Problems

## INFECTIONS AND INFLAMMATIONS

Inflammatory problems and infections of the pharynx are commonly seen in children, but they also affect adults more frequently than anticipated. The treatment of pharyngitis in adults accounts for approximately 40 million visits to physicians annually in the United States.

### Oral Cavity

Oral cavity structures can be involved with bacterial and viral infections, but most symptoms are related to infections of the oropharynx rather than the oral cavity. The bacteria and viruses that can cause infections are discussed in the section on the oropharynx. However, there are certain inflammatory and infectious processes that are primarily limited to the oral cavity.

#### Median Rhomboid Glossitis

The term *median rhomboid glossitis* is a misnomer in that no inflammation is a part of this entity, although it has the appearance of inflammation. In the embryo, the tuberculum impar, which occupies the middle third of the tongue, becomes depressed below the surface as the two lateral halves of the tongue join each other. Occasionally, when there is a minor developmental abnormality, the tuberculum impar persists as a surface structure. The absence of papillae permits the underlying blood vessels to shine through the mucosa, and the tongue looks red and slick.

#### Geographic Tongue

*Geographic tongue* is a term used interchangeably with *migratory glossitis*. In this situation, areas of the dorsal surface of the tongue are depapillated (Fig. 13–1). This exposes the underlying thin epithelium, revealing the reddish areas of the tongue musculature, which gives the appearance of inflammation. These papillae undergo alternating regeneration and desquamation, causing the shining area to change location—thus the term *migratory*. Some information suggests that this represents an actual inflammation because sections have shown infiltration of the depapillated epithelium with leukocytes. Most patients with migratory glossitis have no symptoms, and no treatment is needed.

#### Hairy Tongue

*Hairy tongue* gives the appearance of hair growth on the dorsal surface of the tongue. Actually, the "hair" is nothing more than elongated filiform papillae (Fig. 13–2). The pigmentation is caused by the superimposed organisms. Poor oral hygiene and smoking are believed to be the primary stimulants for this condition. Yeast organisms have been seen within the keratin of these elongated filiform papillae. The surface epithelium is usually inflamed. A variety of treatment programs have been recognized, though none have provided uniform success. Local cleansing measures such as brushing the surface of the tongue with a toothbrush or applying oxidizing solutions have been recommended. Some even advocate cauterizing the papillae.

#### Nicotine Stomatitis

*Nicotine stomatitis* is present primarily on the surface of the hard palate mucosa. The orifices of the minor salivary glands become inflamed, and erythema is noted about them. The concomitant edema causes them to become umbilicated (Fig. 13–3). In patients with extended histories of

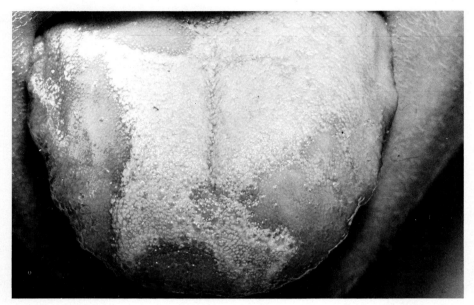

**FIG 13–1.**
Geographic tongue (migratory glossitis). Compare the denuded areas with those in Fig. 12-4.

cigarette smoking, the entire palatal mucosa has a more whitish color. This is thought to be related to hyperkeratosis. Cessation of smoking will usually improve the overall color of the palatal mucosa, but the situation does not always resolve completely.

### Pyorrhea

*Pyorrhea* is a form of periodontitis. This condition is slowly progressive and can cause significant regression of the gingiva from the teeth, exposing more of the roots of the teeth (Fig. 13–4). If enough exposure occurs, the teeth loosen and fall out. The extreme form of this condition can even cause dissolution of alveolar bone. This bone destruction is associated with a pathogenic bacterial invasion. Pyorrhea is usually preceded by gingival erythema and edema, and dental evaluation should be sought as early as possible.

### Herpes Simplex Virus

The oral cavity mucosa can be infected with *herpes simplex virus*. This produces multiple vesicles within the mucosa of the oral cavity and also on the lips. Early in the course of this infection, fever and painful cervical adenopathy develop in addition to pharyngitis and malaise. Whitish ulcerations replace the vesicles following rupture, and these can be quite painful. After the

acute phase, the virus can remain in the tissue in a latent state, which can periodically revert to an acute situation. Treatment for this condition is usually directed at providing symptomatic relief of the pain and control of any systemic symptoms. No antiviral medication is routinely used for herpetic stomatitis. Antibiotics serve no purpose in the treatment of this disease.

### Histoplasmosis

*Histoplasmosis* is a systemic fungal disease. However, it can involve the oral cavity, with the tongue being the primary site of predilection in addition to the larynx. Other areas in the pharynx can also be involved. The lesions are not typical in appearance, but multiple nodular ulcers are not uncommon. There are usually systemic components of the infection, and these are especially related to respiratory illness, with nonspecific symptoms such as cough and shortness of breath being common. The diagnostic evaluation of any patient with oral ulcerations and abnormal respiratory symptoms should include a chest radiograph. Antifungal treatment for histoplasmosis is currently available when appropriate.

### Osteomyelitis

*Osteomyelitis* of the mandible or maxilla also can occur. It can be caused by many microorgan-

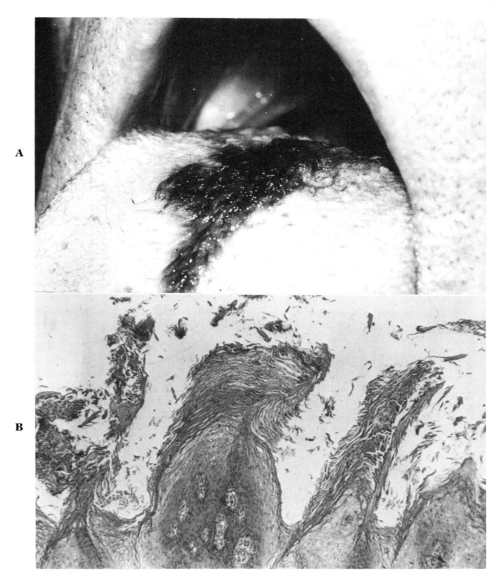

**FIG 13–2.**
**A,** black hairy tongue, cause unknown. **B,** hairy tongue. Note great keratinization.

isms but is most commonly related to bacteria. It is frequently seen in patients with bone exposure from erosive oral cancers or subsequent to complications of radiation therapy. In the acute phase of this disease, there are signs of systemic toxicity with high fever. The purulence noted in the area of infection is invariably deep to the periosteum, which deprives the underlying bone of its primary blood supply. Necrosis is not uncommon, and sequestration of bone fragments is noted. Sinus tracts with draining pus invariably form over the involved bone. Treatment of the acute phase of

the disease involves adequate drainage, débridement, and a course of antibiotics. In chronic osteomyelitis, the drainage and induration persist for a protracted period and more extensive surgical débridement is required.

## Oropharynx

Pharyngitis can have either a bacterial or a viral etiology. Considerable attention has been paid to streptococcal bacterial etiology because of its relationship to rheumatic fever. However, only

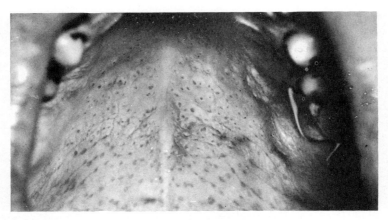

**FIG 13–3.**
Nicotine stomatitis.

about 15% to 20% of pharyngeal infections are caused by β-hemolytic streptococcus. A viral etiology is much more common. It was formerly believed that bacterial pharyngitis would cause symptoms suggestive of a more severe systemic toxicity than a viral infection, but that has not been found to be a reliable indicator. It is clear that the presenting symptoms and signs do not provide enough accuracy to distinguish bacterial from viral etiology. However, the severity of the symptoms sometimes is suggestive and helpful to the clinician in deciding appropriate therapy.

### Presenting Symptoms and Signs

Most patients with any type of pharyngeal infection will have a sore throat. However, patients with severe sore throats accompanied by fever are more likely to have infections of bacterial origin. Patients with this degree of severity will also have dysphagia and odynophagia. Pharyngeal erythema and possibly even an exudate will be found on examination. Sometimes children will have an associated scarlatinal rash. Many patients with this set of symptoms and signs have bacterial infections, usually group A β-hemolytic streptococcus. Some children will also complain of concomitant systemic signs such as gastrointestinal upset and headache. Edema of the soft palate and uvula with tender upper jugular adenopathy is occasionally present.

If the patient's symptoms are not as severe but still include fever and erythema, streptococcus is

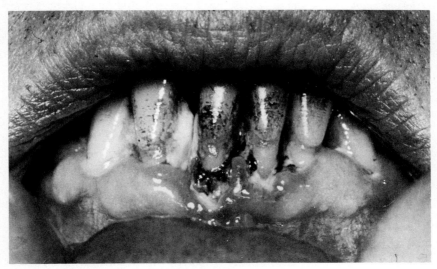

**FIG 13–4.**
Advanced pyorrhea.

less likely to be the cause. Viral illnesses are more common in patients who have moderate pharyngitis. In this situation, cervical adenopathy is rare. Hoarseness is more commonly seen in this group of patients and is consistent with a viral infection.

In patients with sore throats and pharyngeal erythema but no fever or exudate, the percentage of viral cases dramatically increases to 85% to 90%. These patients frequently have associated rhinorrhea. In patients with infections of viral etiology, there are no distinguishing symptoms or signs to identify an infection caused by a particular virus. The only slight exception to that generalization is in *herpangina*. This type of pharyngitis is caused by the coxsackievirus A and has characteristic vesicles with subsequent superficial ulcerative areas that are seen in the pharynx.

It should be emphasized that there are no groups of symptoms and signs that will specifically identify the origin of an infection, whether it be bacterial or viral. Therefore, microbiologic culture remains an important component of the patient's evaluation.

### Diagnostic Evaluation

The most important aspect of the diagnostic evaluation is the culture. The principal bacterial cause of pharyngitis is group A *Streptococcus pyogenes*. The other groupable streptococci (groups C and G), *Neisseria gonorrhoeae*, *Staphylococcus aureus*, *Diplococcus pneumoniae*, and *Corynebacterium diphtheriae*, can also cause pharyngitis. Cultures can accurately detect approximately 90% of children with group A streptococci when the culture and plating are performed properly.

The frequency of diphtheria has dramatically decreased as a result of immunization. However, even in some parts of the United States it continues to be a problem. Between 200 and 300 new cases are reported each year in the United States, most involving children younger than 10 years of age. The toxin released by *C. diphtheriae* results in inflammation, necrosis, and the eventual development of exudate. This exudative membrane adheres to the underlying tissue, and its removal causes bleeding. This adherence is a helpful diagnostic sign in contrasting the exudative membrane of diphtheria with that caused by other microorganisms.

*Neisseria gonorrhoeae* has been increasingly implicated in episodes of pharyngitis. This infection causes physical findings that are more impressive than the usual presenting symptoms. It is important that a pharyngeal swab from a patient suspected of having gonococcal pharyngitis be planted immediately in chocolate agar plates to increase the chances of obtaining a successful growth and diagnosis.

It is even possible for anaerobic bacteria to cause pharyngitis. They are abundant in the endogenous flora of the oropharynx. In a recent report a rather heavy growth of anaerobes was noted from specimens removed during a routine tonsillectomy. Cases of pharyngitis that are culture negative may actually have either viral or anaerobic bacterial etiologies.

A variety of viral infections of the pharynx are associated with other abnormalities. So-called *pharyngoconjunctival fever* includes the usual fever and sore throat of a pharyngitis episode, but conjunctivitis, usually caused by an adenovirus, is also present. Other viruses that can cause pharyngitis are herpes simplex, rhinovirus, and parainfluenza. Treatment for these infections is symptomatic. Patients with *acute lymphonodular pharyngitis* present with more systemic symptoms, including malaise and headache. Coxsackievirus A is characterized by the presence of whitish yellow lesions in the posterior pharyngeal mucosa.

### Treatment

In culture-positive pharyngitis infections originating from group A β-hemolytic streptococcus, oral buffered penicillin G or benzathine penicillin given intramuscularly represents the treatment of choice. The oral penicillin is usually administered for 10 days. In patients who are sensitive to penicillin, a 10-day course of erythromycin is advisable. The microbiologic antibiotic sensitivities derived from the patient's bacterial growth should provide the direction for the use of antibiotics in bacterial infections other than group A β-hemolytic streptococci. When there is no evidence of pathogenic bacterial growth on culture, by exclusion the diagnosis is believed to be viral.

Certain supportive measures are used in addition to antibiotics. Frequent pharyngeal irrigations help to clear inspissated mucus or exudative membranes from the inflamed pharynx. An enema bag filled with saline solution that is directed into the pharyngeal walls provides an effective irrigation system (Fig. 13–5). Gargling is usually not as effective because the self-protective mechanism of the gag reflex prevents the solution from coming into contact with the posterior pharyngeal mucosa. Depending on the severity of the symptoms, these irrigations can be done at hourly intervals while the patient is awake.

Acetaminophen can be used as an analgesic. However, some type of local anesthetic is often more effective in severe cases. Some of the lidocaine (Xylocaine) viscous preparations are so strong that they can cause a profound anesthesia when taken at full strength. This is often more uncomfortable to the patient than the pain of the pharyngitis. Dilution of the full-strength solution initially is recommended. The concentration can then be progressively increased until a suitable level of anesthesia is achieved.

The goal of treatment for diphtheria is to neutralize the unbound toxin. An antitoxin of equine origin is available, but can produce severe allergic reactions. In addition to the antitoxin, penicillin or erythromycin is also used.

Gonococcal pharyngitis is usually responsive to either penicillin given in conventional doses or tetracycline. Current treatment recommendations are usually available from local public health agencies, and should be followed.

### Infectious Mononucleosis

Infectious mononucleosis can cause rather profound pharyngitis with severe symptoms. There is some relationship between the Epstein-Barr virus and mononucleosis. Sore throat is usually accompanied by an exudative membrane that is seen in the oropharynx. Fever and cervical adenopathy are also present. Frequently there is evidence of systemic involvement, with splenomegaly being noted and some component of hepatitis with occasional jaundice. This disease is self-limited. The diagnosis is made serologically. Heterophil agglutination is the diagnostic test performed to confirm the clinical suspicion. Changes noted in the peripheral blood smear also support the diagnosis. These changes include the presence of a large atypical lymphocyte and also an elevated peripheral white blood cell count.

Mononucleosis is a self-limited disease. However, symptomatic treatment in the form of a topi-

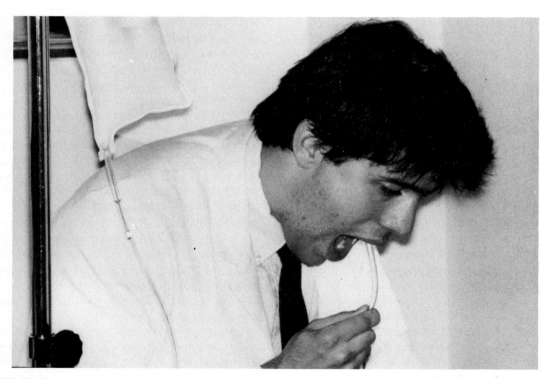

**FIG 13–5.**
Using an enema bag filled with saline solution for irrigation of the throat is a more effective means of delivering fluid to the posterior oropharynx than gargling.

cal analgesic is frequently necessary for the severe sore throat. Antipyretics are used. In addition, the hepatitis component of the disease mandates abstinence from alcohol for an extended period.

It is possible for chickenpox and measles to cause pharyngitis. With measles, small white lesions known as Koplik spots are noted on the buccal mucosa. Once again, the treatment is symptomatic for all of these viral etiologies.

Sometimes a localized viral infection can cause papillomatous growths in the pharynx. These papillomas most commonly involve the tonsillar pillars, the free margin of the soft palate, or the uvula. They usually have a narrow pedicle and are treated by surgical excision if the patient desires.

### Fungal Pharyngitis

*Candida albicans* can cause pharyngitis. It affects both extremes of the age spectrum, namely newborns and the elderly. It is somewhat of an opportunistic infection in the sense that its frequency is increased in those who are immunocompromised or severely debilitated. It can become clinically significant in patients who are on extended courses of antibiotics.

The presenting symptoms of fungal pharyngitis include not only sore throat but also dysphagia because the disease process often extends to involve the esophageal mucosa. The physical examination of these patients reveals the usual pharyngeal erythema but with noticeable absence of edema. Whitish deposits are seen throughout the oral cavity and pharyngeal mucosal surfaces. The diagnostic evaluation includes a microscopic examination, which permits identification from pharyngeal scrapings and microbiologic culture using Sabouraud's medium. Fungal infection is treated with nystatin, which can be given to both adults and children.

Some information suggests that *Chlamydia trachomatis* may be a pathogen capable of causing the usual signs and symptoms of pharyngitis. This particular infection usually responds to erythromycin.

### Vincent's Angina

Vincent's angina is characterized by a sore throat and dysphagia, accompanied by pharyngeal ulcerations and membrane formation. Poor oral and dental hygiene appears to contribute to this problem. What is usually described as a dirty grayish membrane covers the tonsils and can even adhere to the palate. Halitosis is present, as well as tender cervical adenopathy and a low-grade fever.

The diagnostic evaluation relies on microbiologic culture and usually shows a combination of a fusiform bacillus and a long, thin spirochete. There is some debate as to whether these organisms are truly pathogenic. When they are cultured concurrently, this combination is usually considered to cause the previously mentioned symptoms.

Treatment is usually penicillin for 10 days. For the individual sensitive to penicillin, tetracyclines are sometimes used. Diluted hydrogen peroxide used as an irrigant is a helpful adjunct to the antibiotic therapy. The patient must understand that, although the disease is self-limited, it is highly contagious.

### Other Causes of Pharyngitis

A number of systemic diseases can cause inflammation of the oropharynx. Drug-induced agranulocytosis produces sore throat and even malaise and moderate fever. Ulcerations eventually can develop. The diagnostic evaluation shows secondary bacterial invasion of the usual oral flora. However, the blood count and blood smear are particularly remarkable in diagnosing this problem. If the condition is drug related, prompt discontinuation of the drug often can cause a reversal of the problem and resolution of the symptoms. Leukemias and their treatment can also cause a similar picture.

A rare source of sore throat causing pharyngitis is *pemphigus*. This is a slowly progressive disorder that involves the skin and the mucous membranes. The vesicles develop and ultimately burst, forming painful ulcerations. A fibrinous exudate is noted in the area of the palate and posterior oropharyngeal wall. After these vesicles have ruptured, the pain seems to increase and may be a function of the secondary infection of the ulcerations. A variety of immunologic assays are now available to establish the diagnosis of pemphigus. Steroids are the main component of treatment and usually provide a rather prompt resolution of symptoms.

Uncommon causes of pharyngitis are *erythema multiforme* and *Stevens-Johnson syndrome*. Patients with these disorders initially develop rather impressive papules within their oral mucous membranes, which then progress to vesicles that ultimately rupture. The center of the lesion begins to heal, and then other lesions can cause overlapping, which results in unusual configurations of ulcerative areas within the oral cavity and pharynx. Stevens-Johnson syndrome is a more severe form of erythema multiforme and usually includes the abrupt onset of a severe stomatitis in addition to conjunctivitis and skin eruptions similar to the mucosal problems. Steroids are used in the management of both conditions.

## Nasopharynx

Although infection of the nasopharyngeal lymphoid tissue is usually associated with the tonsils and adenoids, it is possible for the nasopharyngeal mucosa, and even the lymphoid tissues, to be infected independent of the palatine tonsillar tissue. The etiology is most commonly viral and is frequently associated with rhinitis or some form of upper respiratory involvement of a viral flu syndrome. However, this infection infrequently causes localized symptoms because it is out of the usual pathway of solid food or liquids, minimizing contact with inflamed tissue. The main symptoms are usually related to edema created near the orifice of the nasopharyngeal end of the eustachian tube. Therefore, a patient with significant nasopharyngeal mucosal infection or inflammation will have symptoms and physical findings suggestive of eustachian tube dysfunction, such as a feeling of fullness or even decreased hearing on the involved side. Physical examination may even reveal decreased mobility of the tympanic membrane or possibly the development of a middle ear effusion. The resolution of the edema within the nasopharynx usually results in improvement of eustachian tube function, which eventually leads to improvement of the otologic symptoms and middle ear physical findings.

### Fascial Space Infections

The fascial spaces of the head and neck are potential spaces and are identified as such only when they are filled, for example, with pus in an abscess or with a neoplasm.

The retropharyngeal space contains lymph nodes in children. These ultimately atrophy during young adulthood, but they can be the source of extension of a pharyngeal infection. If the infection is not reversed, one or more nodes can be overwhelmed by infection and ultimately undergo necrosis with the development of pus. This problem is seen primarily in children and infants. Any accumulation of pus in the retropharyngeal space will compromise the airway, and stridor will eventually develop (Fig. 13–6). The hypopharyngeal extension of the retropharyngeal abscess also will ultimately alter the quality of the voice and the patient's cry. Physical examination reveals a red, bulging posterior pharyngeal wall. Lateral radiographs show the marked increased thickening of the soft tissue of the retropharyngeal space. Treatment for this problem is incision and drainage after endotracheal intubation and general inhalation anesthesia. The airway must be protected from aspiration of the purulent contents of the abscess.

### Pharyngomaxillary Space Infections

The pharyngomaxillary space is located between the superior constrictor musculature medially and the internal pterygoid muscle laterally. It is an important area in that it contains the contents of the carotid sheath. Posteriorly and laterally it lies against the fascia of the parotid gland. In addition to the carotid sheath contents, cranial nerves IX and XII are both located within this space (Fig. 13–7). It connects superiorly with the retropharyngeal space and continues along the vessels into the superior mediastinum. One can suspect a pharyngomaxillary space infection by noting a medial fullness behind the vertical ramus of the mandible during the oropharyngeal examination. It sometimes causes a medial displacement of the lateral wall of the oropharynx. Trismus is frequently present because of the irritation of the internal pterygoid muscle. Because of the variable position of the carotid artery within this abscess, incision and drainage are performed through an external skin incision to improve exposure and ensure complete drainage of the abscess.

### Masseter Space Infection

Abscess of the masseter space is deep to the periosteum of the mandible and is invariably secondary to dental infection. Once again, trismus is common because of the irritation of the masseter

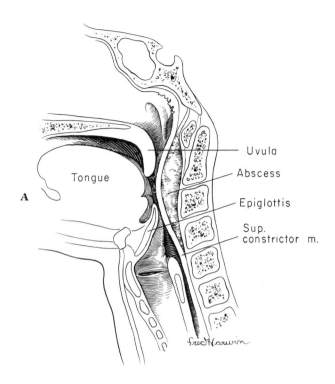

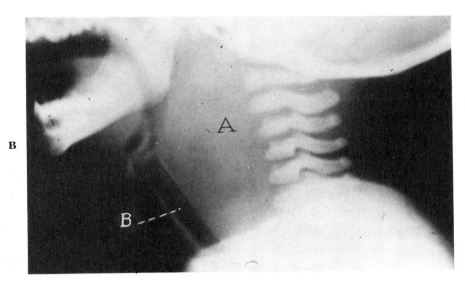

**FIG 13–6.**
**A,** retropharyngeal abscess. **B,** roentgenogram of a retropharyngeal abscess, showing *A,* the abscess and *B,* the displaced tracheal air column.

and even the internal pterygoid muscle with this abscess. The nondistensible elevated periosteum usually results in the physical examination showing no true fluctuation. Once again, surgical treatment is necessary, with incision and drainage through an external incision. The infected tooth causing the abscess is frequently extracted at that time.

### Ludwig's Angina
Ludwig's angina is an abscess involving the fascial spaces of the floor of the mouth (Fig.

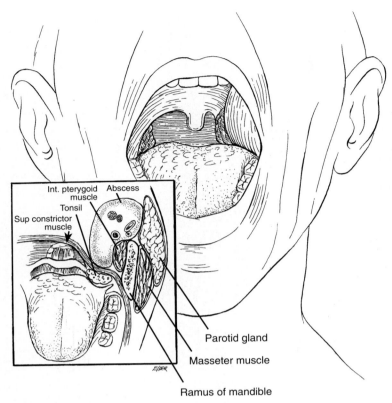

**FIG 13–7.**
Pharyngomaxillary (parapharyngeal) space infection. Note the external swelling as well as swelling in the pharynx. This condition often produces severe trismus, so that the patient cannot open his or her mouth. (Mouth is open here for illustrative purposes.)

13–8). This causes an upward displacement of the tongue and can ultimately compromise the airway. Once again, the abscess is invariably dental in origin. The actual fluid collection can occur either above or below the geniohyoid muscle. Surgical drainage is necessary and is performed through an external skin incision. Tracheotomy is commonly necessary to protect the airway.

## Tonsils and Adenoids

The lymphoid tissue included in Waldeyer's ring can become infected by both bacterial and viral organisms. Although bacteria most commonly cause an exudative infection, it is even possible for some viruses, especially the adenovirus, to cause an exudative reaction. Therefore, microbiologic cultures are critical in identifying the organism causing clinical symptoms. The bacterial infections are usually caused by β-hemolytic streptococci, pneumococci, or staphylococci. They oc-

cur most frequently in either children or young adults.

### Palatine Tonsillitis

The onset of an acute streptococcal tonsillitis is often quite sudden. Chilling and hyperpyrexia are indicative of the systemic effect. Small children are especially vulnerable to rather quick deviations in temperature, and febrile convulsions can occur. Odynophagia is common. Ear pain is also frequently part of the symptom complex because of the common sensory innervation of the pharyngeal and middle ear mucosa through the glossopharyngeal nerve (cranial nerve IX). Normal eating and drinking habits are usually disrupted. In addition to general malaise, joint pain is also common. Some children will even have abdominal distress. Nasal discharge and obstruction may also occur. The obstruction may be caused by the adenoid edema.

Physical examination reveals erythematous and

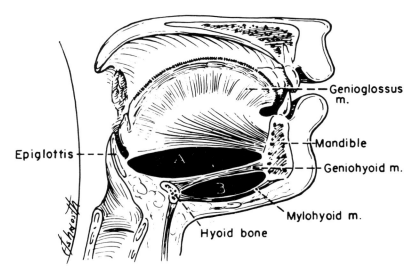

**FIG 13-8.**
Ludwig's angina. The black areas *(A and B)* indicate potential spaces in which infections may start. This condition is a phlegmon rather than an abscess.

edematous tonsils, with a yellowish exudate and some palatal erythema and edema (Fig. 13-9). Posterior oropharyngeal lymphoid patches may also be inflamed, and exudate on these islands of lymphoid tissue may be present. There is usually bilateral, tender upper jugular cervical adenopa-thy. Trismus is common because of the inflammation of the internal pterygoid muscles. Examination of the nasopharynx will reveal inflamed adenoids. Exudate can be present on the adenoids, as well as on the palatine tonsils. The lingual tonsils can also be involved.

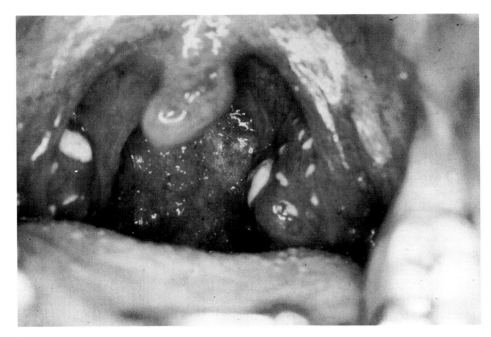

**FIG 13-9.**
Acute tonsillitis is associated with erythema and edema of the tonsils with exudative membranes over both palatine tonsils.

When the patient has these classic symptoms and physical findings, it is not uncommon to obtain a throat culture and to proceed with antibiotic therapy before the culture results are known. If the bacterial etiology is questionable and the patient does not have severe symptoms, it is probably better to await the culture results and plan the antibiotic therapy according to the patient's microbiologic sensitivities. Penicillin is used for tonsillitis in the same manner as outlined for streptococcal pharyngitis in Chapter 10. The other adjunctive measures using saline solution irrigations are also helpful. Control of the fever and the use of topical analgesics are also important adjuncts.

### Scarlet Fever

Scarlet fever, sometimes known as scarlatina, also results from a group A β-hemolytic streptococcal infection. Erythrogenic toxin is released. This exotoxin, which is liberated only by a particular strain of the streptococcus, causes a rash that is generalized over the entire body and punctiform and more evident in the skin folds. This rash follows the onset of sore throat within 2 days. The patient develops systemic signs such as high fever and headache and even some gastrointestinal upset. Oral examination shows a punctate rash over the palate and the usual inflammation on the tonsils and adenoids. The papillae of the tongue also become erythematous and large and give a characteristic appearance referred to as "strawberry tongue." Penicillin is the treatment of choice, and patients usually respond readily. Despite proper antibiotic therapy, however, there is a possibility that the patient will become a streptococcal carrier. Tonsillectomy may be indicated to resolve the carrier state. Poststreptococcal complications such as glomerulonephritis are rare because of antibiotics and medical and public awareness.

### Lingual Tonsillitis

The lingual tonsils can also become infected independent of the palatine tonsils and adenoids. The possibility of lingual tonsillitis may be increased in patients who have previously had the palatine tonsils and adenoids removed. A patient with lingual tonsillitis often has a milder sore throat than that experienced with the usual palatine tonsillitis but will complain of the sensation of a lump in the throat, which causes frequent swallowing. This sensation may be caused by the edematous tonsillar tissue at the tongue base. Treatment for lingual tonsillitis is identical to that for palatine tonsillitis, involving antibiotics and irrigations. If tonsillitis becomes recurrent, lingual tonsillectomy can be performed. The carbon dioxide laser is useful for this procedure because it helps to reduce bleeding.

### Relationship to Ear Disease

It was formerly believed that a close relationship existed between the status of the tonsils and adenoids and the frequency and severity of middle ear infections. It was not uncommon to treat a patient having recurrent ear infections with tonsillectomy and adenoidectomy or possibly with adenoidectomy in addition to some otologic procedure, such as myringotomy alone or myringotomy with placement of a tympanostomy tube. It appears, however, that the incidence of and effective treatment for ear disease are usually independent of the disease status or actual size of the tonsils and adenoids. Currently, otologic problems are being managed independent of tonsil and adenoid considerations and vice versa.

### Complications of Tonsillar Infections

The major complication of tonsillar infection is the development of a peritonsillar abscess, a collection of pus located between the tonsil and the pharyngeal constrictor musculature (Fig. 13–10). The person with a peritonsillar abscess typically has had acute tonsillitis for 8 to 10 days that has not responded well to the usual antibiotic therapy. The patient will present with some drooling because it hurts to swallow. There will also be some alteration in voice quality because of the profound pharyngeal edema. This is frequently characterized as "hot potato voice." Standard treatment in the past has been incision and drainage. However, over the past 10 years there has been considerable interest in removing the tonsils during an acute situation to fulfill the twofold purpose of draining the pus and removing the tissue that may predispose to recurrence. Several studies have documented the safety and efficacy of tonsillectomy in this setting.

### Tonsillectomy and Adenoidectomy

Removal of the palatine tonsils and adenoids continues to be frequently performed. It has un-

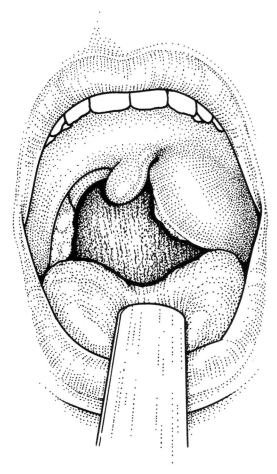

**FIG 13–10.**
Pus from a peritonsillar abscess is trapped between the tonsil and the pharyngeal constrictor musculature.

dergone considerable discussion in both the medical and lay literature. The realization that Waldeyer's ring participates in the immunologic reaction to disease has prompted active discussion about the advisability of removing the tonsils and adenoids.

Clearly, patients benefit from tonsillectomy and adenoidectomy in certain situations. In the young child with tonsillar hypertrophy large enough to cause airway obstruction, it has been well documented that right ventricular hypertrophy and cor pulmonale can result. Tonsillectomy and adenoidectomy will benefit those children having considerable difficulty swallowing because of the massive size of the tonsils and adenoids (Fig. 13–11) and those individuals in whom massive adenotonsillar hypertrophy causes sleep disorders. However, the debate centers on the rela-

tive value of surgical removal for the individual who is having recurrent streptococcal tonsillar infections. It is important to assess initially that the infections are bacterial and especially streptococcal in origin and that they are involving the tonsils and not the pharynx. If it is documented that the cause of the patient's recurrent sore throats is streptococcal tonsillar infections, the frequency of these tonsillar infections becomes the main consideration. There is no absolute number used to determine when surgery is appropriate; however, a general guideline involves the assessment of the frequency of the streptococcal tonsillar infections and the impact on the individual's normal daily activities. If a child is missing an inordinate amount of school because of the inability of antibiotics to resolve the recurrent episodes, tonsillectomy and adenoidectomy represent a reasonable alternative. If an adult is missing considerable work time, tonsillectomy and adenoidectomy should be considered.

There are also special circumstances that develop, especially in children, that would prompt consideration of tonsillectomy and adenoidectomy. A child who has had a febrile seizure as a result of acute streptococcal tonsillitis may benefit from the operation to prevent another case of tonsillitis. Likewise, the individual who has had a peritonsillar abscess may benefit from tonsillectomy and adenoidectomy to prevent recurrence.

Adenoidectomy is performed with the patient under general anesthesia. The adenoid tissue is curetted out of the nasopharynx, and hemostasis is achieved with packing of the nasopharynx for a few minutes. Some of the lower areas of the nasopharynx can actually be directly visualized by retracting the soft palate. Electrocautery can be used to control bleeding after the packs are removed.

The most common complication following adenoidectomy is bleeding. This bleeding can go undetected for a prolonged period because the patient, who is supine in bed, swallows the blood. Eventually massive hematemesis occurs, and hypotension may develop. Frequent postoperative nursing examinations of the area of the posterior pharyngeal wall are advisable.

Tonsillectomy can be performed with either local or general anesthesia. There are numerous alternative techniques for removal of the tonsils, including use of the Sluder guillotine and incision

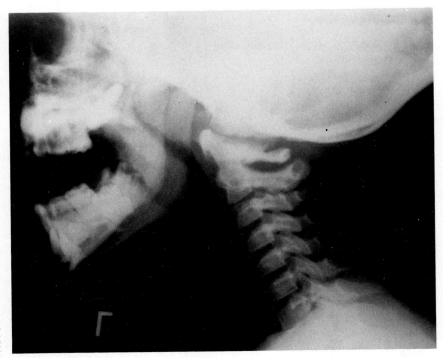

**FIG 13–11.**
A lateral soft tissue radiograph is useful to evaluate the size of the adenoids and the nasopharynx.

of the mucous membrane and dissection of the tonsils away from the underlying constrictor muscles. Bleeding vessels can be ligated, cauterized, or stopped with pressure. The carbon dioxide laser has been advocated by some for tonsillectomy.

Bleeding is the most common complication. Close postoperative monitoring by nurses is important. Sore throat, low-grade fever, and ear pain are common. The glossopharyngeal nerve is the origin of the referred pain. Maintaining adequate hydration and using nonaspirin-containing analgesics help to reduce the throat discomfort.

Tonsillectomy and adenoidectomy is not a minor procedure and is characterized by a substantial blood loss and the development of tissue edema within the aerodigestive tract. Therefore, the potential for airway compromise exists. The advisability of tonsillectomy and adenoidectomy should not be casually decided by any health professional.

# TRAUMA

Trauma to this region can generally be classified according to whether injuries involve bony or soft tissue structures. Trauma to the cervical vertebrae will be discussed in the section on the neck. Therefore, the only remaining bony structure in this region is the mandible. The mandible is second only to nasal bones in frequency of fractures occurring in the head and neck. It is not unusual for it to be fractured at multiple sites. The vectors of force occurring with compression to the mandible invariably are transmitted throughout the mandible and result in stress to multiple regions in addition to the site of impact. A thorough history and physical examination frequently will permit an accurate diagnosis before radiographs are taken. Soft tissue injuries are common. It is important to understand the potential consequences of lacerations involving the soft tissue in certain regions and their relationship to the adequacy of the patient's airway.

## Mandibular Fractures
### *Presenting Symptoms*
In patients who have sustained trauma to the mandible, pain is usually localized to the site of the fracture. This pain is intensified by mandibular movement. It is important to ask the patient about any alterations in dental occlusion follow-

ing the mandibular injury. The patient frequently can identify minor changes in occlusal relationships that may not be easily noted by the examining physician. If there has been an inferior blow to the mandible, the patient may also complain of either unilateral or bilateral ear pain as a result of the mandibular condyles traumatizing the anterior wall of the ear canal with the transmission of the force from an inferior to a superior direction. The patient may also complain of numbness to the chin if the inferior alveolar nerve has been transected by a fracture of the mandible.

### Presenting Signs

The patient should be asked initially to put his or her teeth together so that the examiner or patient can note any alterations in occlusion. The entire course of the mandible, including the temporomandibular joint area, should be palpated; any local tenderness or crepitation may help to locate a fracture. The mobility may also be noted

with palpation. If there is suspicion of one or more fractures involving one side of the mandible, the patient should be asked to bite on a group of five or six tongue blades on the contralateral side of the mandible (Fig. 13–12). The stress of this biting action on the fracture site invariably causes localized pain and helps to confirm the diagnosis. Even though one fracture site has been identified, the entire course of the mandible must be examined because of the common occurrence of multiple fractures. Check the mobility of the fractured elements by gently moving them. Certain fracture locations can affect the safety of the airway.

When the examination suggests bilateral parasymphyseal mandibular fractures, the patient has a potential airway problem. The genioglossus muscle of the tongue attaches to the midline tubercle on the inner surface of the mental portion of the mandible. If there is enough mobility of this central portion following bilateral parasymphyseal fractures, the tongue could conceivably prolapse with retrodisplacement of the central mandibular fragment and oppose the posterior pharyngeal wall when the patient is supine, resulting in airway obstruction (Fig. 13–13). Depending on the mobility of the central fragment and the patient's overall condition, tracheotomy may

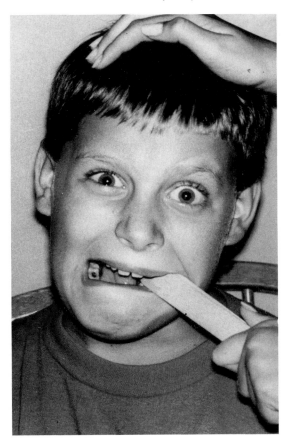

**FIG 13–12.**
Biting on tongue blades will cause pain, which localizes to the site of a mandibular fracture.

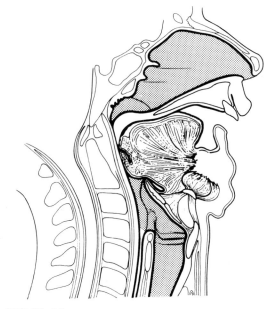

**FIG 13–13.**
Bilateral parasymphyseal fractures permit posterior displacement of the tongue so that it can obstruct the upper airway.

be advisable to protect the airway until the mandible is placed into intermaxillary fixation.

### Methods of Evaluation

Radiographs are invariably taken to confirm the findings at the time of physical examination. Mandibular Panorex radiographs provide excellent views of all portions of the mandible except the symphyseal and parasymphyseal regions (Fig. 13–14). Oblique views of the mandible provide the exposure needed to evaluate the symphyseal and parasymphyseal regions. This combination of radiographs usually represents the initial evaluation.

In patients with multiple facial fractures, computed tomography is another useful means of evaluating the position of the facial bones (Fig. 13–15). However, computed tomography is not considered a mandatory examination on all patients with mandibular trauma. The indications for its use must be individualized according to the medical factors involved with each patient.

### Treatment

There is usually no need to consider the correction of a mandibular fracture an emergency. Often it is better to allow some resolution of the patient's edema and other injuries before proceeding with the definitive repair. The timing of the repair must be individualized according to the myriad factors considered for each patient.

The pain resulting from the mandibular fracture can be reduced by supporting and somewhat stabilizing the mandibular fragments before surgery with the use of an elastic dressing placed about the mandible and around the top of the head. An alternative technique is to use a soft cervical collar to provide support and reduce mandibular movement.

Mandibular fractures require a period of immobilization similar to that for bony injuries involving other parts of the body. Many mandibular fractures now are managed by essentially reducing the fragments in the proper position and immobilizing them with the application of Erich arch bars. These are metallic bands secured by wires to the maxillary and mandibular dentition and connected with rubber elastic bands to maintain the mandible in proper occlusion. Mandibular fractures treated in this fashion usually need to be immobilized for 5 to 8 weeks.

A mandibular fracture at an angle that would predispose the fragments to slip out of their reduced position because of the pull of the masticatory muscles is referred to as an "unfavorable" fracture (Fig. 13–16). Interosseous wiring is usually necessary to maintain proper reduction of the fragments in an unfavorable fracture. When interosseous wiring is applied, the patient must still be placed in intermaxillary fixation with arch bars for a similar period of immobilization.

The counterpart to an unfavorable fracture oc-

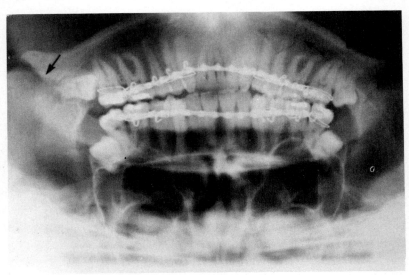

**FIG 13–14.**
Panorex radiograph showing left mandibular angle and right mandibular body fractures.

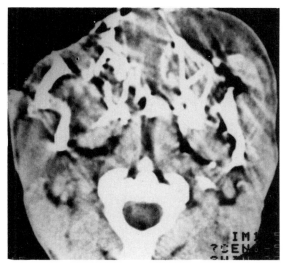

**FIG 13–15.**
Computed tomogram of a patient sustaining multiple comminuted fractures of the midface permits detailed analysis of altered bony relationship.

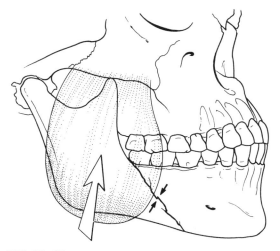

**FIG 13–17.**
The "favorable" fracture does not result in displacement of the bony fragments with contractions of the masticatory muscles.

curs when the masticatory muscles actually help to keep the fragments in proper alignment. A "favorable" fracture (Fig. 13–17) exists when this muscular action promotes correct contact of the mandibular fragments. In this situation, interosseous wiring is usually not needed and intermaxillary fixation is the only treatment.

Immobilization is stressful to the patient. It is uncomfortable and obviously requires a drastic change in nutrition, which inevitably leads to sub-

stantial weight loss. Because of the disadvantages of intermaxillary fixation, there has been renewed interest in the use of small dynamic compression plates (Fig. 13–18), which are metallic plates applied to each side of the fracture that pull the fracture elements together and do not require intermaxillary fixation. However, the use of dynamic compression plates is restricted by the location of the fracture.

## Soft Tissue Injuries
### Presenting Symptoms

The oral cavity and oropharyngeal mucosa have numerous sensory nerves, and any soft tissue injury, whether it be a contusion, abrasion, or

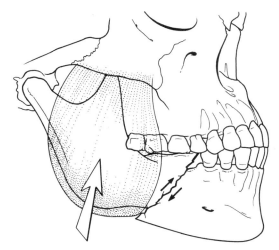

**FIG 13–16.**
Masticatory muscle pull. "Unfavorable" mandibular fracture displaces the mandibular fragments.

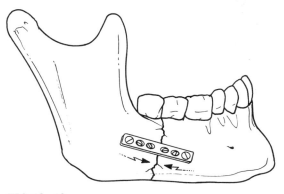

**FIG 13–18.**
Dynamic compression plates provide effective stabilization for certain mandibular fractures.

laceration, will result in pain. The lingual nerve, which provides sensation to the ipsilateral side of the tongue, runs in the floor of the mouth's submucosal tissues. Because it is deep in this area, a laceration would have to be quite deep to transect the lingual nerve, which would result in tongue numbness. The hypoglossal nerves enter the tongue in the deep portion of the musculature, and it would be unusual for a laceration of the floor of the mouth to transect the hypoglossal nerve. If there is a contusion to the soft tissues that results in a hematoma or edema, the patient's voice quality may become muffled.

### Presenting Signs

It is important that the examiner evaluate all areas of the oral cavity, oropharynx, and nasopharynx. This is usually best done by using two tongue blades simultaneously, one in each hand, to spread the tissues for good visualization (Fig. 13–19). Excellent lighting is mandatory. The buccal surface should be examined and the opening of the parotid duct orifice checked for any abnormal secretions or drainage. Blood from the parotid duct orifice, for example, might indicate a parotid duct injury. The floor of the mouth and the entire tongue surface should be inspected. That requires indirect mirror examination of the base of the tongue with either a flexible fiberoptic endoscope or a rod prism instrument. If such

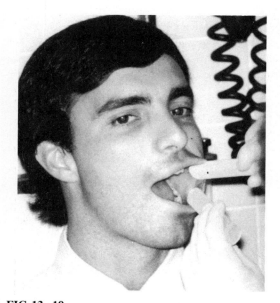

**FIG 13–19.**
The use of two tongue blades provides maximal exposure of soft tissue structures in the oral cavity.

equipment is not available, the tongue base should be palpated to determine if any lacerations are present. Tongue mobility should be checked to rule out possible injury to the hypoglossal nerves.

### Methods of Evaluation

Soft tissue injury to the oral cavity and oropharynx generally does not require any radiographic examinations. Nor is submandibular sialography usually necessary to evaluate a possible laceration to the submandibular duct because these lacerations seldom require reanastomosis of the duct; laceration of the submandibular duct creates a drainage point at a new location. The only possible exception might be the use of computed tomography to evaluate the extent of a hematoma resulting from a contusion.

### Treatment

The oral cavity and oropharynx are areas of the human body that contain multiple gram-positive and gram-negative bacteria as resident nonpathogenic organisms. Therefore, most superficial lacerations are not closed because of the high probability of infection. However, if the laceration involves the free border of the tongue or palate, it is usually advisable to reestablish the normal anatomic relationships with sutures to the free edges but to keep the remaining length of the laceration open for drainage purposes. As stated, a laceration involving the submandibular duct does not require reanastomosis.

It is necessary to consider the location of a hematoma or edema and anticipate its potential impact on the adequacy of the patient's airway. Once again, computed tomography can be helpful with this evaluation. Hematomas should be incised and drained. The submucosal tissue of the oral cavity and oropharynx can become quite edematous rapidly because of the loose planes of muscular tissue. However, the edema can also rapidly subside if the patient's head is kept elevated to at least 45 degrees and preferably closer to 60 or 70 degrees. Once again, any intraoral tissue edema must be closely monitored for potential airway problems.

### Electrical Burns of the Lip

Electrical lip burns resulting from children's attempts to bite electrical cords frequently involve the corner of the mouth (Fig. 13–20). These elec-

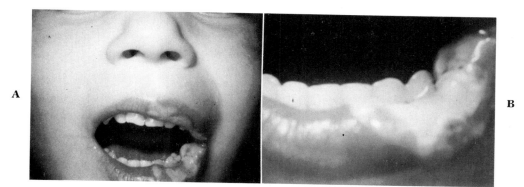

**FIG 13–20.**
Appearance of electrical burn. **A,** to the corner of the mouth in a young boy who has sustained. **B,** a third-degree burn of the vermillion portion of the lower lip.

trical burns can be classified as either arc or contact burns. An arc burn causes charring of the soft tissues. Contact burns occur at the entry and exit sites. Most electrical burns are of the arc type. They are characterized by delayed necrosis with loss of more tissue than what is acutely evident. This delayed necrosis can sometimes cause profuse bleeding from one or both labial arteries as the necrotic fragment becomes detached. The outpatient management of any child with an electrical burn of the lip must include parental awareness of this possibility and instruction as to how to manage the occurrence of such bleeding. This can be done by compressing the lip with the index finger and the thumb. Lip clamps are also available to stop the bleeding.

Local wound care will decrease the chance of infection and reduce the amount of tissue destruction. Treatment usually is conservative and produces satisfactory results. If the child has dentition that will permit attachment of a retainer (Fig. 13–21), it will help to maintain the position of the commissure and prevent contraction with resultant rounding. If this is not possible, the child is followed over a protracted period until the damaged portion of the lips can be reconstructed (Fig. 13–22). Reconstruction can involve numerous techniques, including grafts and flaps (Fig. 13–23).

# NEOPLASMS

Tumors involving the oral cavity, oropharynx, and nasopharynx cause different signs, symptoms, and behavior. Neoplasms of these three anatomic sites are discussed separately.

## Oral Cavity
### Presenting Symptoms

The oral cavity is that portion of the mouth from the lips to the anterior tonsillar pillar. A tumor involving the oral cavity, whether benign or malignant, can cause symptoms. Even a benign tumor, such as a mucous retention cyst of the buccal area, can be traumatized with the teeth and produce pain. Whenever a tumor causes disruption of the surface epithelium within the oral cavity, the combination of contaminants from food, coupled with the irritation from the acidic pH of the saliva, invariably causes pain. This pain can secondarily affect other oral cavity functions, such as eating and talking, with the expected results of weight loss and speech alteration. It is not unusual to discover patients who will change their normal eating patterns to decrease the pain, such as drinking beverages at room temperature to

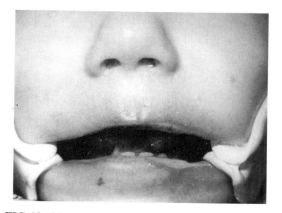

**FIG 13–21.**
An oral retainer fixed around the back of the head can be used to prevent contraction of the oral commissures following a burn to the lips.

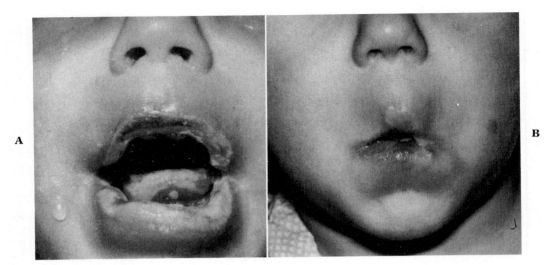

**FIG 13–22.**
Appearance of an acute burn. **A,** soon after electrical cord injury to the upper and lower lips and tongue and, **B,** appearance after wound contraction occurred following unsuccessful attempts to use an oral retainer to prevent contractions.

avoid temperature extremes that would stimulate an ulcerative area within the oral cavity.

It is possible for an oral cavity tumor to affect the sensory innervation so that the patient has either anesthesia or paresthesia within the area. The symptoms indicating neurologic dysfunction are most commonly seen with malignancies that have actually invaded nerve tissue.

### Presenting Signs

The physical findings associated with oral cavity tumors will provide some useful diagnostic information to indicate whether the lesion is benign or malignant. Benign tumors commonly present as submucosal masses (Fig. 13–24) that have a slow pattern of growth. They are usually firm, nontender lesions that do not compromise physiologic or neurologic functions.

In contrast, malignant tumors invariably cause mucosal disruption within the oral cavity (Fig. 13–25). They appear as an indurated mass with ulceration of the overlying epithelium. It is possible for them to be superficial ulcers with no underlying induration. If the ulceration involves the

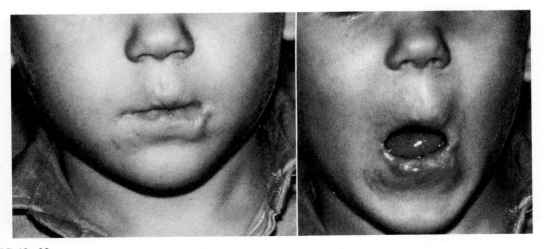

**FIG 13–23.**
Same child as shown in Fig. 13–22 following multiple reconstructions that reestablished the circumference of the mouth and reconstructed the commissures.

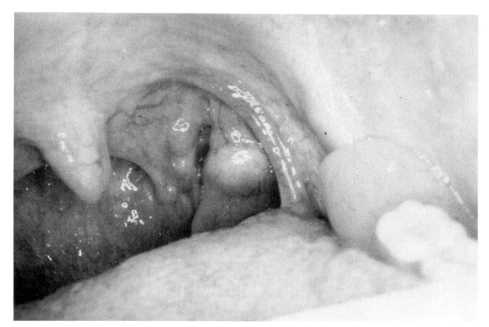

**FIG 13–24.**
This benign tumor of the tonsillar fossa has normal overlying mucosa.

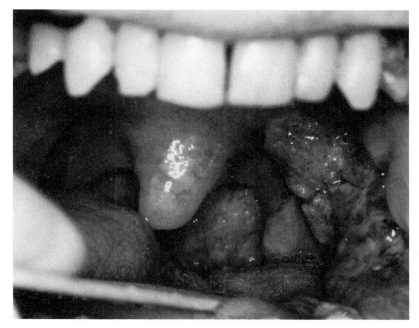

**FIG 13–25.**
Malignancies usually arise from the surface and cause disruption of the normal appearance.

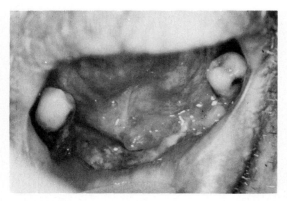

**FIG 13–26.**
Loose teeth in an adult with no history of trauma should be considered suspicious for underlying malignancy.

gingiva, the patient will have loose teeth with no history of previous dental trauma (Fig. 13–26). The ulcerative areas can be red, white, or possibly even a dull yellow. Redness reflects the erythematous component of inflammation that is ubiquitous with any ulcerative area within the oral cavity. The white appearance usually indicates an accumulation of debris over the ulcerative area. A yellow color is consistent with superficial infection causing an exudative membrane that has developed over the ulcer.

### Tumor Types

Some benign tumors involve the oral cavity. The *mucous retention cyst* is the most common and is predominantly located on the mucosal surface of the lips, especially the lower lip. These cysts are asymptomatic, and excision is not mandatory unless malignancy is suspected or their size compromises oral cavity function. Incision and drainage or needle aspiration invariably results in recurrence of the cyst.

A *fibroma* (Fig. 13–27) can involve the oral cavity and seems to have a special predilection for either the buccal mucosa or the tongue, suggesting an etiologic relationship to injury. Fibromas invariably are firm and nontender. However, a clinical distinction from malignancy is not possible, and excisional biopsy for histologic description is recommended.

A *salivary tumor* involving the minor salivary glands can also present as an oral cavity submucosal induration. It is usually asymptomatic and nontender with a slow growth history. Histologic diagnosis is advisable because of the potential for malignancy.

*Granular cell myoblastoma* is a benign tumor arising from the musculature of the tongue and presents as an asymptomatic submucosal induration that is often better palpated than seen. It can

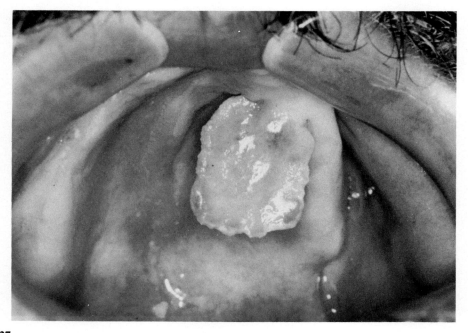

**FIG 13–27.**
Fibromas are usually the result of some trauma to the oral cavity, as seen with this fibroma arising from the maxillary aveolar ridge in an edentulous patient with poor fitting dentures.

occur in other areas of the head and neck, but the tongue is the most common site. Complete surgical excision is usually curative.

Most oral cavity tumors are malignant. In fact, the oral cavity is the second most common site of primary tumors involving the head and neck. The most common histologic cell type is *squamous cell carcinoma,* representing approximately 90% to 95% of all cancers in this area. Other malignancies include those arising from the glandular elements. *Adenoid cystic carcinoma* and *adenocarcinoma* can arise from the minor salivary glands within the oral cavity. *Sarcomas* are rarely seen.

### Risk Factors

There are no particular risk factors that identify a patient population more susceptible to developing benign tumors in the oral cavity. However, the opposite is true for malignancies. Most patients with squamous cell carcinoma are male and in the sixth and seventh decades of life. Recent reports suggest that the frequency of squamous cell carcinoma among women is increasing. Betel nut chewing, a common practice in India, produces a high incidence of oral cancers involving the sites of salivary drainage through the oral cavity, namely the floor of the mouth and buccal areas.

People who smoke have approximately a sevenfold greater chance of developing an oral cavity malignancy than do nonsmokers. The renewed popularity of smokeless tobacco is also having an impact. Buccal and other oral cancers are being noted in this segment of the tobacco-using population.

Individuals who consume alcoholic beverages on a regular basis also have a sevenfold greater chance of developing oral cancers than do nondrinkers. In patients who both smoke and consume alcoholic beverages, there is a fifteenfold increase in the incidence of malignancies when compared with that of the nonsmoking population.

Other risk factors have been identified, such as syphilitic involvement, loose dentures, and poor oral hygiene. However, these factors currently are only minimally important in contrast to alcohol use and smoking.

**History and Physical Examination.** It is imperative to determine if the patient's life-style involves any of the previously mentioned risk factors. This information helps to determine the probability of neoplastic involvement. It is also important to ascertain the duration of the patient's problem and what has occurred with the lesion during that period with special reference to size and symptoms. It is not unusual for patients with nonspecific complaints to have been treated previously with an antibiotic by another physician for the same problem. Questioning the patient about response to the antibiotic may provide useful information about the possibility of an inflammatory cause. It would be expected that a patient with a tumor would experience some decrease in the tumor's size after antibiotic therapy. It is important not to misinterpret this response and to continue to maintain a high index of suspicion of malignancy with oral cavity ulcers.

The accuracy of physical examination of the oral cavity is improved with palpation. The subcutaneous tissue in this area is occupied by salivary ducts, nerves, arteries, veins, vessels, and lymphatics. The loose planes among these structures increase the chances for submucosal extension of the neoplastic process. The true extent of the tumors cannot be determined by visualization alone. In addition, it is imperative for the examiner to remember that the head and neck region is commonly the site of multiple synchronous carcinomas. Therefore, a thorough examination of the entire region, including the hypopharynx and larynx, is mandatory to rule out the possibility of an occult secondary neoplasm. The examination of the neck is also critical because of the frequent involvement of the cervical nodes.

### Malignant Tumor Behavior

**Primary Tumor Site.** The most common site of malignant tumors of the oral cavity is the *lips,* with the lower lip being most involved. This frequency is related to the greater sun exposure to the lower lip. These lesions can be treated with surgery or irradiation. As the tumor grows (Fig. 13–28), the chance of metastases to the neck nodes, especially to the submental and submandibular area, also increases.

Cancer of the *tongue* is the second most common oral cavity tumor and most frequently involves either the lateral edge (Fig. 13–29) or the undersurface. The posterior one-third (base of tongue) can also undergo malignant degeneration. There is a great potential for submucosal exten-

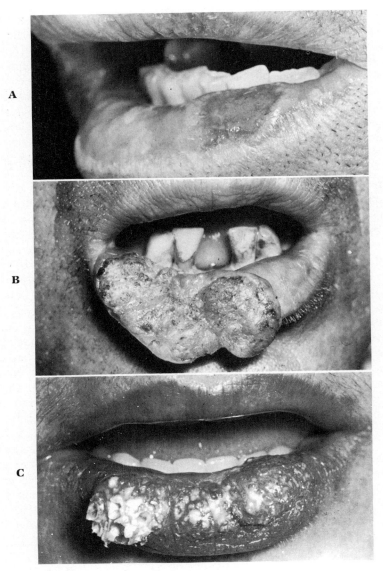

**FIG 13–28.**
**A,** early squamous cell carcinoma. **B,** far advanced squamous cell carcinoma. Bilateral cervical metastases were present. **C,** superficial squamous cell carcinoma.

sion with tongue cancers because of the multiple muscular planes within the intrinsic tongue muscle. The lymphatics, especially in the tongue base, are abundant. The initial drainage occurs to either the submandibular or jugular nodes (Fig. 13–30). Lymphatic drainage can occur to either side of the neck when a tongue cancer involves the midline of the tongue.

The *floor of the mouth* is a "silent" area that is not routinely examined. It is the horseshoe-shaped area of mucosa underneath the tongue, with the

mandible representing the lateral border. Delayed diagnoses are not uncommon. Once again, metastases to neck nodes are common and often involve the submental, submandibular, or jugular nodes. As the tumor grows, it can involve adjacent structures such as the tongue or the gingival ridge of the mandible.

The *buccal mucosa* is another site of oral cancer affecting users of snuff and other smokeless tobaccos. The buccal area is also the most common site of verrucous carcinoma, which appears

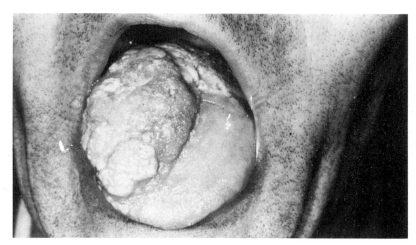

**FIG 13–29.**
Squamous cell carcinoma of the tongue. Treatment consisted of partial glossectomy and radical neck dissection.

clinically as a white filamentous exophytic growth (Fig. 13–31) rather than as an ulcerative lesion. This clinical appearance, coupled with the histologic description of a well-differentiated squamous cell carcinoma, is the combination necessary to make the diagnosis. Verrucous carcinoma

has a more favorable prognosis because of infrequent nodal and distant metastases.

**Neck Nodes.** The regional nodes on either side of the neck are the most common site of metastases from oral cavity carcinomas. The two

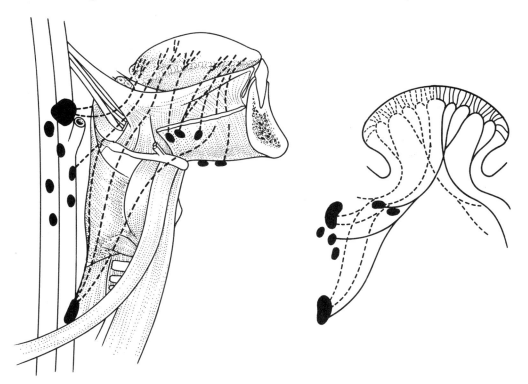

**FIG 13–30.**
Lymphatic drainage from the tongue goes primarily to either the submandibular or jugular lymph nodes. (Redrawn after Hollinshead W: *Anatomy for surgery,* vol 1, ed 3, Philadelphia, 1982, Lippincott. Used by permission.)

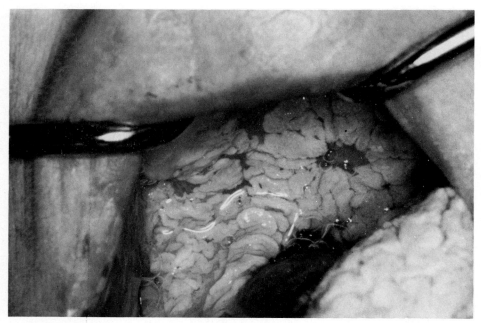

**FIG 13–31**.
This patient had verrucous carcinoma involving the buccal, palatal, and tongue mucosa.

nodal groups routinely involved are the submandibular and jugular nodes. The submental nodes can also be involved, especially in more central midline lesions. The frequency of nodal metastases is related to the size and extent of ulceration of the primary tumor. For certain oral cavity cancers, such as cancer of the tongue base, there is a high incidence of microscopic involvement of metastatic neck nodes in the absence of any palpable adenopathy. This propensity for occult metastatic nodal disease with some types of tongue cancers is the reason for treating some nodal groups even in the absence of palpable adenopathy.

**Distant Metastases.** The combination of radiation therapy and surgery for oral cancers has improved control of the primary tumors and neck nodes. However, 5-year survival rates have not dramatically improved because patients treated in this fashion live long enough to develop and ultimately succumb to distant metastases. Thus the belief that oral cavity cancers rarely undergo distant metastases does not appear to be valid.

**Treatment.** Treatment of oral cavity cancers depends on the primary tumor size, status of the neck nodes, presence or absence of metastatic disease, and the patient's overall health. In patients with relatively small lesions who have no evidence of neck nodal disease or distant metastases, surgical excision and curative doses of radiation therapy have comparable survival rates. Excision with the carbon dioxide laser is a useful modality for superficially invasive, small cancers of the oral cavity. The laser has some hemostatic benefits, and the patients appear to experience less pain.

As the lesions grow, combined therapy programs such as surgery with radiation therapy are used. Recently, chemotherapy has been added to treatment programs for advanced-stage disease. Newer chemotherapeutic agents such as cisplatin and bleomycin act against squamous cell carcinoma of the head and neck and have been incorporated into chemotherapeutic regimens with methotrexate and other agents, such as vincristine and 5-fluorouracil. Response rates as high as 90% have been reported with some chemotherapeutic regimens (Fig. 13–32). It has not been determined whether these regimens will improve the percentage of cured patients.

## Oropharynx

The pharynx is divided into the nasopharynx, the oropharynx, and the hypopharynx. The oro-

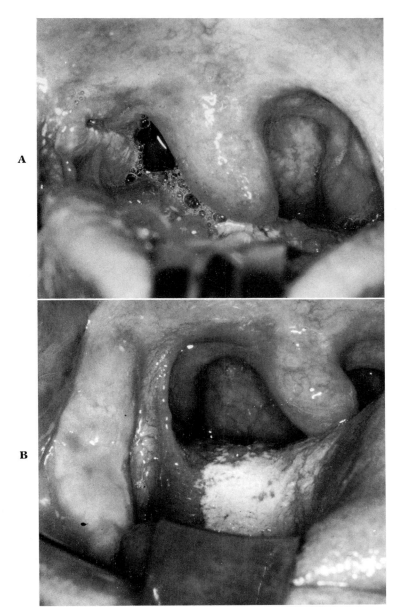

**FIG 13–32.**
**A** indicates stage IV tonsillar carcinoma involving palate and extending down to the tongue base. **B** indicates complete disappearance of this cancer following three courses of cisplatin, vincristine, and methotrexate and bleomycin.

pharynx is that portion which can be seen by looking into the mouth. It is bounded by the level of the free edge of the palate superiorly and the top of the epiglottis inferiorly.

### Tumor Types

Benign tumors of the oropharynx are primarily mucous retention cysts. They commonly involve the oropharynx and are especially common on the tonsillar pillars. Once again, they are often asymptomatic. However, any history of progressive growth or symptoms justifies excision for a histologic description.

*Papillomas* (Fig. 13–33) can occur and present as pedunculated lesions, frequently arising from the free edge of the palate at the base of the uvula or on a tonsillar pillar. Surgical excision is not mandatory unless there is a history of docu-

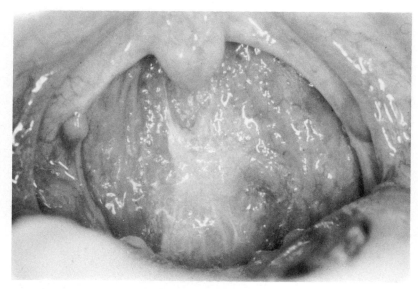

**FIG 13–33.**
This papilloma involves the posterior tonsillar pillar.

mented growth or if the patient's anxiety warrants a histologic diagnosis. These small lesions can also be resected transorally by using the carbon dioxide laser.

Squamous cell carcinoma is the predominant histologic malignant cell type. Both adenocarci-noma and adenoid cystic carcinoma involving the minor salivary glands can present as oropharyn-geal lesions. A deep lobe parotid tumor may also present as a submucosal oropharyngeal mass by causing displacement of the lateral wall of the oropharynx (Fig. 13–34).

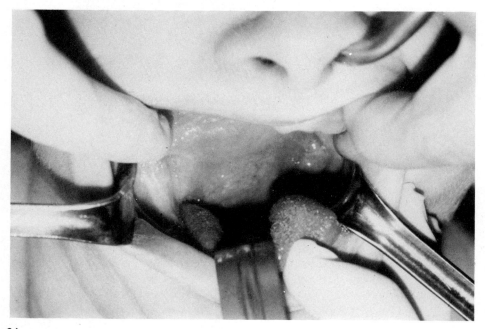

**FIG 13–34.**
This patient had a large tumor involving the deep lobe of the parotid gland that displaced the lateral oropharynx medially and the palate interiorly.

## Risk Factors

The understanding of the risk factors associated with oropharyngeal cancer is changing. Previously they were understood to be similar to those associated with oral cavity cancers in that most such cancers occurred in older males. Recently, it has been noted that younger people and more women are developing oropharyngeal neoplasms. There is the usual association with smoking and alcohol, with the combination having a potentiating effect.

**History and Physical Examination.** The examiner should determine the time interval in which the ulcerative or exophytic lesion appeared within the oropharynx and note any response to previous courses of antibiotics. If there is a history of rather slow but progressive growth without any identifiable association with inflammation, a malignancy should be considered. If an ulcerative lesion or submucosal induration is noted on examination it should be palpated. This examining technique provides information about fixation or involvement of underlying structures. The patient should be instructed to open the mouth widely so that the physician can determine if any component of trismus is present. An otologic examination to look for serous otitis media is also necessary to rule out the possibility of eustachian tube involvement. When *unilateral* middle ear fluid is noted, it should warn the examiner that a nasopharyngeal mass may be obstructing the eustachian tube orifice. Thorough palpation of the neck to detect metastatic adenopathy is critical. Once again, an examination of the upper aerodigestive tract is advisable to rule out the possibility of a synchronous secondary neoplasm.

## Malignant Tumor Behavior

**Primary Tumor Site.** The most common primary tumor site within the oropharynx is the *tonsil*. Neck nodal metastases are encountered frequently, especially when the primary tumor is relatively large. The jugular nodes are commonly involved, and the retropharyngeal nodes are another common site of metastatic involvement from tonsillar carcinomas. Cancers of the *soft palate* are also encountered but are not as common as the tonsillar lesions. The soft palate has many lymphatics that frequently drain to both sides of the neck.

**Neck Nodes.** The jugular nodes represent the most common drainage site for oropharyngeal cancers. The submandibular nodes are not as frequently involved with primary tumors of the oral cavity. One therapeutic consideration involves the relatively frequent metastases to the retropharyngeal nodes (Fig. 13–35), which are surgically inaccessible. As oropharyngeal cancers approach the midline, lymphatic drainage to either or both sides of the neck is not uncommon. Occult microscopic metastases in the absence of palpable adenopathy with oropharyngeal cancers is common.

**Distant Metastases.** The rate of distant metastases is similar to that for oral cavity lesions in that the recent improvement of regional disease control has been associated with an increased frequency of distant metastases.

**Treatment.** Radiation therapy plays a key role in the treatment of oropharyngeal cancers. Tonsillar lesions especially appear to be exquisitely radiosensitive. However, as neck nodal disease becomes involved with advanced-stage tonsillar cancer, the effectiveness of radiation therapy decreases—hence the popularity of com-

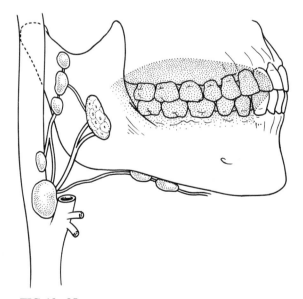

**FIG 13–35.**
The retropharyngeal nodes are often initially involved with tonsillar carcinomas. (Redrawn after Shumrick D, Gluckman I: Cancer of the oropharynx. In Suen I, Myers E: *Cancer of the head and neck,* New York, 1981. By permission of Churchill Livingstone. Used by permission.)

bined therapy programs using both surgery and radiation.

The significant challenge of rehabilitating the patient following palatal resection is the primary reason for the use of radiation therapy instead of surgical resection for small palatal cancers. Once again, larger lesions usually are treated with a combination of therapy programs.

Chemotherapy has also been evaluated for oropharyngeal carcinomas, and the results are similar to those for oral cavity tumors.

## Nasopharynx
### *Presenting Symptoms*

Tumors in the nasopharynx cause somewhat different symptoms from those in either the oral cavity or the oropharynx. Whereas both the oral cavity and oropharynx are in the direct food pathway, the nasopharynx is free from that stimulation. Therefore, an ulcerative lesion in this region frequently does not cause pain. However, there are other symptoms.

The location of the eustachian tube orifice within the nasopharynx plays a critical role in the symptoms of tumors arising in this region. If a mass occludes the eustachian tube orifice or if the mass causes venous or lymphatic obstruction that produces edema of the eustachian tube orifice so that it cannot open, the pressure differential and other factors result in the secretion of a transudate within the middle ear cleft that results in otitis media with effusion. The patient who has fluid within the middle ear experiences a sense of fullness in that ear and mild to moderate reduction of hearing. Pain is rare unless the fluid becomes secondarily infected.

Adolescent males are a special group at risk for developing a nasopharyngeal tumor. In this group, when there is a history of nasal obstruction associated with recurrent nosebleeds, it is imperative that the nasopharynx be thoroughly examined to rule out the possibility of a *nasopharyngeal angiofibroma* (Fig. 13–36).

The occurrence of *unilateral* serous otitis media in an adult mandates a thorough nasopharyngeal examination to rule out some mass effect in the form of either a benign or malignant tumor.

### *Physical Signs*

Unless the mass is huge, a nasopharyngeal tumor is rarely identified through an anterior nasal examination. Examination of the nasopharynx is necessary in any patient complaining of nasal ob-

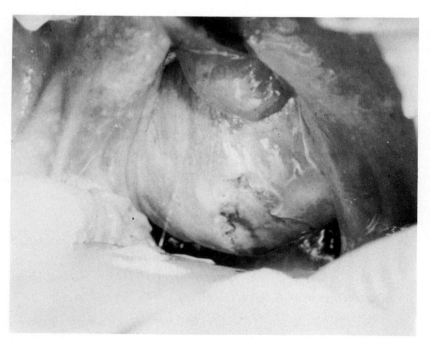

**FIG 13–36.**
Large nasopharyngeal angiotibroma extending below the free edge of the soft palate.

struction or a sensation of ear fullness. The positive findings can range from a mere ulcer to a large submucosal mass. It is important to remember that, although adenoids usually atrophy by the time an individual is 10 or 11 years of age, they sometimes persist into adulthood. Normal adenoid tissue should therefore be considered in the differential diagnosis of a nasopharyngeal mass.

### Tumor Types

The most common benign tumor of the nasopharynx other than adenoid tissue is the *nasopharyngeal angiofibroma,* which occurs almost exclusively in adolescent males. These children will typically have a history of recurrent nosebleeds and nasal obstruction. The diagnosis is confirmed by angiography documenting a vascular mass (Fig. 13–37). This is a histologically benign tumor; however, the anatomic location and proclivity for local recurrence warrant an aggressive therapeutic approach similar to that selected for a malignancy.

The most common malignancy involving the nasopharynx is, once again, *squamous cell carcinoma.* The behavior of this particular epidermoid carcinoma is dramatically different from that of tumors arising in other anatomic regions. It has a

marked predominance among Chinese people and is one of the most common cancers in China. Some evidence suggests a possible relationship to the Epstein-Barr virus.

### Risk Factors

The sex and age predilections for nasopharyngeal angiofibromas have been previously mentioned. There appears to be no special relationship between nasopharyngeal cancer and either smoking or alcohol. However, there is a high incidence of this cancer among Chinese people from the Kwantung province. There may be a correlation with dietary intake of a particular salted fish that is a common component of the southern Chinese diet.

**History and Physical Examination.** The symptoms of a nasopharyngeal tumor are often subtle, and the physical examination of this area is difficult. There is a dangerous potential for delay in diagnosis of these tumors, whether benign or malignant. It is critical for all physicians to remember that certain warning signs and symptoms should increase suspicion of serious problems so that appropriate examinations can be performed. The combination of nasal obstruction and recur-

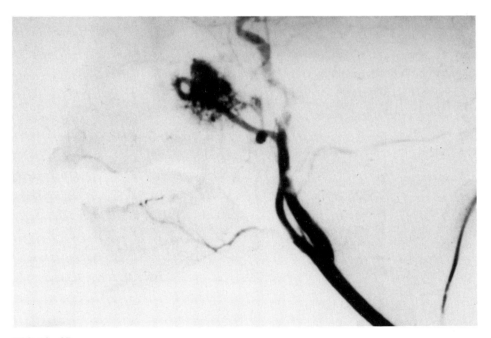

**FIG 13–37.**
Arteriography will demonstrate a highly vascular lesion with a nasopharyngeal angiofibroma.

rent epistaxis in an adolescent male and the presence of unilateral serous otitis media in an adult are both warning signs that should prompt a thorough examination of the nasopharynx.

The technique of examining the nasopharynx with a small mirror using indirect lighting restricts the examination of this region to those specialists who have expertise with this method. However, the recent development of flexible fiberoptic nasopharyngoscopes and rigid rod telescopes with prisms permits even the occasional examiner to obtain a good view of the nasopharynx. Such methods increase the accuracy of diagnosing these tumors in this relatively inaccessible anatomic location.

### Malignant Tumor Behavior

**Primary Tumor.** The nasopharynx is a relatively small area. A lesion of any size often causes an alteration of one or both eustachian tube orifices, causing symptoms and physical findings discussed earlier. For malignant lesions, the numerous lymphatic drainage pathways make nodal metastases commonplace.

**Neck Nodes.** Nasopharyngeal malignancies also differ in their metastatic pattern. Whereas most tumors arising in the head and neck involve the ipsilateral jugular nodal chain, nasopharyngeal cancers almost exclusively involve the posterior triangle nodes and frequently exhibit contralateral or bilateral nodal metastases relatively early in the course of the disease. The jugular nodes are only occasionally involved in nasopharyngeal carcinoma.

**Distant Metastases.** Distant metastases can occur in a fashion similar to other primary tumor sites in the head and neck. Pulmonary metastases appear to be the most common.

**Treatment.** For patients with nasopharyngeal angiofibromas, surgical excision remains the primary mode of treatment in the United States. This is sometimes preceded by embolization of the arteries that have been radiographically identified as the major blood supply to the tumor. Embolization has the potential for reducing the blood loss at the time of surgical resection, which can be massive because of the considerable vascular component of this tumor. The alternative to surgical resection is radiation therapy, which has been used in Canada. However, physicians in the United States are reluctant to use radiation therapy for a benign disease process because of the concern that the patients will develop radiation-induced malignancy later in life.

Most malignancies of the nasopharynx are surgically inaccessible, and radiation therapy is the primary treatment modality. Recent clinical cancer trials are evaluating the role of chemotherapy as an adjunct to radiation. Surgical intervention of the primary tumor is performed only occasionally when combined otolaryngologic-neurosurgical procedures are undertaken to resect a portion of the skull base for recurrent disease. Neck surgery is performed in patients who have either persistent or recurrent neck nodal disease in the absence of any disease within the nasopharynx.

## SLEEP DISORDERS

Sleep disorders have recently been the focus of considerable attention by the medical profession and the public. The previous notion that the sleeping state represented a protracted period of physiologic inactivity has unequivocally been demonstrated to be inaccurate. Certain sleep disorders were described many years ago. Carbon dioxide narcosis in markedly obese patients (pickwickian syndrome) has long been recognized as a medical problem, but only recently has the medical profession been aware of a group of people who experience multiple apneic episodes during sleep. The physiologic stress of these apneic periods can result in a myriad of organ system failures.

### Sleep Apnea

Certain terms associated with sleep disorders must be strictly defined. Significant apnea during sleep is considered to be a total cessation of air flow for more than 10 seconds in an adult. This cessation must exceed 15 seconds in a full-term baby and 20 seconds in a premature infant to be considered a significant apneic episode. Diagnosis of sleep apnea syndrome requires the documentation of 30 or more apneic episodes occurring during a 7-hour period of unsedated sleep. Irrespective of age, the patient who meets this definition is considered to have sleep apnea.

People with sleep apnea syndrome can be grouped according to the mechanism of the apneic episodes. In a patient who has *central* apnea, there is the cessation of air flow through either the nasal or oral cavities in conjunction with absence of any thoracic or other respiratory movement. Patients with *obstructive* sleep apnea will also have no nasal or oral air flow, but will exhibit this persistent and vigorous thoracic and other respiratory efforts. Some people will have both types of apnea, and this is termed *mixed* sleep apnea. In this situation, there is cessation of air flow with absence of respiratory efforts initially. Subsequently, respiratory efforts resume and air flow is reestablished. The obstructive type of sleep apnea is the most common form. In patients with mixed sleep apnea, the obstructive component is usually more prevalent.

### Risk Factors

Current information indicates a strong sexual predilection. The male to female ratio of persons with sleep apnea is 10:1. This ratio may change as awareness increases and more people are diagnosed. There appears to be no particular age predilection; both children and elderly adults have been diagnosed with this problem. Some researchers speculate that sudden infant death syndrome (SIDS) may sometimes be explained on the basis of an infant with sleep apnea syndrome.

Frequency among obese people appears greater. This is especially true when obesity involves the cervical anatomy. Therefore, the obese patient with a short neck (Fig. 13–38) appears to be at greater risk for developing sleep apnea than the obese patient whose subcutaneous fat deposits do not particularly involve the cervical region and who has a long neck. It must be emphasized that this syndrome does not occur exclusively among obese people. This factor is what distinguishes sleep apnea from the other sleep disorders such as the pickwickian syndrome. The patient in Fig. 13–39 was thin with a long neck yet had one of the most severe cases of obstructive sleep apnea recorded at the Ohio State University Sleep Disorder Center. Although sleep apnea is frequently seen in obese patients, especially males, it can also be noted in thin persons and can affect any age group.

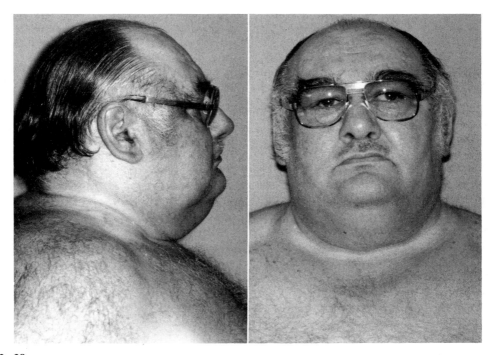

**FIG 13–38**.
This gentleman has a short and thick neck with oral cavity and pharyngeal anatomy that predispose to airway obstruction while asleep.

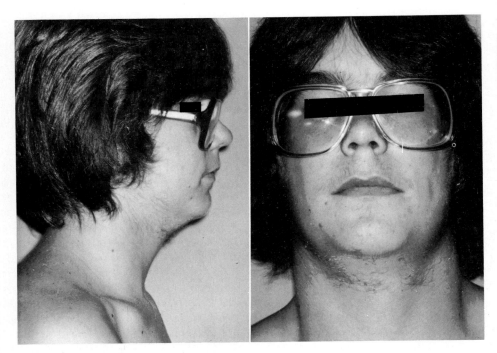

**FIG 13–39.**
Sleep disorders do not occur exclusively in obese people, as evidenced by this thin individual who had severe sleep apnea.

### Possible Mechanism of Obstruction

Although the sleep apnea syndrome is a relatively new entity, a variety of possible etiologies have been described in an attempt to define the mechanism of obstruction. These hypotheses can basically be subdivided into those dealing with *static* anatomic abnormalities and those involving *dynamic* anatomic alterations.

A group of *static* anatomic changes has been noted or proposed in patients with obstructive sleep apnea. Obstruction of the nasal air flow secondary to septal deviation and/or hypertrophic turbinates can be severe enough to force oral breathing. If this nasal obstruction is accompanied by adenotonsillar hypertrophy, the patient may have problems with exchange through either the nasal or oral cavities.

A recessed mandible (retrognathia) can also reduce the volume of the oral airway so as to compromise respiratory exchange during sleep. Other static obstructions include an abnormally enlarged tongue (microglossia), vocal cord dysfunction, and masses of the hypopharynx. Any occult cyst of the supraglottic larynx or other abnormalities such as congenital laryngeal anomalies may compromise the air flow during the sleep state. Al-though such anatomic abnormalities theoretically can result in sleep apnea, it is not common to demonstrate an isolated problem that lends itself to surgical correction that ultimately will totally resolve the patient's sleep disorder.

There has been interest in hypotheses that deal with *dynamic* changes occurring within the laryngopharynx that may cause airway obstruction during sleep. Repetitive glottic spasms, soft palate appositions to the posterior pharyngeal wall, genioglossus muscle inhibition with resulting tongue prolapse, passive prolapse of the hypopharynx, and active hypopharyngeal contraction have been proposed as dynamic mechanisms that could cause airway obstruction.

One uniform area of the upper airway appears to consistently represent the level of obstruction. Video recordings (Fig. 13–40) of the dynamic alterations in the oropharynx and laryngopharynx during the sleep state suggest that some patients experience obstruction at the level of the hypopharynx just superior to the laryngeal inlet (Fig. 13–41). The vocal cords remain abducted throughout these events. However, other evaluations have shown that many patients experience the initial obstruction at the level of the orophar-

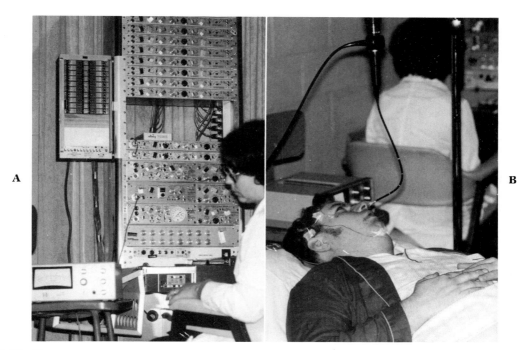

**FIG 13–40.**
**A,** a patient undergoing an evaluation of a sleep disorder in a sleep laboratory, which simultaneously measures the numerous parameters during sleep including even the possibility of **B,** visualizing changes in laryngopharyngeal anatomy during sleep.

ynx. Obstruction can probably occur at a variety of levels; the accurate determination of the level of obstruction is important in the choice of treatment.

As mentioned, it is unusual for a patient with obstructive sleep apnea to have a singular anatomic abnormality that could be surgically corrected to the extent that it totally cures the patient of the sleep disorder. However, it has been noted that one patient can have a variety of anatomic abnormalities that collectively result in reduction of the volume of the upper airway. Abnormalities such as an abnormally large tongue, retrognathic mandible, long palate, shallow pharynx, hyperactive gag reflex, short neck, and floppy epiglottis can contribute to "disproportionate anatomy" that results in a decreased oral and hypopharyngeal volume and predisposes to airway obstruction while the patient is in a supine position during sleep.

### Presenting Symptoms

There are no symptoms that are pathognomonic of sleep apnea. However, certain symptoms can be considered suggestive of a sleep dis-

order and the need for further evaluation. One initial clue is that the patient has excessive daytime somnolence. The person who has difficulty maintaining a job because of inability to stay awake may be experiencing sleep apnea. In addition, sleep apnea appears to have some relationship to restless sleep activity and loud snoring. Patients who are experiencing sleep disorders will frequently have impaired sexual activity. The patient's sleep mate may notice periods of apnea while the patient sleeps and difficulty in arousing the patient from the sleep state. It is not uncommon for patients with sleep apnea to have to be struck in order to be awakened and resume breathing.

### Presenting Signs

When examining the patient who has symptoms suggestive of a sleep disorder, one should look at anatomic features that might result in compromise of the upper airway. Therefore, an evaluation of the length and width of their neck and the amount of subcutaneous tissue within the neck is important. It then becomes critical to evaluate the volume of the oral cavity, orophar-

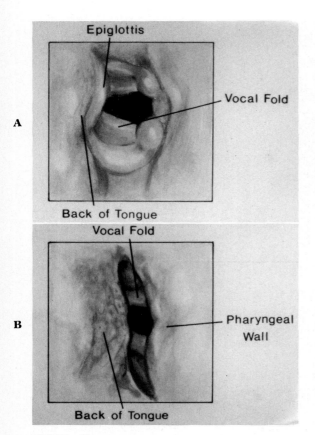

**A**

**B**

**FIG 13–41.**
**A,** appearance of laryngopharynx during nonobstructed sleep and **B,** collapse of hypopharyngeal soft tissue superior to the larynx which results in airway obstruction during apnea.

ynx, and hypopharynx. When present, those anatomic deviations previously described as disproportionate anatomy, such as an abnormally large tongue, narrow mandibular arch, recessed mandible, shallow pharynx, long uvula and/or palate, hyperactive gag, adenotonsillar hypertrophy, and floppy epiglottis should all be noted. Three or more of these features may constitute disproportionate anatomy, which is frequently seen in people with obstructive sleep apnea (Fig. 13–42).

### Method of Evaluation

Although the symptoms and physical signs can help to identify a group of people who have sleep apnea, the diagnosis of this disorder cannot be made yet by any isolated radiographic or other diagnostic evaluation. The patient must undergo a comprehensive evaluation in a sleep laboratory that involves multisystem monitoring over a protracted period of sleep. This is accomplished with the polysomnograph, which allows for multichannel evaluations of electroencephalogram, electrocardiogram, intercostal electromyogram, ear oximetry, nasal air flow, oral air flow, and even video endoscopic recordings if desirable. After this multisystem recording is completed, it is analyzed and the frequency and type of apneic episodes are noted. It ultimately permits the diagnosis on the basis of quantifiable objective data. The generation of these data also permits the mechanism for evaluating response to therapy.

### Treatment

Sleep apnea can be treated with either medical or surgical approaches. The nonsurgical approach usually involves the use of certain respiratory stimulants such as the tricyclic antidepressants. L-tryptophan has also been used with some success either alone or in combination with other medications. Other adjunctive approaches such as adjusting the position of a patient can provide supplemental benefits. Patients seem to have less obstruction when they are sleeping in a lateral rather than a supine position. One way in which the patient can maintain a lateral position during sleep, for example, is to place tennis balls in the pockets on the back of the pajamas. This helps prevent the patient from rolling into the supine position. Nasopharyngeal or other types of airway expanders have not met with uniform success in the nonsedated patient because of patient intolerance. Weight reduction programs are an important adjunct to the nonsurgical treatment, but are rarely effective enough to resolve the sleep apnea problem.

The surgical approaches attempt to bypass the level of obstruction. One form of surgical treatment has been tracheotomy. Because of the anatomic peculiarities common to this patient population (i.e., short necks with considerable layers of adipose tissue), standard surgical approaches and tubes have seldom been applicable. It has become necessary to modify the standard surgical approaches to tracheotomy in addition to using different equipment (Fig. 13–43).

In addition, other surgical treatment has been described. Uvulopalatopharyngoplasty is an operation that is intended to remove redundant mucosal folds in the area of the oropharynx. The op-

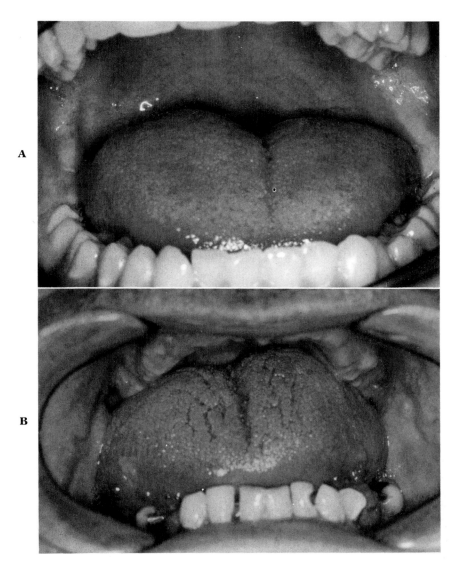

**FIG 13–42.**
**A,** example of normal oral cavity and pharyngeal anatomic relationships in a patient with no obstructive sleep apnea and **B,** obstructive sleep apnea patient who has disproportionate anatomy characterized by an unusually narrow mandibular arch, large tongue, flat palatal arch, and shallow pharynx.

eration, which effectively expands the air-containing volume of the oropharynx, is successful in a certain percentage of patients with obstructive sleep apnea. It probably reflects that group of patients whose obstruction is occurring at the level of the oropharynx rather than the hypopharynx. The advantage of this operative approach is that it avoids the need for permanent tracheotomy. This operation has also helped patients with severe snoring problems with or without sleep apnea.

Information concerning sleep apnea continues to increase rapidly. It is anticipated that more patients will be diagnosed as having sleep apnea as the medical profession becomes more familiar with it. Refinements in diagnosis and treatment will inevitably follow this greater awareness.

## SPECIAL CLINICAL CONSIDERATIONS

A number of observable changes in this section of the upper aerodigestive tract are not strictly

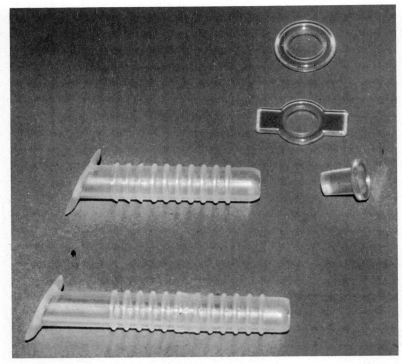

**FIG 13–43.**
The tracheal cannula is a means of providing access to the trachea that bypasses the obstruction during apnea but permits vocalization and nasal breathing while awake.

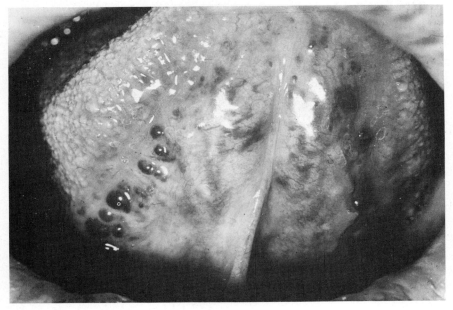

**FIG 13–44.**
Lingual varicosities.

A

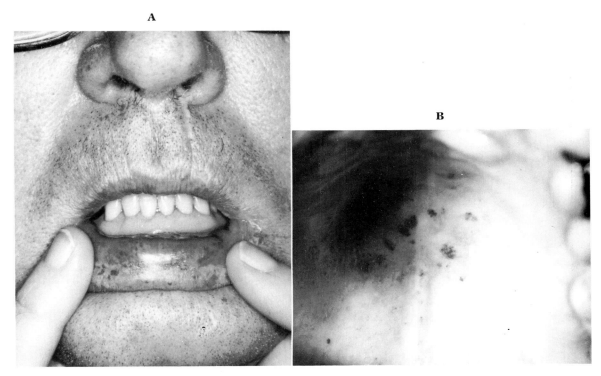

**FIG 13–45.**
Patient with hereditary hemorrhagic telengectasia has lesions present on **A,** the lip, nose, and **B,** hard palate.

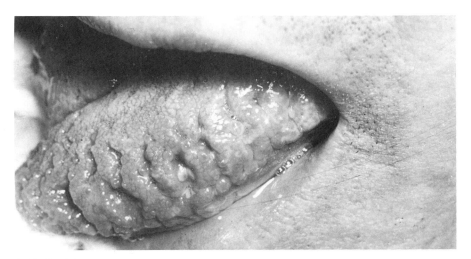

**FIG 13–46.**
Fissured tongue, asymptomatic.

considered to be tumors or the results of any inflammatory process.

### Varicose Veins

Varicose veins can develop on the ventral surface of the tongue (Fig. 13–44). This is especially common in the elderly. Varicosities are also noted in the valleculae and sometimes over the surface of the tongue base. They appear as bluish bulges under the mucosa. They rarely are the site of bleeding or the cause of symptoms, and no treatment is necessary.

### Hereditary Hemorrhagic Telangiectasia

Telangiectasia of Rendu-Osler-Weber disease involves any of the oral cavity structures as well as other surface areas of the oral mucosa. It is rare for telangiectases within the oral cavity and pharynx to cause significant bleeding (Fig. 13–45). This observation is in sharp contrast to the fragility of these lesions in the nasal mucous membranes, which can be the site of massive epistaxis. The telangiectases are submucosal, and the nasal mucous membrane's thinness permits frequent trauma to the underlying telangiectases, which appear to contain arterial blood. Removing the nasal mucous membranes containing the telangiectases and applying a skin graft (septal dermoplasty) are effective treatment.

### Fissured Tongue

Fissured tongue refers to the appearance of deep furrows along the lateral edges of the tongue (Fig. 13–46). It is considered to be a familial disorder, but it is not always congenital. Food particles can occasionally become entrapped within the fissure, causing localized glossitis. No treatment is necessary for a fissured tongue except for any infections caused by trapped food.

### Prominent Lingual Frenum

A prominent lingual frenum can impair the normal mobility of the tongue. This was formerly believed to be the cause of a child's misarticulations. Incising this frenum was a common prac-

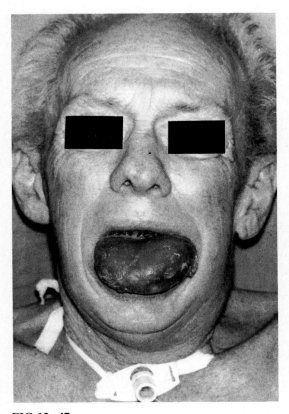

**FIG 13–47.**
Massive tongue edema occurred as a result of obstruction of lymphatics by large tongue base cancer.

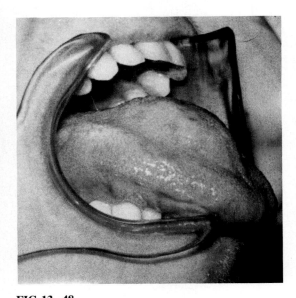

**FIG 13–48.**
This patient developed an abcess within the tongue musculature following accidental puncture wound with a pencil.

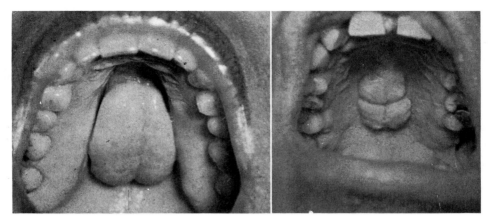

**FIG 13–49.**
Large tori palatini.

tice to correct the speech problem. However, it has since been demonstrated that if the tongue can touch the anterior dentition, mobility is adequate for the development of normal speech. In those rare situations in which the frenum significantly impedes the tongue excursion, Z-plasty of the frenum is preferable to a simple incision. Incision of the frenum can result in the development of a thick nondistensible scar contraction band that might actually cause more restricted movement than the original frenum.

### Macroglossia

Some individuals have larger tongues than others. There are racial differences between the size of the tongue relative to the other oral cavity structures. Some clinical conditions can also cause this situation, namely lymphangioma, amyloid deposits, and lymphedema (Fig. 13–47). Allergic reactions, such as angioneurotic edema, can result in enlargement of the tongue for several hours before it subsides. This clinical situation can also be caused by submucosal tumors and even by hematomas or abscess formation (Fig. 13–48). Understanding the etiology is critical to determining appropriate therapy.

### Torus Palatinus

Torus palatinus is a bony exostosis located in the midportion of the hard palate, which is cov-

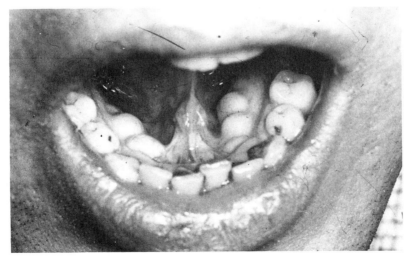

**FIG 13–50.**
Multiple mandibular tori. Large growths like these are unusual, but smaller ones are common.

ered by the palatal epithelium (Fig. 13–49). The mass is usually solitary and located in the midline. There is no increased potential for malignant degeneration. Excision is advisable only when it is necessary for proper fitting of a maxillary denture.

## Torus Mandibularis

Toris mandibularis is similar to torus palatinus except that it is attached to the mandible and frequently occurs bilaterally with attachment on the lingual aspect of the mandible near the midline (Fig. 13–50). For the uninformed, it represents a diagnostic challenge. It is rare that any type of treatment is necessary except for surgical contouring to improve denture fittings.

## Bifid Uvula

The bifid uvula as an isolated entity rarely has any clinical significance (Fig. 13–51). However, it is sometimes associated with submucous cleft palate. Submucous cleft palate exists when there is mucosal continuity of the soft palate but discontinuity of the palatal musculature and loss of the posterior nasal spine (Fig. 13–52). The palatal musculature participates in elevating and tensing the palate during swallowing and talking. Because of the possibility for hypernasal speech in a child who undergoes adenoidectomy in the presence of a submucous cleft palate, it is imperative that every individual with a bifid uvula be exam-

ined for the presence of a submucous cleft palate before nasopharyngeal surgery such as adenoidectomy is performed. The removal of this pad of lymphoid tissue in the nasopharynx coupled with a submucous cleft palate that has compromised palatal movement may be enough to cause inadequate closure of the palate to the posterior pharyngeal wall, resulting in hypernasal speech.

## Gingival Hyperplasia

Gingival hyperplasia can result from a long-standing irritation. It could be localized or diffuse with upper and lower jaw involvement (Fig. 13–53). Patients who have been receiving phenytoin for seizure control may develop gingival enlargement as a result of connective tissue proliferation. In addition, it is sometimes seen in patients with leukemia. Poor-fitting dentures can even cause gingival hyperplasia.

## Epulis

A giant-cell epulis usually occurs near an infected tooth root that has caused an area of local-

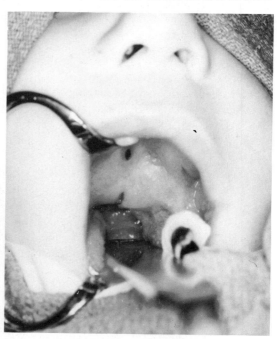

**FIG 13–52.**
This child has a discontinuity of the soft palate musculature, which creates a "blue line" in the midline of the soft palate up to the point where there is actual dehiscence at the posterior edge of the hard palate.

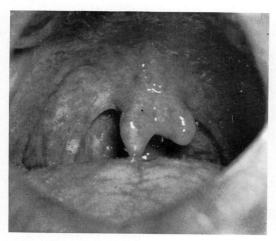

**FIG 13–51.**
Bifid uvula.

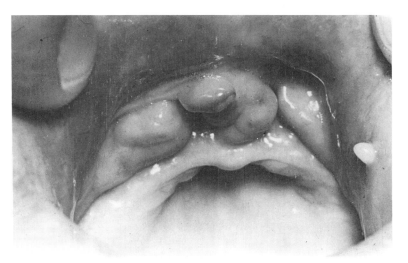

**FIG 13–53.**
Gingival hyperplasia caused by an ill-fitting denture.

ized osteomyelitis (Fig. 13–54). Treatment involves the extraction of the infected tooth and excision of the epulis. Sometimes an epulis develops during pregnancy, and treatment is deferred until after delivery. Removal during pregnancy is marked by a high recurrence rate.

### Amalgam Tattoo

Amalgam tattoo is a common cause of confusion. It is a deposit of silver amalgam inadvertently implanted during filling of a dental caries. It can also result during an extraction and become incorporated into the submucous tissue layer. It appears as a pigmented lesion (Fig. 13–55) and

can be confused with malignancies such as melanoma.

### Fordyce Spots

Fordyce spots are sebaceous glands located in the submucosal tissue of the buccal area. They appear as yellow spots that are not elevated (Fig. 13–56). Fordyce spots are part of the normal anatomy and need no treatment.

### White Lesions

White lesions are frequently the source of confusion among clinicians. Most are not malignant

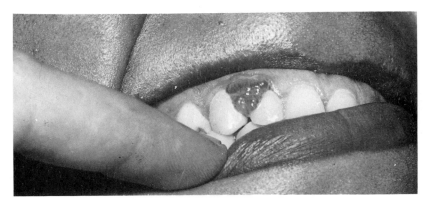

**FIG 13–54.**
Giant cell epulis.

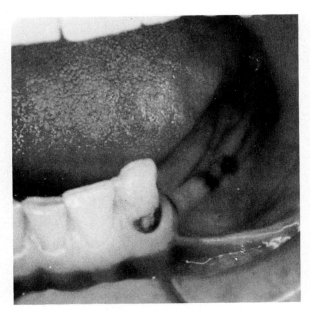

**FIG 13–55.**
Amalgam tattoo occurs as a result of filling material gaining access to beneath the mucosa.

and are not even considered premalignant changes. The only exception is leukoplakia, which will be discussed later.

### Lichen Planus

Lichen planus is actually a dermatologic disease that can involve the oral mucous membranes. In fact lichen planus can be present only in the oral cavity without causing skin changes. When there is involvement of the skin, it is usually on the flexor surface of the arms and legs. The lesions appear as purple papules, and they can be pruritic. The oral lesions present as fine filamentous white lines that are arranged in a lacelike pattern predominantly in the buccal mucosa (Fig. 13–57). They are white because there is increased keratin production in this area. The cause is unknown. Lichen planus usually causes minimal symptoms, and the patient is often unaware of its existence. No treatment is necessary. There

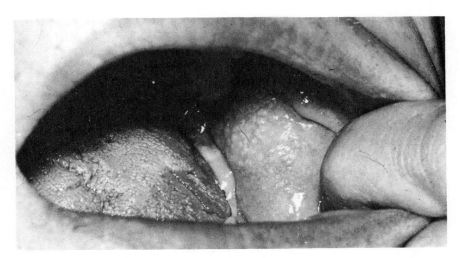

**FIG 13–56.**
Fordyce spots—normal sebaceous glands just under the buccal mucosa. They are seen in every adult.

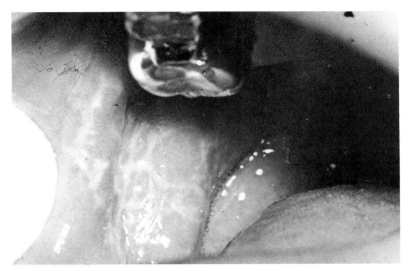

**FIG 13-57.**
Lichen planus in the buccal mucosa. Note the lacelike pattern. No skin lesions were present. The patient recovered without treatment, except reassurance, and then relapsed. He had no symptoms.

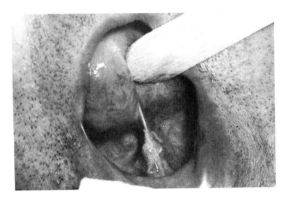

**FIG 13-58.**
Hyperkeratosis. This condition must be distinguished from leukoplakia and cancer.

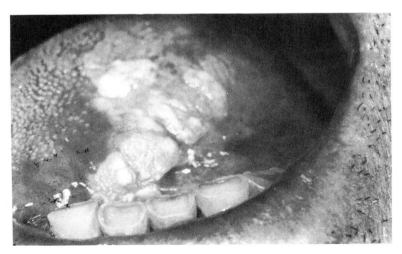

**FIG 13-59.**
Leukoplakia, side of the tongue. Tissue diagnosis was necessary to differentiate the condition from cancer.

is no increased potential for premalignant change or malignant degeneration.

### Hyperkeratosis

Hyperkeratosis can involve any portion of the oral cavity. However, its sites of predilection are the buccal mucosa and the tongue (Fig. 13–58). It can result from a local irritant. There rarely are any symptoms. Histologic examination reveals nothing to suggest premalignant degeneration.

### Linea Alba

As the redundant buccal mucosa becomes traumatized between the molar teeth, linea alba can form a thickened line that runs horizontally from the posterior portion of the buccal mucosa forward to the first molar. Once again, it is white as a function of the increased keratin content. It is so common that it is actually considered to be a variant of normal. No treatment is necessary.

### Leukoplakia

Leukoplakia is considered to be a premalignant change. It presents as a white lesion within any areas of the oral cavity (Fig. 13–59). However, histologically there are epithelioid changes suggestive of premalignant degeneration. These lesions are thick and plaquelike. No suggestion of a fine pattern is seen in lichen planus. The lesions can be the result of irritation from ill-fitting dentures or a jagged tooth. Surgical excision is advisable and will provide both therapeutic and diagnostic results.

# PART IV
# Salivary Glands

# 14

# Anatomy and Physiology

## ANATOMY

Understanding of the basic gross anatomy of the salivary glands facilitates comprehension of their pathology. These glands are intimately associated with numerous critical nerves and vessels in the head and neck area. Any abnormalities involving the salivary tissue have the potential to compromise the functions of these structures. Although there are literally thousands of minor salivary glands throughout the upper aerodigestive tract and the paranasal sinuses, this discussion focuses on the major salivary glands. There are three paired major salivary glands that account for most of the salivary production: the parotid, submandibular, and sublingual glands.

## Parotid Gland

The *parotid gland* is located in the preauricular area. Although a portion of its anterior component overlies the vertical ramus of the mandible, a substantial amount of the gland is between the vertical ramus of the mandible and the external ear canal (Fig. 14–1). The tail of the parotid gland extends inferiorly and somewhat posteriorly to lie below the mandible. Masses in the tail sometimes are confused with the upper cervical lymph nodes. The gland itself is covered by skin and a relatively thin layer of subcutaneous fat.

The facial nerve is deeply embedded within parotid tissue and not protected by any facial or other layers. In addition to the facial nerve, the greater auricular and auriculotemporal nerves are related to the parotid gland. There are also several veins coursing about the gland. The external carotid artery, internal maxillary, and superficial temporal arteries are intimately related to its deep portion.

The parotid duct courses anteriorly from the gland, crosses the masseter muscle, and then turns deep to penetrate the buccinator muscle, where it enters intraorally through the buccal mucosa opposite the maxillary second molar. The horizontal plane of the duct is generally considered to be on a line drawn from the bottom of the ear canal to a point just above the oral commissure. The medial extent of the parotid gland comes to lie adjacent to the lateral oropharyngeal wall. It is conceivable for neoplasms arising within the deep lobe of the parotid gland to cause medial displacement of the oropharyngeal wall, which is detected not by external examination but by intraoral inspection and palpation (Fig. 14–2). It is important also to recognize that there are lymph nodes adjacent to the capsule of the gland and within the substance of the gland itself.

The parotid gland is divided into multiple small compartments by strong fibrous septa. These septa account for the lack of noticeable fluctuation with the development of a parotid abscess.

## Submandibular Gland

The *submandibular gland* is the second largest of the major salivary glands. It lies just inferior to the body of the mandible and slightly anterior to the angle, being located in the submandibular triangle, which is bound by the anterior and posterior bellies of the digastric muscle (Fig. 14–3). In children, this gland is frequently not palpable because it is located along the medial aspect of the mandible. As supporting fascial structures relax

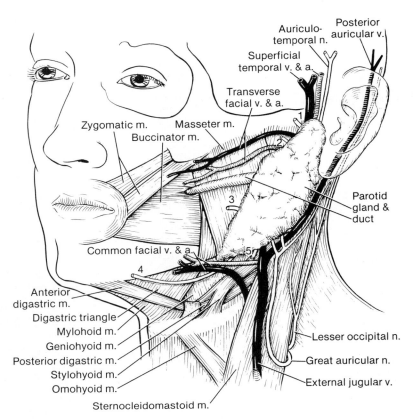

**FIG 14–1.**
Normal anatomy of parotid glands.

with age, the gland assumes a lower position in the neck. It is not uncommon for this gland to be a source of confusion to the clinician examining the elderly patient, in whom it may be palpable below the body of the mandible. The deep surface of the gland is against the mylohyoid muscle and also the hypoglossus muscle. The facial artery, which is a branch of the external carotid system, traverses the gland, initially entering in the posteroinferior portion of the gland, coursing obliquely, and exiting superiorly as it joins the facial vein to course over the mandible heading toward the corner of the mouth. The submandibular (Wharton's) duct runs from the anterior portion of

**FIG 14–2.**
This intraoral photograph shows a tumor of the deep lobe of the parotid gland, which has medially displaced the lateral pharyngeal wall to the extent that it has caused ulceration of the overlying mucosa.

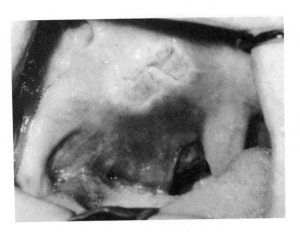

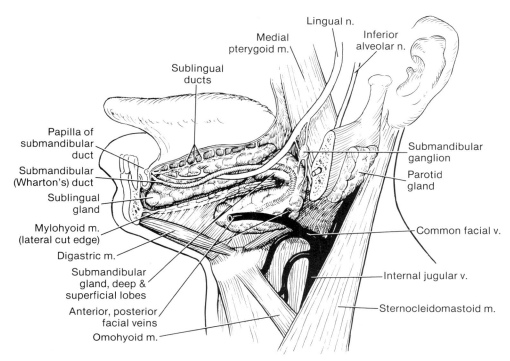

**FIG 14–3.**
Normal anatomy of the submandibular gland.

the gland deep to the mylohyoid muscle, heading toward the anterior floor of the mouth and entering it adjacent to the lingual frenulum near the midline.

The hypoglossal nerve (cranial nerve XII) courses deep to the gland along the floor of the submandibular triangle. The lingual nerve, which provides the route of parasympathetic innervation, is located superior to it and is actually attached to the gland through the submandibular ganglion. The marginal mandibular branch of the facial nerve, as it courses toward the corner of the lip, drops below the body of the mandible and runs over the submandibular gland lateral to the facial artery and vein and then curves superiorly toward the corner of the mouth. Multiple lymph nodes are located about the submandibular gland. It is rare for a lymph node to be located within the substance of the gland, as is the case with the parotid gland.

### Sublingual Gland

The *sublingual gland* is the smallest of the three major salivary glands and lies deep to the mucosa of the anterolateral floor of the mouth (Fig. 14–4). It actually rests on the mylohyoid musculature. Instead of there being a single duct, multiple ducts exit the gland from its superior surface and enter the floor of the mouth at multiple sites. In contrast to the other two glands, just a few lymph nodes are associated occasionally with the sublingual gland.

## PHYSIOLOGY

The physiology of the major salivary glands involves primarily the types of secretions and the mechanism of stimulation. The parotid secretions are largely serous in consistency. This is in contrast to those of the submandibular gland, which are both serous and mucous secretions. The fact that there is a substantial mucous component that needs to be drained through a duct coursing from an inferior to a superior orientation explains some of the problems noted with calculi involving this gland. The sublingual gland produces a primarily mucous secretion. The minor salivary glands do not produce one predominant type of secretion.

The secretion of the major and minor salivary

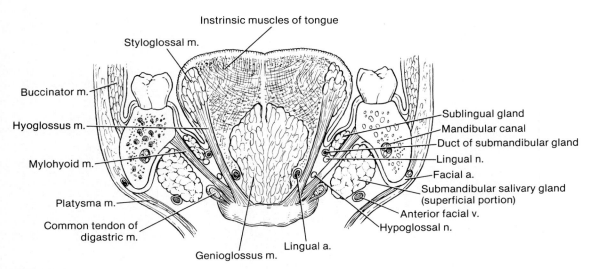

**FIG 14–4.**
Normal anatomy of sublingual gland.

glands is controlled by the physical stimulation of food or other matter in the oral cavity. However, there is also a psychic component of stimuli arising from the taste, smell, or even vision. These stimuli are mediated primarily through the autonomic nervous system. The paraganglionic parasympathetic innervation to the parotid gland actually traverses the middle ear en route to the otic ganglion, which is suspended from the auriculotemporal branch of the third division of the trigeminal nerve (cranial nerve V) (Fig. 14–5). The sympathetic component arises from the carotid plexus traveling with the carotid artery. The preganglionic parasympathetic fibers going to the submandibular gland also traverse the middle ear through a branch of the seventh nerve, the chorda tympani (Fig. 14–6). After exiting the middle ear, it joins the lingual nerve, also from the third branch of the trigeminal nerve, where its fibers synapse in the submandibular ganglion, which is

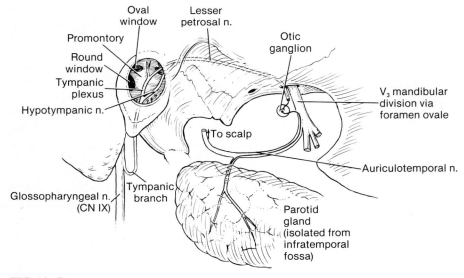

**FIG 14–5**.
Parasympathetic innervation to the parotid gland is by means of the otic ganglion.

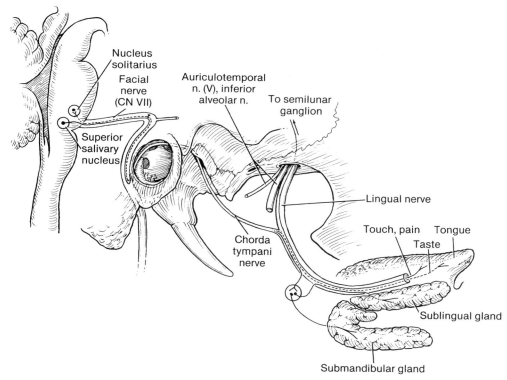

**FIG 14–6.**
Parasympathetic innervation to the submandibular gland via the submandibular ganglion.

attached to the submandibular gland. Once again, the sympathetic fibers travel by way of the carotid plexus to the submandibular gland.

The actual rate of salivary flow is highly varible and strongly dependent on stimuli. Production appears to be markedly reduced early in the day, progressively increasing throughout the day. During sleep there is essentially no salivary production. Although the actual total daily volume of salivary production cannot be accurately determined, it is estimated to be approximately 500 mL. About 90% of the total salivary production comes from the parotid and submandibular glands, with the remainder being produced by the minor and sublingual glands.

Saliva serves many functions. Its lubricating function aids the production of a food bolus. It also has a dental protective mechanism because there are minerals within the saliva that help the maturation of the teeth. The bicarbonate and phosphates within saliva also have a certain amount of antibacterial activity. Secretory IgA is present in saliva, and this appears to facilitate bacterial phagocytosis. Lysozymes are also present within the saliva to help in bacterial cell wall destruction. Numerous factors, such as radiation therapy, medications, and systemic diseases, can all affect not only the quantity but also the quality of salivary production.

# 15

# Special Diagnostic Procedures

Diagnostic evaluation of salivary gland disease relies heavily on the patient's presenting symptoms and physical findings. However, additional diagnostic procedures can provide supplemental information, although they frequently do not represent an alternative to obtaining a tissue diagnosis, especially in the case of neoplasms. Procedures with some adjunctive potential benefit are sialograms, radioisotope scanning, computed tomography, and fine-needle aspiration.

## SIALOGRAMS

Sialograms, which have been used for a number of years, involve the insertion of a small catheter through the duct of either the parotid or the submandibular gland and the injection of a small amount of radiopaque dye. This allows evaluation of the nature and position of the ductal system (Fig. 15–1). The caliber and length of the main duct can be studied as well as the configuration of the small ductules. The sialogram can be used to evaluate patients with recurrent inflammatory disease of the salivary glands or to evaluate ductule or duct displacement or gland destruction as a result of neoplasm. Sialectasia can be noted in some of the connective tissue disorders and therefore is a helpful radiographic determination. Most information obtained from sialography, once again, is supportive of a diagnosis but not pathognomonic for a particular disease state.

## RADIOISOTOPE SCANNING

Radioisotope scanning of the salivary glands has been performed using primarily technetium.

Uptake is increased following intravenous injection of the radioisotope, and the gland to be studied is scanned several minutes later. In those glands which have been chronically inflamed over a protracted period, the uptake is generally decreased. Because of the amount of variability in uptake among patients, it is best to compare uptake within the same patient by using a noninvolved counterpart gland as the control. Radioisotope scanning is usually not valuable for nonneoplastic pathology of the salivary glands. It has some usefulness in evaluation of salivary neoplasms. It can confirm the presence of a mass and indicate its size and position (Fig. 15–2). Those neoplasms with increased uptake usually represent a benign process. Two lesions that classically produce the appearance of a "hot" nodule are the Wharton's tumor and the oncocytoma.

Malignancies usually result in some destruction of a portion of the gland, and this can be visualized on the scan. However, none of these findings are consistent enough to permit diagnosis of any particular disease process.

## COMPUTED TOMOGRAPHY AND MAGNETIC RESONANCE IMAGING

Computed tomography has proved a helpful, noninvasive means of identifying the position and size of a salivary mass (Fig. 15–3). It is replacing sialography and radioisotope scanning as the imaging procedure of choice for salivary gland pathology.

Magnetic resonance imaging represents an exciting technique that does not require irradiation and provides impressive soft tissue detail (Fig.

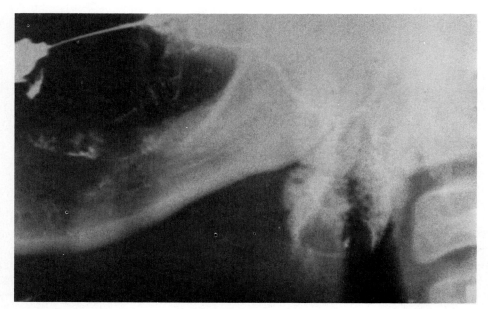

**FIG 15–1.**
This parotid sialogram shows a normal duct with the normal parotid duct and a lacy ductal system.

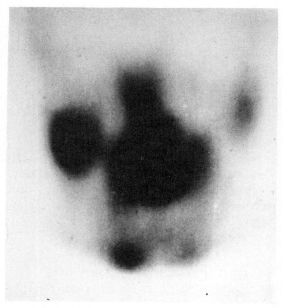

**FIG 15–2.**
A large tumor of the parotid gland.

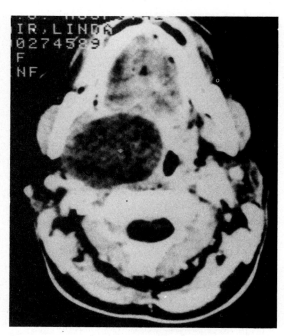

**FIG 15–3.**
This computed tomogram demonstrates the location of a large mixed tumor involving the deep lobe of the parotid gland and medially displacing the lateral wall of the oropharynx.

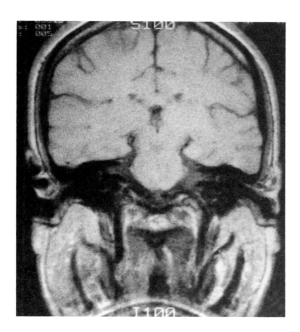

**FIG 15–4.**
Magnetic resonance image of a patient shows normal anatomy of the parotid gland.

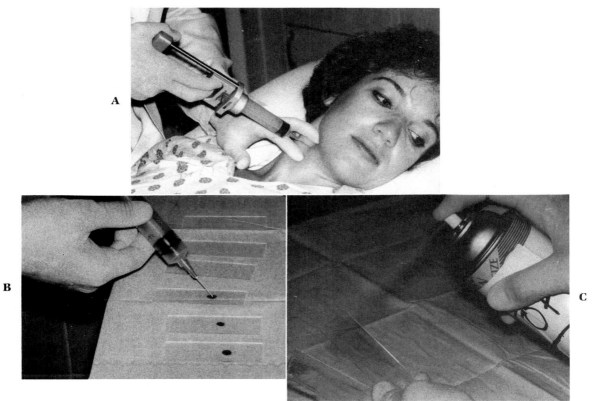

**FIG 15–5.**
**A,** fine-needle aspiration is accomplished by stabilizing the mass between the fingers of one hand while the needle is inserted into the tumor. Aspiration follows. **B,** immediately after aspiration, the contents of the syringe are transferred to a glass slide and smeared. **C,** the slide is quickly sprayed with a fixative to prevent air drying of cellular contents.

15–4). There is no question that computed tomography still is a useful imaging technology
when bony detail is required. However, magnetic
resonance imaging is proving to be extremely useful for soft tissue analysis of salivary gland problems. As the sophistication of computed tomography and magnetic resonance imaging increases
their diagnostic capabilities, conventional sialography and radioisotope scanning have become less
frequently used.

## FINE-NEEDLE ASPIRATION

Fine-needle aspiration biopsy is used in an attempt to obtain a histologic diagnosis of a neoplasm. This technique is probably safer when
used on the submandibular gland than on the parotid gland, where blind insertion of a needle may
traumatize one of the branches of the facial nerve.
A 21-gauge needle is inserted into the mass, and
negative pressure removes some cells (Fig.
15–5). The cells are immediately placed on slides
and fixed. The staining that follows permits histopathologic examination. Total familiarity with
the technique and expertise by the surgical pathologist are required. Extensive experience is
necessary for the pathologist to make a definitive
diagnosis with a limited amount of cellular material. For these reasons, fine-needle aspiration has
not received widespread acceptance yet.

It is evident that there are currently no noninvasive diagnostic procedures with enough specificity to permit a tissue diagnosis for the patient.
For this reason, biopsy of salivary gland neoplasms is usually necessary. This approach will
be discussed in subsequent chapters on neoplasms.

# 16

# Infections, Inflammations, and Neoplasms

## INFECTIONS AND INFLAMMATIONS

Infectious and inflammatory diseases of the salivary glands are common. They most frequently involve the major salivary glands, and the parotid gland seems especially vulnerable. The glands can be infected by either bacteria or viruses. In fact, the clinical symptoms can be grouped according to the etiology of the infection and its time course.

### Acute Bacterial Sialoadenitis

Acute bacterial sialoadenitis primarily involves either the parotid or submandibular glands. The history will relate a rather short onset of edema of the gland, which causes marked pain. There is also edema of the tissue about the infected gland. Fever and elevation of the white blood cell count in the peripheral blood are not uncommon. On physical examination, the involved gland will be enlarged, tender to palpation, and indurated. Pressure on the gland usually releases purulent fluid from the involved gland's duct orifice (Fig. 16–1).

In the past, most of these cases, especially those involving the parotid gland, were seen in postoperative patients. Although less common now than in the past, surgical parotitis still occurs. It seems especially prone to occur in patients whose overall health is compromised by poor nutritional status, dehydration, or an imbalance in fluid and electrolytes. However, most recently this disease appears to be especially common in immunocompromised patients with malignancies or those who are candidates for organ transplantation.

Coagulase-positive *Staphylococcus aureus* is the most common pathogenic bacteria seen from cultures of the infected salivary secretions. Cultures should be obtained as soon as possible depending on the degree of systemic illness. Blood cultures are sometimes taken. If the patient is severely ill, often antibiotics are given before culture results are available. Usually an antibiotic is used that is appropriate for penicillinase-resistant *Staphylococcus*. When there is septicemia, some of the broader-spectrum antibiotics that have antistaphylococcal properties are used. Usually, with proper antibiotic management and attention to the fluid and electrolyte balance, there is prompt improvement in the symptoms and physical findings. However, if patients do not show any improvement on physical examination, they may be developing abscesses. Fluctuance is usually detectable if the sialoadenitis involves the submandibular gland, but because of the septations throughout the parotid gland that were previously mentioned, it is not possible to palpate fluctuance in the parotid gland. Rather than one abscess, there are usually multiple small abscesses.

In the absence of clinical improvement, the presumptive diagnosis is a parotid abscess, and formal drainage must follow. However, because of the presence of the facial nerve, incision and drainage are complicated. The procedure usually requires a general anesthetic. Skin flaps are elevated away from the parotid gland, and a series of superficial incisions are made, followed by blunt probing of the parotid gland to drain the multiple abscesses that are usually encountered.

Acute viral infections also are possible. Mumps is the most common viral cause of sialoadenitis, this primarily affecting children and

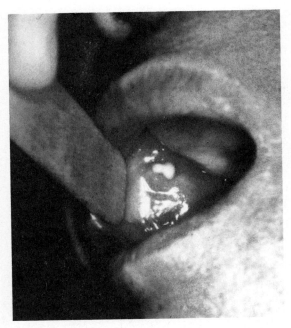

**FIG 16–1.**
External pressure on the parotid gland of this patient with acute bacterial sialadenitis produced pus at the parotid duct orifice.

young adults. The patients have a rather sudden onset of fever, systemic symptoms such as headache, and ultimately swelling of both parotid glands. The swelling progresses rather quickly and then decreases over a longer period of time. The distinction between a bacterial and a viral etiology is that the salivary drainage is clear with a viral problem. Sometimes secondary suppuration can follow a viral sialoadenitis. Other phenomena are associated with mumps sialoadenitis, such as the possibility of development of a sensorineural hearing loss. Coxsackievirus A and echovirus have also been identified as causing a viral sialoadenitis. As expected, there is no specific treatment for this type of infection.

## Chronic Sialoadenitis

There are times when an acute sialoadenitis does not totally resolve and predisposes to chronicity in the sense of causing recurrent inflammatory episodes. When this problem is bacterial in origin, most frequently the parotid gland is involved. There are many hypotheses about the cause of the chronic state. However, some component of ductal obstruction appears to be critical to the ongoing situation.

In addition to a bacterial etiology, other causes have been considered. Some anticholinergic medications may cause persistent decreased salivary outflow, with resultant secondary inspissation of the saliva, which predisposes to chronic sialadenitis. With chronic sialoadenitis, there appears to be not only an alteration in the amount of salivary flow, but also some retention leading to stasis of the secretions. The quality of saliva also seems to change with this condition. In short, a rather complex interrelationship among events causes compromised salivary gland function in the presence of bacterial infection.

The history documents repeated episodes of glandular enlargement and mild to moderate tenderness, which is potentiated by eating. The gland is not as tender to palpation or as indurated as the acutely infected gland. However, it is not unusual for some purulent fluid to be noted exiting the ductal orifice. The intent is to promote salivary flow with the use of sialagogues. To decrease the chance of salivary stasis, patients are asked to massage the gland to decompress it. None of the treatment programs recommended are consistently successful. It is important to assess whether there are any anatomic reasons for outflow obstructions of the main ductal system such as a stone in the duct or strictures. Surgical removal of the gland is indicated only when conservative management programs have failed to control the problem. Surgery for chronic salivary inflammatory disease is extremely difficult, especially the dissection and preservation of the facial nerve because of the amount of fibrosis associated with long-standing inflammation.

A gland that has been recurrently infected and persistently inflamed may develop sialectasia (Fig. 16–2). These patients have swelling of the involved gland that slowly worsens.

## Fungal Sialoadenitis

It is possible for the salivary glands to contract a fungal infection, but this occurs infrequently.

Actinomycosis has been noted, and it usually follows some dental manipulations. Patients will experience trismus and even have some systemic symptoms. Involvement of the parotid gland is

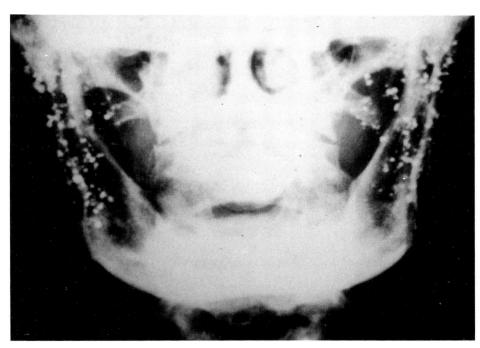

**FIG 16–2.**
The sialogram of a patient with chronic sialoadenitis shows a pooling of dye in the expanding of ducts, which prevents drainage of secretions.

from contiguous spread from the infected tooth and is not hematogenous. The clinical picture is one of parotid abscess, and the need for surgical drainage is not uncommon. In addition to requiring surgical drainage, these patients frequently need high dosages of penicillin for protracted periods of time. The administration of antibiotics can last for months. Patients with recurring actinomycotic infections sometimes need penicillin therapy for years.

### Granulomatous Sialoadenitis

The salivary glands can be involved with granulomatous processes. Although tuberculosis used to be common it is less frequently encountered now. It primarily involves the parotid glands and is seen in young adulthood. This diagnosis is made by means of tissue examination. The acute phase is not distinguishable from other bacterial or viral etiologies. However, rather than resolving, the acute phase frequently progresses to a chronic stage in which localized induration develops. Occasionally drainage of the involved gland is necessary. However, antituberculous chemo-

therapy is the treatment of choice when possible. Atypical mycobacterial infections sometimes occur, and these are usually diagnosed and managed by excision of the involved tissue. Sarcoidosis is another granulomatous process that can involve salivary glands, sometimes in combination with other organ systems. An example is Heerfordt's disease, which is characterized by involvement of the salivary glands in addition to the lacrimal apparatus and the uveal tract. Once again, this is a tissue diagnosis, and it has no particularly distinguishing clinical findings. Sarcoid sialoadenitis is usually diagnosed by means of tissue examination rather than by a distinguishing set of clinical circumstances, except for the involvement of other organs as previously mentioned. Cat scratch disease is another example of a granulomatous problem that can involve the salivary glands secondary to primary nodal involvement. The parotid gland is most susceptible.

### Salivary Calculi

The complex interrelationships that occur with acute and chronic inflammatory disease of the salivary glands can predispose to formation of calculi within the ducts of primarily the submandibular and parotid glands. Any condition that causes stasis or alters the quality of the salivary secretions can secondarily result in the development of a calculus. The submandibular duct is most commonly involved with calculi because this gland produces inspissated mucous secretions that have to traverse a duct that is oriented superiorly heading toward its orifice. Therefore, any stasis or slight stricture of the duct or tendency of the secretions to become more inspissated will increase the chances for calculus formation, initiated by precipitation of the minerals within the saliva. Although less common, parotid duct stones are also seen. The salivary calculi are different from real calculi in that most salivary calculi are radiopaque (Fig. 16–3).

The patient describes a history of intermittent swelling associated with firmness and tenderness in the area of either the parotid or submandibular glands. A distinguishing feature that should make one suspect a stone is increased swelling and tenderness of the involved gland whenever the patient encounters a stimulus for salivary production, such as eating. If the obstruction is partial, the patient will state that the gland gradually decreases in size. There may be a secondary suppurative process, and palpation of the gland will cause pus to exit the duct orifice. Sometimes neither the submandibular nor parotid stones are palpable by digital manipulation. Dental occlusal radiographs often confirm the clinical suspicion by identifying a radiopaque stone. If the diagnosis is not made with this radiograph, sialography can be done. However, sialography is not advisable while a gland is acutely inflamed because of the irritative potential of the dye injected into the gland. After the acute inflammation has been treated with antibiotics, sialography can be more safely performed and the diagnosis can be established.

The treatment of salivary gland calculus is its removal. Often dilation of the duct orifice and the duct with lacrimal probes will extrude the stone. If this is not possible, the duct can be opened under local anesthesia and the stone removed manually. If the stone is located within the hilus of the gland, such relatively conservative measures may not be successful. The decision about excision of

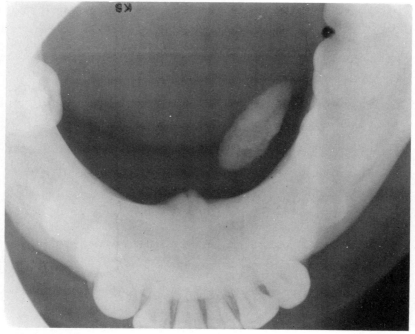

**FIG 16–3**.
This radiograph demonstrates a radiopaque submandibular duct stone.

the gland is made based on the severity and frequency of symptoms caused by the calculus.

## Sialoadenitis Caused By Extrinsic Factors

As mentioned, the pattern of salivary outflow obstruction or stasis of or alteration in the secretions can sometimes be caused by intrinsic factors such as drug effect. Most notable in a group of drugs predisposing to this are the antihelimergic agents. Derivatives of phenothiazine create an antihelimergic effect with subsequent stasis and possibly sialadenitis. Discontinuation of the medication usually resolves the problem.

Radiation therapy can alter the amount of salivary flow, causing secondary xerostomia. It can also alter the content of the saliva being produced by the gland that received radiation therapy. The degree of damage to the salivary gland is directly related to the dosage of the radiation therapy. It appears that the serous-secreting components of the glands are more susceptible to the radiation effect than are the mucous glands. Atrophy of the gland will ultimately occur, with resultant decreased salivary production and its secondary adverse effects on the oral mucosa and dentition (Fig. 16–4).

## NEOPLASMS

Neoplasms can involve any of the major or minor salivary glands. These usually appear as painless swellings within the gland (Fig. 16–5). Sometimes malignant neoplasms cause disruption and destruction of surrounding important structures, such as the facial nerve or skin, which will then add to the presenting symptoms in the form of pain and nerve dysfunction or fixation of surrounding structures to the tumor. The presence of a progressively enlarging, painless, discrete induration in any of the salivary glands should be considered a neoplasm until proved otherwise. It is necessary to remember that lymph nodes are intimately associated with the parotid, submandibular, and sublingual glands. There are also lymph nodes *within* the parotid gland. These can be the source of confusion as to the identity of a mass in these anatomic regions (Fig. 16–6).

Certain generalizations are helpful to guide the

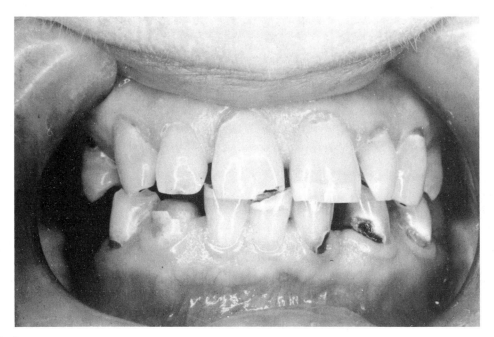

**FIG 16–4.**
This patient sustained severe damage to the teeth as a result of altered salivary production following radiation therapy.

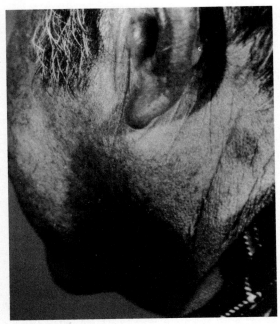

**FIG 16-5.**
This patient has a tumor of the parotid gland that has produced an asymptomatic enlargement of the tail of the parotid gland.

clinician in the assessment of a painless, progressively growing tumor involving any of the salivary glands. Approximately 25% of all parotid neoplasms are malignant. There is a greater chance of malignancy in the submandibular gland, where about 50% of neoplasms are malignant. The biologic behavior of a malignancy arising in a minor salivary gland is usually more aggressive than that of an identical cell type occurring in a major salivary gland.

## Benign Tumors
### Pleomorphic Adenoma

The most common of the benign neoplasms involving the salivary glands is the *pleomorphic adenonoma* (benign mixed tumor). This tumor has a slow growth pattern and can occur in any portion of the parotid gland, submandibular, or sublingual glands. It is a firm, discrete mass that is usually nontender to palpation. These tumors occur less frequently in the submandibular gland than they do in the parotid gland. Although they can be encapsulated, it is not unusual for them to have pseudopod-type extensions into the normal salivary tissue.

Past treatment involved an incision of the skin over the mass with enucleation in an effort to minimize injury to the critical structures associated with the salivary glands, especially the facial nerve. However, this technique was associated with an unacceptably high recurrence rate. The realization that these fingerlike extensions were probably being transected and left in situ explains the reason for the failure of this approach.

Resection of the entire gland or at least the lobe of the gland involved with the tumor is now the treatment of choice, and this requires a formal dissection of the facial nerve to avoid injury (Fig. 16-7). No noninvasive diagnostic studies are accurate enough to avoid the need for tissue examination. Fine-needle aspiration is an alternative, but the possible danger of injury to a branch of the facial nerve has limited its acceptance.

It is important for benign mixed tumors to be completely resected because of the potential for recurrence. There are rare instances in which these tumors, although having a benign histologic appearance, behave in a locally aggressive fashion similar to that of a malignancy. Complete surgical resection is necessary to decrease the chances that this unfortunate set of clinical circumstances will occur.

### Papillary Cystadenoma Lymphomatosum (Warthin's Tumor)

Papillary cystadenoma lymphomatosum is a benign tumor that occurs primarily in the parotid

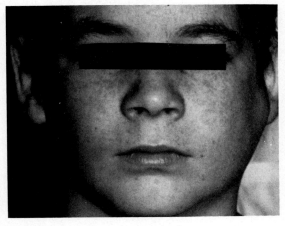

**FIG 16-6.**
This boy developed a painless, firm, discrete mass within the parotid gland, which parotid lobectomy showed to be an intraparotid lymph node.

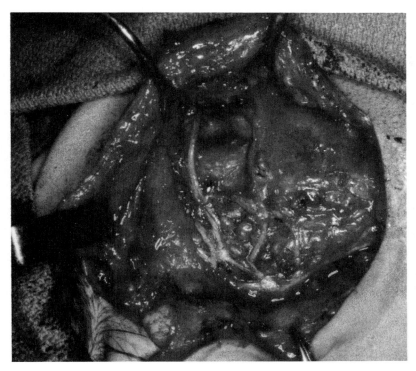

**FIG 16–7.**
This figure demonstrates the appearance of the facial nerve following lateral parotid lobectomy with formal dissection of the facial nerve.

gland, is much more common in males than in females, and involves primarily older age groups. It characteristically involves a mass over the tail of the parotid gland and can be bilateral (Fig. 16–8). Surgical resection with dissection and preservation of the facial nerve is the treatment of choice, and the recurrence is limited.

### Acidophilic Cell Adenoma (Oncocytoma)

Acidophilic cell adenoma is a benign tumor believed to arise from the epithelium forming the ducts. The clinical presentation is similar to that of the benign mixed tumor in that it has a slow growth pattern with a paucity of symptoms. It can occur in the submandibular gland and the parotid gland. Surgical excision, with preservation of the critical structures, is the treatment of choice.

There are a variety of other less common benign salivary tumors such as the *acinic cell adenoma*. Most of these can involve either the parotid or submandibular gland. Once again, surgical excision is the treatment of choice.

## Malignant Tumors
### Mucoepidermoid Carcinoma

Mucoepidermoid carcinoma presents as a progressively growing mass with a variable growth rate. There are actually two histologic subtypes: a low grade and a high grade. The low-grade mucoepidermoid carcinoma has a rather indolent biologic behavior. Complete surgical excision usually results in 5-year cure rates in excess of 95%. Some even consider this type of behavior to be more consistent with that of a benign rather than a malignant tumor.

In contrast, the high-grade mucoepidermoid carcinoma has a more aggressive behavior pattern with a strong propensity for local recurrence, regional nodal metastases, and distant metastases. This malignancy frequently involves critical structures such as the facial nerve, and its complete resection often includes intentional sacrifice of a part or all of the facial nerve (Fig. 16–9). The survival rates are not good with high-grade mucoepidermoid carcinoma. Combined therapy programs using surgery and postoperative radiation therapy and sometimes even chemotherapy have

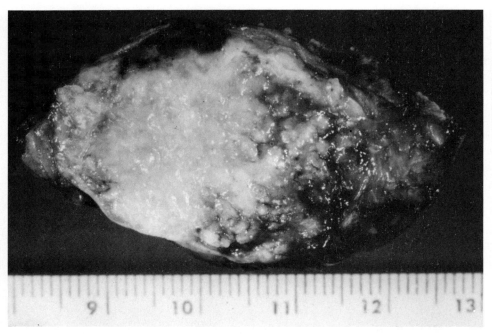

**FIG 16–8.**
A Warthin's tumor has a typical gross appearance characterized by spongy consistency and mucoid type of fluid seen from a cut surface.

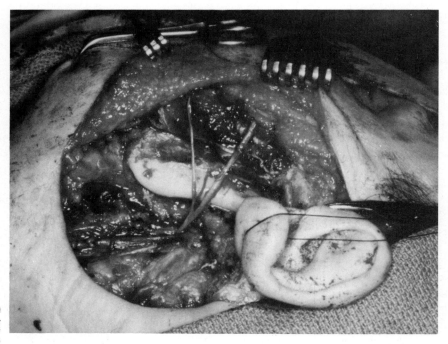

**FIG 16–9.**
This patient underwent total parotidectomy, including a section of the facial nerve, followed by a graft of the great auricular nerve to the cut ends of the facial nerve.

been used to attempt to improve locoregional control.

### Adenoid Cystic Carcinoma (Cylindroma)

Adenoid cystic carcinoma can involve any of the major or minor salivary glands. The outlook is better if the tumor arises in the major salivary glands. Cylindroma shows an affinity for perineural extension (Fig. 16–10). It also is characterized by a rather indolent but prolonged course. Five-year cure rates are not an accurate assessment of the success of treatment, because it is not unusual for patients to be disease free for protracted periods of time and then develop local recurrences and/or distant metastases. Patients who develop distant metastases from an adenoid cystic carcinoma also have a surprisingly long survival in the face of metastatic disease. This biologic behavior distinguishes adenoid cystic carcinoma from any other salivary malignancies. A variety of treatment programs have relied primarily on complete surgical excision. Depending on the age of the patient and the site of the malignancy, adjunctive treatment with irradiation and/or chemotherapy is sometimes used.

### Malignant Mixed Tumors

Some benign mixed tumors undergo degeneration into a malignant mixed tumor, and aggressive treatment, usually surgical, is indicated because of the high local recurrence rate and the potential for distant metastatic disease. Complete surgical resection of benign mixed tumors is important to prevent this potential malignant degeneration.

### Squamous Cell Carcinoma

Squamous cell carcinoma is believed to arise from metaplastic changes of the ductal epithelia. It is again found more in the parotid than in the submandibular gland. The facial nerve seems to be compromised by squamous cell carcinoma arising in the parotid gland more than by any of the other cell types. Metastases to the cervical lymph nodes occur routinely. Distant metastatic

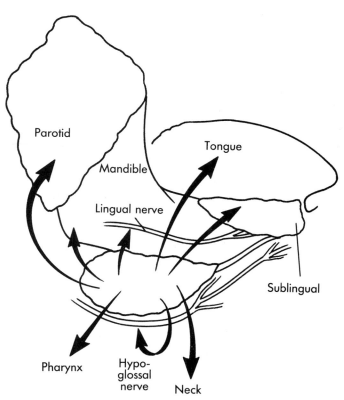

**FIG 16–10.**
Adenoid cystic carcinoma has an affinity for perineural extension.

disease also can occur. The 5-year survival rates are poor for this disease, and combined therapy programs rely heavily on surgical resection of the primary tumor and the regional nodal drainage bed. If the facial nerve is intentionally resected with tumor ablation, nerve grafting or some other facial rehabilitation technique is routinely used.

It is important to understand that other neoplasms can occur in the salivary tissue. *Lymphomas* can arise in any of the major salivary glands. Lymphomas and *congenital cysts* can present as neoplasms. Once again, no noninvasive diagnostic studies are available to enable the tissue diagnosis to be made without tissue excision.

## Salivary Gland Neoplasms in Children

Salivary gland neoplasms in children are uncommon. However, they deserve mention because their behavior is somewhat different from that of other tumors. Most children with these benign and malignant tumors have a favorable outlook. The tumors can be subclassified as vascular neoplasms and benign and malignant tumors.

### Vascular Neoplasms

Vascular tumors include hemangiomas and lymphangiomas. The hemangiomas are classified according to their histologic features and can be categorized as capillary, cavernous, or mixed. The tumor itself is usually confined to the intracapsular portion of the gland. It can result in rather markedly disfiguring tumors in the child

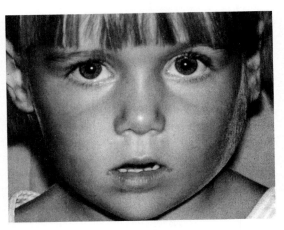

**FIG 16–12.**
The same child as seen in Fig. 16–11 has a marked reduction in the size of the hemangioma 3 years later.

(Fig. 16–11), which can cause considerable concern among parents. However, both hemangiomas and lymphangiomas often undergo spontaneous resolution (Fig. 16–12), and many totally disappear without the need for any surgical intervention (Fig. 16–13). This is more commonly seen with hemangiomas than lymphangiomas.

However, there still is some potential for regression with lymphangiomas, and conservative treatment is advocated unless the lymphangioma is located in a salivary gland that could potentially cause airway obstruction if the lymphangioma were to rapidly enlarge. Current treatment for benign vascular salivary neoplasms in children centers on the conservative attitude of watchful waiting.

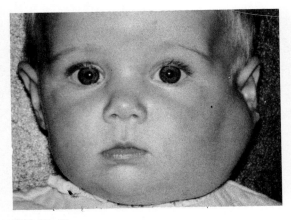

**FIG 16–11.**
This hemangioma involves the left parotid gland in this infant.

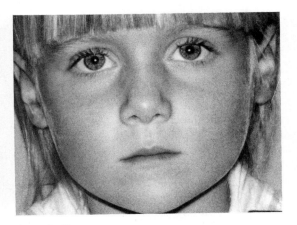

**FIG 16–13.**
The hemangioma has now completely disappeared by 5 years of age. No surgical intervention was needed.

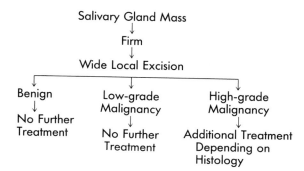

**FIG 16–14.**
This schema depicts a recommended therapeutic approach to salivary gland tumors in children.

### Benign Neoplasms

The benign tumors seen in children are similar in frequency to those noted in adults. The benign mixed tumor is the most common. These present in an identical fashion. Unfortunately, the chances of a parotid mass being an intraglandular lymph node are greater in children than in adults. There is still no diagnostic study to permit diagnosis without tissue excision.

### Malignant Neoplasms

The *potential* for malignancy of a firm asymptomatic mass within the parotid gland of a child is actually greater in children than it is in adults. About 60% of these masses in children are malignant. The most common malignancy is the low-grade mucoepidermoid carcinoma, and this has a favorable outlook. Once again, the treatment of choice is surgical excision. If the histologic diagnosis is low-grade mucoepidermoid carcinoma or any other of the low-grade histologic malignant cell types, the excision of the tumor, usually accompanied by facial nerve preservation, represents adequate treatment (Fig. 16–14). In children who have high-grade salivary gland malignancy, the outlook is poor, and adjunctive treatment using radiation therapy and/or chemotherapy is advisable.

# PART V
# Larynx and Hypopharynx

# 17

# Anatomy and Physiology

## ANATOMY

The anatomic relationship of the larynx to the hypopharynx is intricate. The normal anatomy allows for separation of the food from the air passageways. Any pathologic states that will alter either the anatomy or physiology of this area could significantly challenge the safety of the airway.

The larynx occupies the central compartment of the neck. It is located more superiorly in the child than in the adult. The cricoid cartilage in the child is at the level of the fourth cervical vertebral body in contrast to that in the adult, which is at the level of the sixth vertebral body. The carotid sheath (carotid artery, vagus nerve, and internal jugular vein) is located in each lateral compartment of the neck and is adjacent to the larynx. It is not unusual for pathologic processes of the larynx, such as a malignancy, to involve the contents of the carotid sheath because of this anatomic intimacy. The trachea is attached to the cricoid cartilage and courses inferiorly and posteriorly into the mediastinum. Overlying the trachea is the isthmus of the thyroid gland (Fig. 17–1). The thyroid has an extensive venous drainage system that exits the isthmus inferiorly. The level of the horizontal plane of the isthmus is variable and can be as low as the fourth or fifth tracheal ring and as high as the cricothyroid membrane. It is rarely over the cricothyroid membrane in the adult.

The rigid framework of the larynx is a system of cartilages and one bone (Fig. 17–2). The hyoid represents the only bone within the airway. Therefore, it is the only radiopaque structure within the larynx. The remaining rigid structures are all cartilaginous. The larynx comprises a thy-roid cartilage below the hyoid bone and the cricoid cartilage inferior to the thyroid cartilage. The tracheal rings are attached to the cricoid cartilage. It is important to recognize that the cricoid cartilage is the only rigid circular structure in the airway. The tracheal "rings" should probably be more accurately referred to as the tracheal "horseshoes." They are absent in the posterior tracheal wall (Fig. 17–3). The hyoid bone is connected to the thyroid cartilage by the thyrohyoid membrane, and the cricoid cartilage is connected to the thyroid cartilage by the thyrohyoid membrane.

There are two general groups of muscles associated with the larynx. The extrinsic laryngeal muscles are involved with moving the larynx as a unit. Most of the extrinsic muscles are attached to the hyoid bone and are referred to as the suprahyoid group, which elevates the larynx, and the infrahyoid muscles, which depress the larynx. The suprahyoid muscles comprise the musculature of the floor of the mouth. The infrahyoid muscles are primarily the strap muscles, which originate from the hyoid bone superiorly and the sternum and scapula inferiorly.

The intrinsic laryngeal muscles are involved with vocal cord mobility. The term *intrinsic* does not refer to their position within the larynx. All of these muscles are located within the larynx except for the cricothyroid muscle, which runs from the cricoid to the posterior portion of the thyroid external to the larynx (Fig. 17–4). Multiple intrinsic laryngeal muscles are involved with moving the true vocal cords. All of the intrinsic laryngeal muscles cause the true vocal cords to move toward the midline (adduct) except for the cricoarytenoid muscle, which causes the vocal cords to separate (abduct). The motor innervation of the

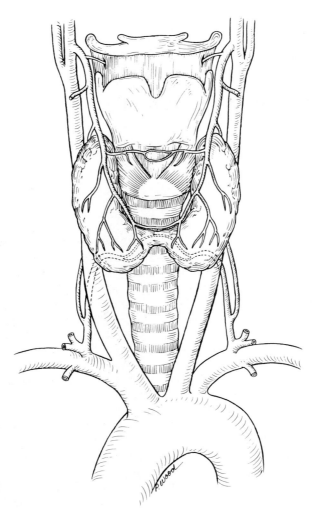

**FIG 17–1**.
Anatomic relationship of the thyroid gland with the trachea.

intrinsic laryngeal muscles is via the recurrent laryngeal nerve (cranial nerve X). The only exception is the cricothyroid muscle; it is innervated by the external branch of the superior laryngeal nerve, which is also a branch of the vagus nerve (cranial nerve X).

The internal branch of the superior laryngeal nerve enters the endolarynx via the thyrohyoid membrane and provides sensation of the laryngeal mucosa from the level of the vocal cords superiorly. The recurrent laryngeal nerve provides sensation to the lower portion of the larynx.

The arytenoid cartilages sit on top of the posterior portion of the cricothyroid cartilage. Each arytenoid has a body, a muscular process, and a vocal process. The vocal process is attached to the inner surface of the thyroid cartilage by the vocal ligament (Fig. 17–5). Some of the intrinsic muscles are attached to the vocal ligament.

The laryngeal musculature and cartilage are covered by respiratory epithelium—ciliated pseudostratified columnar epithelium. However, there are some areas of squamous metaplasia, and these areas usually represent the points of the larynx that have frequent physical contact with either food particles or another portion of the larynx. The tip of the epiglottis, aryepiglottic folds, and the free edge of the true vocal cords have squamous epithelium. It is important to understand that the vocal fold is much more than mucosa over muscle. The anatomy of the vibratory margin includes not only the epithelium but also

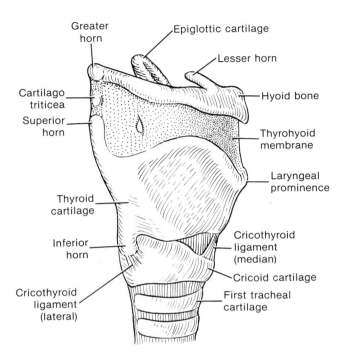

Greater horn

Epiglottic cartilage

Lesser horn

Cartilago triticea

Hyoid bone

Superior horn

Thyrohyoid membrane

Laryngeal prominence

Thyroid cartilage

Cricothyroid ligament (median)

Inferior horn

Cricoid cartilage

Cricothyroid ligament (lateral)

First tracheal cartilage

**FIG 17–2.**
The hyoid bone is the only bone within the rigid components of the larynx and trachea.

**FIG 17–3.**
The tracheal "rings" resemble horseshoes with no rigid support posteriorly.

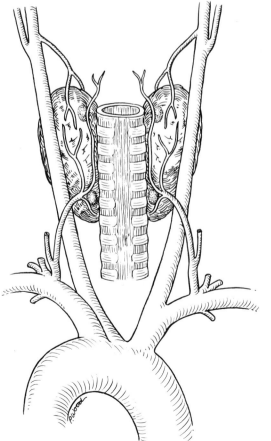

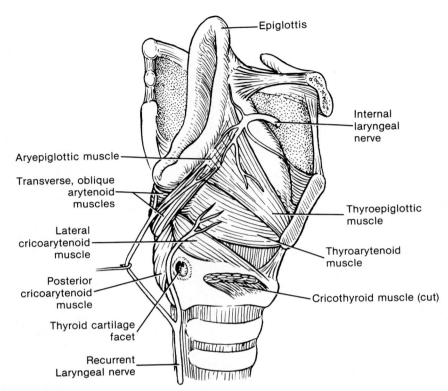

Epiglottis

Internal laryngeal nerve

Aryepiglottic muscle

Transverse, oblique arytenoid muscles

Thyroepiglottic muscle

Lateral cricoarytenoid muscle

Thyroarytenoid muscle

Posterior cricoarytenoid muscle

Cricothyroid muscle (cut)

Thyroid cartilage facet

Recurrent Laryngeal nerve

**FIG 17–4.**
All of the intrinsic laryngeal muscles are within the larynx except for the cricothyroid muscle.

three layers of lamino propria and the intrinsic laryngeal muscle.

Just superior to the true vocal cords is a recess referred to as the laryngeal ventricle. Immediately superior to the ventricle is another set of vocal cords, the false vocal cords, which are more rounded, blunted protrusions located on a plane superior to the true vocal cords (Fig. 17–6). They contain minimal musculature but are rich in glandular structures. A fold of mucosa, the aryepiglottic fold, connects the epiglottis with the arytenoid cartilages. Extending inferiorly from the vocal ligament to the inferior border of the cricoid cartilage is a tough, fibrous band called the triangular membrane or conus elasticus laryngis.

The larynx is compartmentalized into supraglottic, glottic, and subglottic portions. The supraglottic larynx extends from the tip of the epiglottis down to the laryngeal ventricle. The glottic larynx essentially includes the true vocal cords and extends for about 5 to 7 mm inferior to the vocal ligament. The subglottic portion of the larynx extends from the inferior portion of the glot-

tis down to the inferior edge of the cricoid cartilage.

The larynx is located within the hypopharynx. The lateral pharyngeal recesses on each side of the larynx are the pyriform sinuses (Fig. 17–7). They are the primary route for food passage into the cervical esophagus.

## PHYSIOLOGY

The physiology of the larynx involves several areas. The primary activity of the larynx is to protect the airway from the entrance of food particles and other nondesirable elements. This is accomplished by a series of reflex events that occur subconsciously in the normal individual during the act of swallowing. However, any alterations in the anatomy can affect this sequence drastically.

The airway is protected through a sequence of events initiated when a bolus of food comes into contact with either the tip of the epiglottis or the aryepiglottic folds. The sensory reflex arm of this

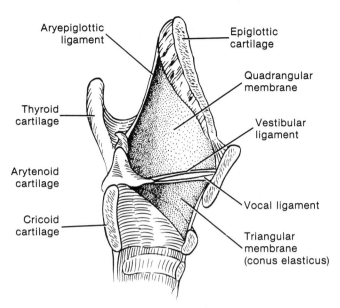

**FIG 17–5.**
The vocal ligament provides rigid support to the free edge of the true vocal cords.

arch is the glossopharyngeal nerve (cranial nerve IX). The motor arch is mediated via the vagus nerve. The initial occurrence with this stimulation is the inhibition of inspiration. The true vocal cords then forcefully close, which secondarily causes closure of the false vocal cords. Subsequent to this, the aryepiglottic folds are drawn medially, posteriorly displacing the epiglottis. While these events are occurring with the intrinsic laryngeal musculature, the extrinsic laryngeal muscles are also active. The suprahyoid extrinsic muscles are stimulated at the same time that the infrahyoid extrinsic muscles are inhibited. This stimulation and inhibition cause a superior-anterior vector force on the larynx as a unit, which displaces it under the protective hood of the base of the tongue during the act of swallowing. These sequential events usually are sufficient for the subconscious passage of food beyond the larynx and into the cervical esophagus, where it is transported into the stomach with no danger to the airway.

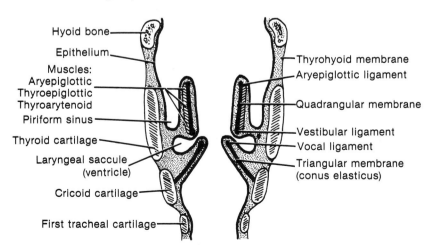

**FIG 17–6.**
The false vocal cords contain no musculature.

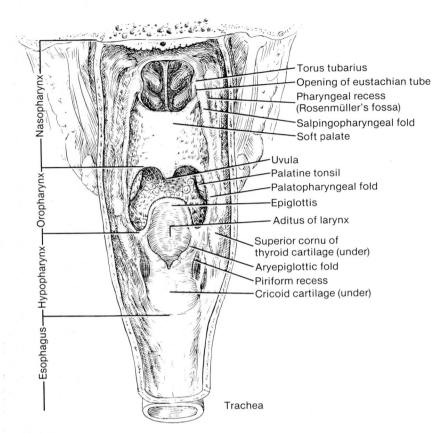

Nasopharynx
Oropharynx
Hypopharynx
Esophagus

Torus tubarius
Opening of eustachian tube
Pharyngeal recess
(Rosenmüller's fossa)
Salpingopharyngeal fold
Soft palate

Uvula
Palatine tonsil
Palatopharyngeal fold
Epiglottis
Aditus of larynx
Superior cornu of
thyroid cartilage (under)
Aryepiglottic fold
Piriform recess
Cricoid cartilage (under)

Trachea

**FIG 17–7.**
The pyriform sinuses are the pathway for feeding into the cervical esophagus.

Phonation is another physiologic function of the larynx. It was formerly believed that the vocal cords opened and closed in an active series of musculature contractions and relaxations. However, it is now believed that phonation results from an initial forceful closure of the vocal cords during the act of expiration. Cord closure increases the intratracheal pressure with expiration. It ultimately results in a pressure that is greater than the closing pressure of the vocal cords, thus forcing them open. However, this opening of the cords causes a rapid reduction of the intratracheal pressure, permitting the vocal cords to close again and effectively pinch off a "puff" of air. This alternating rise and fall of the intratracheal pressure causing the vocal cords to open and close and pinch off boluses of air is responsible for phonation. Any pathologic processes altering the mass of the vocal cords or their ability to close will ultimately affect the quality of the voice. This alteration is collectively referred to as hoarseness.

The larynx also participates in respiratory activity. Inspiration is marked by a stimulation of the recurrent laryngeal nerve, resulting in vocal cord abduction just before phrenic nerve stimulation, which permits air flow into the lungs.

# 18

# Special Diagnostic Procedures

Many physicians fail to master the techniques of examination of the larynx and hypopharynx, despite the considerable number of common pathologic conditions involving this anatomic area. Visualization of this area formerly required the clinician to be comfortable with the use of indirect lighting reflected from a head mirror onto an examining mirror placed in the oropharynx and properly angulated to see the laryngopharyngeal structures. When this technique is mastered, it still provides an excellent view. However, the recent development of reliable flexible fiberoptic nasopharyngoscopes and the rigid rod telescopes, discussed in Chapter 1, allows an excellent view of this area by even the occasional examiner. These instruments enable the examiner to note changes in color, abnormal masses, or abnormal mobility of the vocal cords. However, in certain instances additional information that is not obtained by physical examination is necessary.

## RADIOGRAPHIC EXAMINATIONS

Radiographic examinations have been frequently used for the evaluation of laryngeal disease. The one portion of the larynx that is especially important to evaluate radiographically is the subglottic area because it is not adequately seen on routine physical examination. Even flexible fiberoptic endoscopy does not provide a mechanism for studying the undersurface of the true vocal cords or the possible change in configuration of the subglottic area created by a submucosal mass.

Computed tomography allows imaging of not only the soft tissue but also the bone and cartilage that make up the larynx. It enables examination of multiple levels of the larynx to study the relationship of laryngeal structures with other structures in the neck (Fig. 18–1). Gross destruction of cartilage and bone can often be detected with computed tomography. However, subtle changes are still not within the realm of detectability, even with the newest generation of scanners.

Magnetic resonance imaging (Fig. 18–2) provides a superb means of assessing soft tissue of the endolarynx. The fact that it does not directly visualize cartilage and/or bone means that it does not resolve the limitations of computed tomography in studying laryngeal pathologic processes involving cartilage or bone erosion.

Videostroboscopy is a new technique that uses stroboscopic equipment for more precise analysis of endolaryngeal tissue activity during phonation. This technology allows for more precise study of the wavelike movement of the vocal fold mucosa and how it can be altered by different pathologic processes. Strobovideolaryngoscopy is often coupled with some newer objective means of voice quantification, such as phonatory analysis, to enhance diagnostic capability. The combination of newer radiographic imaging studies and strobovideolaryngoscopy with objective voice quantification—in addition to interdisciplinary input from both otolaryngologist–head and neck surgeons and speech pathologists—has increased diagnostic and therapeutic capabilities for patients with laryngeal disorders.

Radiographic examination of the hypopharynx with contrast material is sometimes used. However, it continues to represent a diagnostic challenge for the radiologist. The intimate relationship between the hypopharynx and the larynx prevents the use of a large amount of barium contrast ma-

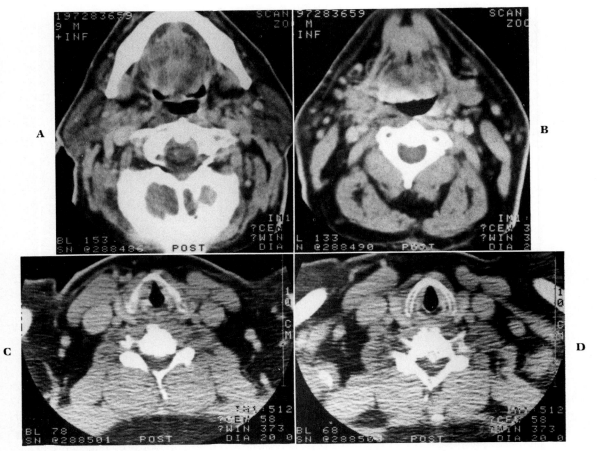

**FIG 18–1.**
This computed tomogram demonstrates different levels of the larynx, including the tip of the epiglottis, **A,** the inferior epiglottis, **B,** the true vocal cords, **C,** and the cricoid cartilage, **D.**

**FIG 18–2.**
This magnetic resonance image shows normal laryngeal anatomy of the true and false vocal cords and laryngeal ventricle.

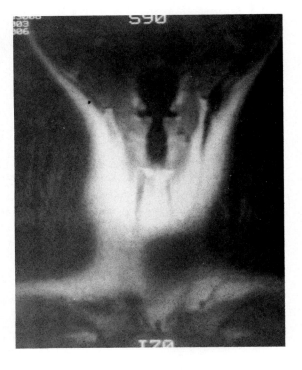

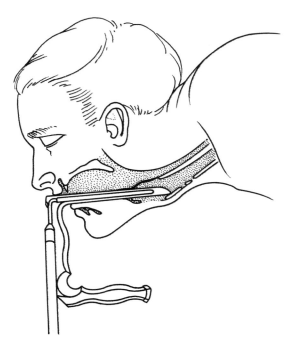

**FIG 18–3.**
The laryngoscope provides transoral visualization of the endolarynx.

terial for fear of aspiration. Sometimes the use of contrast material is restricted because of the fear of aspiration as the result of a particular pathologic process. Some radiologists use a more viscous barium solution to help with the evaluation of this portion of the pharynx. It provides a mechanism for identifying some surface abnormalities, although these are frequently detectable on physical examination if the clinician has either the skills or the equipment to examine the hypopharynx. These contrast studies do have value when fluoroscopy and cine recordings are used to evaluate the movement of the contrast material through the hypopharynx and through the cricopharyngeal sphincter into the cervical esophagus. They have the potential for raising a level of suspicion for any hypopharyngeal motility, pathology, or cricopharyngeal spasm.

In patients who are having difficulty swallowing (dysphagia), physical examination may be normal. Static anatomy is usually not the etiology, but there can be a problem with the dynamic aspects of the hypopharyngeal musculature. Physical examination and many radiographic studies usually do not reveal an abnormality that is evolving over a period of time. In this instance,

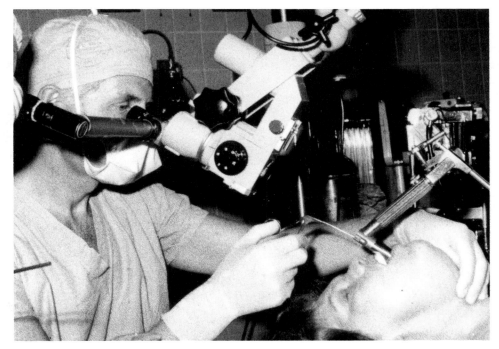

**FIG 18–4.**
Microscopic surgery is routinely used for endoscopic laryngeal surgery.

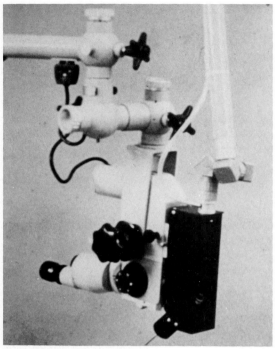

**FIG 18–5.**
The ability to attach the carbon dioxide laser to the microscope has enhanced microlaryngeal surgery.

the barium hypopharyngogram, especially when coupled with fluoroscopic examination, may elicit some level of suspicion. Manometric studies of the esophageal pressure and other motility studies are available to help with the diagnosis of this condition. Consultation with gastroenterologists, who have expertise in motility studies, can be productive in the diagnostic evaluation of patients with dysphagia.

## DIRECT LARYNGOSCOPY

In most cases, the larynx can be thoroughly viewed either with indirect laryngoscopy using la-

ryngeal mirrors and headlight or with the newer flexible fiberoptic equipment described in Chapter 1. In some instances neither provides adequate exposure. There are also times when tissue removal is necessary. Direct laryngoscopy, which shows another view of the larynx, is the most common technique for the endoscopic removal of laryngeal tissue.

Direct laryngoscopy can be performed with use of either local or general anesthesia. If it is being performed primarily for diagnostic purposes with minimal tissue manipulation, local anesthesia can be used. The anesthesia blocks the superior laryngeal nerves and the sensory component of the recurrent laryngeal nerve. Transcutaneous infiltration of a local anesthetic at the lateral portion of the thyrohyoid membrane bilaterally blocks the superior laryngeal nerves, and a transtracheal injection of local anesthetic through the cricothyroid membrane blocks the sensory portion of the recurrent laryngeal nerve. This anesthesia is supplemented by spraying a local anesthetic over the surfaces of the oropharyngeal and the hypopharyngeal mucosa.

The laryngoscope is an L-shaped metallic structure with a hollow shaft. It is inserted through the mouth and advanced to a position just posterior to the epiglottis. In this position, it exposes the endolaryngeal structures (Fig. 18–3). Two fiberoptic light sources run through separate channels down the shaft of the laryngoscope and provide excellent distal illumination. The handle can be attached to a connecting arm used for stabilization, thus freeing the surgeon's hands. The larynx can be examined with the use of a microscope, and endoscopic surgery can be performed with specially designed microlaryngeal instruments (Fig. 18–4). The carbon dioxide laser can be attached to the microscope (Fig. 18–5).

# 19

# Embryology and Congenital Disorders

The anatomic intimacy of the larynx and hypopharynx is readily understandable with an appreciation of certain embryologic facts. The primordial structures that compose the entire respiratory system begin as an outpouching from the ventral surface of the embryonic foregut. This is a depression initially but then continues to develop into an outpouching that will eventually form the larynx, trachea, and lungs. The pouch ultimately develops into the laryngotracheal tube. The cranial end of the tube is the site of the larynx. Mesodermal concentrations in the area of the developing larynx represent the material that ultimately differentiates into laryngeal components. Three main masses of mesoderm are in the area of the developing epiglottis and the two arytenoids. They will fuse to close the opening of the laryngopharynx. Further embryonic development results in recanalization of the lumen. Any alteration of this normal pattern will result in congenital disorders. For example, a failure of the mesodermal condensation may create a partial or total cleft of the laryngopharynx. If the larynx does not totally recanalize, some compromise of the airway could occur, such as laryngeal stenosis or web formation.

There are a variety of congenital laryngopharyngeal disorders. However, the frequency of occurrence is disproportionately distributed. Any condition that alters the size of the laryngeal lumen has the potential to alter the infant's cry or the noises created during respiratory activity. *Stridor* is the term used to describe any noises that are created as a result of airway obstruction. Often, the type of stridor will provide a clue for the clinician concerning the site of the laryngeal abnormality. For example, inspiratory stridor is usu-

ally associated with an abnormality of the supraglottic portion of the larynx. If there is both inspiratory and expiratory stridor, it usually suggests some compromise of the airway below the level of the vocal cords. A more peripheral obstruction, such as in the bronchi, will cause wheezing.

In addition to noting the presence of any stridor, the clinician should listen to the infant's cry. If there is a weak "air-spilling" cry, the child may have a vocal cord paralysis. Another useful clinical tool is to determine if there is alteration in the child's stridor with change in body position. Any neurologic impairment of the larynx may make the airway vulnerable to aspiration, and the child will have feeding difficulties, which are usually associated with frequent coughing spells.

## LARYNGOMALACIA

Laryngomalacia is the most common congenital laryngeal problem. The infant with laryngomalacia typically presents with inspiratory stridor that is considerably worse in the supine than in the prone position. The symptoms appear shortly after birth, persist for a few weeks, and gradually improve and ultimately disappear. Feeding difficulties are rare. The pathophysiology involves laryngeal cartilages that have not yet developed the resilience to provide rigid support of the airway. Therefore, any inspiratory effort that creates negative pressure through the larynx results in medial displacement of the laryngeal tissue, which decreases the caliber of the airway lumen. As the rigidity of the cartilage improves during the ensuing weeks, the child's symptoms eventually disappear. It has been estimated that laryngomalacia accounts for at least 90% of all congenital laryngeal disorders in infants. Strong suspicion for the clinical diagnosis should arise if the history is consistent with what has previously been described and if there is improvement in the child's inspiratory stridor when he or she is in a prone position. The airway distress is rarely such that some type of airway protection is necessary, such as an endotracheal or tracheotomy tube. This disorder is common and usually not associated with severe airway compromise. Often, direct laryngoscopy is not necessary to confirm the clinical diagnosis. If the child's stridor does not improve after a few weeks, laryngoscopy is advisable to rule out other congenital laryngeal disorders.

## VOCAL CORD PARALYSIS

Vocal cord paralysis is the second most common congenital laryngeal problem. Injuries occurring during delivery that stretch the recurrent laryngeal nerve can be the cause. There are also a variety of central neurologic states that cause vocal cord paralysis. Cord paralysis can cause stridor if it involves both vocal cords. If the vocal cord paralysis is unilateral, there is frequently a weak "air-spilling" type of voice or sometimes an absent voice. Children with bilateral vocal cord paralysis have fairly strong cries but more airway distress. The converse occurs for unilateral vocal cord paralysis.

Bilateral vocal cord paralysis sometimes necessitates tracheotomy. However, the paralysis will frequently resolve in the child with Arnold-Chiari malformation after the insertion of a ventriculojugular shunt. It is not uncommon for unilateral vocal cord paralysis to require no treatment during either infancy or adulthood. If there is still some weakness of the voice during adolescence or into adulthood and the patient desires some improvement, endoscopic Teflon injection of the paralyzed vocal cord has potential for improving the voice quality. In cases of bilateral paralysis, some definitive treatment in hopes of decannulation is usually recommended but is deferred until the child is older.

## LARYNGEAL CYSTS

Cysts can arise from any portion of the larynx. Congenital laryngeal cysts most commonly involve the supraglottic larynx (Fig. 19–1), but

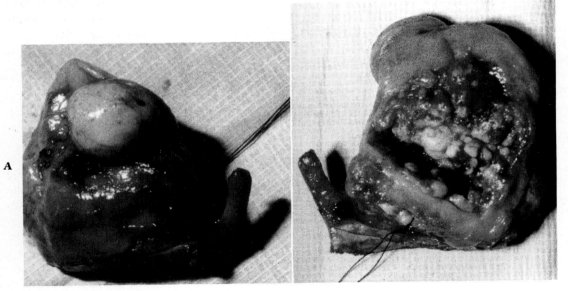

**FIG 19–1.**
**A,** cyst arising from the tip of the epiglottis in a patient with **B,** carcinoma involving the laryngeal face of the epiglottis.

they are rare. They can alter the child's voice and cause inspiratory stridor. If the cyst is on a portion of the supraglottic larynx that interferes with the food passage, feeding difficulties may also be encountered. Laryngoscopic examination usually reveals a freely mobile submucosal cystic structure. These cysts can usually be treated endoscopically with excision using microlaryngeal instrumentation or the carbon dioxide laser. They can be treated by excision of a portion of the wall, followed by pressing the retained mucosa against the underlying tissues with an endotracheal tube for a few days.

Another type of laryngeal cyst is associated with a lymphangioma. These can involve the larynx as direct extensions from a cervical lesion. Once again, this condition is quite rare. Laryngocoeles, which are outpouchings of the laryngeal mucosa into the neck structures that usually exit the endolarynx from the thyrohyoid membrane, have also been described. Once again, compared with laryngeal cysts, the laryngocoele is quite rare.

## LARYNGEAL WEBS

Laryngeal webs result from the failure of complete recanalization of the laryngeal lumen during embryonic development. As a result, fibrous segments partially or totally occlude the laryngeal inlet. Total occlusion is referred to as laryngeal atresia and obviously represents an immediate postpartum emergency. The recognition that no airway exchange is occurring necessitates prompt rupture of the atretic membrane. Otherwise, the infant will not survive, and laryngeal atresia will be a postmortem diagnosis.

The partial failure of recanalization also results in laryngeal webs, and this is considerably more common than complete obstruction. However, laryngeal webs are a less common congenital disorder than either laryngomalacia or cysts. Frequently this web is noted in the area of the anterior commissure connecting the true vocal cords and produces a blunting of the glottic chink anteriorly (Fig. 19–2). In addition to exhibiting respiratory distress with stridor, the child will have alteration in the quality of the cry and may even be aphonic. These webs can be endoscopically re-

moved with microlaryngeal instrumentation or the carbon dioxide laser.

## SUBGLOTTIC STENOSIS

Congenital subglottic stenosis is a difficult problem. This narrowing of the subglottic larynx produces both inspiratory and expiratory stridor, which is noted soon after birth. If it is severe, the child may need protection of the airway with either an endotracheal tube or a tracheotomy. Because the cricoid cartilage is the only circumferential rigid structure in the airway, it is understandable how some narrowing of this area prevents any opportunity for the tissue to expand. Many infants with subglottic stenosis undergo expansion of this area as they grow, and no further treatment is necessary. For children who do not outgrow the problem, the treatment continues to be a major challenge to the otolaryngologist–head and neck surgeon. Although a variety of techniques have been proposed to treat this problem, none are consistently successful.

## SUBGLOTTIC HEMANGIOMAS

Hemangiomas in infants are not uncommon. These benign vascular tumors can also involve the subglottic area, where they are usually not large enough to create stridor at birth. However, several weeks later, the child does develop inspira-

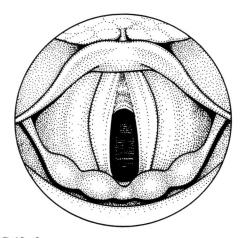

**FIG 19–2.**
Some thin congenital webs can be vaporized with the carbon dioxide laser attached to the microscope.

tory and expiratory stridor. About half of children with subglottic hemangiomas will also have additional cutaneous hemangiomas. In the child with delayed development of stridor, it is advisable to examine for any evidence of cutaneous hemangiomas. Diagnosis is made by direct laryngoscopy. Once again, many hemangiomas, including the subglottic variety, spontaneously regress with time. There have been some preliminary encouraging reports describing the use of a variety of types of lasers to resect these vascular tumors endoscopically.

## LARYNGOESOPHAGEAL CLEFT

Laryngoesophageal cleft represents a failure of a portion of the pharyngotracheal wall to close embryonically. Children with this disorder present with symptoms suggestive of aspiration. They will also have weak cries because the cleft extends up through the lamina of the cricoid cartilage between the arytenoid cartilages. The treatment of this rare condition is surgical closure, which is a formidable undertaking.

# 20

# Clinical Problems

## INFLAMMATION

### Conditions in Children

The larynx is frequently involved with inflammatory processes in all age groups. It can be the focus of an isolated infection or a disease process involving multiple organs. In children two inflammatory processes are commonly encountered.

#### Laryngotracheobronchitis

Laryngotracheobronchitis, frequently referred to as "croup," primarily affects children 2 years of age and younger. There is no sex predilection. The child often has a symptom complex suggestive of a flu syndrome. However, a nonproductive "barking" cough is a major symptom. Sore throat is common, and if there is progression of the disease, stridor can develop. The symptoms change within a relatively short period of time, measured in hours.

The physical examination will reveal a child who appears to be systemically ill, being febrile and complaining of malaise. Nasal congestion and clear rhinorrhea are usually present, as is inspiratory or expiratory stridor. The child's lung fields are usually clear to auscultation, however. If the respiratory obstruction is severe, it is not uncommon to encounter suprasternal, substernal, or intercostal retractions and extension of the head with inspiration.

Laryngotracheobronchitis usually has a viral origin. Adenovirus is a common etiology. Others such as echovirus and coxsackievirus have been isolated. It is usually not possible to visualize the child's larynx because of lack of cooperation and amount of airway distress. The larynx undergoes rather profound changes in the laryngeal compart-

ments. The supraglottic and glottic areas are relatively noninflamed. However, erythema and edema of the subglottic larynx can both result in airway compromise (Fig. 20–1). The trachea may have some secondary edema, but not as pronounced as the subglottic inflammation. It is important to understand that the edema involves the mucosa over the cricoid cartilage, which is the only level in the entire airway that is restricted by a circumferential, rigid cartilaginous structure. This area has no potential to expand as do other areas of the airway.

The assessment of the child suspected of having laryngotracheobronchitis depends on obtaining an accurate account of the chronology of symptoms. The fear of laryngeal spasm prompted by the manipulation of a mirror during examination or some other attempt to visualize the larynx usually precludes such evaluation, especially in the anxious child who has significant airway compromise. If the child's airway status will permit, the physical examination is usually supplemented by radiographs to assess the size of the epiglottis and also of the chest to rule out the possibility of pneumonic infiltrates.

Once the diagnosis is established, the treatment is based on the severity of symptoms. Most children have self-limiting disease that is only mild or moderate in terms of airway distress. It is often resolved with exposure to a well-humidified environment or with the use of a vaporizer, which helps to relieve the compromise caused by the copious inspissated secretions. Antibiotics have little value unless there is some suspicion of a secondary bacterial infection. In children with more severe airway distress, racemic epinephrine aerosols have been found to reduce the edema, ei-

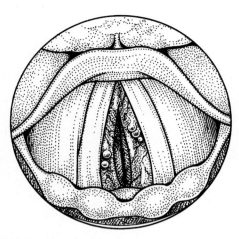

**FIG 20–1.**
Laryngotracheobronchitis is accompanied by narrowing of the subglottic portion of the larynx as a result of edema.

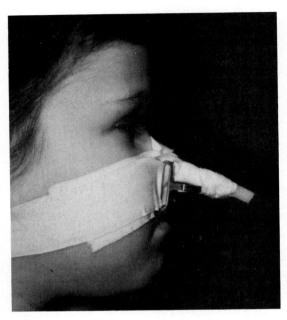

**FIG 20–2.**
The nasotracheal tube is found to be an effective and safe way of treating severe airway obstruction in epiglottitis and laryngotracheobronchitis.

ther permanently or transiently improving the airway distress. It is not unusual for repeated racemic epinephrine aerosols to be administered. However, a certain percentage of children will require more vigorous treatment to manage the airway distress.

In the past, a child with a compromised airway secondary to laryngotracheobronchitis almost always underwent tracheotomy. Today, the realization of the risks of tracheotomy in children has resulted in the use of endotracheal intubation as a means of securing the airway (Fig. 20–2). This has been found to be an effective means of treating the compromised airway. The only possible exception is in young children under 1 year of age, whose larynx is so small that the use of the endotracheal tube might create secondary problems such as ulceration of the mucosa, fibrosis, and stenosis. Most children can be successfully extubated after a few days and have no permanent clinically significant sequelae from either the disease or the treatment.

Because laryngotracheobronchitis can be caused by many different viruses, it is not unusual for a child to have more than one episode. Each episode results in antibody production only to the specific viral strain causing that particular infection.

### Epiglottitis
Epiglottitis is another laryngeal inflammatory process that primarily affects children. The pre-

senting symptoms are similar to those of laryngotracheobronchitis, but there are some differences (Fig. 20–3). Epiglottitis occurs in an older age group, involving primarily 2- to 4-year-old children. One major difference is the rate of symptom development. The progression of edema with epiglottitis is more rapid, and thus airway distress also occurs more quickly. Once again, there is usually a concomitant upper respiratory symptom complex that also includes sore throat. With epiglottitis, it is not unusual for the child to have some difficulty swallowing. There is alteration in the voice quality with airway distress, which progresses quite rapidly, occurring in minutes rather than hours. In severe cases requiring treatment in the emergency department, it is not uncommon for children to have some changes in their level of awareness as a result of the airway compromise.

The physical examination will reveal a child who appears to be systemically ill with malaise and respiratory distress. A child who is having significant airway compromise will often assume a posture that improves the airway. This is characterized by flexing the trunk and extending the back while flexing the neck and extending the

Epiglottitis

■ Croup

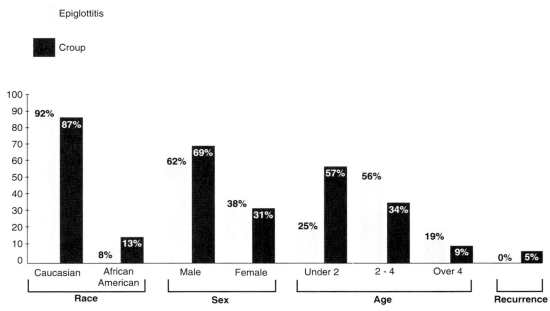

**FIG 20–3.**
The multiple viral origins of croup are the reason there is a greater chance for recurrence than with epiglottitis.

head in an effort to straighten the airway and facilitate air movement (Fig. 20–4). Drooling is common because of the increased production of saliva and the reluctance to swallow because of pain. Because the larynx is relatively high in the neck of a child, it is not unusual to be able to identify an edematous and erythematous epiglottis, which is markedly enlarged, just by opening the child's mouth and inspecting the oral cavity and oropharynx. The use of a tongue blade is generally not recommended for fear of inadvertently touching the inflamed epiglottis, which may precipitate a laryngospasm and total airway obstruction. After the diagnosis of epiglottitis has been established on the basis of clinical findings, it is imperative to respect the natural history of the rapid progression of airway compromise and to have medical personnel closely attending the child in the event of a sudden airway obstruction. A lateral soft tissue radiograph can be helpful in identifying an epiglottis that has become enlarged as a result of the inflammation (Fig. 20–5).

The etiology of epiglottitis is bacterial rather than viral. *Haemophilus influenzae* is the most common pathogen. Antibacterial therapy is possible and usually effective. Ampicillin used to be the most frequently prescribed antibiotic, but the increased frequency of ampicillin-resistant strains

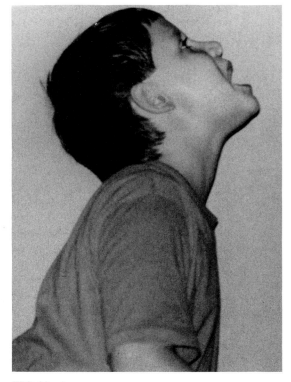

**FIG 20–4.**
Typical positioning of a person with partial airway obstruction who is trying to straighten the upper airway in an effort to facilitate air exchange.

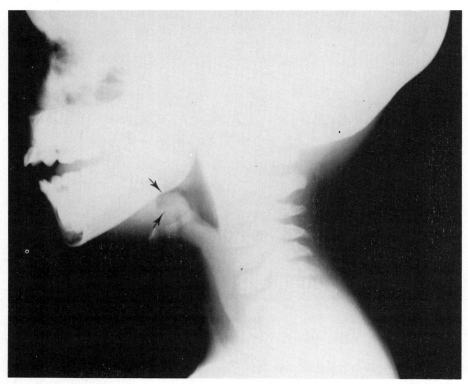

**FIG 20–5.**
Lateral soft tissue radiograph has demonstrated the blunted and enlarged epiglottis seen in a child with epiglottitis.

of *H. influenzae* has prompted the need for chloramphenicol in certain instances. Vaporization is also part of the treatment program.

As mentioned, it is critical to respect the natural history of the disease, which includes rapid progression of airway distress. Some advocate securing the airway with either tracheotomy or intubation in every child who has epiglottitis. The incidence of needing airway intervention for epiglottitis is considerably higher than it is for laryngotracheobronchitis. In a group of children with laryngotracheobronchitis at Columbus Children's Hospital, the incidence of endotracheal intubation was about 6% as compared with 60% for those children with epiglottitis. If airway obstruction is determined to be severe, either tracheotomy or endotracheal intubation can be used. Endotracheal intubation has been found to be an effective, safe approach, and tracheotomy is no longer used as frequently.

The pathologic changes with epiglottitis involve profound edema and erythema of all of the supraglottic structures, specifically the epiglottis,

aryepiglottic folds, and false vocal cords. In fact, some have suggested that a more accurate name for epiglottitis would be *supraglottitis*. The glottic and subglottic compartments of the larynx are relatively uninvolved and appear normal.

The clinical course is characterized by rapid improvement to the point that often the airway is much improved within 48 hours and the endotracheal tube is no longer necessary. Because this disease is bacterial in origin, involving primarily one genus, the incidence of recurrence is negligible.

## Conditions in Adults
### Acute Laryngitis

Acute laryngitis is primarily viral in etiology and often occurs in conjunction with an upper respiratory infection involving additional sites. Although viral acute laryngitis can be seen in children, it is more common in adults. In addition to the usual symptoms of an upper respiratory infection, there is hoarseness. As discussed, any physical changes in the vocal cords that interfere with their normal mass and impede their ability to close totally during phonation will alter the normal voice quality. The hoarseness is usually constant in duration. It is rare for it to be intermittent. Indirect laryngoscopy reveals that the true vocal cords are erythematous and edematous (Fig. 20–6). Vascular injection of the vocal cord mucosa is also commonly seen. It is not unusual to see some component of erythema in the supraglottic portion of the larynx, but it is most pronounced in the glottis. It is rare for viral acute laryngitis to cause edema that compromises the airway. There is no impairment of vocal cord mobility. The process is usually self-limited, with spontaneous improvement. However, voice rest (to prevent further irritation of the inflamed vocal cords) and vaporization help to expedite recovery, as does the removal of any irritants such as cigarette smoke or other environmental agents.

### Chronic Laryngitis

If the acute laryngitis does not completely resolve, the process progresses to a chronic inflammatory state. The tissue changes are more consistent with those of chronic inflammation than with those of acute infection. The true vocal cords are edematous, and there is a minimal amount of either vascular injection or erythema. Once again, treatment is supportive; management is directed at trying to minimize the stress to this inflamed tissue with the use of voice rest, vaporization, cessation of smoking, and avoidance of environmental irritants. This treatment usually results in a gradual improvement. However, some patients do not improve and undergo further tissue changes.

### Polypoid Corditis

Polypoid corditis is a form of chronic laryngitis that is characterized by persistent hoarseness without other symptoms. Indirect laryngoscopy demonstrates vocal cords with rather profound tissue edema without erythema (Fig. 20–7). This mucosal edema can be so extensive that the true vocal cords appear to be "water bags." At this stage, conservative treatment is usually not successful. It is advisable to encourage the patient to develop an ongoing program of smoking cessation, avoidance of irritants, and nonstressful use of the larynx. Definitive therapy is primarily surgical. This is done endoscopically and involves the removal of the edematous tissue to allow for regeneration of the normal vocal cord mucosa. The tissue can be removed using microlaryngeal instruments or the carbon dioxide laser.

### Vocal Cord Nodules

Vocal cord nodules typically result from a localized chronic inflammation created by vocal abuse. Vocal nodules cause hoarseness and are seen in both children and adults. They are the result of stress to the larynx and are frequently seen in children who do a considerable amount of screaming and in adults who stress their larynges with frequent yelling or singing. Parents and chil-

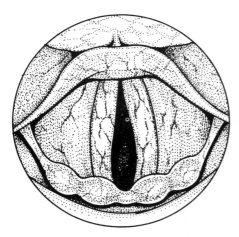

**FIG 20–6.**
The true vocal cords are uniformly erythematous and edematous in acute laryngitis.

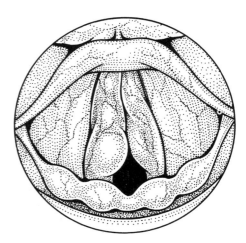

**FIG 20–7.**
Polypoid corditis is characterized by profound edema, giving the true vocal cord mucosa a baggy appearance.

dren who are members of large families in which yelling for disciplinary or attention-drawing reasons is frequent seem to be especially at risk for developing nodules. The nodules are usually not painful and cause no problems with swallowing. The hoarseness is persistent and not intermittent.

The physical examination reveals a protrusion on both true vocal cords, usually at the junction of the anterior and middle one-third of the cord (Fig. 20–8). The protrusions develop initially from submucosal hemorrhages resulting from an impact injury between the vocal cords. The blood is ultimately replaced by fibrous tissue that eventually matures into a firm nodule. These vocal cord nodules do not have a pattern of progressive growth. They do not create airway problems and have no realistic potential for malignant degeneration.

When the diagnosis is established, treatment is directed primarily at correcting the stressful vocal behavior that resulted in the creation of the nodules. Therefore, voice therapy plays a prominent role in most treatment programs. After the abusive behavior has stopped, it is not unusual for the nodules to resolve completely without the need for any specific surgical intervention. If the vocal behavior has been corrected and the nodules persist, surgery is advisable. Excision is performed endoscopically using suspension microlaryngoscopy. These nodules can be removed with either instruments or the carbon dioxide laser. Vocal rest is important following the surgery to permit mucosal regeneration over the areas of the resected nodules.

### Vocal Cord Polyps

Another extension of the same type of pathophysiology seen in polypoid corditis is the development of more discrete mucosal swellings giving the clinical appearance of polyps (Fig. 20–9). The symptom complex is similar, namely, persistent and painless hoarseness. Conservative treatment is usually not effective, and endoscopic surgical excision is advisable.

### Vocal Cord Granulomas

Vocal cord granulomas develop over the vocal process of the arytenoid cartilages and represent ulcerations on the free edge of each vocal cord (Fig. 20–10). They can be the result of mechanical stress to the larynx from an endotracheal tube during an operative procedure. They may also be seen in professionals with considerable voice demands, such as teachers and singers. Vocal cord granulomas can develop from an ulcerative stage into granulation tissue within the ulcer forming a spherical mass of tissue (Fig. 20–11). In addition to the usual persistent hoarseness, some pain may be present, resulting from secondary infection of the granulation tissue composing these granulomas.

Numerous treatment programs have been proposed, but none are universally successful. Conservative treatment involving voice rest and steroid inhalers has been tried with variable success. Some believe that these granulomas may be associated with esophageal reflux and advocate treatment programs including antacids, head of bed elevation, and other antireflux measures. Surgical

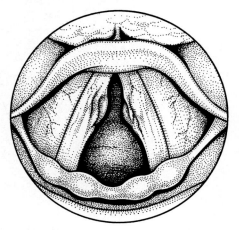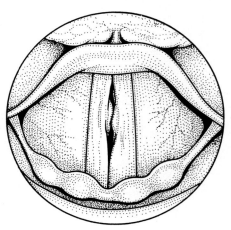

**FIG 20–8.**
Vocal cord nodules are typically seen at the junction of the anterior and middle thirds of the true vocal cords.

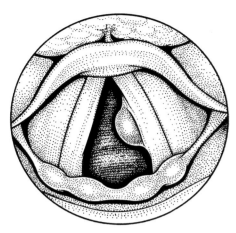

**FIG 20–9.**
Vocal cord polyps are a manifestation of localized mucosal edema.

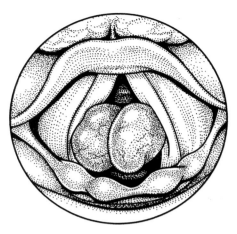

**FIG 20–11.**
Vocal cord granulomas are accumulations of granulation tissue in an area of ulceration.

programs involving resection of the granulomas with endoscopy or the carbon dioxide laser followed by steroid injections to the base have also only been intermittently successful. Vocal cord granulomas continue to be a major therapeutic challenge, and patients must be informed before treatment that they have a problem that is often difficult to resolve and may recur.

### Diphtheria

Diphtheria can involve the larynx. It causes hoarseness and can ultimately develop into respiratory distress with a thick exudative membrane that occludes the glottis. Tracheotomy is some-

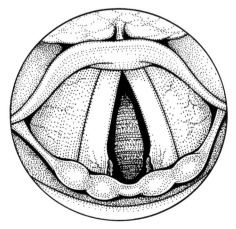

**FIG 20–10.**
Breakdown of the epithelium over the vocal processes of the arytenoid cartilages creates pain with inflammation.

times necessary. Treatment is identical to that for diphtheria involving other portions of the upper aerodigestive tract. Diphtheria is currently an extremely rare problem in the United States.

### Tuberculous Laryngitis

Tuberculosis can infect the larynx secondary to either the pulmonary disease causing passage of infected secretions through the larynx or as a primary infection independent of any pulmonary components. Although it was formerly believed that most abnormalities were seen in the posterior portion of the larynx, it has now been demonstrated that any location within the larynx can be involved. Nontender hoarseness occurs and is not associated with a cough unless there is pulmonary involvement. The endolaryngeal mucosa is usually erythematous and edematous. Superficial ulcerations are common. The diagnosis is made by noting the presence of caseating granuloma, by taking tissue biopsies, and by correlating the biopsy results with the culture and skin test results. Treatment is with currently advised antituberculous agents.

### Professional Voice Users

Professional singers and actors have an obvious need for a normally functioning larynx. Even the slightest alteration in laryngeal anatomy can be responsible for changes that could significantly detract from the individual's professional talents. But there are also others whose professions are heavily dependent on optimal laryngeal function.

Teachers, politicians, clergy, and others whose effectiveness is linked to verbal communication skills also need optimal laryngeal function. The emergence of more sophisticated radiographic imaging studies as well as strobovideolaryngoscopy and objective mechanisms for quantifying voice production have provided the technologic means of increasing diagnostic and therapeutic capabilities. When this technology is accompanied by an interdisciplinary approach that involves an otolaryngologist–head and neck surgeon and a speech pathologist, there is certainly the potential to improve on changes in vocal function that are significant to the professional voice user. The pathologic condition can range from subtle anatomic changes to alterations in extrinsic laryngeal muscle tension or even psychologic conditions that can affect the quality of voice. Often therapy does not involve surgical intervention. It is important to understand the often complex therapeutic needs of this special population.

## TRAUMA

Laryngeal trauma is usually the result of blunt trauma to the neck. Motor vehicle accidents are the most common cause. The symptoms and physical findings can be deceptively unalarming. However, it is not unusual for slow, progressive airway compromise to occur. If the clinician is not knowledgeable about the symptoms and signs of significant trauma to the larynx, it is conceivable that such airway obstruction could occur after the patient has been discharged following an initial evaluation.

The individual who has sustained a fracture of the larynx will not always have a neck skin laceration. The rather rapid development of laryngeal edema usually causes an alteration in the voice quality soon after the incident. The patient may even complain of tenderness with swallowing as a result of the vocal cord adduction during the act of swallowing. Airway obstruction may not be present as an acute condition but can develop several hours after injury as edema advances.

The physical examination begins with inspection of the neck. If the usually protruding thyroid notch (Adam's apple) is absent, the examiner should suspect a fracture with displacement (Fig. 20–12). The physical examination of the neck may reveal some edema over the larynx. The patient who has had a laryngeal fracture will typi-

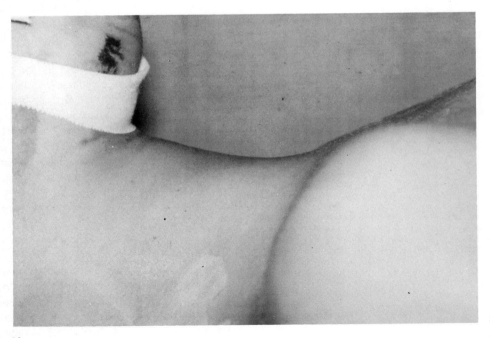

**FIG 20–12.**
The usual protusion of the thyroid notch is absent in this patient who was found to have a displaced comminuted laryngeal fracture.

cally have rather exquisite tenderness over the fracture site. It is critical for the clinician to recognize that vigorous palpation may move the fragments of the laryngeal cartilage. This may potentiate the degree of airway obstruction, thus converting a partial into a total obstruction. The examiner should only lightly palpate the larynx. The intent of palpation is not so much to identify the actual fracture lines but rather to determine the existence of localized tenderness, which would increase the index of suspicion that the fracture exists.

Palpation will also determine if there is any evidence of subcutaneous crepitation. If this is present in combination with localized tenderness, there is a strong chance that a laryngeal fracture has lacerated the laryngeal mucosa and permitted air to escape into the soft tissue of the neck. With more severe injuries, the subcutaneous crepitation can be so extensive that it involves the entire neck and extends down into the mediastinum and up into the face. Indirect laryngoscopy usually reveals an edematous and ecchymotic larynx. The examiner must try to identify the existence of any lacerations and/or exposed fragments of laryngeal cartilage. Vocal cord mobility should also be assessed. Most laryngeal fractures in adults are not single but usually include multiple fracture lines (Fig. 20–13).

If the patient's airway is stable, radiographic examinations can help to determine the extent of the injury. However, these are not absolutely essential if the clinical suspicion of fracture exists. When there is a strong clinical suspicion of laryngeal fracture, tracheotomy with surgical exploration of the larynx is recommended. When there have been notable lacerations of the laryngeal mucosa, exploration, reduction, and fixation of the fracture should be undertaken as soon as the patient's general condition will permit. Early surgical intervention in this clinical situation seems to decrease the incidence of postoperative infection, which can have disastrous effects on the outcome.

In the individual who has sustained blunt trauma to the neck and has subcutaneous crepitation but no localized tenderness of the larynx and no voice abnormalities, the examiner should suspect a laceration of the hypopharynx. Endoscopic evaluation is essential, followed by exploration and surgical drainage of the neck and possibly even an attempt at closure of the laceration if one is identified.

The successful management of laryngopharyn-

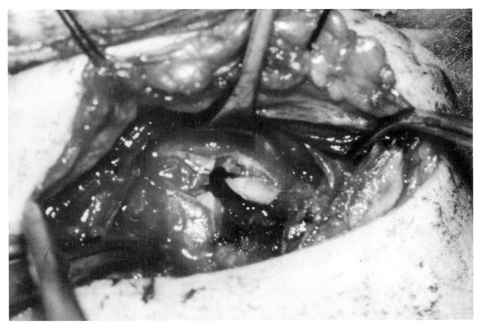

**FIG 20–13.**
Operative photograph of a patient who has sustained a comminuted laryngeal fracture.

geal trauma depends on the awareness of the clinician involved in the initial evaluation of the patient. Often the area is not examined in a patient who has other serious injuries to organ systems. It is only several days later, when the patient's other problems have stabilized, that otolaryngologic consultation is obtained to evaluate a problem that may have been managed more effectively if diagnosed and treated earlier. Greater awareness of these subtle symptoms and physical findings should result in earlier diagnosis and improved treatment results.

## NEOPLASMS

The presenting symptoms of a laryngeal neoplasm, whether it be benign or malignant, are indistinguishable from those of any pathologic condition that alters the mass and/or mobility of endolaryngeal structures. A patient will have a change in voice quality, referred to as hoarseness. However, in sharp contrast to the hoarseness associated with inflammatory conditions, the hoarseness of a patient with a laryngeal neoplasm will persist for as long as the neoplasm is present because it impairs the normal closure of the true vocal cords (Fig. 20–14). The key, therefore, is to note the duration and persistence of the hoarseness. *In an adult, and especially one who smokes, hoarseness that is present for 2 weeks or longer demands a complete examination of the larynx.*

At times laryngeal neoplasms arise from structures of the endolarynx that are away from the free edges of the true vocal cords. An example of this would be cancer arising in the supraglottic portion of the larynx, such as on the epiglottis. In this situation, there is no impairment of vocal cord closure during phonation and the patient is not hoarse. However, the patient usually complains of sore throat and sometimes odynophagia. Laryngeal neoplasms arising in areas that do not cause hoarseness are particularly troublesome. Invariably, they result in nondescript symptoms that usually are not considered to be significant by a primary care physician. Often, that physician does not have the skills to do a thorough laryngeal examination, and an unfortunate delay in diagnosis occurs, which can have an adverse effect on the outcome of treatment. The hypopharyngeal area must be examined with a laryngeal mirror

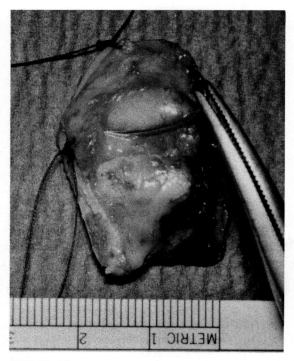

**FIG 20–14.**
A photograph of the right side of the larynx following removal of a true vocal cord cancer seen below the suture needle, which is positioned in the laryngeal ventricle.

and/or flexible fiberoptic instrument relatively early, especially in ethanol-consuming and cigarette-smoking patients, who have an increased risk for the development of laryngeal neoplasms.

The physical examination of the larynx has been previously described. The neoplasm will appear as either an exophytic or ulcerative mass that has disrupted the normal surface epithelium. The examiner must be able to identify the exact limits of the neoplasm and then assess its impact on normal vocal cord mobility and laryngeal function. The skilled examiner of the larynx can obtain considerable information from these office examining techniques, although they are inevitably followed by a more thorough examination using direct laryngoscopy performed under either a local or general anesthetic. This type of examination can provide definitive information about all parts of the laryngopharyngeal complex except the subglottic region. It does not allow adequate exposure of this region.

The current radiographic test more frequently

used to study laryngeal neoplasms is computed tomography, which was discussed in Chapter 16. Contrast laryngograms have been used but do not provide the specificity that can be obtained with computed tomography. The primary purpose of radiographic studies is to examine the subglottic region, which cannot be adequately evaluated with the other approaches. Radiographic tests usually precede direct laryngoscopy because biopsy may alter the anatomic relationships as a result of the development of edema at the biopsy site. The biopsy invariably results in the histopathologic diagnosis, and appropriate treatment can be planned.

## Benign Neoplasms

There are some benign tumors that can involve the larynx in children. *Hemangiomas* and *lymphangiomas* are the most common. They show a predilection for the subglottic region of the larynx. The presenting symptoms are voice alteration and ultimately airway distress. A substantial percentage of children with cutaneous hemangiomas will also have an associated subglottic hemangioma or lymphangioma. Tracheotomy is often necessary to preserve an adequate breathing passage. As with cutaneous hemangiomas, a conservative approach is emphasized because of the marked propensity for these vascular benign tumors to undergo spontaneous resolution to the extent that no surgical excision is required.

Some advocate the use of the carbon dioxide or Nd:Yag laser to decrease the volume of the hemangiomas to allow earlier tracheal decannulation. Such an approach, if proved to be reliable and effective, might be attractive because it would shorten the duration of an indwelling tracheotomy tube in an infant or young child. Tracheotomy in children causes substantial morbidity and even mortality because of the difficulty of maintaining its position and patency.

Laryngeal papilloma (Fig. 20–15), although relatively rare, can have a devastating impact on the physiologic function of the larynx and the psychologic stability of the patient. It is believed to be viral in origin. The papillomas present as papillary growths that arise from any portion of the endolarynx. Papillomas can occur in either sex and can initially occur at any age. If papillomatous growths are present on the true vocal

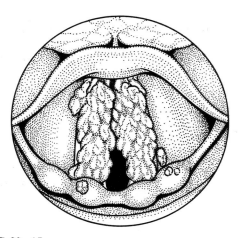

**FIG 20–15.**
The presumed viral origin of laryngeal papilloma is believed to be the reason for multiple recurrences, which are commonplace.

cords, hoarseness is the primary complaint. If papillomas are located in other portions of the endolarynx, such as in the supraglottic larynx, the individual may have other symptoms such as sore throat and/or airway distress.

These papillomatous growths can become large enough to cause significant airway obstruction. The presumed viral etiology suggests a potential for infecting other sites of the airway. Tracheotomy is avoided if at all possible because of the fear of implanting papillomas at the tracheotomy site or in the distal tracheobronchial airway. Emergent direct laryngoscopy with removal of the papillomas is the preferred treatment for the obstructed airway rather than tracheotomy.

These papillomas have a marked propensity for recurrence. The carbon dioxide laser is a precise means of vaporizing the papillomas and minimizing the damage to noninvolved epithelium, reducing the potential for scarring. However, it does not decrease the frequency of recurrences. Some patients with papillomas will eventually enter a quiescent state and no longer have recurrences. It is not unusual for patients to require numerous operations extending from infancy to adulthood. There are even reports of papilloma infiltrating not only the distant tracheobronchial tree but also the lung parenchyma.

There are a variety of other tumors that involve the larynx but do not occur frequently. About 50% of all *granular cell* tumors arise in some portion of the head and neck. They most commonly involve the oral cavity but can arise within the larynx. These tumors were initially believed to be of muscular origin, but recent evidence suggests that they are neurogenous in origin. The histopathologic findings can be confused with those of squamous cell carcinoma. These benign tumors can occasionally be successfully removed endoscopically.

*Oncocytic* laryngeal tumors also occur. They appear as a bluish submucosal cyst. These lesions almost exclusively involve the supraglottic larynx. Once again, endoscopic excision appears to be an effective form of treatment.

*Paragangliomas* or other neurogenic tumors can also involve the larynx. However, they are rare and have no distinguishing clinical findings but are usually identified solely by histopathologic examination. If the excised tumor is found to be a neurofibroma, there is the potential for multiple site involvement.

*Lipomas* are another form of a rare laryngeal tumor. The supraglottic larynx has the greatest amount of subcutaneous fat and therefore represents the most frequent site of origin of a lipoma. They present as submucosal yellowish masses. Endoscopic removal is feasible for small lipomas.

*Chondromas* can involve the larynx, and most originate from the cricoid cartilage. They occur predominantly in males. Endoscopic removal can occasionally be successful but an external approach is more commonly used. Sometimes it is possible to remove only a portion of the larynx, avoiding total laryngectomy and the stress created by loss of laryngeal speech.

Other extremely rare conditions, such as *pleomorphic adenoma, nodular fasciitis,* and *fibrous histiocytoma* can involve the larynx. However, the improved sophistication of microlaryngeal technology, especially since the advent of the carbon dioxide laser, has dramatically increased the endoscopic capabilities of excising these benign laryngeal tumors.

## Malignant Neoplasms

Squamous cell carcinoma is overwhelmingly the most frequent malignancy involving the larynx. Approximately 90% of all laryngeal malignancies are epidermoid carcinomas. It was formerly believed that the degree of histologic differentiation had prognostic significance for the pa-

tient, but recent evidence suggests that such a relationship is not as reliable as was thought. Adenoid cystic carcinoma can also arise from the larynx, although it is considerably less common than epidermoid cancer. Chondrosarcoma is the malignant counterpart of the benign chondroma. Many chondrosarcomas have a favorable outlook, and this observation has prompted greater use of operative procedures that leave part of the larynx rather than remove it totally when the malignancy is not sensitive to radiation therapy. Such procedures are termed *conservation surgery*. Lymphomas can also originate from laryngeal structures, although they are quite rare.

The larynx sometimes is a metastatic site for certain cell types. Both adenocarcinomas and malignant melanomas not only arise from laryngeal structures but also metastasize to the larynx from other primary locations.

The biologic behavior of laryngeal malignancies is closely related to their site of origin within the larynx. The *supraglottic* larynx is a region rich in lymphatics. It is also a region where a primary tumor frequently can enlarge substantially before it causes any bothersome symptoms (Fig.

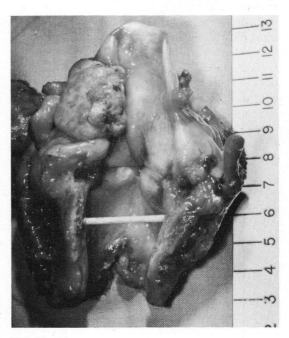

**FIG 20–16.**
This large carcinoma involved the aryepiglottic fold. It caused minimal symptoms until it became so large that it prolapsed into the glottic chink and caused sudden airway obstruction.

20–16). For these reasons, neck nodal metastases are common either as detectable palpable nodes or as microscopically metastatic normal-sized nodes.

In contrast, the *glottic* portion of the larynx has only a few lymphatic channels. Nodal metastases are rare for glottic cancers. In addition, glottic cancers produce hoarseness early in their course. A laryngeal cancer that involves the free edge of the true vocal cord and is as small as 2 or 3 mm in diameter will cause hoarseness that should alert the patient and the physician to the need for a thorough laryngeal examination. The combination of sparse lymphatics and the onset of hoarseness early in the course of the disease results in a favorable outlook for patients whose malignancies involve the glottic portion of the larynx.

The *subglottic* region is rarely the site of origin of a laryngeal primary cancer, but it is not unusual for it to be involved secondarily from inferior extension of a cancer arising from the glottic region. Lymphatics are abundant in this region and can involve not only the lateral neck nodes but also the paratracheal neck nodes.

The *hypopharynx* is a bothersome region for the development of malignancies because the loose submucosal tissues allow considerable submucosal extension of tumor that is not detected by physical examination. In addition, the hypopharynx is rich in lymphatics to the lateral neck nodes. As a hypopharyngeal lesion approaches the midline, the possibility also exists for neck nodal metastases to both sides. Hypopharyngeal lesions typically do not cause any distinguishable symptoms until they are quite large and start interfering with swallowing or speech. Early in their course, they usually cause some odynophagia and dysphagia.

The treatment of laryngeal and hypopharyngeal cancers is a function of the extent of the disease. For an early-stage laryngeal cancer in which there is no evidence of neck nodal involvement, surgery and radiation therapy provide an equal chance for cure. Radiation therapy will frequently allow better voice quality than surgery. However,

the advent of the carbon dioxide laser has brought some surprisingly excellent voice quality results with no apparent compromise in the potential for cure. It is anticipated that laser usage for early-stage laryngeal cancers will increase.

As laryngeal cancers become larger, the effectiveness of either surgery or radiation therapy decreases. Patients often receive planned, combined therapy in which surgery and irradiation are both used. There is recent evidence to suggest that some laryngeal cancers can be treated using chemotherapy with radiotherapy. This preserves the larynx without compromising chances for survival. There has been considerable interest in adding adjunctive chemotherapy to these combined therapy programs as a means of trying to treat the distant metastatic disease. As the use of surgery combined with radiation therapy became more popular, it became apparent that the local and regional disease was being better controlled. However, patients were not living any longer because they were developing distant metastases and dying of the uncontrolled distant disease. As with other head and neck cancers, it appears that the combined therapy programs have not actually improved the survival rate but have changed the pattern of how the treatment programs fail. The major change in surgical treatment of laryngeal cancers is the increasing frequency of operations that do not totally remove the larynx. This matter will be discussed in more detail in Chapter 21.

The treatment of hypopharyngeal cancers basically mirrors the approach for the treatment of laryngeal malignancies. However, the more aggressive biologic behavior of the hypopharyngeal lesions is reflected in the use of planned combined therapy for some of the earlier-stage lesions. Only the small primary tumors that have no evidence of neck nodal involvement are treated with either surgery or radiation therapy alone. The overwhelming majority of tumors are treated with some sort of planned, combined therapy. Even with this approach, the control of hypopharyngeal cancers remains a major problem.

# 21

# Laryngeal Reconstruction and Rehabilitation

Few things are as disabling as the impairment resulting from total loss of laryngeal speech. The impact of the total removal of the larynx is so dramatic that it can even affect the patient's decision regarding treatment. Even though the total surgical removal of the larynx may provide the greatest chance of successfully controlling a malignancy, it is not unusual for a patient to knowingly compromise a chance for cure by choosing another form of treatment that would result in preservation of the larynx and the ability to speak. Ever since the first total laryngectomy was performed more than 100 years ago, surgeons have been trying to develop modifications either to preserve a portion of the larynx or to create a technique that would allow some type of vocalization following total laryngectomy. There has been considerable progress, and procedures have been developed to preserve adequate portions of the larynx to permit laryngeal speech without compromising the quality of the patient's cancer resection.

One of the most dramatic developments in otolaryngology and head and neck surgery is vocal restoration for the patient who has undergone total laryngectomy. The speaking mechanism can be reconstructed in the patient whose larynx was totally removed many years ago. The procedure can also be done during a total laryngectomy. Blom, Singer, and Panje developed this safe, effective reconstructive technique for vocal restoration.

The techniques used for laryngeal reconstruction can be classified according to the etiology of the injury. The surgical approaches to these major etiologic groupings (trauma, cancer, neurologic)

differ. In the trauma patient, laryngeal reconstruction is designed to use as much remaining laryngeal structure as feasible. This is in contrast to the technique for the patient who has a laryngeal malignancy in which a portion of the larynx is removed and a defect has to be closed. Patients with neurologic injuries involving the larynx demand special reconstructive considerations, and these are usually directed at the mechanisms of preventing the possibility of aspiration.

## RECONSTRUCTION FOLLOWING TRAUMA

It is important for the patient to understand the expectations of surgery for laryngeal reconstruction following trauma. It is rare for voice quality to be restored to normal in patients who have sustained significant injury to the larynx. The goals of reconstruction in the trauma patient are to provide an adequate airway so that a tracheotomy tube is not necessary and a voice quality suitable for usual communication.

The management of the acute laryngeal injury is critical to the chances for success. Because the larynx is part of the upper airway, any laryngeal mucosal lacerations will be subject to secondary bacterial infections. It is usually best to perform laryngeal reconstruction of the acutely injured larynx as soon as the patient's other injuries will permit.

This promptness minimizes the amount of edema and also decreases the chances of wound infection. The surgery involves restoring soft tissue structures to their normal anatomic position. If laryngeal soft tissue has been lost, it must be replaced with mucosa. The buccal mucosa is often a useful donor site for a graft. After soft tissue continuity has been restored, the rigid framework needs to be reconstructed. If there is no loss of cartilaginous structures, these fragments of fractured cartilage can be wired to provide support required to maintain an adequate airway. If this is not possible, a soft Silastic stent is inserted into the larynx to maintain configuration as wound healing progresses (Fig. 21–1). However, the type of material for and the duration of stenting remain controversial.

In the patient who has a long-standing laryngeal injury following trauma, it is necessary to define whether soft tissue needs to be augmented and/or rigid support is necessary. A multitude of mucosal grafts, local skin flaps, and osseomuscular flaps have been used to meet these needs (Fig. 21–2), but none of them are uniformly successful.

Once again, it is important for the patient to have realistic expectations about the outcome of reconstruction. The first priority is to create an adequate airway, and the second priority is to provide a voice quality that is useful for meaningful communication.

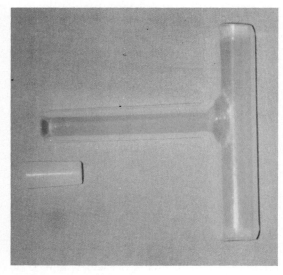

**FIG 21–1.**
The soft Silastic tracheal T tube provides a means of stenting the trachea following repair while maintaining a safe airway.

# RECONSTRUCTION FOLLOWING LARYNGEAL CANCER SURGERY

With laryngeal cancer surgery the emphasis is on the preservation of enough of the larynx so that it sustains its usual functions. It becomes critical for the treating physician to have the diagnostic skills to accurately assess the extent of cancer involvement of the larynx. Only with this information can a proper decision be made regarding the extent of excision. Laryngeal resections that result in preservation of a portion of the larynx are referred to as *conservation* laryngeal surgery. The proper term is *conservation,* not *conservative surgery;* the surgical approach is anything but conservative. The conservative approach for treating a laryngeal cancer would be to remove the entire larynx and, it is hoped, ensure adequate margins of resections. As stated previously, though, it is now well documented that one can remove less tissue when excising a laryngeal cancer and not compromise the oncologic safety of the operation.

For patients who have malignancies involving one true vocal cord or one true vocal cord and a portion of the other, a form of conservation laryngeal surgery referred to as hemilaryngectomy can be performed. A synonym for this operation is *vertical partial laryngectomy.* It refers to the removal of one half or possibly more of the larynx in the vertical plane (Fig. 21–3). This operation is usually well tolerated by the patient. Difficulty in swallowing is minimal postoperatively. Although the patient's voice quality is altered, it is usually adequate for meaningful communication, even over the telephone.

When cancer involves the supraglottic portion of the larynx, another type of conservation laryngeal surgery, referred to as a supraglottic laryngectomy, can be performed. A synonym for this operation is *horizontal partial laryngectomy.* In this surgery, the supraglottic portion of the larynx is removed. The procedure usually entails the removal of endolaryngeal structures from the tip of the epiglottis down to and including the laryngeal vertical (Fig. 21–4). After this operation, the patient's voice quality is often excellent. In fact, it is not unusual for the voice quality to be unaltered. The main reason for this excellent voice quality is that the true vocal cords have been pre-

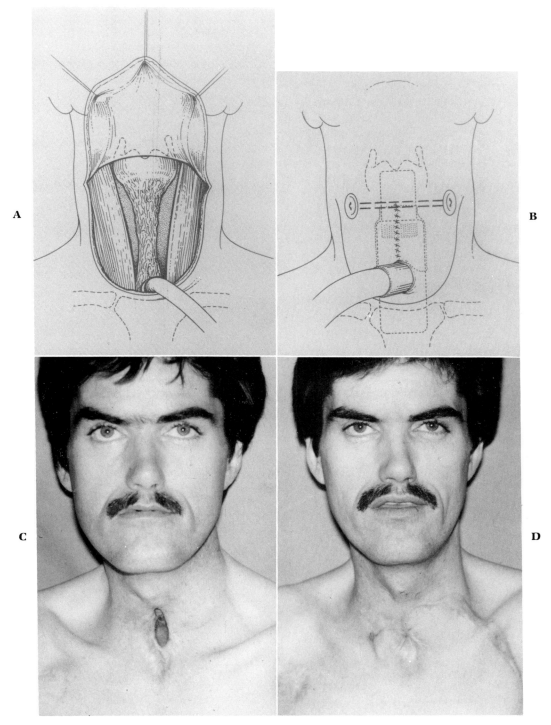

**FIG 21–2.**
**A,** diagrammatic representation of a total loss of the lower half of the larynx and cervical trachea following a gunshot injury. Stage reconstructions were done to **B,** reestablish continuity of the pharynx with the thoracic trachea. Subsequent reconstruction involved **C,** numerous flaps, grafts, and stents, which eventually **D,** restored the airway in this patient who has now had a safe airway for 8 years with only minimal restrictions in physical activity.

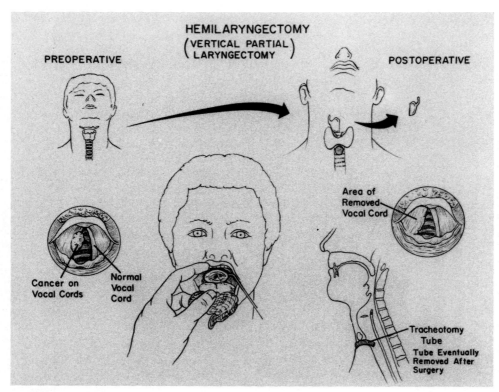

**FIG 21–3.**
The technique of hemilaryngectomy.

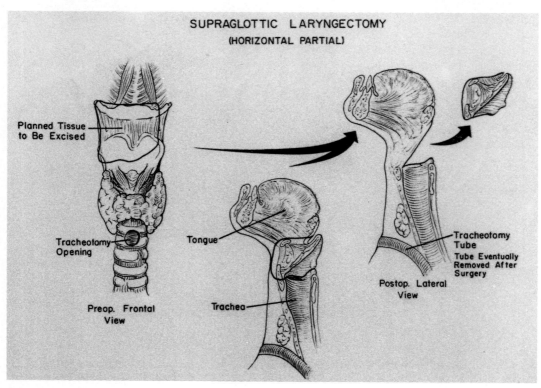

**FIG 21–4.**
The technique of supraglottic laryngectomy.

served. However, the challenge to patients undergoing this operation relates to their ability to swallow without aspiration. This particular operation can create aspiration problems because the major reflex arc that causes closure of the larynx is initiated by the sensory receptors in the supraglottic larynx. Patient selection is important. The patient must have an adequate pulmonary reserve. These patients need special swallowing training postoperatively. Although the speed of satisfactory rehabilitation is variable, it is rare to have a patient who is permanently unable to take adequate feedings by mouth.

In patients in whom it is not oncologically safe to perform one of the conservation procedures, total laryngectomy is done. After this procedure, the patient is obviously no longer able to communicate with laryngeal speech. In the past, communication depended on whether the patient had the anatomic capabilities and motivational reserve to develop esophageal speech. However, the popularity of combined therapy programs that use surgery and postoperative irradiation has decreased the success rate of patients trying to learn useful esophageal speech. The tissue fibrosis that occurs subsequent to this vigorous treatment program adversely affects the ability to develop esophageal speech.

It is in this category of patients that vocal restoration using the tracheoesophageal puncture technique has achieved considerable success. This can be performed on patients who have previously undergone total laryngectomy or who undergo restoration during laryngectomy. The surgical aspects of vocal restoration are technically not difficult. The operation involves creation of a tracheoesophageal fistula with a puncture large enough to permit ultimate insertion of the valve prosthesis. The prosthesis is simple in design. It is a hollow tube open at the tracheal end and closed with a horizontal slit at the hypopharyngeal end (Fig. 21–5). The air pressure opens this closed end during phonation, permitting air to enter the hypopharynx. With cessation of talking, the hypopharyngeal end closes and prevents saliva from draining into the trachea. The success of this vocal restoration depends heavily on the expertise and energy level of the speech pathologist who is part of the vocal restoration team. Variables associated with vocal rehabilitation following tracheoesophageal puncture technique are discussed in

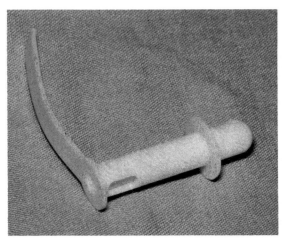

**FIG 21–5.**
This vocal prosthesis allows for the passage of air from the trachea into the hypopharynx but prevents the opposite flow of saliva.

Chapter 22. The quality of voice is excellent, and speech is easily understood over the telephone. Some patients can even sing with tracheoesophageal valve speech.

## RECONSTRUCTION FOLLOWING NEUROLOGIC LARYNGEAL INJURIES

A vocal cord can be paralyzed from a variety of infectious, metabolic, traumatic, and neoplastic processes. However, transection of the recurrent laryngeal nerve during thyroidectomy remains the most common cause.

The patient who has sustained a unilateral vocal cord paralysis will frequently experience an air-spilling type of hoarseness initially. Over several weeks, this can improve to the point that the voice quality is actually normal despite persistence of the paralysis. This phenomenon usually results from the paralyzed vocal cord assuming a more midline position as scarring of the intrinsic laryngeal muscle occurs so that the functioning vocal cord can fully approximate it and produce a normal voice (Fig. 21–6). The patient with a unilateral vocal cord paralysis usually does not have any airway problems and, in the compensated state, does not have problems with aspiration. If the patient cannot completely close the glottis, aspiration is possible.

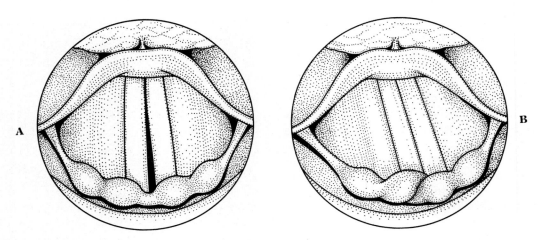

**FIG 21–6.**
**A,** sketch of uncompensated vocal cord paralysis that eventually will **B,** compensate as the functioning cord crosses the midline to touch the paralyzed cord.

In the patient who has bilateral vocal cord paralysis, voice quality is usually excellent. In fact, there may be no detectable abnormality. The reason for this paucity of physical findings is that the true vocal cords usually become fixed at a point relatively close to one another. Therefore, the alterations in air flow are not dramatic and are not reflected in an alteration in the voice.

A great potential for airway obstruction exists in this situation, however. In the patient with normal noninflamed bilateral vocal cord paralysis, the airway is usually adequate so that the patient can maintain a sedentary life-style. Airway compromise is encountered with any sort of vigorous activity that increases the respiratory rate. Any inflammatory process that involves the larynx, however, can have emergent consequences with just a minimal amount of mucosal edema. The most important measure for a patient with bilateral vocal cord paralysis is to provide a safe airway as soon as possible. This usually requires tracheotomy. After the airway is protected with tracheotomy, the options for laryngeal construction can be discussed with the patient.

The patient with unilateral vocal cord paralysis who has not undergone compensation will have air-spilling hoarseness and possibly even aspiration problems. The endoscopic injection of Teflon paste into the paralyzed cord, which increases the cord's bulk and results in medial displacement, is an effective procedure that can be performed with the use of local anesthesia. The improvement in voice quality can be dramatic, and patients are usually extremely satisfied.

There are some options for the patient with bilateral cord paralysis. Once again, it is important that the patient be fully informed of the consequences of surgical reconstruction. The standard reconstructive technique for bilateral paralysis involves removal of one arytenoid cartilage (arytenoidectomy). This increases the separation between the vocal cords and provides a safer airway. The disadvantage to this approach is that voice quality is sacrificed. This must be explained to the patient so that he or she can make an informed decision regarding surgery.

Because of the drawbacks of arytenoidectomy, surgical alternatives have been investigated. One procedure involves the transfer of a pedicle of muscle attached to one of the end branches of the ansa hypoglossi into the body of the posterior cricoarytenoid muscle in an effort to reinnervate that paralyzed muscle so that the vocal cord can abduct. Early enthusiasm for this procedure has been tempered somewhat by more extended experience. It does not always restore enough motor function to provide a safe airway.

In patients who have severe central neurologic disorders that render the larynx totally incompetent with bilateral vocal cord abduction, steps must be taken to prevent life-threatening aspiration in an already compromised individual. Procedures to close the glottic inlet by suturing the vocal cords to prevent aspiration have been developed that are reversible in case of neurologic improvement.

# 22

# Diagnosis and Treatment of Speech Disorders

**Michael Trudeau, Ph.D.**

This chapter is intended to provide an overview of the role of the speech-language pathologist (hereafter, clinician) in the management of patients with communicative dysfunction as sequelae to otolaryngologic disorders. Four areas of dysfunction are described and the communication goals of therapy are outlined. The chapter covers resonance disorders, benign voice problems, problems associated with head and neck cancer, and disorders of swallowing. Whatever the disorder, the clinician's goal is to improve the communicative skills of individuals with speech and language problems in order to facilitate normal social, emotional, and intellectual functioning.

For the type of patient discussed in this chapter, a physician's referral for speech-language therapy is mandatory. The initial medical evaluation is necessary for two reasons. First, anomalies or diseases of the upper respiratory system can be life threatening. By acting on the basis of competent referral, the clinician ensures that medical treatment has been initiated and that speech therapy will not interfere with medical treatment. Second, in many cases (e.g., cleft palate) correction of speech patterns cannot be successful until structural abnormalities have been corrected or modified.

Therapy for any of the various communicative disorders follows a general plan. The first stage is an overall evaluation of the patient's communication skills. Although this evaluation may emphasize the disorder specified in the referral, it should assess all other areas of possible communicative dysfunction as well. From the evaluation, the clinician establishes the nature of the patient's com-

munication problem or problems, gauges the severity of involvement, and determines appropriate short-term and long-term goals for therapy. Once goals are set, the clinician uses the principles of behavioral psychology, applied through techniques specific to the patient's disorder, to move the patient incrementally toward normal communicative abilities. Important points here are that the clinician modifies behavioral patterns and that this modification typically takes time.

## RESONANCE DISORDERS

The vocal tract has three resonating chambers: the pharynx, oral cavity, and nasal cavity. Adjustments in the size and coupling of these chambers are intrinsic in the differentiation of vowels and in distinguishing the nasal consonants (*m, n, ng*) from their nonnasal cognates (*b, d, g*). The preponderance of disorders of resonation is attributable to the selective coupling of the nasal cavity with the other two chambers. Although the result frequently is hypernasality (too much nasal quality), hyponasality (too little nasal quality) can also occur, and some patients may display both.

The etiology of the disorder may be functional, with no identifiable physical cause, but more often is associated with incompetence or absence of the velopharyngeal port.

The child with a cleft palate best exemplifies this condition, not only because of the evident cause-and-effect relationship, but also because of the vulnerability of such a child to numerous other communicative disorders. This patient cannot isolate the nasal cavity from the rest of the vocal tract and so produces severely hypernasal speech. Additionally, the production of certain consonants, such as *t* and *s,* creates high intraoral pressure, which the absent or incompetent velopharyngeal port cannot contain. Air, therefore, is audibly ejected through the nares, producing nasal emission and interfering with clear articulation. The articulation of consonants often is further disrupted by the patient's use of abnormal articulatory movements to compensate for the hypernasality and nasal emission and by the structural abnormality itself, which can create other defects of the oral cavity, such as poor dentition and malocclusion.

Another threat to the patient's communicative development is the widespread occurrence of hearing impairment in this population. The hearing loss can result from genetic malformation of the auditory system or, more commonly, from the extremely high incidence of otitis media in individuals with craniofacial anomalies. The otitis media threatens the child's health and impairs the main channel (audition) for learning language, producing delays in language development.

Incorrect laryngeal valving to produce voice also characterizes patients with cleft palates. The voices of these patients are described variously as hoarse, hyperfunctional, too loud, too soft, and monotonic. These symptoms probably arise as misdirected compensatory strategies for controlling nasality. As such, they are unsuccessful and tend only to exacerbate the patient's communicative disability.

In dealing with patients with cleft palates, the clinician confronts deficits in resonance, phonation, articulation, language, and audition. The clinician's role in habilitation can be both direct and indirect. In the direct role, the clinician devises a therapy program focusing on the individual patient's specific problems, then implements this program through direct clinical contact with the patient and/or the patient's parents. In the indirect role, the clinician functions on an interdisciplinary team as an advocate and resource person for the patient's communicative development. By providing the perspective on the normal development of linguistic skills, the clinician influences the cleft palate team's overall habilitation plan for a patient. The goal is to engender normal communicative patterns to the degree possible and to prevent the appearance of insidious compensatory behaviors.

## VOICE DISORDERS

A convenient taxonomy for dealing with the effects of laryngeal disorders on voice is to classify the disorder as influencing either the mass or the normal approximation of the vocal folds. Mass-related effects predominantly arise from increases in the size of the folds created by such problems as contact ulcers and edema. Because a speaker's fundamental frequency (pitch) is a function of vocal fold mass (increasing mass, decreasing pitch) and vocal fold tension (increasing tension, increasing pitch), mass-related problems typically lower pitch and limit the speaker's range of pitch variability, frequently producing a monotonic voice. Disorders of approximation often are related to disorders of mass, in that the mass derives from an alteration of the folds, which prevents proper adduction as with vocal polyps. Poor adduction of the vocal folds yields inefficient use of the pulmonary air stream, producing a breathy voice, often with a choppy phrasing. The two extremes in disorders of approximation are hysterical or functional aphonia, in which no adduction occurs during speech, and adductor-type spastic dysphonia, in which adduction is so forceful that phonation is strained or interrupted.

Advantages in technology have greatly altered the role of the clinician in the diagnosis of voice disorders. In the past, the clinician's main purpose in assessing the voice of the dysphonic patient was to establish the degree of the dysphonia and to focus therapy. These goals remain important, particularly when voice therapy is the primary treatment for a given patient. With the availability of sophisticated, often computer-assisted instruments with which to measure the acoustic and aerodynamic characteristics of voice and to image the phonatory mechanism by means of video recording, stroboscopy, and electroglottography, the clinician can provide the otolaryngologist with significantly more and relevant information with which to establish a valid diagnosis and to plan surgical or medical treatment. Though these advances potentially benefit any patient with a voice problem, they are particularly germane in the case of the so-called "professional voice user." This is the individual whose profession places extremely high value on clear vocalization—for example, the opera singer, the lawyer, and the cleric. These patients demand high accountability from their physicians, as inappropriate treatment, delays in treatment, or improperly prolonged treatment have long-term vocational and financial implications. By completing a balanced battery of tests (minimally including videolaryngostroboscopy, aerodynamic analysis of phonation, and acoustic analysis of the voice) the clinician can provide the otolaryngologist with a comprehensive description of the patient's laryngeal dysfunction. In many cases this additional information greatly aids the otolaryngologist in establishing the correct diagnosis and in fine-tuning treatment.

After evaluating voice, the clinician interviews the patient and/or patient's parents to identify mannerisms, habits, and situations that may promote or exacerbate the voice disorder. Voice therapy generally has three foci. First, therapy is symptomatic in nature. If the patient has monotonic pitch, the clinician assists the patient in expanding pitch range. If the patient's voice is strained and harsh, the clinician trains a more relaxed, less forceful phonation. The underlying premise is that in restoring more normal-sounding phonation, the clinician is also developing patterns of normal laryngeal function in the patient.

Second, just as the clinician trains the patient in awareness and elimination of idiosyncratic dysfunctional vocal behaviors, the clinician also aids the patient in monitoring and controlling environmental factors (e.g., pollutants and loud social gatherings) that threaten normal phonation. These goals are beneficial even when additional medical management is necessary because they reduce recidivism. An example is the person with vocal nodules. This disorder often responds to voice therapy alone; however, for some patients the nodules require surgical removal. In this instance, voice therapy removes the phonatory behaviors that produced or sustained the nodules and establishes more normal, less abusive patterns.

Frequently voice therapy must include a third, intangible focus—vocal self-image. Many patients with voice disorders ranging from chronic

abuse to contact ulcers have developed ingrained vocal habits and have a strong psychologic identification with their voices. These patients approach therapy with a conscious commitment to change but with a subconscious predisposition to maintain their pathologic voice patterns. The clinician must assist these patients in shifting their vocal self-image from their former voices to their rehabilitated voices, in recognizing the differences between the two, and in responding immediately to instances of relapse. This process, which requires a strong rapport between patient and clinician, is difficult to assess objectively, yet is fundamental to successful treatment.

## HEAD AND NECK CANCER

Patients referred to the clinician after or during treatment for cancer of the head and neck typically present with speech defects in three areas: resonation, articulation, and phonation. These patients have suffered damage to the components or innervation of the speech mechanism, limiting or eliminating certain functions and creating speech marked by such symptoms as hypernasality, nasal emission, misarticulations, and aphonia. The goal for these patients is to achieve the maximum speech intelligibility possible within the constraints of remaining structure and function or to devise an alternative mode of expression when functional speech is infeasible. Successful therapy must assist the patient in accepting the goal of greatest restoration attainable as opposed to return to normalcy. Failing in this, the clinician faces a patient whose participation in therapy will be superficial and whose generalization of trained skills to the social and vocational environments will be poor.

Therapy seeks to enhance and retrain remaining function and supplant lost function. Patients will attempt to use remaining functions to sustain premorbid speech patterns. This effort requires direction so that the patient does not degrade intelligibility further, as with the patient who continues to use a normal rate of speech (160 to 180 words per minute). For the patient with a defect of the velopharyngeal port, such a rapid rate may interfere with proper valving. For the patient with a partial glossectomy, a normal rate of speech may produce slurred articulation because lingual movement has been impaired. By slowing the rate of speech, the clinician may allow delayed velopharyngeal valving to occur, elicit more precise enunciation, and permit the patient's listeners more time to adjust to the deviant nature of the speech. In some cases, simply increasing habitual voice intensity proves a great aid to listeners. The clinician evaluates the patient not only to assess degree of deficit but also to estimate the usefulness of residual functions in improving intelligibility.

When function has been lost (e.g., in palatal resection), prosthetic management may be beneficial. Residual function remains important to rehabilitation, but training in new skills becomes prominent. The palatal lift and the prosthetic tongue are new devices for the patient, who has no experience with such appliances. The clinician designs a therapeutic plan that builds the patient's skills from a rudimentary level, such as single sound production through intermediate stages (multisyllabic words or short phrases), to conversational speech.

The cancer patient most commonly referred to the clinician is the laryngectomee. For speech, the obvious result of total laryngectomy is the loss of phonation. However, a second equally basic deficit is the loss of pulmonary air as the power source for speech. The airway exits the body via a tracheostoma and is no longer joined to the vocal tract. Voice restoration must provide a vibratory body and a means of energizing the vibratory body. The three approaches currently employed are voice with an artificial larynx, esophageal voice, and surgical-prosthetic voice restoration.

Although pneumatic artificial larynges are available, the electronic devices are more prevalent. The power source is an electric battery, and the vibratory body is an electromechanical vibrator. The vibrations enter the vocal tract either by transmission through the soft tissue of the neck or through a tube inserted into the oral cavity. Selection of type depends on the needs of the patient. Whichever type is used, most patients require a period of speech therapy to learn to use the device correctly. Typical problems are the timing of phonation with speech, failure to transfer the vibrations into the vocal tract, production of increased background noise, and attempts to speak too rapidly. The main advantages are speed of training and generally good intelligibility. The main disadvantages are reliance on an external speech aid and the perceptual effect of a mechanical-sounding voice.

Esophageal voice has long been the mainstay in alaryngeal voice therapy. The pharyngoesophageal sphincter serves as the site of vibration, powered by air trapped in the esophagus. The primary difficulty in acquiring this form of voice is the controlled inflation of the esophagus, which usually involves a modified swallow at rapid speed. Some patients lack the physical ability to produce such control. For patients who will be successful, speech therapy is a lengthy undertaking (6 to 15 months). As with most forms of speech therapy, the clinician progresses in discrete steps from the simple—mere eructation from the esophagus—to the complex—pairing esophageal voice with connected speech. The principal advantages are that the patients use their own existing physiology to produce voice and that perceptually the vocal result is generally preferred to voice with an electrolarynx. The principal disadvantages are that a sizable number of laryngectomees (40% by some sources) fail to acquire useful esophageal speech, that acquisition is a lengthy process, and that intelligibility declines rapidly in noisy environments.

Surgical-prosthetic voice restoration focuses on attempts to reconnect the pulmonary airstream to the vocal tract, obviating the need for trapping air in the esophagus or for the electrolarynx, while avoiding aspiration of food and fluids. These attempts were largely unsatisfactory until 1980, when Singer and Blom and Panje introduced their respective restoration procedures and prostheses. With these and subsequent improvements and modifications, the otolaryngologist can reestablish the pulmonary air stream as the power source for speech to energize the pharyngoesophageal sphincter as the voicing source. Because the air is diverted from the trachea into the esophagus, this form of speech is referred to as tracheoesophageal speech.

The clinician's role in this rehabilitation program encompasses two areas: care of the prosthesis and use of the prosthesis to speak. Patients or their families should be able to remove, clean, and reinsert the voice prosthesis independently and rapidly to forestall fistula stenosis. These skills must be acquired, although many patients approach them with great reluctance.

Voice therapy trains correct timing between stomal occlusion and speech and the development of abdominal breathing to support fluent, connected speech. Voice therapy for the patient experiencing difficulty in voicing is a matter of isolating and correcting the factor or factors creating the difficulty. These include airtight closure (spasm) of the pharyngoesophageal sphincter or insufflation, excessive tension, and improperly sized prosthesis. Some of these problems are amenable to the clinician's efforts alone. Others may require joint efforts by the clinician and otolaryngologist.

Once the goals of independent self-care and fluent speech are achieved, the patient may be a candidate for a supplemental appliance, the tracheostoma valve. This device, which is placed over the stoma, allows for normal respiration but responds to the increase of expiratory air pressure associated with speech production by closing. The valve occludes the stoma, freeing the patient from the need to provide digital closure. The clinician assists in evaluating the patient's potential for success with this device and trains the patient in proper use.

The experience with tracheoesophageal speech at the Ohio State University is over one decade long. The advantages noted over that time have been speed of vocal restoration (particularly when the fistula is created at the time of the laryngectomy), speech that is perceptually more pleasing than speech with an electronic larynx, and speech that is closer to normal in rate and phrasing than esophageal speech. Tracheoesophageal speech also appears to pose a more viable means of voicing for patients with flap reconstruction of the pharynx and pharyngoesophageal segment, in that the reconstructed segment may be too flaccid to allow for trapping of air in the esophagus. Disadvantages include reliance on a prosthesis, the need to care for and change a prosthesis, and the requirement for stoma occlusion to produce speech.

None of the three methods described in this section is effective in restoring voice in all cases. If the goal is the return of functional speech, the responsible professional selects the method or methods that most benefit the patient in regaining speech. Biases toward one method to the exclu-

sion of others do not serve the patient. The three methods are in no way mutually exclusive, and some patients find it useful to employ two or even three of them.

## DISORDERS OF SWALLOWING

Increasingly the clinician is dealing with patients who display disorders of swallowing. The rationale for such referrals is that the anatomy and physiology underlying correct swallowing also underlie correct speech production; therefore, the clinician's training provides the expertise to deal with both areas. Additionally, patients who suffer from swallowing disorders, or dysphagia, are referred from populations normally served by the clinician, such as head and neck cancer patients, patients with neurologic disease or trauma, and patients with neuromuscular development disorders.

The goals of swallowing therapy are to improve the patient's nutritional capabilities and to avoid or eliminate swallowing patterns that produce aspiration. The clinician's concerns are with the oral and pharyngeal phases of swallowing because the musculature involved in controlling the bolus during chewing, moving the bolus into the pharynx, and contracting the pharynx to force the bolus into the esophagus generally subserves speech as well.

The therapy program for the dysphagic patient may focus on the act of swallowing itself, in which case the patient and clinician use food and fluid in adapting the patient's swallowing. For many patients, however, therapy begins by improving function in the area that is impaired. The clinician will direct the patient in exercises and activities to increase control over oral musculature or valving of the larynx and velopharyngeal port or to heighten the swallowing reflex. Frequently the therapy program involves speech and swallowing, but some dysphagic patients evidence no defects of speech or language while having considerable swallowing problems.

## CONCLUSION

The focus of this chapter has been on the communicative problems likely to occur in the otolaryngologic patient population and the role of the speech-language pathologist in dealing with those problems. Although the activities of the speech-language pathologist were stressed, effective management of such cases should be interdisciplinary in nature, with the speech-language pathologist contributing to an overall plan developed by a professional team. In no sense was this discussion definitive. Literally volumes have been written on each of the communicative disorders described herein. The intent was to acquaint the medical practitioner with the scope of the speech-language pathologist's functions so that appropriate referrals can be made and more complete patient care can be given.

# 23

# Laser Surgery

Although lasers are currently being used in a variety of settings in otolaryngology and head and neck surgery, the most frequent application is to the larynx. Current clinical use of the laser and any future applications are based on years of investigations. In fact, the earlier investigations were somewhat discouraging. In the 1960s, the neodymium glass laser was tried by Jako and Polyani. This laser caused difficulty with creating a circumscribed site of damage. In view of the laser's small absorption, high-power pulses were necessary to destroy tissue, and these often created somewhat violent tissue reactions. It was only when the carbon dioxide laser was developed by Patel at the Bell Telephone Laboratories that some encouraging results were obtained. This laser operated at a wavelength of 10.6, which is located in the infrared region of the spectrum. The electromagnetic radiation for this wavelength is normally absorbed by tissues. For example, the 1-micron radiation of the neodymium glass laser requires a distinction length of the energy of 60 mm. In contrast, the 10-micron radiation of the carbon dioxide laser has a distinction length of only 0.3 mm. This rapid distinction rate explains the well-circumscribed areas of tissue destruction that are possible with the carbon dioxide laser. Subsequent research and refinements to the carbon dioxide laser ultimately led to its use in humans and now have clearly established it as an effective clinical surgical instrument (Fig. 23–1).

The word *laser* is actually an acronym for *l*ight *a*mplification by *s*timulated *e*mission of *r*adiation. Basically, when an electron drops from a high energy level (and a molecule to a lower energy level), light is emitted. This light is a photon that, when dropped to a second lower level, releases a second photon with the same wavelength, direction, and phase as the initiating photon. A chain reaction called a photon cascade is created as the light bounces back and forth between mirrors. A mirror at the end of the focusing chamber has a small aperture that allows the escape of only some light beams that are traveling parallel to the long axis of the chamber (Fig. 23–2). Such laser light leaves its source in a narrow, parallel bundle with a narrow band and with wave forms in phase.

This beam can then be focused with a lens to increase its power. Various types of lasers have been constructed to destroy tissue in varying widths or depths by means of proper control of the beam. The energy produced by lasers is converted to heat in the tissue. This heat vaporizes the cellular water and ignites the remaining flammable tissue, causing a shallow charred crater. The heat results in closure of the transected capillaries and other small vessels. Vessels larger than 0.5 mm in diameter, however, are not effectively sealed with the carbon dioxide laser.

Wound healing is affected by the use of the carbon dioxide laser. Studies have demonstrated a difference in healing in wounds created by the laser instead of scalpel incisions. A laser wound tends to have a tensile strength that is weaker early in the healing phase than that of a similar wound created with a scalpel. However, the rate of increasing tensile strength with the laser wound is ultimately faster than with the scalpel wound, and the plateau for maximal tensile strength is similar for both wounds (Fig. 23–3). There is no

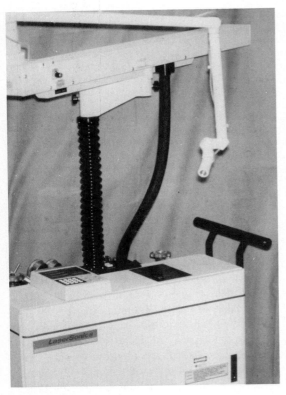

**FIG 23–1.**
The carbon dioxide laser has an articulating arm that permits use as a hand-held "scalpel" or attachment to a microscope.

appreciable difference in the types of collagen fibers that are formed in laser and scalpel wounds. Healed wounds several months after laser and scalpel incisions are clinically indistinguishable (Fig. 23–4).

Laser wounds appear to have less edema postoperatively, possibly because the laser seals vessels and lymphatics that prevent extravasation of fluid into the surgical wound. This lack of edema may be a partial explanation for the reduced postoperative pain in people undergoing laser surgery compared to what would be expected with conventional techniques. This phenomenon may be a function of the sealing of fine sensory nerve endings with the laser.

The advantage of the carbon dioxide laser in otolaryngologic–head and neck surgery is associated with the capabilities of "no touch" surgery. This is especially valuable in surgical procedures in which the anatomy restricts exposure to the surgical field. The ability to remove tissue coupled with the specificity of tissue destruction and decreased morbidity make it an attractive technology. As might be expected, however, there are potential disadvantages, and it is imperative that both the clinician and the patient be informed of these potential risks.

The carbon dioxide laser creates the tissue reaction on a thermal basis. The carbon dioxide la-

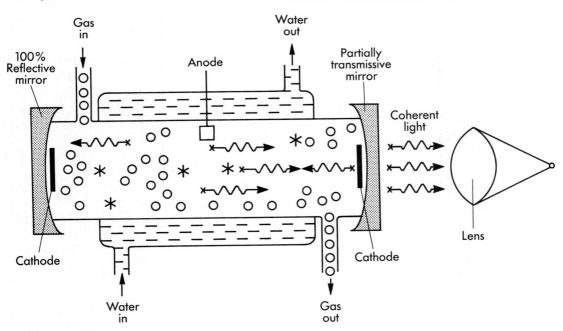

**FIG 23–2.**
The focusing chamber of the laser permits alignment of light beams parallel to the lung axis.

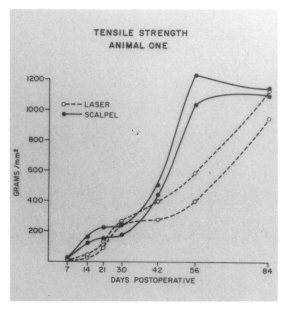

**FIG 23–3.**
This experience with animals demonstrated that the tensile strength of the laser wound ultimately approximated that of the scalpel wound.

ser has the capability of burning skin, surgical drapes, and endotracheal tubes. Although the amount of tissue removed in laryngeal laser surgery is small compared with that in intraabdominal laser surgery, for example, the risks of laryngeal laser surgery are far greater. These risks center on the potential for the laser igniting combustible materials and burning the tracheobronchial tree, which is a potentially life-threatening complication. Several precautions are necessary to avoid this risk. Obviously, no combustible anesthetic gases can be used with laser surgery. If the laser beam touches any combustible material that is dry, it will ignite. However, moist combustible materials do not burn when exposed.

The anesthetic endotracheal tube presents the biggest potential hazard. The polyvinyl chloride endotracheal tubes are combustible and usually are not used. Using the red rubber endotracheal tube wrapped by a self-adhesive aluminum tape is one of the more frequently used approaches (Fig. 23–5). However, several alternatives now exist. It should be emphasized that none of them offer total protection. The laser surgeon must under-

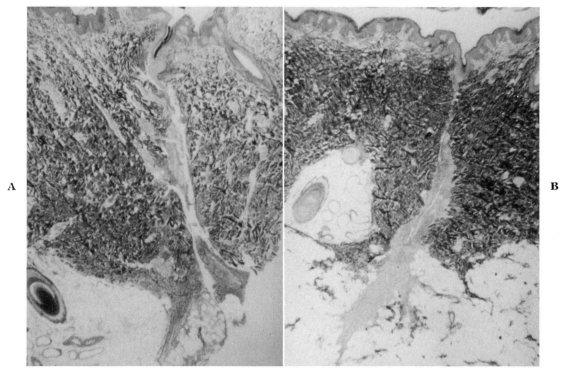

**FIG 23–4.**
The histopathologic appearance of **A,** the scalpel wound when compared with that of **B,** the laser wound is indistinguishable.

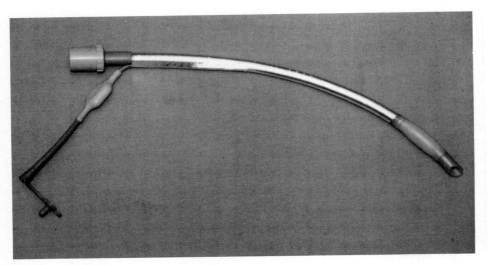

**FIG 23–5.**
The red rubber endotracheal tube wrapped with metallic tape decreases but does not totally prevent the chance of laser ignition.

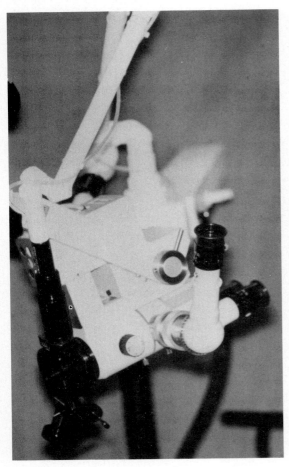

**FIG 23–6.**
Microlaser surgery allows cutting or vaporizing of tissue without the need for instrumentation at the site of tissue alteration.

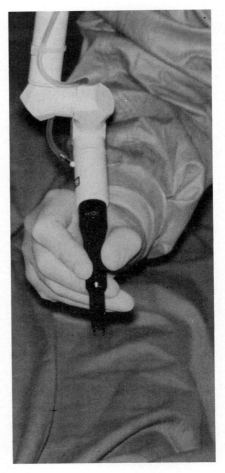

**FIG 23–7.**
The hand-held carbon dioxide laser can be used like a scalpel that has cutting and some coagulating potential.

stand these risks and how the complications can be minimized.

The current major otolaryngologic indication for the use of the laser is laryngeal abnormalities. A number of benign laryngeal lesions have been effectively treated with the carbon dioxide laser. There is some concern that the removal of lesions on the vibratory margin of the vocal fold with the laser may produce deleterious results. One needs to be cautious in this clinical situation. One of the most difficult laryngeal problems that seems to have benefited from laser technology is recurrent juvenile laryngeal papilloma. These papillomas involve primarily the larynx but can also involve any portion of the tracheobronchial tree. The laser increases the specificity of papilloma removal while minimizing damage to normal laryngeal mucosa. Although it was previously speculated that the laser might decrease the frequency of papilloma recurrences, that does not appear to be the case. However, it certainly minimizes the amount of scarring because of its tissue-destroying specificity, and this is an important consideration and advantage for the person who is anticipating multiple procedures to control the problem. This type of laser laryngeal surgery is done with the carbon dioxide laser attached to the microscope, providing the advantages not only of microscopic surgery but also of the "no touch" technique (Fig. 23–6).

The carbon dioxide laser has been used in the management of some laryngeal and tracheal stenosis problems. It appears to be most effective for thin bands of scar tissue. When scarring becomes appreciably thick, the value of the laser is decreased.

The use of the carbon dioxide laser in the management of multiple benign tumors of the vocal cords is now well documented. It is an excellent technique for the removal of vocal cord nodules, polyps, areas of hyperkeratosis, and edematous mucosa. Although the laser has been used to remove vocal cord granulomas, it does not ensure that these granulomas will not recur, which is the primary challenge to the patient.

The laser has also been used in managing certain laryngeal carcinomas, mostly selected small cancers of the true vocal cords. Although some advocate more aggressive use of the laser and its application to larger malignancies of the larynx, these have yet to be established as oncologically

safe approaches. In patients who qualify for laser surgery for small vocal cord cancers, the results of treatment are most impressive. The larynx frequently heals so that it is indistinguishable from the appearance of a normal larynx, and there is virtually no alteration in the patient's voice quality.

The carbon dioxide laser has been used for a variety of otolaryngologic procedures that do not involve the use of the microscope. In these situations, the hand-held arm of the carbon dioxide laser is used (Fig. 23–7). The carbon dioxide laser has also been used to remove benign and some small malignant tumors of the oral cavity and oropharynx. The advantage in this setting relates to the hemostatic effect of laser surgery and the decreased postoperative morbidity. The laser has been found to be an effective contouring mechanism in the surgical excision of rhinophyma (Fig. 23–8). One can achieve excellent sculpting of the nose with the laser, at the same time minimizing the amount of bleeding during the procedure. This represents a distinct advantage over the conventional scalpel approach. Both benign and malignant cutaneous lesions have been excised and vaporized with the carbon dioxide laser.

Some modifications of lasers are already being used clinically. One modification of the carbon dioxide laser is the development of a bronchoscopic attachment for management of lesions of the tracheobronchial tree. Once again, this bronchoscopic coupler enables the "no touch" surgical approaches in an area where exposure is limited.

Another laser now undergoing clinical evaluation is the Nd:Yag laser. Whereas the carbon dioxide laser is primarily considered to be a cutting unit with some coagulating capabilities, the Yag laser is primarily considered to be a coagulating unit with some cutting capabilities. Its use has been evaluated in the control of gastrointestinal bleeding from ulcers and tumors. In otolaryngology it is currently being evaluated in the control of certain vascular tumors such as hemangioma and certain vascular abnormalities such as telangiectasia.

The argon laser has been used in some middle ear surgeries such as stapedectomy and in some otologic procedures for chronic otitis media. It has also received considerable attention for the management of "port-wine" hemangiomas. The argon laser is activated by pigment and can pen-

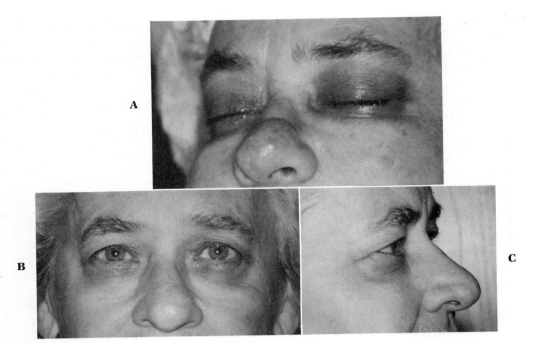

**FIG 23–8.**
**A,** preoperative photograph of a patient with rhinophyma treated by carbon dioxide vaporization. **B,** and **C,** two-year postoperative appearance.

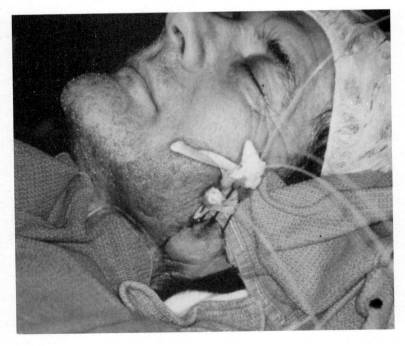

**FIG 23–9.**
This patient is receiving photodynamic therapy by having the fibers from a laser inserted through large-bore needles inserted into the tumor mass.

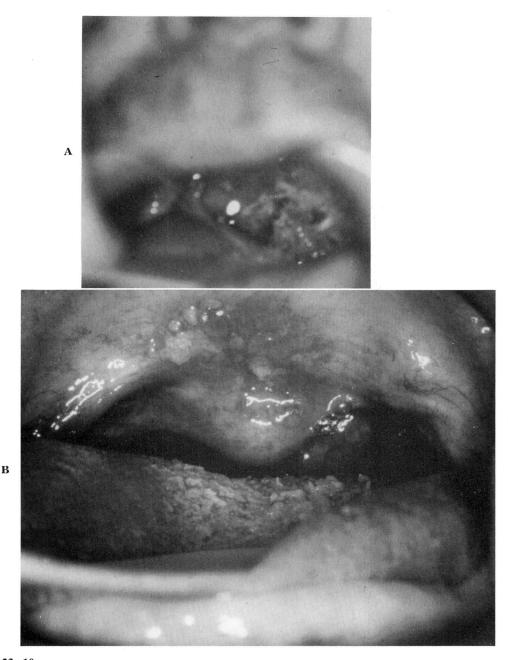

**FIG 23–10.**
**A,** this patient underwent photodynamic therapy of a recurrent palatal carcinoma 24 hours previously, and it is now edematous and partially necrotic. **B,** the same patient is free of disease 20 months after receiving photodynamic therapy.

etrate intact epithelium and cause the tissue interaction that changes the coloration of the pigment.

Another interesting form of laser surgery involves the treatment of malignancies with photodynamic therapy. With this approach, hematoporphyrin derivative is injected intravenously. It has been demonstrated that this derivative selectively localizes in tumor-containing tissue. When this tumor is exposed to light from a tunable dye laser at a certain wavelength (630 mm), a photodynamic reaction occurs that destroys only those cancer cells which contain the hematoporphyrin derivative (Fig. 23–9). This is an especially attractive form of cancer therapy because it is cancer specific and avoids removal or impairment of normal surrounding tissue (Fig. 23–10). Although the clinical use of photodynamic therapy is in its infancy, it is expected that this area of cancer therapy will undergo evaluation, modification, and advances in the future.

Laser surgery is a rapidly expanding field in otolaryngology and head and neck surgery. The advancements are at different phases for each type of laser. The carbon dioxide laser is clearly established as an effective tool and is now receiving widespread use in humans. The Nd:Yag and argon lasers, although receiving less attention than the carbon dioxide laser, still have been shown to be effective adjuncts to the treatment of certain pathologic conditions. The use of the tunable dye laser in photodynamic therapy for malignancies is an exciting new aspect of laser technology that may be beneficial in otolaryngology–head and neck surgery.

# PART VI
# Trachea and Esophagus

# 24

# Anatomy and Physiology

## ANATOMY

The diagnosis and treatment of diseases of the trachea and esophagus have changed considerably as a result of improved instrumentation available to evaluate these two structures. Flexible fiberoptic instruments are available that permit excellent visualization with minimal discomfort and risk to the patient.

The trachea connects the laryngopharynx with the lungs. Its length is variable, being somewhat greater in men than in women. Approximately one half of the trachea resides in the neck, and the lower half is located in the superior mediastinum. It is a hollow, midline structure in the neck that assumes a course to the right of midline as it descends through the mediastinum. Its walls are a combination of cartilage and muscle. The anteroposterior diameter is somewhat shorter than the transverse diameter. The average transverse diameter in an adult is about 18 mm. Because the trachea is an elastic structure that is not fixed in one location, the position of the larynx varies depending on how the patient positions the head and neck.

It is important to remember the fact, discussed in Chapter 17, that the tracheal cartilages are deficient in the posterior tracheal wall. The tracheal lumen is lined with pseudostratified ciliated columnar epithelium. This epithelium is rich in goblet cells. There are approximately 18 tracheal cartilages that provide rigid support to the anterior and lateral walls. The posterior wall is entirely muscular, composed primarily of the trachealis muscle.

Inferiorly, the lowest tracheal ring produces a notable ridge, which is referred to as the carina. The right and left main-stem bronchi are also supported with tracheal cartilages. The right main-stem bronchus not only is longer but also has a greater transverse diameter than the left one (Fig. 24–1). The right main-stem bronchus has a smaller angle of deviation from the trachea, which is clinically important concerning the location of bronchial foreign bodies. Foreign bodies in the right main-stem bronchus are more common than those in the left bronchus. Cartilaginous support of the distal bronchi ultimately disappears close to lung parenchyma. It is in the small bronchi that the muscle of the walls becomes more prominent. The smooth muscle composing the walls of the distal bronchioles in the periphery has clinical relevance.

The lungs are divided into lobes, with three on the right and two on the left. The right lobes are referred to as the upper, middle, and lower lobes, and the left side of the lung is divided into the upper and lower lobes. The upper lobe of the left lung is subdivided into the upper and lower divisions. Figure 24–2 illustrates the tracheobronchial tree, showing endoscopic views along different levels with the subdivisions of the lungs.

The esophagus is also not fixed to any rigid adjacent structures. It is the narrowest part of the digestive tract and is the alimentary continuation of the laryngopharynx to the stomach. Although the esophagus starts as a midline structure, it quickly assumes a position somewhat to the left of the midline in the lower portion of the neck. It is narrowest at the points of attachment to the hypopharynx and the stomach. The configuration of the esophagus is purely a function of its relationship to the rigid adjacent structures. Therefore, any protrusions from the vertebral bodies, such as osteophytes, can alter its normal configuration

Bronchial tree

RIGHT LUNG                    LEFT LUNG

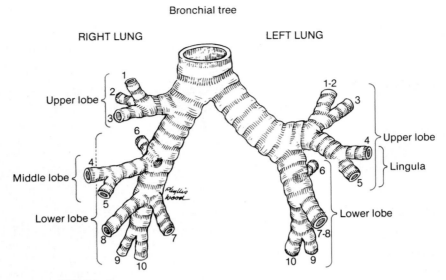

**FIG 24–1.**
The right main-stem bronchus is larger and longer than the left one.

and position. It also is affected by the mediastinal vasculature and is routinely narrowed at the level of the fourth and fifth thoracic vertebrae by the arch of the aorta (Fig. 24–3). The left main-stem bronchus is another structure that can cause some compression of the esophagus.

The esophagus is divided into cervical, thoracic, and abdominal portions. The anterior wall is in contact with the posterior muscular wall of the trachea. The lateral groove created between the esophagus and trachea in the cervical portion is the location of the recurrent laryngeal nerve. The cervical portion of the esophagus laterally is also closely related to the lobes of the thyroid gland. Posteriorly it is adjacent to the vertebral fascia.

The thoracic portion of the esophagus is also in contact with the trachea until the bifurcation. Just superior to this point, the arch of the aorta and the left main-stem bronchus cross the esophagus and can normally cause some compression. Below the arch of the aorta, the esophagus is enveloped by the pleural sacs of the lungs. The abdominal portion, which is only about 2 cm long, is below the level of the diaphragm.

The esophagus measures about 23 to 25 cm in length from the takeoff point at the cricopharyngeal area to its junction with the stomach. It is lined by stratified squamous epithelium. However, it is not unusual to encounter intermittent is-

lands of gastric mucosa along the surface of the esophagus. As with other portions of the alimentary tract, the esophagus has an inner circular and an outer longitudinal muscular layer. In the upper third of the esophagus, the musculature is voluntary striated muscle. The middle third contains both striated and involuntary smooth muscle, and the lower third is entirely made of smooth muscle. The cricopharyngeal area is composed of a sphincter located at the entrance to the esophagus at the level of the cricoid cartilage and another sphincter distally is located at the entrance into the stomach. The walls of the esophagus are delicate and can be easily perforated with any kind of endoscopic equipment.

The blood supply of the esophagus originates from a variety of arteries in the neck, thorax, and abdomen. Most arterial inflow in the neck comes from the inferior thyroid arteries. The motor nerve supply is derived from the vagus nerves, which contribute to the esophageal plexus at the level of the hili of the lungs.

## PHYSIOLOGY

The physiologic function of the trachea is primarily to continue the warming, humidifying, and cleansing process that was begun in the nasal passages. Warming is accomplished by the contact of

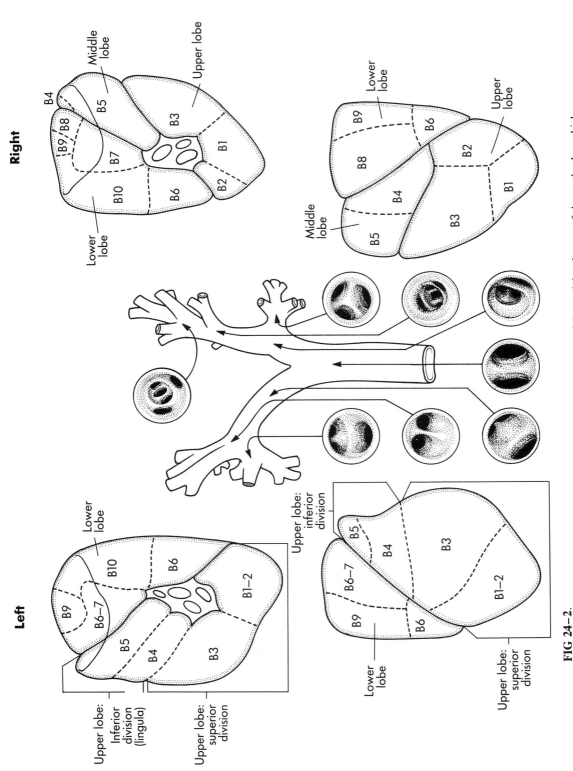

**FIG 24–2.**
Flexible fiberoptic bronchoscopy has permitted evaluation of more of the peripheral parts of the tracheobronchial tree than what was previously possible with rigid endoscopes. (Redrawn after Ballenger: *Diseases of the nose, throat, ear, head, and neck*, ed 13, Philadelphia, 1985, Lea & Febiger. Used by permission.)

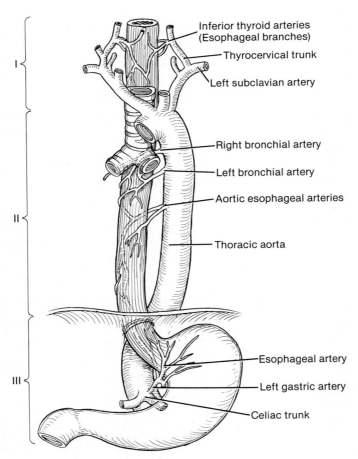

I

Inferior thyroid arteries
(Esophageal branches)

Thyrocervical trunk

Left subclavian artery

II

Right bronchial artery

Left bronchial artery

Aortic esophageal arteries

Thoracic aorta

III

Esophageal artery

Left gastric artery

Celiac trunk

**FIG 24–3.**
The esophagus can be narrowed at multiple levels by extrinsic pressure under normal conditions.

the air with the anatomic structures, which are at normal body temperature. The humidification is involved with the mucus-secreting glands in the tracheal mucosa. The cleansing is accomplished by the mucous blanket, which is directed by the ciliated epithelium to exit the airway via the larynx and to be either swallowed or expectorated.

The physiology of the esophagus involves passage of food into the stomach. This is referred to as the esophageal phase of swallowing. It is initiated by a marked decrease in pressure of the cricopharyngeal area when there is a pharyngeal contraction directing the bolus of food into the proximal esophagus. This swallowing act stimulates a series of sequential contractions within the esophageal musculature that courses distally rather rapidly in the upper striated portion, but then it slows in the lower portion, which contains the smooth muscle with the esophageal wall. Distally, there is a high-pressure zone of the esophagus at the gastroesophageal junction. When this pressure decreases, food enters the stomach; an increase of pressure in this area follows promptly to prevent food reflux.

# 25

# Embryology and Congenital Disorders

The trachea and esophagus develop from an outgrowth from the ventral wall of the foregut. This is initially seen in the 26-day-old embryo (Fig. 25–1). The laryngotracheal groove is located immediately below the pharyngeal arches. The trachea is the pulmonary component of the outgrowth of this tube, and it soon becomes separate from the esophagus, as noted in the diagram. There is some controversy as to the development of this independence. Some embryologists believe a septum develops between the trachea and the esophagus. Others think that the separation is merely a function of outgrowth and elongation. The blind end of the trachea proceeds to develop into the main-stem bronchi, and ultimately there is connection with the lungs. The esophagus continues to elongate and differentiate into connections with the remaining alimentary tract.

It is the elongation of the trachea and esophagus with this subsequent separation that provides the basis for the most common congenital anomalies, namely congenital atresia of the esophagus with tracheoesophageal fistula. The symptoms of this problem are noted soon after birth. The child appears to produce an excessive amount of saliva and has episodes of choking and cyanosis that increase with attempts to feed. The most common tracheoesophageal fistulas are illustrated in Figure 25–2. Surgical correction of this problem is necessary because it is not compatible with life.

Tracheal and esophageal webs are sometimes encountered but not frequently. A congenital shortness of the esophagus that places a portion of the stomach within the thoracic cavity can also develop. This can present problems with the lack of adequate distal sphincter, creating an inadequate mechanism with resultant reflux.

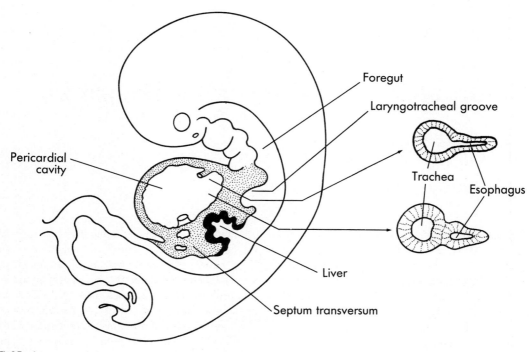

**FIG 25–1.**
An extension from the ventral wall of the foregut eventually leads to the tracheoesophageal complex. (Redrawn after Davies J: *Embryology of the face, palate, nose, and paranasal sinuses.* In *Paparella M, Shumrick, D* eds: *Otolaryngology,* vol 1, Philadelphia, 1980, WB Saunders. After Streeter: *Developmental horizons and human embryos,* 1942. Used by permission.)

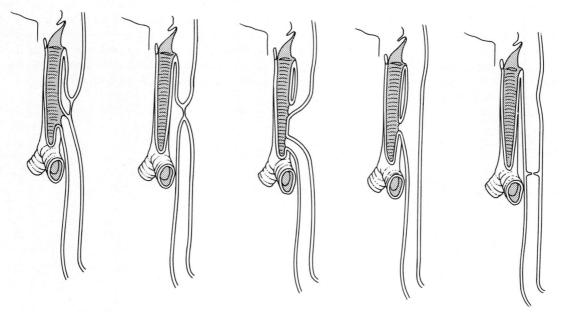

**FIG 25–2.**
These sketches depict multiple presentations of tracheoesophageal fistulae.

# 26

# Special Diagnostic Procedures

Bronchoscopy has undergone considerable changes. The advent of flexible fiberoptic instrumentation has permitted more thorough evaluations of the distal tracheobronchial tree and better patient tolerance. Most patients will tolerate a flexible fiberoptic bronchoscopic examination with just the use of a mild sedative and topical anesthetic. The flexible bronchoscope has a shaft that is approximately 6 mm in diameter (Fig. 26–1). The shaft of this instrument contains glass fibers for visualization and illumination, one lumen for the insertion of biopsy instruments, and another lumen to allow simultaneous aspiration of secretions or instillation of an additional anesthetic agent. This instrument can be passed through the nose into the trachea or through the mouth after placement of an orotracheal tube. The latter approach is well tolerated by patients and provides a greater opportunity for atraumatic removal and reinsertion of the bronchoscope than does the transnasal route.

Flexible fiberoptic bronchoscopy is used primarily for diagnostic purposes when visualization of the tracheobronchial structures is important. Information received from the examination can be enhanced with the use of biopsy forceps and small brushes that can be placed through the instrument to take samples of tissue (Fig. 26–2). The flexible fiberoptic bronchoscope can also be used to remove inspissated secretions.

The rigid open bronchoscope was the mainstay of bronchoscopy for several years until the development of flexible fiberoptic equipment. However, it is by no means an obsolete instrument; it continues to be valuable for the rapid removal of inspissated secretions, endobronchial tumors, and foreign bodies (Fig. 26–3). The rigid broncho-

scope is not as well tolerated with local anesthesia as the flexible fiberoptic instrument.

The esophagoscope has undergone the same evolutional changes as the bronchoscope. The open, rigid esophagoscope has been used for the past 100 years. In the mid-1960s, the flexible fiberoptic esophagoscope was introduced, and this has dramatically changed the field of esophagology. Once again, the flexible fiberoptic esophagoscope is well tolerated by patients under local anesthesia. Its flexibility reduces the risk of perforation and permits the examination of people with limited neck motion. It is an excellent instrument, similar to the bronchoscope, for visualizing esophageal mucosa and for removing small pieces of tissue. This diagnostic technique can be used in the evaluation of not only malignancies but also inflammatory processes and trauma-related injuries such as strictures from ingestions.

Mediastinoscopy is another specialized diagnostic procedure and is used to examine tissues of the mediastinum. Its greatest value is with diseases that can involve paratracheal and carinal lymph structures. There are currently two main indications for mediastinoscopy: the evaluation of mediastinal adenopathy and determination of resectability in lung cancer to avoid the need for thoracotomy.

Mediastinoscopy is usually performed using general anesthesia to eliminate the possible risk of mediastinal emphysema and air embolism. The mediastinoscope, which resembles the laryngoscope, is introduced beneath the pretracheal fascia to allow for advancement down to the carina and behind the major vessels (Fig. 26–4). Mediastinoscopy continues to be a valuable adjunctive diagnostic procedure with a low complication rate.

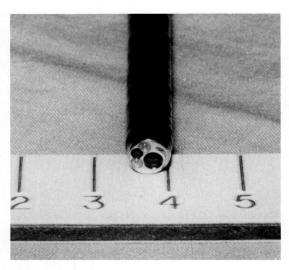

**FIG 26–1.**
The small diameter of the flexible fiberoptic broncho-scope enhances patient comfort and provides greater vi-sualization of the peripheral tracheobronchial tree.

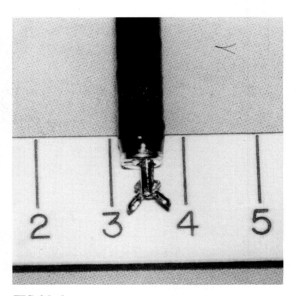

**FIG 26–2.**
Channels through the flexible bronchoscope allow the advancement of small biopsy forceps.

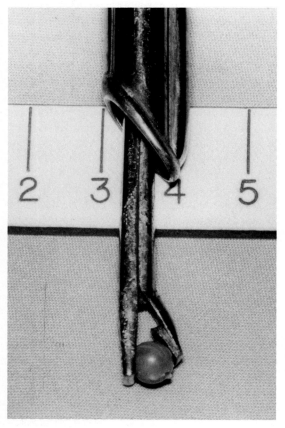

**FIG 26–3.**
Rigid bronchoscopes continue to be the safest approach for removal of bronchial foreign bodies.

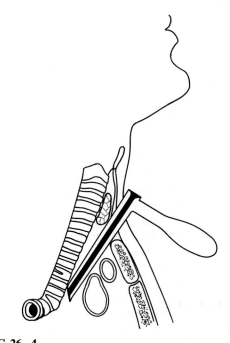

**FIG 26–4.**
Mediastinoscopy permits the identification of abnormal mediastinal anatomy such as metastatic lymph nodes.

# 27

# Clinical Problems

## TRACHEA

### Infections and Inflammations

#### Acute Tracheitis

Acute tracheitis is often associated with upper respiratory infections. This can involve any age group. It tends to be a self-limiting problem, and in most cases is viral in origin. There can be a productive cough because of the increased mucus resulting from the inflamed tracheal mucosa. Rarely does it cause airway compromise. The mucus produced is invariably clear in color unless a secondary bacterial infection changes the color to yellow or greenish yellow.

#### Chronic Tracheitis

Chronic tracheitis can occur from environmental irritants such as air pollution and cigarette smoke. The patient usually has a nonproductive cough, but it can be productive depending on the amount of mucus being produced by the tracheal mucosa. Symptoms can usually be improved by avoiding the irritant and by increasing humidification and the patient's fluid intake.

#### Acute Bronchitis

Acute bronchitis is similar to tracheitis because it involves all ages and is frequently seen in combination with an upper respiratory infection. There is usually a self-limited viral origin. However, bacterial infection can occur, and it is appropriate to obtain sputum cultures when the sputum is not clear.

Increasing the level of airway humidification and fluid intake will decrease the symptoms arising from the inspissated secretions. Airway compromise occurs only rarely in adults. However, the amount of mucus produced in children can become a problem that sometimes necessitates bronchoscopic aspiration to clear the airway.

#### Chronic Bronchitis

Chronic bronchitis is becoming a common condition resulting from prolonged exposure to airway irritants originating from either smoking or environmental pollutants. Other factors such as allergy have also been implicated. The patient is bothered with a cough that, once again, can be productive. Coloration of the sputum is an indication of possible bacterial infection, and cultures should be obtained. Avoidance of airway irritants and improved airway humidification and fluid intake help to minimize the symptoms. However, airway clearance with bronchoscopic aspiration is sometimes necessary.

### Trauma and Foreign Bodies

Although there are some inflammatory processes that can cause tracheal scarring with formation of stenosis, currently the most common cause of tracheal trauma is endotracheal intubation. The endotracheal tube provides positive-pressure ventilatory support and a mechanism for an efficient pulmonary toilet in patients who require such treatment. The ciliated respiratory epithelium of the trachea can be damaged with compromise of its blood supply from the endotracheal tube. Destruction of this ciliary transport system impairs the normal clearance of the mucous blanket, predisposing to infection.

The endotracheal tube has an inflatable cuff (Fig. 27–1) that seals the trachea to permit positive-pressure ventilation and also to protect the airway from aspiration. If the pressure within the

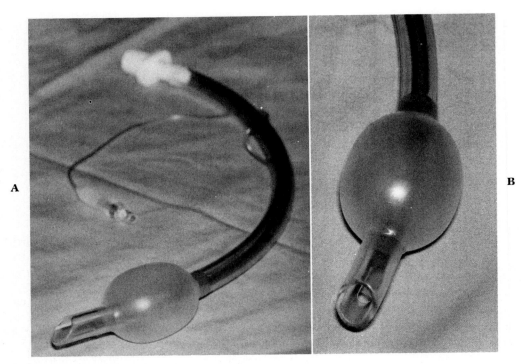

**FIG 27–1.**
**A,** endotracheal tubes have an inflatable cuff to seal the airway. **B,** this cuff usually has a high-volume low pressure to minimize the chances of injury to the tracheal mucosa.

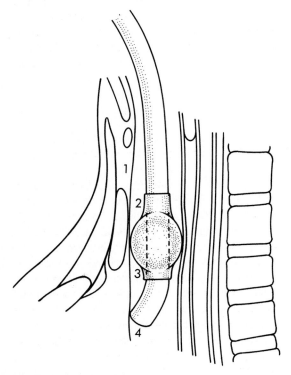

**FIG 27–2.**
This sketch illustrates the different levels at which the mucosa can be traumatized by an endotracheal tube.

cuff of the endotracheal tube is greater than the arterial pressure supporting the tracheal mucosa in that area, the blood supply will be halted and necrosis of the tracheal mucosa will occur. Inflammation will be initiated, with the potential for scarring and ultimately stenosis. The tracheal mucosa can also be traumatized by the tip of an endotracheal tube rubbing against the tracheal wall (Fig. 27–2). This rubbing action of the tip of the endotracheal tube can also disrupt the mucosal surface, with the similar pathophysiology occurring. Any hurried intubations that might inadvertently lacerate the mucosa can also have the same effect.

The patient with a significant tracheal stenosis will have airway compromise following endotracheal tube extubation. This will manifest itself as both inspiratory and expiratory stridor. If the condition is severe enough, emergent tracheotomy is necessary. Treatment is planned according to the degree of stenosis. A relatively thin web of tracheal stenosis can often be effectively managed endoscopically with vaporization by the carbon dioxide laser. However, more extensive stenosis requires reconstructive procedures using one or a combination of grafts, flaps, composite

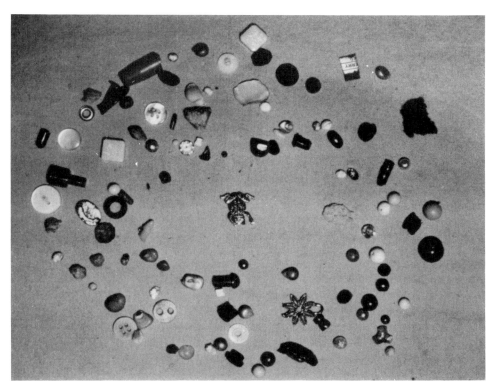

**FIG 27–3.**
An array of bronchial and esophageal foreign bodies successfully removed, including a plastic frog noted in the center.

bone flaps, and a variety of other techniques.

Foreign bodies in the trachea are most commonly found in children under the age of 2. Although nuts are the most common foreign body aspirated, the types of foreign bodies are limited only by the ingenuity of the child (Fig. 27–3). In the discussion of tracheal foreign bodies, it is important to initially mention certain generalizations that apply to prevention. Parents must recognize that the young child's neuromuscular coordination is not as good as the adult's. Generally, it is advisable for children under the age of 6 not to attempt to chew gum or to eat foods that contain peanuts or other nuts. Children should be cautioned about playing while eating. Parents should be careful not to place potential airway foreign bodies in locations accessible to children.

Most tracheobronchial foreign bodies have rounded edges. Sharp objects tend to become stuck in certain areas of the oropharynx or hypopharynx before being able to pass through the larynx into the trachea. The relatively straight course of the right main-stem bronchus predisposes it to be the most common location of a foreign body.

A child who aspirates a foreign body usually develops a persistent, nonproductive cough. If the foreign body is large enough or if some laryngospasm is associated with the initial event, there may be a transient episode of severe airway distress, which may even include some associated perioral or fingernail cyanosis. Once the foreign body is within the lumen of the trachea, a variety of changes can occur. Most foreign bodies are not large enough to completely obstruct the trachea. If that rare event occurs, it obviously represents a life-threatening emergency. In the case of a nonobstructing foreign body in the airway, the patient will present with audible respirations and may have inspiratory and expiratory stridor (Fig. 27–4). As the tracheal mucosa in the area of the foreign body becomes irritated and edematous, the air flow pattern will change. With inspiration, the normal tracheal diameter decreases. The development of any mucosal edema around the tracheal foreign body obstructs the exit of air through the bronchus containing the foreign body (Fig. 27–5). This leads to the clinical situation referred to as obstructive emphysema. The lung

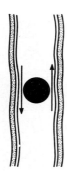

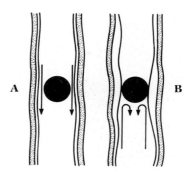

**FIG 27–4.**
A nonobstructing foreign body will still alter air currents to produce audible respirations.

**FIG 27–5.**
**A,** air can enter the lungs with inspiration as a result of expansion of the diameter of the bronchus, but the decreased circumference of exhalation, **B,** obstructs the exit of air.

becomes hyperinflated, and therefore breath sounds on that side appear to be more distant. The radiographic appearance is also that of a hyperinflated lung (Fig. 27–6).

If a foreign body persists in the same location for an extended period, the trapped air in the lung begins to become absorbed and obstructive emphysema converts to atelectasis. That lung begins to undergo atelectatic changes. The radiographs

show increased opacity of the part of the lung corresponding to the blocked bronchus and a shift of the mediastinal structures toward the obstructed side (Fig. 27–7). This is in contrast to the patient with obstructive emphysema, in whom the mediastinal structures on radiographic appearances are shifted away from the obstructed side.

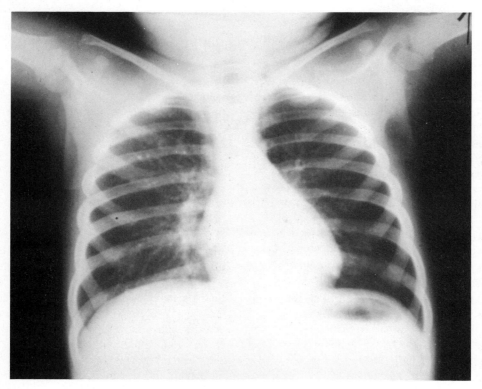

**FIG 27–6.**
This radiograph shows a child who has obstructive emphysema as a result of occlusion of the left main-stem bronchus.

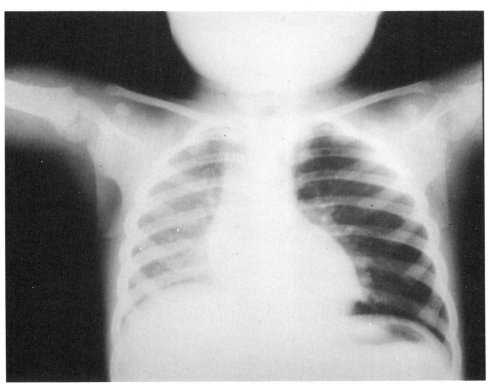

**FIG 27–7.**
This radiograph shows a child who has a foreign body in the right main-stem bronchus that has produced right atelectasis and a shift of the mediastinum to the right.

A foreign body should be suspected initially when a child presents with a nonproductive and persistent cough. The clinician should seek any information in the history suggestive of an obstructive episode, such as the development of cyanosis or the child's activity before the event. For example, if the child was playing with a plastic toy in the mouth and then had an episode suggesting obstruction, that is useful information. The physical examination primarily involves auscultation of the chest. The child with a bronchial foreign body who has obstructive emphysema will have more distant breath sounds over the obstructed lung. If there is atelectasis, the breath sounds appear more prominent. After the history and physical examination are completed, chest radiographs are obtained if the child's airway is stable. The standard radiographs ordered are inspiratory and expiratory anterior and posterior views of the lungs. The radiographic appearance of obstructed emphysema involves not only the hyperaerated lung with a shift of the mediastinal

contents away from the side of the foreign body, but also a flattening of the hemidiaphragm on the side of the hyperinflated lung. In contrast, the atelectatic lung will have increased opacity on the side of the foreign body, with a shift of the mediastinal contents toward the obstruction and an elevation of the hemidiaphragm on the side of the foreign body. There will be times when the usual physical and radiographic findings are not present. However, if the history documents a definite episode of significant airway compromise, bronchoscopy is usually advisable to rule out a possible foreign body of the airway.

### Primary Tracheal Tumors

Primary tracheal tumors are rare. The trachea is more commonly involved secondarily with esophageal cancers. There are some tracheal tumors that can occur, such as chondromas, chondrosarcomas arising from the tracheal cartilage, and leiomyomas arising from the musculature.

Primary tracheal cancers are extraordinarily rare and carry an ominous prognosis because they often are not diagnosed until far advanced.

## ESOPHAGUS

### Infections and Inflammations

The esophagus is subject to a variety of inflammatory diseases. However, primary infections of the esophagus are rare in the United States. The one notable exception is fungal esophagitis occurring in patients who are immunocompromised, such as those receiving transplants or undergoing cancer chemotherapy.

Esophageal inflammatory problems are relatively common and seen primarily in adults. They usually result from the inability of normal anatomic and physiologic mechanisms to protect the esophageal mucosa from exposure to the acidic gastric contents. Any mechanical problem, such as a hiatal hernia, that interferes with the distal sphincteric mechanism will permit reflux that can

potentially inflame the esophageal mucosa. The symptoms usually involve "heartburn" as a result of the inflammation. This often is readily managed with antacid therapy and a bland diet. The more severe problems can result in the inflammation causing formation of fibrous tissue with scarring and ultimate stricture of the esophagus. This may cause dysphagia to the point that it might require surgical intervention. Esophageal ulcers and varices are often seen in long-time abusers of ethanol.

### Trauma and Foreign Bodies

The esophagus, being a thin structure, is subject to lacerations and complete tears during compression injuries to the thorax. The esophagus rarely undergoes spontaneous rupture in this distal portion. More commonly, esophageal perforation can occur in chronic ethanol abusers who are experiencing a protracted period of forceful vomiting (Mallory-Weiss syndrome). This condition is also a surgical emergency. The potential for con-

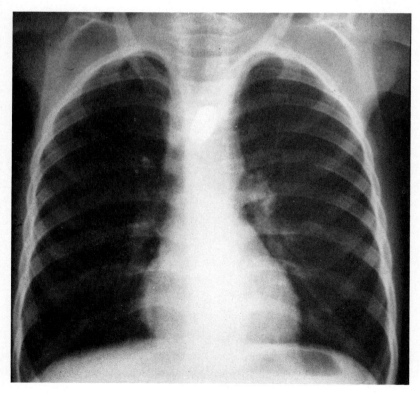

**FIG 27–8.**
This child swallowed a coin, which passed beyond the cricopharyngeal area and became lodged in the mid-esophagus.

tamination of the mediastinum with such an injury obviously demands immediate surgical intervention. One of the more common traumatic injuries of the esophagus relates to scar formation and stricture development from ingestion of caustic agents. Lye is an example of the most caustic agent. Lye causes liquefying necrosis, which allows for a deeper injury and more extensive damage. This is in contrast to acids, which cause a coagulative necrosis, in which the coagulum of the mucosa tends to inhibit any deeper tissue destruction. Caustic ingestions, if diagnosed acutely, can be managed quite effectively with conservative measures such as antibiotics, steroids, and serial dilatations. These measures often prevent the development of a significant stricture that would require costly and dangerous esophageal reconstructive surgery.

Foreign bodies in the esophagus are frequently encountered in children. They do not represent as great a danger as foreign bodies in the trachea. Coins are the most common esophageal foreign body. The level of the cricopharyngeal area is a frequent site (Fig. 27–8). The potential for aspiration of an esophageal foreign body to develop into an airway emergency is the concern that prompts most physicians to remove the object as soon as the diagnosis is established. Rigid esophagoscopy is the preferred technique for removing foreign bodies. It is imperative that the patient be observed for several hours after removal of a foreign body to determine whether esophageal injury has occurred. This observation should be done before the patient is fed by mouth.

## Tumors

Benign tumors of the esophagus are rare. Some of the benign tumors, such as lipomas or fibromas, arise from mucosal abnormalities, and some, such as leiomyomas, arise from the wall of the esophagus. Most of these tumors are asymptomatic unless they totally obstruct the esophagus. They occasionally can bleed. Surgical excision is usually recommended.

Malignancies of the esophagus are most commonly squamous cell carcinomas. They are usually classified as arising in the upper, middle, and lower thirds of the esophagus.

Malignancies of the upper third of the esophagus occur more frequently in women than in men. Dysphagia, hoarseness, and even ear pain are frequently seen with a lesion of the upper third of the esophagus. The evaluation usually involves radiographic studies and endoscopy, with the diagnosis established by biopsy. The intimate relationship of the proximal esophagus with the laryngopharynx often means that treatment will necessitate removal of the larynx. The prognosis for advanced-stage upper esophageal lesions is grave. Therapy involving surgery, radiation therapy, and even chemotherapy is frequently recommended.

The middle third of the esophagus is the second most common area of esophageal cancers. Once again, dysphagia, pain, and even regurgitation of food are the presenting symptoms. Radiographic and endoscopic evaluations are indicated for patients with these symptoms. Combined therapeutic approaches are used for this disease. The outlook is also poor for this group of patients.

The most common site of esophageal cancer is the lower third of the esophagus. Squamous cell carcinoma arising in this portion of the esophagus can be quite extensive. There are instances in which adenocarcinomas arising in the upper portion of the stomach actually involve the distal esophagus with submucosal extension. Once again, combination therapy is recommended. However, the outlook remains poor.

# 28

# Airway Management

The diagnosis of a patient with *complete* airway obstruction is not difficult. The patient will have an apprehensive facial expression and will demonstrate vigorous chest wall movement with no evidence of air exchange. As hypoxia develops, the patient will become excitable, uncooperative, and even combative. Anoxia will ultimately result in loss of consciousness. *Partial* airway obstruction is more difficult to assess, especially by those health professionals who are not routinely involved with managing the airway; this inexperience often increases the difficulty of determining the relative severity of a particular patient's airway compromise.

The patient with partial airway obstruction will have stridor. The stridor is usually inspiratory when the obstruction is at the level of the hypopharynx. When the stridor is both inspiratory and expiratory, the trachea may be the site of obstruction. One of the most important assessment tools is to question patients about the adequacy of their breathing passages. The patient will provide information that is useful because it defines how he or she is reacting to the severity of the obstruction. The history of the development of the partial obstruction is also useful and should be obtained if possible. The time sequence is important, as is mechanism of the injury if it was related to neck trauma. Whenever there is a history of trauma, the physical examination can provide useful information. A physical examination with vigorous palpation may inadvertently convert a partial airway obstruction to a total one. The assessment of the patient with laryngeal trauma has been discussed in Chapter 19.

In the patient with partial airway obstruction, positioning can often improve the airway. Al-though most patients are not familiar with the relevant anatomy, they instinctively posture themselves to improve the airway. This usually is characterized by the awake patient leaning forward, straightening the back, flexing the neck, and extending the head with protrusion of the mandible. All of these maneuvers result in straightening of the air route into the tracheobronchial tree.

Unconscious patients provide a different challenge. They cannot help themselves. Besides the airway obstruction, there is the potential for additional insult with aspiration. When encountering an unconscious patient with airway obstruction, the clinician should initially place the patient on his or her side to facilitate clearance of any food contents that may have been regurgitated into the hypopharynx. In the absence of specialized medical equipment, any maneuver to straighten the airway will help to alleviate the obstruction (Fig. 28–1). If the airway is not adequate, emergency cricothyroidotomy is advisable.

Cricothyroidotomy is performed by initially making a generous vertical skin incision, with the midpoint located directly over the cricothyroid membrane. The incision continues sharply through the underlying subcutaneous tissue. Depending on the urgency of the situation, it is not necessary to specifically identify the cricothyroid membrane but just to have an appreciation for its location. An incision is made through the cricothyroid membrane into the airway (Fig. 28–2). The lamina of the cricoid cartilage is usually directly opposite the incision into the airway and protects the esophagus from injury if the patient were to suddenly move forward while the knife or scalpel is in the lumen. After the airway is en-

315

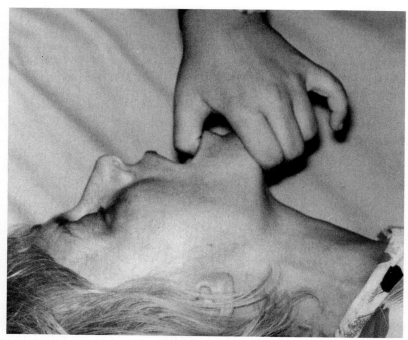

**FIG 28–1.**
Demonstration of how the airway can be improved by elevating the mandible, which displaces the tongue base away from the posterior pharyngeal wall and straightens the airway.

tered, the end of the knife or scalpel can be placed through this incision and turned 90 degrees to open the cricothyroid membrane (Fig. 28–3). This position can be held until assistance arrives, and an endotracheal or tracheotomy tube is inserted to maintain the airway. After the airway has been secured with insertion of a tube, the subcutaneous bleeders can be stopped with packing about the tube until the patient can be stabilized and taken to an operating room, where the cricothyroidotomy will be converted to a tracheotomy.

Airway management involves understanding the relevant anatomy along with an appreciation for certain crucial factors, which have been described previously. It must be emphasized that the most conservative steps to achieve resolution of the airway obstruction are to be attempted first. Often this involves simple positioning of the patient. In the event of complete airway obstruction, endotracheal intubation provides the safest, quickest, and most efficient approach. Only when endotracheal intubation cannot be done or is not indicated should one consider cricothyroidotomy.

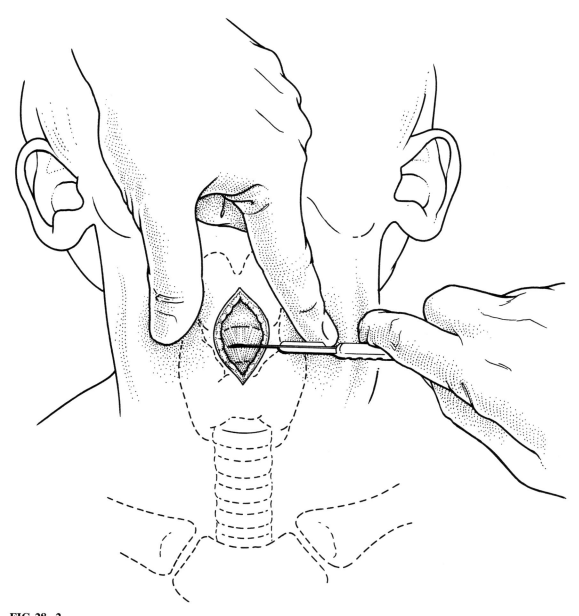

**FIG 28-2.**
Access to the airway can be quickly established by incising through the cricothyroid membrane. (Redrawn after Montgomery W: *Surgery of the upper respiratory system*, Philadelphia, 1973, Lea & Febiger. Used by permission.)

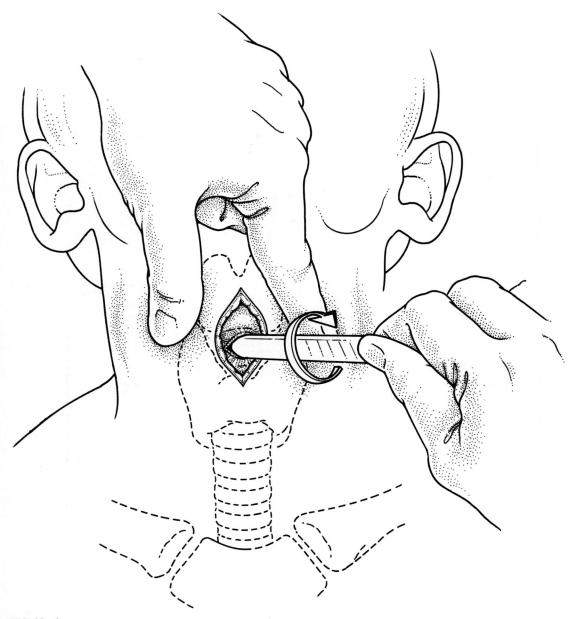

**FIG 28–3.**
The opening of the cricothyroid membrane can be maintained by holding something in place to keep the edges separated. (Redrawn after Montgomery W: *Surgery of the upper respiratory system*, Philadelphia, 1973, Lea & Febiger. Used by permission.)

# PART VII
# Neck

# 29

# Anatomy

The anatomy of the neck is both complex and fascinating. Within this relatively small area resides a myriad of structures that are intimately related to one another. This chapter is intended to provide a basic understanding of the anatomy for individuals dealing with health problems in this area.

It is important to be aware of certain prominences of the neck surface because they represent key anatomic landmarks. Surface anatomy can be helpful in detecting presence of disease. In the individual with a long, thin neck, an oblique prominence runs from the ear region down to the clavicle. This represents the sternocleidomastoid muscle (Fig. 29–1). In the upper midline of the neck, the "Adam's apple," the protrusion caused by the thyroid notch of the larynx, is palpable. Approximately 2 to 3 cm inferior to the thyroid notch in the midline is a slight prominence, which represents the arch of the cricoid cartilage. The clinician should be able to identify this surface landmark quickly because of its importance to airway management. In elderly individuals, a prominence in the skin of the neck is frequently noted about 3 to 4 cm below the body of the mandible. This is usually bilateral and symmetric. Rather than representing adenopathy, most of the time these are the submandibular glands, which have descended into the neck as a result of relaxation of the connective tissue support that normally retains them in the submandibular triangle. It is even possible to note pulsations in the lateral portion of the neck at times. These pulsations can be the result of vascular tumors, aneurysmal dilatations, or tortuous carotid arteries seen especially in the elderly (Fig. 29–2).

Deep to the skin of the neck and a variable-thickness layer of subcutaneous fat is a broad sheet of platysmal muscle (Fig. 29–3) that covers almost the entire lateral neck. It attaches to the upper thoracic cage musculature and then superiorly narrows to form bands that contribute to the mimetic muscles (muscles of facial expression). The medial edge of the platysma muscle creates the "wattles" seen in the elderly (Fig. 29–4). Deep to the platysma, the sternocleidomastoid muscle runs obliquely from the mastoid process to the clavicle in the manubrium (Fig. 29–5). Anatomists traditionally have used this to arbitrarily divide the cervical structures into the anterior and posterior triangles.

The laryngeal compartment is in the anterior triangle, as is the submandibular triangle. The submandibular triangle is actually bound by the anterior and posterior bellies of the digastric muscle inferiorly and the mandible superiorly. The lingual nerve runs superiorly in the submandibular triangle, and the submandibular parasympathetic ganglion is attached to this nerve and the gland. The muscles of the submandibular triangle include some of the muscles of the floor of the mouth. The major structure within is the submandibular gland, whose duct courses anteriorly and superiorly to empty into the oral cavity near the midline of the anterior floor of the mouth. The marginal mandibular branch of the facial nerve runs deep to the platysma and lateral to the facial artery and vein in the submandibular triangle and is vulnerable to injury from trauma, from neoplastic involvement, or during surgery in this region.

The posterior triangle contains a variable amount of subcutaneous fat, lymph nodes, and the spinal accessory nerve coursing toward the trapezius muscle (Fig. 29–6).

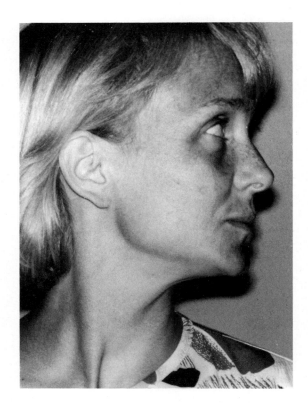

**FIG 29–1.**
The sternocleidomastoid muscle is easily seen as an oblique structure on each side of the neck.

Deep to the sternocleidomastoid muscle is the carotid sheath, which contains the common, external, and internal carotid arteries, the internal jugular vein, and the vagus nerve. Intimately associated with the internal jugular vein is the jugu-lar nodal chain. The hypoglossal nerve courses over the internal and external carotid arteries at a variable level ranging anywhere from the carotid bulb to as high as 5 cm superior to it. Anteriorly, it passes deep to the digastric muscles and

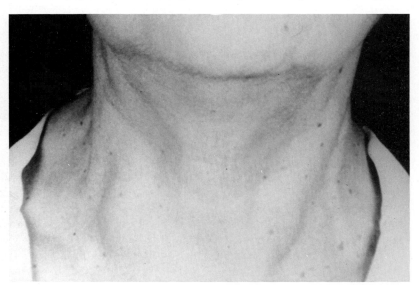

**FIG 29–2.**
This patient has bulges in the lower portion of each side of the neck. They were found to be the result of tortuous carotid arteries.

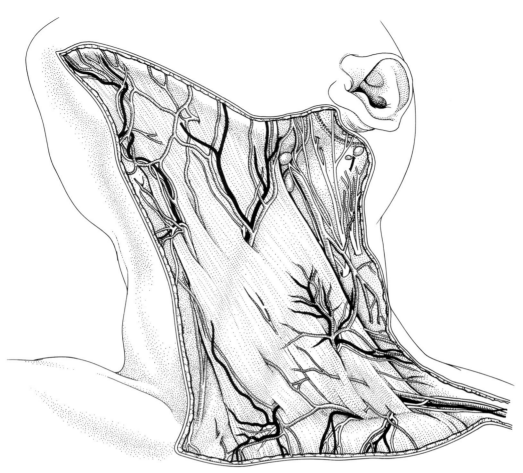

**FIG 29–3.**
Platysma is a broad sheet of muscle covering the deep structures of the lateral neck. (Redrawn after Pernkopf E: *Head and neck,* vol 1. In Helmut F, ed: *Atlas of topographic and applied human anatomy,* ed 2, Baltimore-Munich, 1980, Urban & Schwarzenberg. Used by permission.)

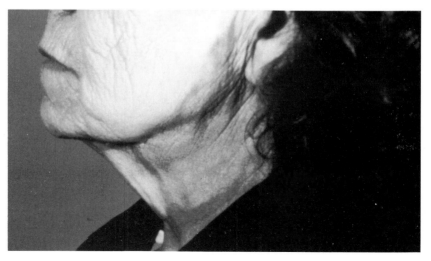

**FIG 29–4.**
The "wattles" seen in this patient are the medial edge of the platysma.

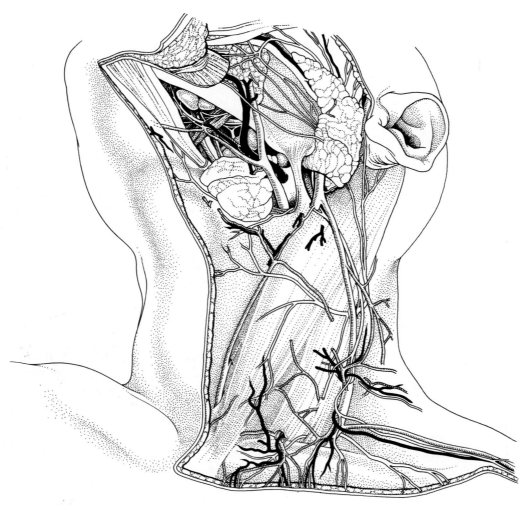

**FIG 29–5**.
Sternocleidomastoid muscle is responsible for head movement resulting in turning the head away from the side of the muscle. (Redrawn after Pernkopf E: *Head and neck,* vol 1. In Helmut F, editor: *Atlas of topographic and applied human anatomy,* ed 2, Baltimore-Munich, 1980, Urban & Schwarzenberg. Used by permission.)

traverses the submandibular gland en route to the tongue musculature (Fig. 29–7).

The posterior cervical triangle is bounded by the sternocleidomastoid muscle anteriorly, the trapezius muscle posteriorly, and the clavicle inferiorly. It contains a variable amount of subcutaneous fat, lymph nodes, and the spinal accessory nerve (cranial nerve XI) coursing from the sternocleidomastoid muscle to the trapezius muscle.

Basic awareness of the cervical nodal anatomy is important to the understanding of head and neck oncology. It is estimated that approximately 40% of all lymph nodes in the body are in the neck. All of the structures of the head and neck have lymphatic channels that involve the cervical nodes. These nodes are arranged into certain drainage groups, such as the internal jugular, spinal accessory, and transverse cervical nodes (Fig. 29–8). An understanding of this cervical nodal anatomy helps in the creation of a differential diagnosis when patients present with neck masses.

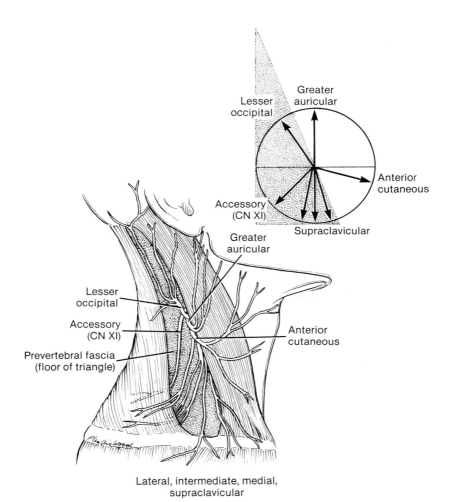

**FIG. 29–6.**
The spinal accessory nerve is an important structure within the posterior cervical triangle.

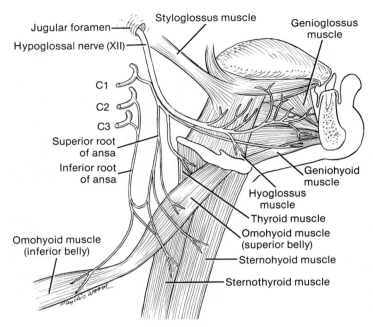

**FIG 29–7.**
The hypoglossal nerve runs deep to the digastric muscles.

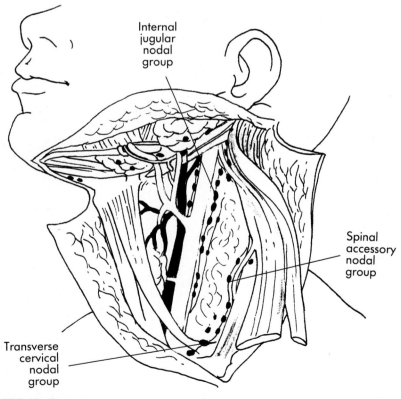

**FIG 29–8.**
This sketch identifies the main nodal groups on each side of the neck.

# 30

# Embryology and Congenital Disorders

The neck is one of the most common sites for congenital disorders. The embryology of the neck helps the clinician understand the location of cysts, sinuses, and fistulas that result from altered embryologic progress.

Neck embryology involves changes associated with the branchial apparatus. These primitive gill slits undergo differentiation in the human embryo and development until they are not identifiable in the 40-week-old fetus. The embryo has paired branchial arches that are separated from one another by four pairs of endodermal pouches and ectodermal clefts (Fig. 30–1). The arches are well-defined units, each of which possesses its own blood supply, skeletal muscle, and connective tissue. Branchial clefts two, three, and four eventually fuse into what is referred to as the cervical sinus of His. The nerves of each of the five arches are the trigeminal (cranial nerve V) for the first arch, acoustic (cranial nerve VIII) for the second, glossopharyngeal (cranial nerve IX) for the third, vagus (cranial nerve X) for the fourth, and spinal accessory (cranial nerve XI) for the fifth. The pouches, clefts, and arches eventually develop into the structures shown in Figure 30–2.

If there is no communication with either the inner mucosa or the outer neck skin, the trapped arch remnant produces a cyst. Cysts are commonly seen in people in the second through fourth decades of life. A branchial sinus refers to a neck mass with a tract that communicates with either the neck skin or the pharyngeal mucosa. A fistula is an epithelial tract that connects the pharynx with the skin. Sinuses and fistulas tend to occur in children more commonly than in adults. The external sinus or fistula often appears as a dimple in the neck skin (Fig. 30–3).

First branchial cleft (Fig. 30–4) sinuses and/or fistulas frequently have one opening in the external auditory canal. The other opening is in the upper neck area, usually inferior to the angle of the mandible. Sometimes the opening is over the parotid gland. The course of anomalies of the first branchial tract is variable through the parotid gland, and there usually is an intimate relationship to the facial nerve. Surgical excision involves a formal dissection of the facial nerve (Fig. 30–5).

The second branchial cleft sinus (Fig. 30–6) is the most common congenital disorder of the neck. It usually is present as a mass in the midregion of the lateral neck. The sinus tract will course superiorly, heading toward the gut, and classically goes between the carotid arteries (Fig. 30–7). If it is a true fistula, it will enter the pharynx in the palatine tonsil area.

The third branchial cleft sinus is not common. It can present as a mass located somewhat lower in the neck than the second branchial cleft sinus. Its tract will usually course superiorly and also posterior to the carotid artery system. It then turns and takes a more inferior direction as it heads towards its pharyngeal destination in the pyriform sinus (Fig. 30–8). A fourth branchial cleft sinus is a theoretic possibility, but its clinical existence has not been documented. This tract would be expected to run into the superior mediastinum and actually enter the gut in the upper cervical esophagus.

Another congenital problem is the thyroglossal duct cyst, which represents an entrapment of some of the epithelium involved with the embryologic descent of the thyroid gland from the tuberculum impar into its normal position in the 40-

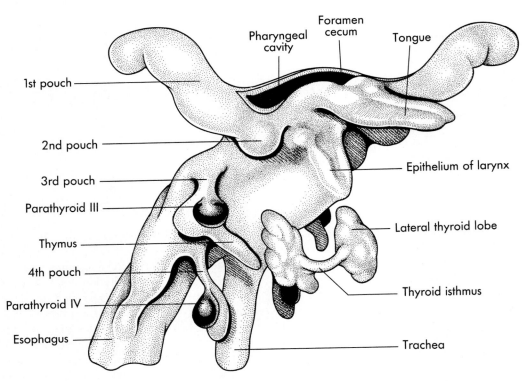

**FIG 30–1.**
The branchial arches are separated from each other by pouches and clefts. (© Copyright CIBA-GEIGY Corporation. Adapted with permission from The CIBA Collection of Medical Illustrations by Frank H. Netter, MD. All rights reserved.)

week-old fetus (Fig. 30–9). Thyroglossal duct cysts usually are detected by the time a person is in the second decade of life. They usually present in the midline at the level of the thyroid membrane. However, they can be located to either side of the midline and can become quite large (Fig. 30–10). Thyroglossal cysts have a propensity for becoming recurrently infected and can even spontaneously develop abscesses and drain with resultant scarring. Such recurrence of infection prompts most physicians to recommend surgical excision.

The embryologic descent of thyroid tissue ne-

cessitates an excision that removes not only the cyst but also tissue in which a tract may be located from the foramen cecum area of the tongue to the cyst through the hyoid bone. Therefore, the excision involves removal of the central portion of the hyoid bone and that tissue up to the foramen cecum of the tongue in order to decrease the chance of recurrence. Before thyroglossal duct cysts are excised, it is important to demonstrate that normally functioning thyroid tissue is in its usual location. Thyroid scans and thyroid function studies are ordered preoperatively.

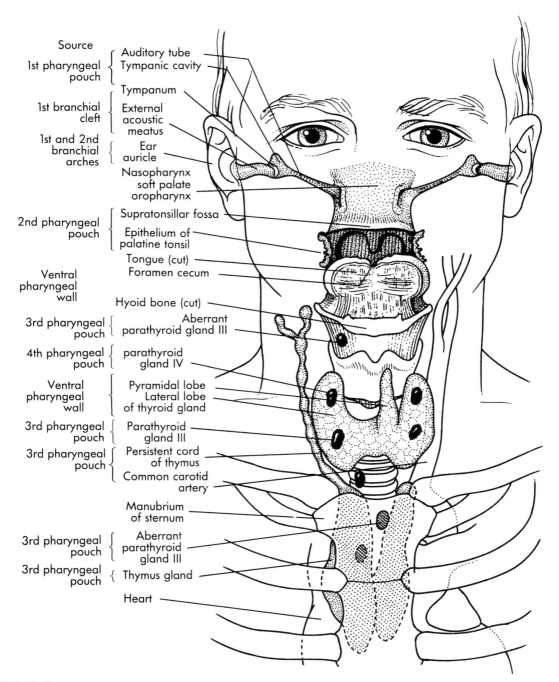

**FIG 30–2.**
This sketch outlines the adult structures and their embryologic derivations. (© Copyright CIBA-GEIGY Corporation. Adapted with permission from *The CIBA Collection of Medical Illustrations* by Frank H. Netter, MD. All rights reserved.)

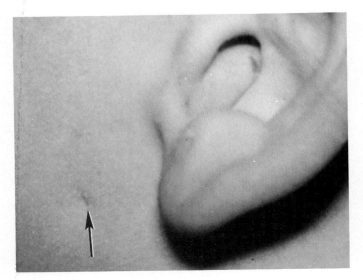

**FIG 30-3**.
A dimple in the skin of the preauricular area is the opening of the first branchial cleft sinus in this child.

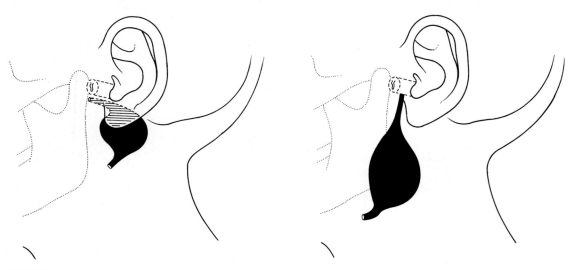

**FIG 30-4**.
These sketches show the different forms of the problem with the first branchial cleft. (From Chandler J, Mitchell B: Bronchial cleft cysts, sinuses and fistulas, *Otolaryngol Clin North Am* 14:175, 1981. Used by permission.)

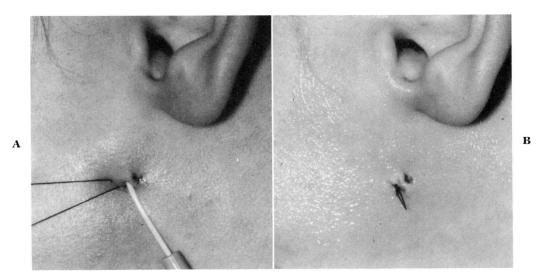

**FIG 30–5**.
The excision of congenital sinus tracts can be facilitated by **A,** injecting radiopaque dye into the sinus tract and **B,** closing it with a stitch to facilitate radiographic and visual identification at the time of surgery, as seen in this child with a first branchial cleft sinus tract.

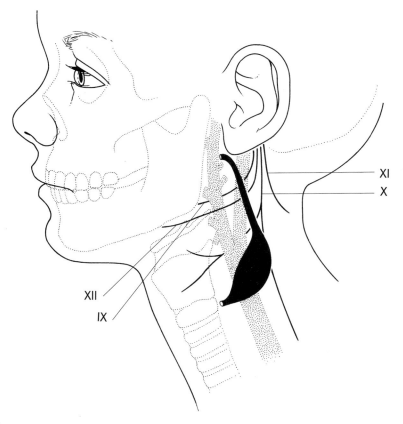

**FIG 30–6**.
Sketch of the course of the second branchial cleft sinus. (From Chandler J, Mitchell B: Bronchial cleft cysts, sinuses and fistulas, *Otolaryngol Clin North Am* 14:175, 1981. Used by permission.)

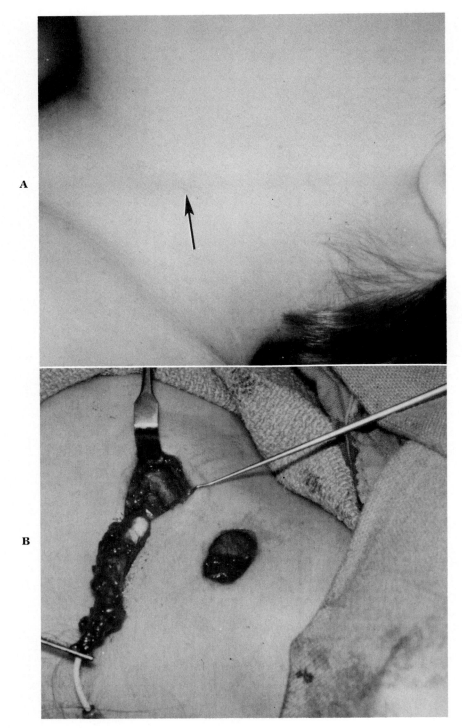

**FIG 30-7.**
**A,** dimple in the midportion of the neck in a child who experienced intermittent drainage from this dimple. **B,** excision of second branchial cleft fistula following injection of dye that courses between the carotid arteries en route to the tonsillar fossa.

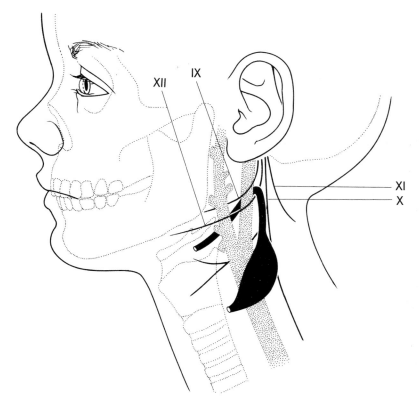

**FIG 30–8.**
The third branchial cleft sinus will open into the pyriform sinus. (From Chandler J, Mitchell B: Bronchial cleft cysts, sinuses and fistulas, *Otolaryngol Clin North Am* 14:175, 1981. Used by permission.)

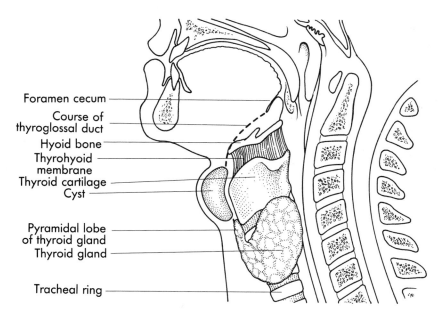

Foramen cecum
Course of thyroglossal duct
Hyoid bone
Thyrohyoid membrane
Thyroid cartilage
Cyst

Pyramidal lobe of thyroid gland
Thyroid gland

Tracheal ring

**FIG 30–9.**
Thyroglossal duct cysts are caused by trapping of epithelium as a result of the descent of the thyroid gland. (From Rood S, et al: *Diagnosis and management of congenital head and neck masses,* Washington, DC, 1981, American Academy of Otolaryngology–Head and Neck Surgery, SiPac; and Schuller D, Krause C: *Cleft lip and palate,* Washington, DC, 1979, American Academy of Otolaryngology–Head and Neck Surgery, SiPac #79400. Used by permission.)

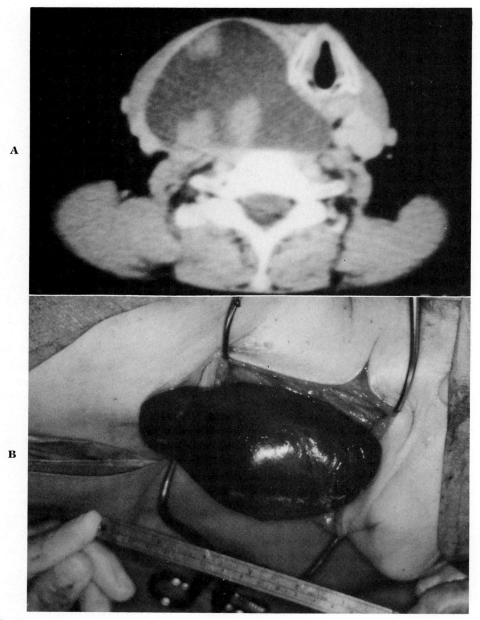

**FIG 30–10**.
**A,** computed tomogram showing a large neck cyst in an elderly woman. **B,** the cyst was surgically resected and found to be a thyroglossal duct cyst.

# 31

# Clinical Problems

## INFECTION AND INFLAMMATION

Infections involving the neck structures can involve both adults and children. Children can develop infections isolated to a single lymph node. Cervical adenitis causes enlargement of the node, which becomes tender to palpation and usually causes some erythema of the overlying neck skin (Fig. 31–1). This nodal infection is usually the result of a primary infectious process occurring somewhere in the lymphatic drainage bed for that particular lymph node chain. Often, the primary source of infection is not identified. In the absence of any fluctuance, antibiotic therapy that includes an antistaphylococcal component will usually cause prompt resolution. However, a smaller percentage of children will continue to have progression of their disease until there is necrosis of the involved lymph node with abscess formation. In this situation, incision and drainage are advisable. There can be a variety of infections involving the neck in adults. Some infections are primary in the sense that they directly involve the neck skin. Systemic antibiotic therapy with local care of a cutaneous infection is effective.

Another common infectious process involving neck structures is the secondary involvement of the nodal lymphatic system following infection originating in the normal drainage pathway for a particular group of nodes. Lymph nodes can undergo hypertrophy, with involvement resulting from either bacterial or viral causes. Inflamed lymph nodes irritate surrounding structures. The patient will not only have tenderness to palpation of the enlarged node but also may even demonstrate some voluntary reduction in neck movement because of the pain. The surrounding musculature may have some component of spasm.

Treatment directed at the primary infection usually results in resolution of the neck nodal involvement. However, in adults it is common for neck nodes that have become inflamed to remain enlarged after the inflammation disappears. This fact often causes concern among adults, who have been sensitized to fears of cancer, and reassurance is necessary.

A genuine infectious threat to the patient's well-being involves the deep neck structures. It is important to understand that the neck has a series of fascial compartments adjacent to the deep musculature. These fascial compartments are potential spaces that are continuous with similar compartments in the mediastinum. The anatomic potential exists for a deep neck infection to become a life-threatening problem with extension into and involvement of the mediastinal structures.

Deep neck infections can actually originate from a variety of processes involving the pharynx, salivary glands, vertebrae, paranasal sinuses, and temporal bone. They can also arise from dental-related infections of the oral cavity.

The development of antibiotics has had a significant positive impact on the seriousness of infectious processes, but it has caused some potential for masking the seriousness of the deep neck infections. The relative infrequency of these problems means that they are less well understood by many health care professionals. The use of antibiotics that might not be curative but rather mask an ongoing acute inflammatory process involving some of the deep neck spaces may allow such an infection to persist and actually progress without the clinician being aware of the worsening clinical situation. It is interesting to note that deep neck infections formerly had the potential to cause

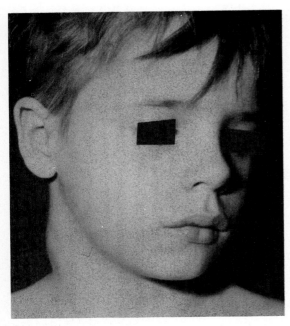

**FIG 31–1.**
This child developed cervical adenitis, which completely responded to intravenous antibiotics.

death related to septicemia. This clinical course has been altered in the postantibiotic era. A cause of death from deep neck infections is bleeding and may result from delayed diagnosis and its adverse effect on the critical structures running adjacent to these fascial compartments within the neck. The intent of this discussion is not to describe the anatomic detail of the fascial compartments, but at least to promote an awareness of it so that the clinician can consider these compartments whenever infectious processes involving the neck are encountered.

The bacteria causing deep neck infections include a variety of organisms. The pyogenic bacteria predominate, with *Streptococcus hemolyticus* being the most common. In fact, *Streptococcus* accounts for approximately 80% of deep neck infections. If an infection originates in the oral cavity, it is not unusual for the spirillum of Vincent's angina to be cultured from a deep neck infection.

It is helpful to understand the primary site of an infection involving the neck. This information can provide hints about the fascial compartment involved in the neck. For example, an infection of the tonsil can cause downward extension into the compartments adjacent to the hypopharynx and larynx. Sinus infections can produce retropharyngeal neck infections.

The deep neck infections can involve a variety of spaces. Whenever a tonsillar infection penetrates the pharyngeal constrictor muscles behind the tonsil, it has gained access to the pharyngomaxillary spaces. In addition to having fever and sore throat, patients will complain of trismus and pain with movement of the neck. As the disease process advances, swelling in the upper lateral neck becomes apparent and local tenderness develops.

An infection of the submandibular area of the neck usually has a dental origin, especially dental extraction. Ludwig's angina is an example of such a process that has extended to involve the sublingual, submaxillary, and submental spaces. It typically becomes evident as long as 4 days after a dental extraction. Swelling of the anterior floor of the mouth and inflammation increase to the extent that the edema causes upward and posterior displacement of the tongue (Fig. 31–2). Because this inflammation spreads through the fascial planes and not through lymphatic channels, there is usually bilateral involvement. All of the inflammation of the upper neck structures makes neck movement, mastication, and deglutition difficult. Eventually, abscess formation occurs, and incision and drainage are necessary. It is not unusual for multiple abscesses involving the submental, submaxillary, and sublingual areas to be involved in one case of Ludwig's angina.

The retropharyngeal space can also become in-

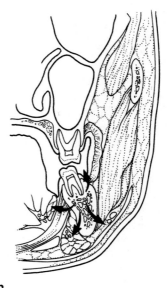

**FIG 31–2.**
If the posterior displacement of the tongue is great enough, airway obstruction can develop.

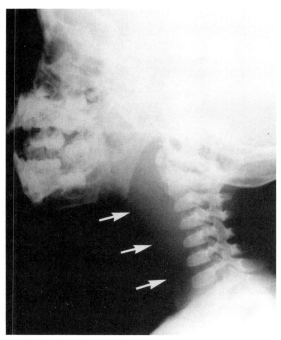

**FIG 31–3.**
This child had a large retropharyngeal abscess with thickening of the soft tissue of the posterior pharynx, as seen on this radiograph.

fected. This is a problem that is more frequently seen in children than in adults. The retropharynx can be involved with infections originating from the nose and paranasal sinuses. It also can occur subsequent to a laceration of the posterior pharyngeal mucosa. The initial event is usually involvement of the lymph nodes, with ultimate necrosis, abscess formation, and downward extension of the infection. The child with this problem typically has trismus and odynophagia. Neck rigidity can be a component because of the inflammation of the prevertebral fascia. As the edema increases, the voice quality can be altered; airway compromise can even result in the more severe cases. Because of the inability to open the mouth widely and the lack of patient cooperation, diagnostic approaches in addition to physical examination are sometimes necessary. The lateral soft tissue cervical radiograph (Fig. 31–3) is helpful because it demonstrates thickening of the retropharyngeal space and possibly even the presence of air. Incision and drainage are recommended.

A variety of other deep neck infections can occur that involve the pretracheal space, the masticator space, and even extension of primary pa-

rotid infections. An awareness of the possibility of these infections is important for any clinician.

## TRAUMA

For patients with penetrating neck injuries, the initial physical examination is important. The decision for exploration is not difficult when there are signs strongly suggestive of an injury to a major vascular structure. Shock, active bleeding, expanding hematoma, abnormal auscultative sounds over blood vessels, and any evidence of abnormal neurologic findings suggesting cerebrovascular insufficiency are all strong indicators of a major vascular injury requiring surgical exploration. However, it has been estimated that as many as 33% of patients who have major vascular injuries have none of the preceding signs. It becomes evident that arteriography is important for any patient being evaluated for a penetrating neck injury in the absence of any of these signs. Not only does the arteriogram help to identify the presence of a vascular injury, but it also locates it so that the surgeon can plan accordingly.

Evaluation of the laryngopharynx, trachea, and esophagus is also important. The presence of any voice alterations indicates laryngeal trauma that may lead to significant airway compromise hours later. The presence of subcutaneous crepitation indicates that either the esophagus or trachea has been lacerated and air has escaped into the soft tissues of the neck. Once again, this is an indication for surgical exploration.

Extravasation of any contrast material into the soft tissue of the neck is also an indicator supporting the advisability of exploration. Endoscopic examinations of the aerodigestive tract are also useful.

If the patient's overall condition is stable, early exploration of the neck is appropriate when any of the aforementioned diagnostic studies indicate abnormalities. The sooner appropriate drainage can be established and/or the pharynx, esophagus, or trachea closed, the less chance there is of salivary contamination of the neck structures and subsequent development of infection.

There is no uniformly applicable generalization for penetrating neck injuries. One needs to be knowledgeable of the pitfalls of the physical examination. Certain important diagnostic radiographic studies such as arteriography must be readily available for the optimal evaluation of the patient with neck trauma. These are discussed in Chapter 32.

## TUMORS

Most neck tumors that originate in structures within the neck are benign. These primary neck tumors can occur in both children and adults, although the majority are seen primarily in adults. They can arise from the subcutaneous fat or vascular, neural, or salivary structures. Lipomas do occur in the neck. They usually present as isolated soft masses that are not adherent to surrounding structures and permit easy excision (Fig. 31–4). There is one disorder, Madelung's disease, that causes impressive deposits of subcutaneous fat tumors throughout the body, primarily involving the neck and occasionally the upper back region (Fig. 31–5). These unfortunate patients have the physical appearance of those with adrenal or steroid metabolism problems. This disease has no relation to the adrenal-pituitary axis. Surgical resection of these fatty tumors is warranted to improve range of motion of the neck and for cosmetic reasons. Complete excision is difficult because of the extensive involvement of all tissue planes.

Vascular tumors involving neck structures do occur. Hemangiomas can involve the deep structures of the neck. They can even result in dis-

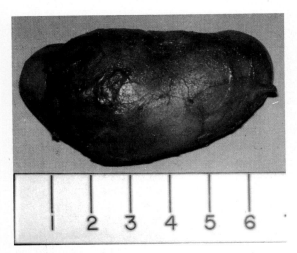

**FIG 31–4.**
A lipoma usually has a well-defined capsule.

placement of the pharyngeal wall. Although the general approach to hemangiomas is conservative because of their propensity for spontaneous resolution, excision is recommended if the hemangioma is located where it may obstruct the airway.

Nonchromaffin paragangliomas can arise from cells within the carotid body at the level of the carotid bulb and the vagal body near the jugular foramen. These two uncommon vascular tumors are referred to as carotid body tumors and vagal body tumors, respectively. These present as pulsatile neck masses. Arteriography is diagnostic and reveals highly vascular tumors (Fig. 31–6). Surgical resection is indicated. However, replacement of the carotid artery may be necessary because of the possibility of damaging the wall of the artery while excising the tumor. When these tumors are suspected, bilateral carotid angiography is usually performed because multiple sites of involvement are common. Surgical excision is usually definitive, with only a small chance for recurrence.

Another form of a vascular tumor is the lymphangioma or cystic hygroma, which involves the proliferation and dilatation of lymphatic vessels. Although the lymphangioma is the lymphatic counterpart of hemangioma, it has less of a chance for spontaneous resolution. Therefore, excision is usually necessary, especially whenever the cystic hygroma involves neck structures that could cause airway compromise. These tumors can enlarge rapidly as a result of infection, which causes rapid increase of fluid within the tumor.

Benign tumors of neural origin, such as schwannomas, can involve any of the nerves coursing through the neck. A preoperative definitive diagnosis is difficult with these tumors. Surgical excision invariably results in the need to resect the nerve of origin. Neurofibromas often are multiple.

Salivary gland tumors can present as neck masses. When a parotid tumor involves the tail of the gland, it will present as an upper neck tumor. Also, a submandibular tumor will cause prominence and alteration of the surface anatomy of the skin overlying the submandibular triangle. Although it is possible for neck masses in this location to be enlarged lymph nodes, one should consider a submandibular primary tumor.

There are other neck tumors that result from spread of primary neoplasms. This relates to cervical adenopathy, seen primarily with tumors aris-

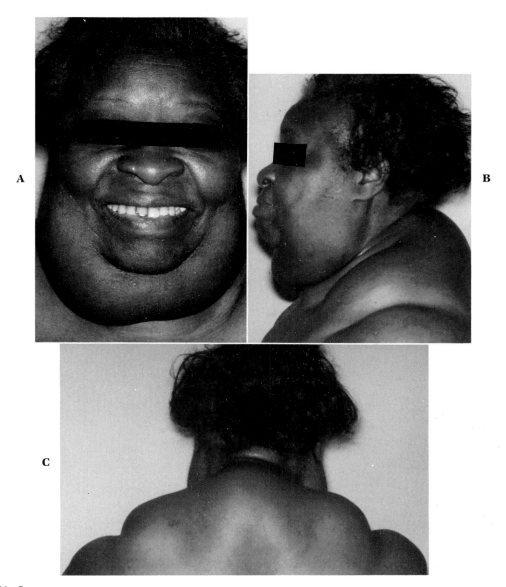

**FIG 31–5.**
Anterior, **A,** lateral, **B,** and posterior, **C,** views of a patient with Madelung disease demonstrate the extensive fat deposits present in this condition.

ing in the upper aerodigestive tract. As mentioned, a solitary firm and nontender neck mass in an adult should be considered a metastatic lymph node until proved otherwise. It has long been urged that excision of such a neck mass is deleterious to the patient. Sound statistical evidence has supported this generalization. Removal of a metastatic lymph node from the neck increases the morbidity and decreases the probability for survival.

The proper approach to such a mass is to search initially for the primary site of the malignancy and, if one is found, to plan appropriate therapy. If such a primary tumor site is not located, management involves an excisional biopsy of the neck node followed immediately by a frozen-section analysis. If the results are positive for metastatic tumor, the patient undergoes a neck dissection immediately during the same operative procedure as the biopsy.

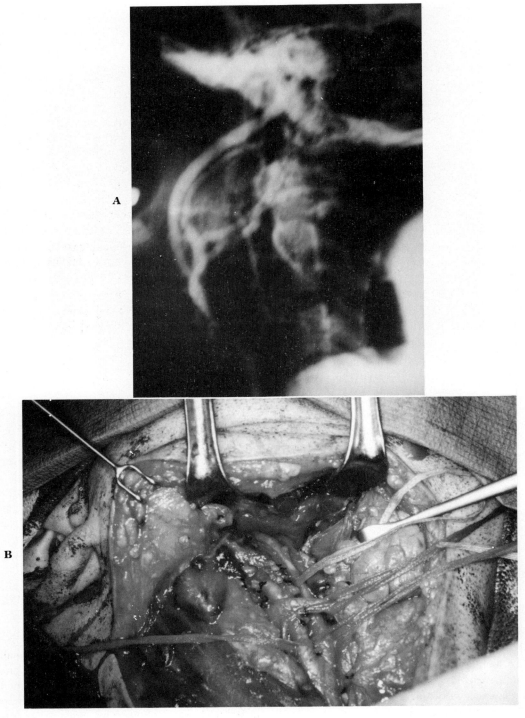

**FIG 31–6.**
**A,** arteriogram shows marked displacement of the carotid arteries as a result of a vagal body tumor that was, **B,** resected with preservation of the carotid artery system.

## Thyroid Tumors

Thyroid tumors continue to represent a diagnostic challenge. The development of thyroid tumors in patients who have previously been irradiated for benign disease in that area, such as for an enlarged thymus, has received considerable publicity. It behooves the clinician to include questions about irradiation as a regular part of a standard interview process with any patient. It is difficult to determine the absolute frequency of benign and malignant thyroid tumors. It has been estimated that as many as 50% of solitary thyroid nodules occurring in children are malignant. Thyroid disease is generally more common in females than in males. Malignant thyroid disease is also more commonly seen in females. A male who has a solitary thyroid nodule is likely to have a malignancy. Most reviews of thyroid malignancies demonstrate that the highest percentage occurs in patients younger than 20 years of age.

Many approaches for examining the thyroid gland have been described previously. Whichever technique is most comfortable for the clinician should be used. It is important to understand that slight flexion of the neck places the platysma, sternocleidomastoid, and strap muscles at rest and allows more accurate palpation of the thyroid gland (Fig. 31–7). If a solitary nodule is hard to palpation, histologic examination is advisable. Any solitary nodules with concomitant ipsilateral cervical adenopathy are also especially suspicious. If there is an ipsilateral vocal cord paralysis associated with a solitary nodule, histologic examination is also advisable.

The results of thyroid scans were formerly believed to have great significance in determining whether neoplasms were benign or malignant. A functioning "hot" nodule (Fig. 31–8) was previously thought to have a lower incidence of cancer than a nonfunctioning "cold" nodule (Fig. 31–9). However, there are reports that refute these findings and demonstrate that a certain percentage of both benign and malignant thyroid nodules are radiographically described as being "hot." Whether the disease is benign or malignant cannot be determined from thyroid function studies. However, the scans provide a useful baseline of information and are usually obtained.

Thyrocalcitonin assays are now considered to be diagnostic for medullary thyroid carcinoma, but are not recommended as part of the screening evaluation because medullary carcinomas are not common. If there is other evidence to cause suspicion of this diagnosis, use of the assays may be helpful before obtaining histologic information. Medullary thyroid cancer can be associated with adrenal pheochromocytoma, parathyroid hyperplasia, or parathyroid adenoma in Sipple's syndrome. These patients usually have paroxysmal hypertension and may even have abnormal serum calcium levels. Medullary thyroid cancer has a mendelian dominant inheritance pattern, and

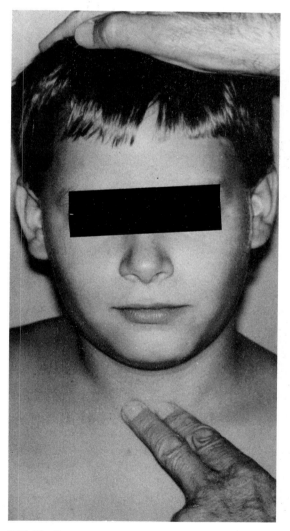

**FIG 31–7.**
An accurate thyroid examination is best accomplished by slight flexion of the neck, which relaxes the platysma and sternocleidomastoid muscles to facilitate deep palpation.

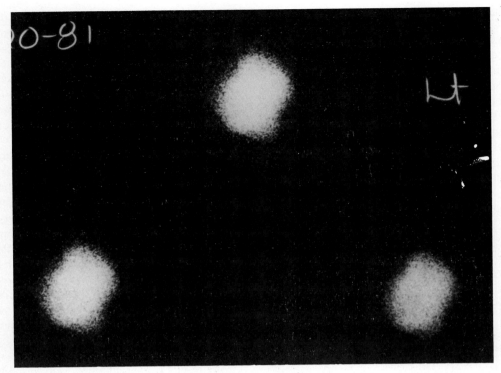

**FIG 31-9.**
A "cold" thyroid nodule as seen in the right lobe on this scan has a higher incidence of malignancy.

families of patients with this problem should be evaluated.

Fine-needle aspiration has provided a useful means of obtaining material for histologic evaluation in patients with suspicious nodules. There is a low incidence of false-positive and false-negative results. However, it is important for pathologists interpreting this material to have experience with fine-needle aspiration.

When the clinical circumstances support the

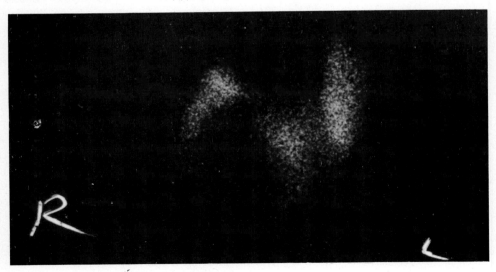

**FIG 31-8.**
A "hot" thyroid nodule has a low incidence of cancer.

removal of a thyroid nodule, a benign adenoma will be the probable diagnosis. If the nodule is malignant, the outlook still is favorable, except for patients with the rare anaplastic thyroid malignancy, for which there is no effective treatment. Papillary and papillary-follicular thyroid carcinomas tend to have multiple sites within the thyroid gland, and this has created some active discussion about the extent of tissue removed surgically versus the use of adjunctive therapy with radioactive iodine. The presence of neck nodal metastatic disease with papillary carcinoma increases the seriousness of the clinical situation. However, the outlook is still favorable. There does not appear to be any increased benefit for the patient with cervical nodal metastatic disease to undergo neck dissection instead of removal of only those palpable nodes.

Parathyroid disorders can also occur. Hyperparathyroidism can be the result of one or more glands undergoing hyperplasia or of an actual parathyroid neoplasm. The parathyroid glands can evolve into a state of hyperparathyroidism with no identifiable cause. In contrast, they can also develop hyperparathyroidism as a result of other organ abnormalities. Patients with renal disease are particularly prone to developing hyperparathyroidism.

The usual symptoms associated with parathyroid dysfunction involve suggestions of problems relating to the kidneys, the gastrointestinal tract, and/or the skeletal system. Recurrent renal stones often are the first indication of parathyroid dysfunction. Decalcification of the bones can cause vague nonspecific discomforts. Recurrent fractures may also be an indicator. The gastrointestinal symptoms are usually associated with peptic ulcer disease. This problem usually does not respond to the typical medical management of ulcers. Pancreatitis may also be a component of the gastrointestinal symptoms. The patients may have central nervous system symptoms such as headache, weakness, and depression. Blood serum levels reveal hypercalcemia. A medical crisis is possible if the serum calcium level is 15 mg/100 ml or higher. When these subjective symptoms are associated with objective hypercalcemia, attempts at localizing the parathyroid hyperplasia or adenomas should be instituted, with the ultimate goal being surgical removal.

# 32

# Evaluation of the Neck Mass

A mass that appears in the neck can have a congenital, inflammatory, or neoplastic etiology. Considerable information about the possible diagnosis can be derived before any tissue is removed for biopsy purposes. In fact, sometimes excisional biopsy is not advisable.

The age of the patient is an initial indicator of the probable diagnosis. In children, inflammatory causes of neck masses are considerably more common than others. Congenital causes are the second most common, and neoplasms occur only rarely. This is in contrast to adults, in whom that order is reversed: Neoplasms are the most common cause, followed by congenital and inflammatory processes. A unilateral neck mass in an adult should be considered a neoplastic process until proved otherwise.

It is important to assess the presence of any concomitant disease in a patient with a neck mass. This is especially critical in the adult. Most adults with unilateral neck masses have a malignancy that invariably does not originate from the neck structures. The primary lesion is most commonly located within the upper aerodigestive tract. Therefore, a thorough search of this area is critical. It is also necessary to evaluate the scalp and facial skin to rule out a cutaneous malignancy that could account for cervical adenopathy. The patient who has received a transplant and other immunocompromised individuals exemplify another group of patients with diseases that could have a bearing on the cause of a neck mass.

The time course of the development of a neck mass is useful information that permits some generalizations. Rapid growth of a neck mass is usually seen in nonneoplastic processes, whereas neoplasms tend to cause a slower, more gradual change in size.

The location of a neck mass is important and becomes more useful to the clinician who has an understanding of basic cervical anatomy. If a lesion is located in the midneck at the level of the hyoid bone, the most likely diagnosis is a thyroglossal duct cyst. This is in contrast to a lateral neck mass in the midportion of the neck, which may be either a midjugular lymph node or a branchiogenic cyst, especially if it is cystic in consistency. Spherical masses in other parts of the neck usually represent adenopathy.

The consistency of a mass determined by palpation has variable specificity. In the individual with a long, thin neck who is easy to examine, one can frequently palpate a neck mass and determine whether it is solid or cystic. A cystic mass speaks strongly in favor of a benign process. Palpation is also important because it assesses whether the lesion is tender. A mass that is tender often indicates an inflammatory cause. Palpation also reveals whether there is any pulsation present.

Auscultation of neck masses can also be informative. It should be performed routinely for any lateral neck masses that are possibly related to one of the major vascular structures, such as the carotid artery system. The presence of any bruits noted with auscultation indicates some disturbance of normal blood flow and is consistent with vascular disease, whether that be aneurysm, arteriovenous malformation, or vascular tumor.

After the history and physical examination are completed, the number of possibilities in the differential diagnosis can usually be reduced. It is

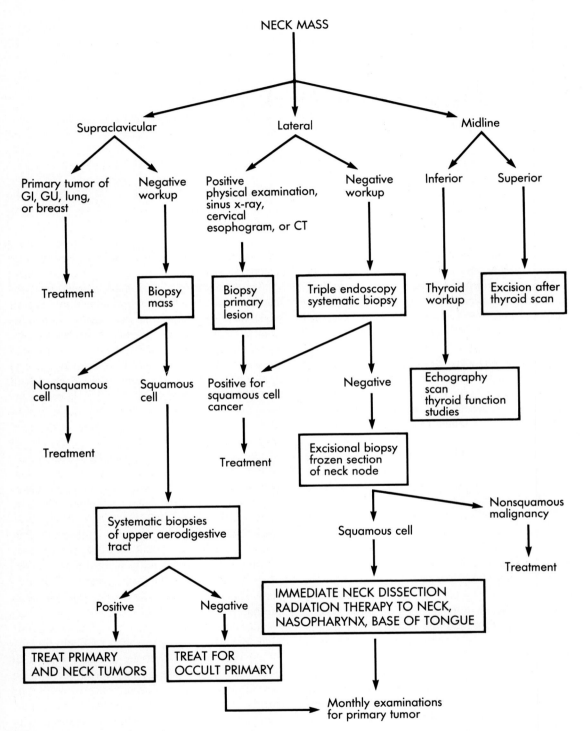

**FIG 32–1.**
This algorithm outlines the sequence of the diagnostic evaluation of a neck mass. (Modified from Schuller D: *Mass in the neck.* In Holt GR, Matox DE, Gates GA, eds: *Decision making in otolaryngology,* Toronto, 1986, BC Decker. Used by permission.)

this differential diagnosis that should direct the clinician to pursue further information with some of the specialized diagnostic techniques. Noninvasive radiographic studies such as computed tomography and echography can help determine the consistency of the mass and its relationship to surrounding structures. If there is any concern about vascular pathology, angiography becomes increasingly important. If histologic information is desirable prior to definite treatment, fine-needle aspiration biopsy is a highly accurate and well-tolerated technique, especially when experienced pathologists are involved with interpretation of the aspirated material.

The decision about whether more extensive tissue removal is warranted must be based on the information derived from fine-needle aspiration biopsy. If there is any concern about a possible malignant cause, any biopsy technique other than fine-needle aspiration as a separate procedure is to be discouraged. Removal of malignant lymph nodes causes seeding of the surgical wound with tumor cells, ultimately leading to increased pa-

tient morbidity and mortality. This is a critical issue, and all clinicians should be aware of the inadvisability of proceeding in this fashion.

It is apparent that numerous factors can potentially provide useful diagnostic information about the cause of a neck mass. All of these considerations can be confusing. This possibility for confusion can be reduced by a diagnostic approach based on the position of the neck mass. If the evaluation is based on whether the mass is located in the supraclavicular, lateral, or midline region of the neck, the diagnostic evaluation becomes easier. An algorithm (Fig. 32–1) can be used to assist in an orderly approach.

The numerous possible identities of a neck mass can be dramatically reduced when age, time of onset, location, and consistency are determined from the history and physical examination. The additional information derived from some special diagnostic procedures can even further reduce the differential diagnosis so that the clinician can plan a rational therapeutic approach.

# 33

# Treatment of Neck Nodal Disease

*Neck dissection* is the term applied to the surgical procedure designed to remove the lymph nodes and lymphatic channels from a patient who has a cancer arising in the upper aerodigestive tract or other anatomic sites within the head and neck. In an effort to completely remove all of the node-bearing tissue, the surgeon resects certain structures that are not nodal tissue but are closely related to nodes. In the classic radical neck dissection, the submandibular salivary gland, sternocleidomastoid muscle, internal jugular vein, and spinal accessory nerve are routinely excised as a means of assuring complete removal of node-bearing tissue. Modifications of this operation that preserve some of these structures have been described (Fig. 33–1). These are referred to as modified, conservative, or functional neck dissections. Such modifications are usually coupled with radiation therapy to increase chances of success. They have the potential advantage of causing less morbidity than a classic radical neck dissection. These patients usually sustain some degree of discomfort as a result of the intentional sacrifice of the spinal accessory nerve and denervation of the trapezius muscle. The modifications of the standard operation are sometimes used in those clinical situations in which neck nodal metastatic disease is not far advanced.

The decision to include neck dissection in the treatment of a head and neck cancer is based on either the clinical presence of enlarged neck nodes or the location and size of the patient's primary tumor. Retrospective analyses have indicated to clinicians that the size and location of certain primary tumors will dramatically increase the probability of the presence of occult metastatic disease in patients who have no palpable adenopathy. Even in the absence of such palpable adenopathy, this type of patient undergoes a neck dissection.

The alternative to neck dissection is radiation therapy to control neck nodal disease. It is generally agreed that occult neck nodal disease can be just as effectively controlled with radiation therapy as it can with surgery. However, as the size of metastatic nodes increases, the effectiveness of radiation therapy decreases and surgery plays a greater role.

Neck dissection for neck nodal disease in patients with head and neck cancer is an important component of proper management. It is critical for the clinician to have a basic understanding of the rationale for such therapy and its consequences to the patient.

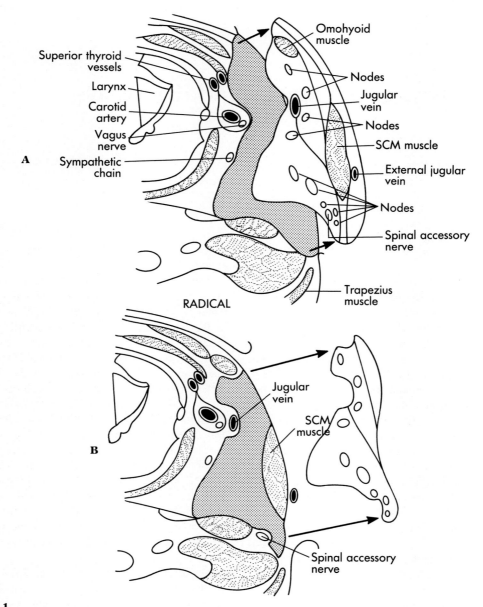

**FIG 33–1**.
This sketch shows the differences in the amount of tissue removed in the standard neck dissection **A,** as compared with the modified neck dissection, **B.**

# PART VIII
# Ear

# 34

# Anatomy and Physiology

## ANATOMY

The external ear consists of the auricle and the external auditory canal.

### Auricle

Cartilage, elastic tissue, and skin make up the entire auricle, except for the dependent lobule, which contains no cartilage (Fig. 34–1). The skin is closely attached to cartilage in front of the ear but is loosely adherent behind and easily separated. The skin of the ear is thinner than skin elsewhere in the body. Because it lacks a protective layer of fat and has essentially only one layer of blood vessels, the auricular skin is more subject to frostbite than any other part of the body. Three small muscles attach the auricle to the head, called the anterior, superior, and posterior auricular muscles. These are innervated by the facial nerve. Lower animals have great control of their auricular muscles and use them to increase their hearing acuity. In humans, however, these muscles serve no practical function and are only of comic social relief.

Lymphatics drain anteriorly, inferiorly, and posteriorly (Fig. 34–2). Lymphadenopathy behind the ear in patients with external otitis or with an infection from the scalp may confuse the examiner in that the ears are pushed forward and the patient may look as though he or she has acute mastoiditis. Also, frequently there is a palpable node just anterior to the tragus that can become involved in infection spreading from an external otitis, and it can become confused with a parotid mass.

Sensory nerve supply of the auricle is derived from four sources: the great auricular nerve, the lesser occipital nerve, the auricular branch of the vagus nerve, and the auriculotemporal nerve from the mandibular division of the trigeminal nerve (Fig. 34–3). It should be noted that the fifth, seventh, and tenth cranial nerves contribute sensation in addition to cervical sources. Thus, disease or trauma to other areas of the mouth, nose, throat, or neck may produce pain in the ear. This is called referred pain or referred otalgia and is important diagnostically.

### External Auditory Canal

The external auditory canal ends at the tympanic membrane. The tympanic membrane is oblique; the exterior canal's superior wall is 5 mm shorter than the anterior-inferior wall. Because the canal bends, it is necessary to straighten it by upward traction on the auricle before the eardrum can be easily examined (Fig. 34–4). The outer half of the ear canal is cartilaginous. The inner half is bony, although in the infant in whom ossification has not occurred the entire canal is cartilaginous. The skin lining the cartilaginous canal is thick and contains fine hairs, sebaceous glands, and cerumen-producing glands. The cartilage of the ear canal is continuous with that of the auricle. The cartilaginous portion of the ear is oval and forms an incomplete circle.

In the adult, the external auditory canal is approximately 24 mm long, the bony canal being somewhat longer than the cartilaginous portion. Seven millimeters from the tympanic membrane, the bony canal forms a constriction known as the isthmus. Inferiorly and anteriorly beyond the isth-

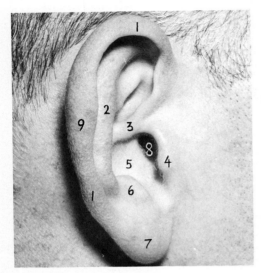

**FIG 34–1.**
Auricle. *1*, Helix. *2*, Antihelix. *3*, Crus of helix. *4*, Tragus. *5*, Concha. *6*, Antitragus. *7*, Lobule. *8*, External auditory meatus. *9*, Darwin's tubercle.

mus, but external to the lower part of the drum, is the tympanic sulcus (Fig. 34–5). Debris often collects here, especially in patients with external otitis. Also, foreign bodies can be lodged in this area and difficult to remove. Occasionally, the anterior portion of the bony canal is prominent and obscures the drumhead. This is a complicating feature when one desires full visualization of the tympanic membrane.

Anterior to the ear canal is the temporomandibular joint, and ear pain is often attributable to abnormalities of this joint. To test this possibility, one should press with the index finger over each temporomandibular joint while the patient's mouth is open and ask him or her to bite down. If there is tenderness in one or both temporomandibular joints with light pressure and the tympanic membrane is normal in appearance, the temporomandibular joint is probably the culprit. Superiorly and posteriorly, the bony canal is thin and directly under the mastoid antrum. This is important in that acute mastoiditis may cause periosteal inflammation and sagging of this portion of the ear canal. In addition, chronic mastoiditis or cho-

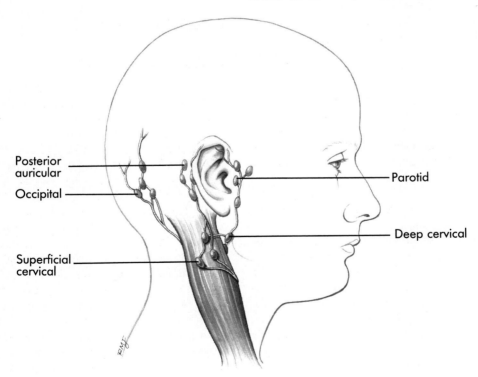

**FIG 34–2.**
Lymphatic supply of the external ear.

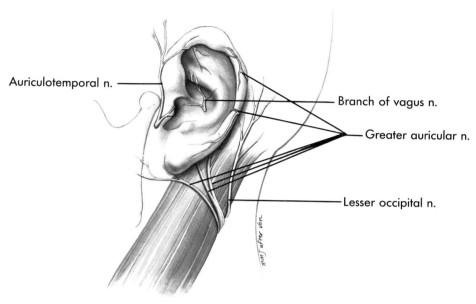

**FIG 34–3.**
Sensory nerve contribution to the external ear. (Redrawn after Shambaugh G Jr, Glassock M II: *Surgery of the ear,* ed 3, Philadelphia, 1980, WB Saunders. Used by permission.)

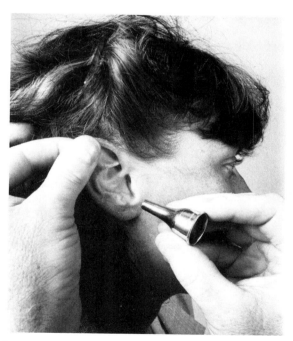

**FIG 34–4.**
Straightening of the external canal by pulling the ear upward and posteriorly.

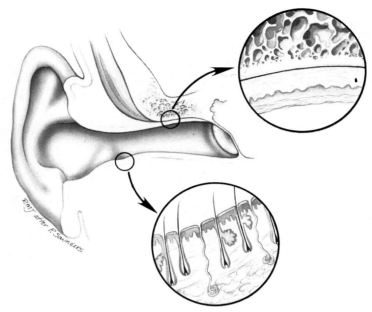

**FIG 34–5**.
External auditory canal. *Upper inset,* cartilaginous ear canal shows hair follicles, sebaceous glands, and ceruminous glands. *Lower inset,* thin epithelium attached to the bone.

lesteatoma may erode this thin, bony plate and appear in the external canal lateral to the anulus of the tympanic membrane. Because the epithelium of the bony canal is delicate, even slight trauma may produce hematoma.

## TYMPANIC MEMBRANE

The tympanic membrane is made of two layers of epithelium, an outer layer of squamous epithelium and an inner layer of cuboidal. There is a central layer of fibrous tissue that is incomplete superiorly bordered by the anterior and posterior malleolar ligaments. The portion of the drum containing the fibrous layers is known as the pars tensa, and the tiny remaining portion (Shrapnell membrane) is called the pars flaccida.

The tympanic membrane is cone shaped like the diaphragm of loud speakers and inclined so that the upper part is more external or closer to the examiner than the lower portion. Both the concavity of the drumhead and its position relative to the ear canal vary and may be altered greatly with disease. The fibers of the tympanic membrane condense peripherally in a fibrocartilaginous ring, called the anulus, which fits into a

sulcus. The anulus is not complete, there being a defect superiorly between the anterior and posterior malleolar ligaments. This deficiency of the ring is known as the notch of Rivinus (incisura tympanica). The portion of the tympanic membrane enclosing this area is the pars flaccida, which is so called because it lacks a fibrous layer.

The primary landmark in an otologic examination of the tympanic membrane is the malleus. The long process and short process of the malleus are embedded in the tympanic membrane. The short portion stands out like a knob at the upper end of the manubrium (long process) (Fig. 34–6). The anterior and posterior malleolar folds are directed upward and outward from the short process. The umbo is at the lower portion of the malleus, and from here the light reflex is directed anteriorly-inferiorly. Occasionally, in some normal ears, the long process of the incus may be seen behind the malleus in the posterior-superior portion of the drumhead. The incus is at a level deeper than the malleus and is not attached to the tympanic membrane under ordinary circumstances. Therefore, it is only seen when the tympanic membrane is not thickened or more translucent than normal. The chorda tympani nerve arches high across the back side of the drumhead

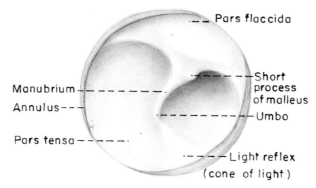

**FIG 34–6.**
Landmarks of the right tympanic membrane. The size of the pars flaccida is exaggerated in this drawing.

and occasionally is visible in the posterior-superior quadrant. There are normal variations in the color of the tympanic membrane, but usually it is described as pearl gray. There may be significant variation of vascularization along the anulus and around the manubrium of the malleolar folds. Occasionally, there is white mottling of the tympanic membrane, making the drumhead look denser or thicker than normal.

## Middle Ear

The middle ear, or tympanic cavity, is roughly an oblong space lined with mucous membrane.

The portion directly behind the tympanic membrane is sometimes called the mesotympanum, and that area above the tympanic membrane is known as the epitympanum or the attic. It is in the attic that the bodies of the incus and malleus are located. The smaller part of the middle ear, known as the hypotympanum, lies below the level of the promontory and round window. Occasionally, the bony floor of the hypotympanum may be dehiscent, and the dome of the jugular bulb may protrude upward into the middle ear space. In those cases, it is seen through the tympanic membrane inferiorly as a bluish shadow or bulge. All the walls of the middle ear except the lateral wall

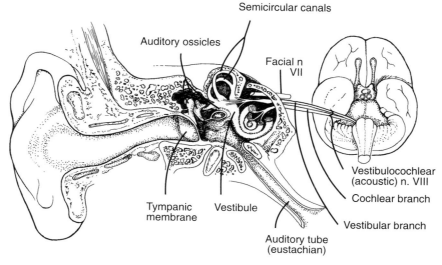

**FIG 34–7.**
Relationship of the external ear, middle ear, and inner ear. Note the ossicles of the middle ear, the relationship of the cochlea and semicircular canals, and the location of the eustachian tube. Note that the head of the malleus and the body of the incus are *superior* to the eardrum. (From Jacobs SW, Francone CA: *Structure and function in man,* ed 5, Philadelphia, 1982, WB Saunders. Used by permission.)

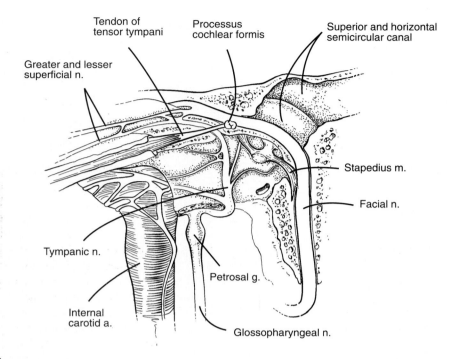

**FIG 34–8.**
Medial wall of the middle ear. Note the tympanic plexus of nerves over the promontory, and the beginning of the vertical course of the facial nerve.

are bony. The part of the lateral wall covering the mesotympanum is the tympanic membrane. Anteriorly, the eustachian tube leads downward and medially to the nasopharynx (Fig. 34–7). Medially opposite the tympanic membrane is a prominence called the promontory, which houses the basal coil of the cochlea. Posteriorly and superiorly, the stapes fits into the oval window, and inferior to this is the round window niche. The seventh cranial nerve crosses the medial wall of the middle ear, passing just above the oval window (Fig. 34–8). The middle ear itself opens posteriorly into the mastoid antrum, the connecting passage being called the aditus ad antrum (Fig. 34–9).

The middle ear contains the three ossicles: the malleus, incus, and stapes. The malleus has a head, neck, handle, and short process. The handle and short processes are embedded in the layers of the tympanic membrane, but the head and neck extend above the upper margin of the drum into the epitympanic space (Fig. 34–10). The head of the malleus articulates with the body of the incus. The articulation is a true joint, with a capsule and supporting ligaments. The incus

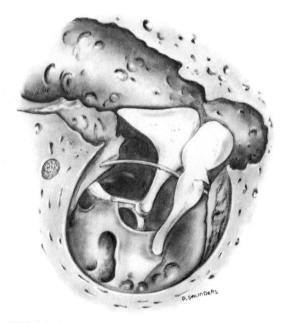

**FIG 34–9.**
Lateral view of the right middle ear after the drumhead has been removed. The chorda tympani nerve passes behind the malleus but in front of the long crus of the incus. The stapedial tendon joins the neck of the stapes.

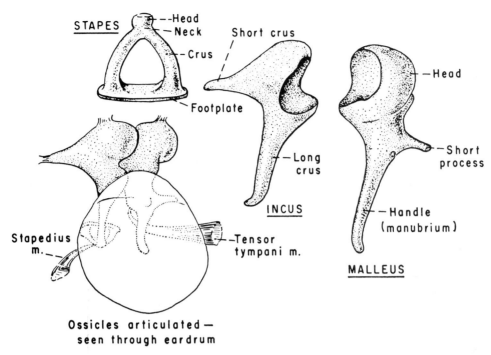

**FIG 34–10**.
Ossicles of the middle ear—separate and articulated. The drawing of the articulated ossicles is of a right ear.

has two crura, one long and one short. The short crus is directed backward, resting on the posterior bony wall, and acts as a fulcrum on which the incus rotates. At the end of the long crus is a short articular facet called the lenticular process connecting to the stapes. The stapes has a head, neck, anterior and posterior crura, and a footplate. The footplate closing the oval window has a surrounding anular ligament allowing mobility of the stapes. Two muscles attach to the ossicular chain. One, called the tensor tympani, originates from the bony canal above the eustachian tube and emerges as a tendon near the neck of the malleus. This tendon turns sharply around the processus cochleariformis to attach to the neck of the malleus. This muscle is supplied by a branch of the fifth nerve. Its action is to tense the tympanic membrane by pulling the handle of the malleus inward and stiffening it. The second muscle, the stapedius, is the smallest muscle in the body and arises from the bony pyramid in the posterior wall of the middle ear. It attaches to the neck of the stapes and is supplied by a branch of the seventh nerve. Its action is to tilt the stapes posteriorly and affix it in the oval window. It is believed to protect the internal ear from sudden loud sounds by

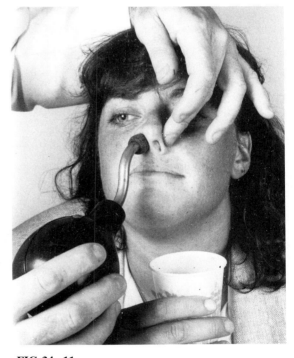

**FIG 34–11.**
Politzerization. With the use of the Politzer bag, air is forced up into the nose and eustachian tube as the patient swallows (which closes the palate).

preventing abnormal excursion at the footplate.

The eustachian tube (pharyngotympanic tube) connects the middle ear to the lateral wall of the nasopharynx just above the plane of the floor of the nose. It is lined with respiratory mucous membrane. The cartilaginous or medial portion of the eustachian tube closest to the nasopharynx is about 24 mm long. The osseous portion extending

from the middle ear is approximately 12 mm long. The diameter is greatest at the nasopharyngeal end, narrowing to an isthmus at the junction of the cartilaginous and bony portions. The function of the eustachian tube is to provide a passage from the nasopharynx to the ear, equalizing the pressure on both sides of the eardrum. If the pressure of the external ear canal is greater than that

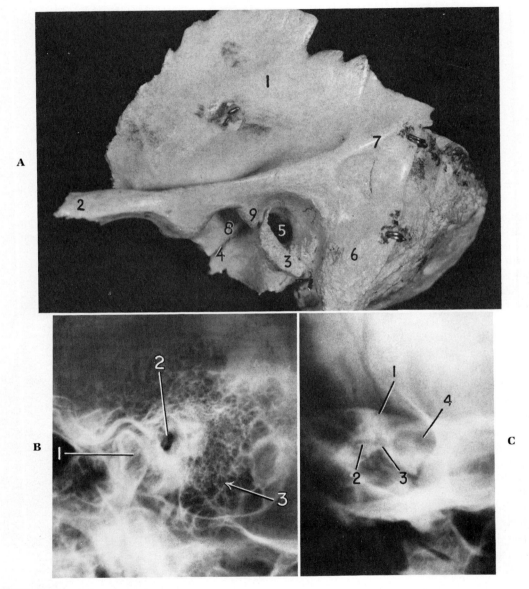

**FIG 34–12.**
**A,** left temporal bone, lateral view. *1,* squamous portion. *2,* zygomatic portion. *3,* tympanic portion. *4,* petrotympanic fissure. *5,* external auditory meatus. *6,* mastoid portion. *7,* linea temporalis. *8,* temporomandibular joint. *9,* articular tubercle. **B,** x-ray film of the left temporal bone, Law position. *1,* mandibular condyle. *2,* external auditory canal. *3,* mastoid cells in the body and tip. **C,** x-ray film of the right temporal bone, Stenver's position. *1,* superior semicircular canal. *2,* horizontal semicircular canal. *3,* vestibule. *4,* internal auditory meatus.

in the middle ear, the eardrum is displaced inward. If the pressure in the middle ear is greater than that of the external canal, the eardrum bulges outward.

The eustachian tube, which is normally closed, is opened by action of the tensor and levator muscles of the palate. It may open briefly for 0.1 to 0.2 second during swallowing, but this is intermittent. Obstruction of the eustachian tube caused by edema and inflammation is a major factor in the development of otitis media and serous otitis. When the eustachian tube is completely obstructed, the purulent matter in the middle ear tends to rupture through the drumhead, rather than drain into the nasopharynx. The eustachian tube can be opened forcefully by increasing air pressure in the nasopharynx. One common way to increase air pressure in the nasopharynx is to attempt to blow air against the resistance of the closed mouth and nose. However, many people are unable to do so. Another method is to occlude one side of the nose and force air into the other nostril as the patient swallows, with swallowing having closed the palate (Fig. 34–11).

The temporal bone is formed by the fusion of several distinct developmental segments of bone (squamous, mastoid, petrous, tympanic portions, and styloid process). The squamous portion is thin bone lying above the temporal line—an important surgical landmark superior to the external auditory canal. The root of the zygoma extends anteriorly from the squamous portion of the temporal bone and forms the articular process of the temporomandibular joint (Fig. 34–12). The mastoid process of the temporal bone provides an attachment for the sternocleidomastoid and digastric muscles. The cortex of the bone covers the honeycomb of interconnecting air cells. The thin mucous membrane of each cell is continuous with that of the middle ear. Mastoid cells are separated from the dura of the temporal lobe and the cerebellum by a thin cortical sheet of bone. During the first few years of life, the diploic bone is gradually replaced by air cells that develop from the mastoid antrum. The mastoid antrum is the largest mastoid air cell and connects directly to the middle ear through a narrowing called the aditus. In the well-pneumatized temporal bone, tracts of air cells extend deep behind the inner ear, deep to the middle ear, and into the petrous portion of the temporal bone, which houses the internal ear. Cells may often extend far anteriorly into the root of the zygoma.

The mastoid is adjacent to the following important intracranial structures: (1) superiorly, the dura of the temporal lobe, (2) posteriorly, the cerebellar dura, the sigmoid sinus (a continuation downward of the lateral venous sinus), (3) inferi-

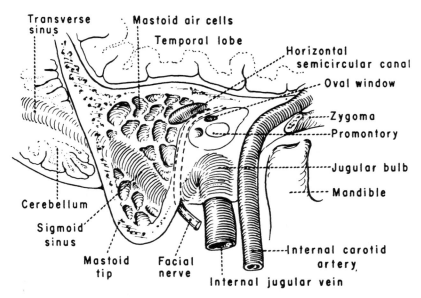

**FIG 34–13.**
Composite drawing of the right ear, showing the relationship between the middle ear, the mastoid, and surrounding structures.

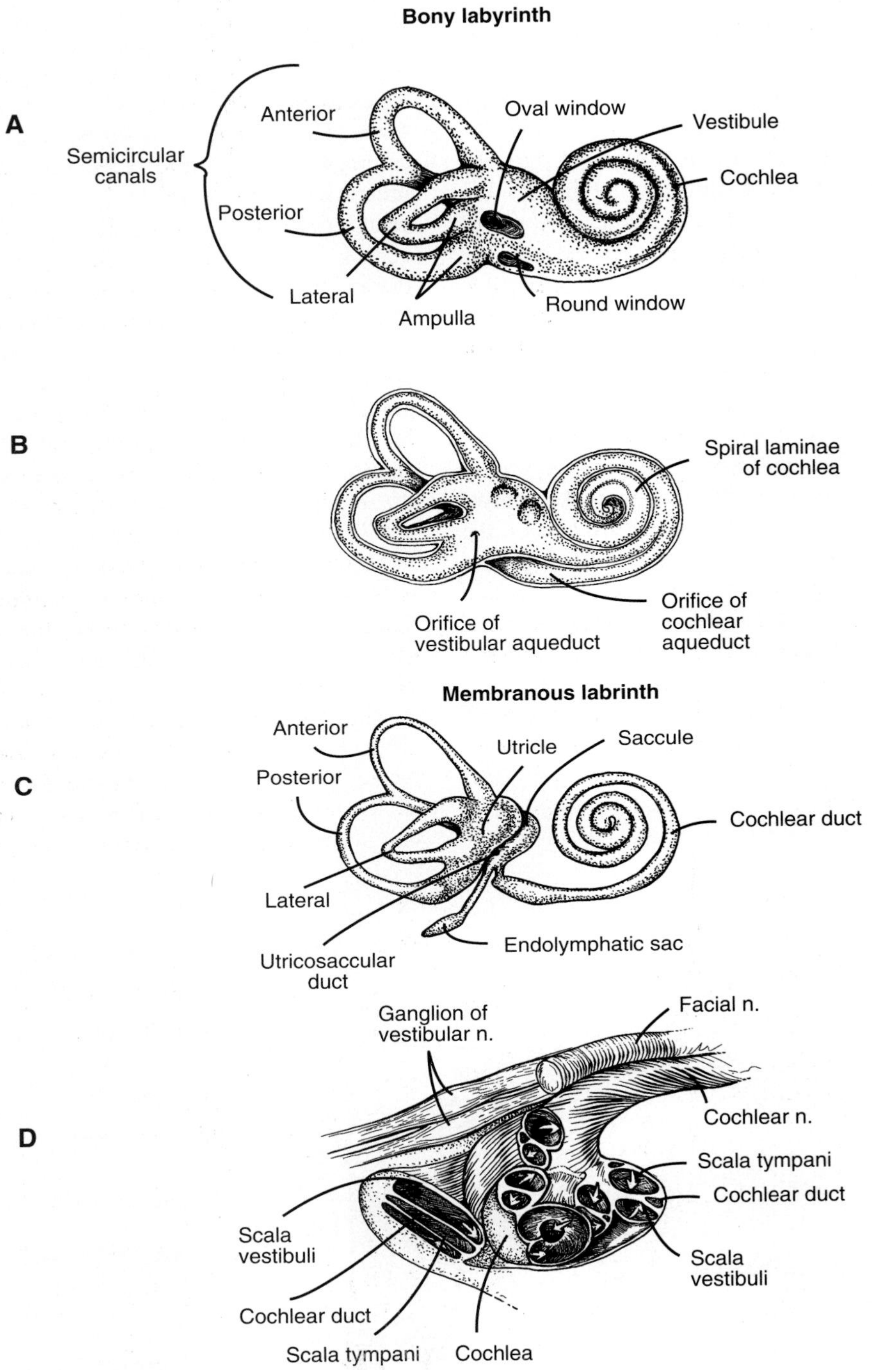

**Bony labyrinth**

**A**

Semicircular
canals

Anterior

Oval window

Vestibule

Posterior

Cochlea

Lateral

Ampulla

Round window

**B**

Spiral laminae
of cochlea

Orifice of
vestibular aqueduct

Orifice of
cochlear
aqueduct

**Membranous labrinth**

**C**

Anterior

Utricle

Saccule

Posterior

Cochlear duct

Lateral

Utricosaccular
duct

Endolymphatic sac

**D**

Ganglion of
vestibular n.

Facial n.

Cochlear n.

Scala tympani

Cochlear duct

Scala
vestibuli

Scala
vestibuli

Cochlear duct

Scala tympani

Cochlea

**FIG 34–14.**
**A** and **B,** bony labyrinth. **C,** membranous labyrinth. **D,** cochlea opened up, with its relationship to the seventh and eighth cranial nerves shown. (From Jacob SW, Francone CA: *Structure and function in man,* ed 5, Philadelphia, 1982, WB Saunders. Used by permission.)

orly, the jugular bulb, and (4) anteriorly, the internal carotid artery passing upward into the cranial cavity medial to the eustachian tube (Fig. 34–13).

The blood supply of the middle ear and mastoid is from branches of the internal maxillary artery, a branch of the external carotid system. The nerve supply of the middle ear and mastoid is from branches of the fifth, seventh, ninth, and tenth cranial nerves. Branches of these nerves form the tympanic plexus on the promontory in the middle ear. The small fibers lie in grooves in the bone of the promontory just beneath the mucosa of the middle ear. The disturbances of other anatomic regions supplied by these nerves (cranial nerves V, VII, IX, X), such as teeth, tongue, tonsils, and larynx, may cause pain to be referred to the ear. The referred pain (in contrast to ear pain, which is usually of a dull, aching variety) is sharp and shooting. The petrous portion of the temporal bone fits into the base of the skull beneath the sphenoid anteriorly and the occipital bones and separates the middle cranial fossa from the posterior cranial fossa. The petrous portion of the mastoid houses the end organs of the auditory and vestibular systems. On its posterior surface is found the internal auditory meatus, which transmits the seventh and eighth cranial nerves.

## Inner Ear

The inner ear is composed of the end organ receptors for hearing (the cochlea) and equilibrium (the labyrinth). Both are contained in the petrous portion of the temporal bone (Fig. 34–14). The bony capsule that surrounds these organs is the most compact bone in the body. These structures are protected from mechanical damage to a greater degree than almost any body structure, for in addition to the hard bone that surrounds the cochlea and labyrinth (called the otic capsule), the membranous end organs are surrounded by fluid, called perilymph. This fluid acts as a cushion against abrupt movements of the head. The membranous cochlear labyrinth literally floats in this fluid. The membranous end organ contains endolymph, a fluid high in $K^+$ content in relation to the surrounding perilymph. Endolymph is thought to be produced by the stria vascularis in the endolymphatic duct. Electrolyte changes within the endolymph are caused by osmotic transfer across the permeable membrane between the endolymph and perilymph. Perilymphatic fluid surrounding the membranous inner ear is continuous with the subarachnoid space through the cochlear aqueduct, a small canal through bone that provides direct exchange of fluid with the spinal fluid. Be-

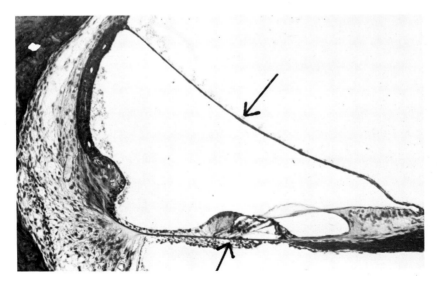

**FIG 34–15.**
High-power view of a cross section of the cochlea (monkey). The *upper arrow* indicates the membrane between the cochlear duct and the scala vestibuli (Reissner's membrane). The *lower arrow* indicates the organ of Corti, resting on the basilar membrane. (From Bredburg G, Ades W, Engstrom H: *Acta Otolaryngol* 301:1, 1972. Used by permission.)

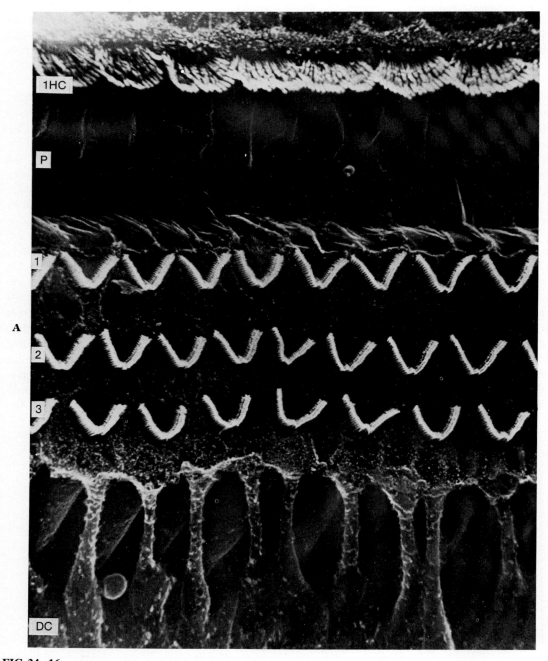

**FIG 34–16**.

**A,** scanning electron micrograph of upper surface of organ of Corti with tectorial membrane removed. Modiolus is toward top of picture. Three rows of outer hair cells *(1, 2, 3)* with their characteristic V- or W-arranged stereocilia and single row of inner hair cells *(IHC)* with slightly curved rows of stereocilia can be seen. Inner and outer hair cells are separated by heads of pillar cells *(P)*. Phalangeal processes of third row of Deiters' cells *(DC)* can be seen by virtue of fact that Hensen's cells have been removed. (Courtesy Dr Merle Lawrence, Ann Arbor, Mich).

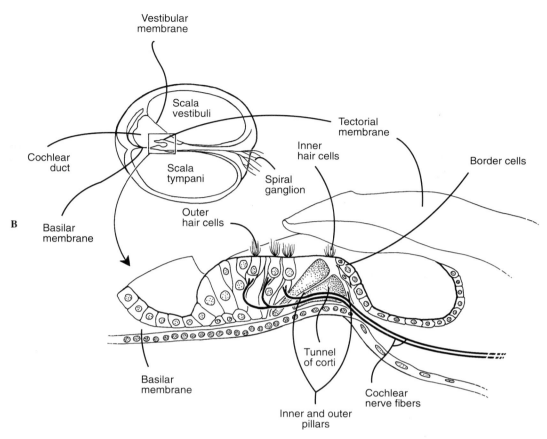

Vestibular
membrane

Scala
vestibuli

Tectorial
membrane

Inner
hair cells

Border cells

Cochlear
duct

Scala
tympani

Spiral
ganglion

**B**

Basilar
membrane

Outer
hair cells

Basilar
membrane

Tunnel
of corti

Cochlear
nerve fibers

Inner and outer
pillars

**FIG 34–16, cont'd**.
**B,** cross section of the cochlea. The organ of Corti is shown in detail.

cause of the lack of barriers between the cochlea and the labyrinth, injury or disease frequently affects both hearing and equilibrium.

### Cochlea

The cochlea is coiled upon itself like a snail shell and makes two and a half turns. It lies in a horizontal plane. The basal end (the largest in diameter) is the medial wall of the middle ear corresponding to the promontory. There are three compartments within the cochlea: two of these, the scala vestibuli and the scala tympani, are associated with the oval and round windows and contain perilymph. The third, the cochlear duct, contains endolymph. The membranous wall upon which rests the delicate end organs of hearing is called the basilar membrane (Figs. 34–15 and 34–16). The membranous cochlear duct connects with the saccule located in the vestibular labyrinth.

The neural end organ for hearing, the organ of Corti, rests on the basilar membrane. The organ of Corti extends along the entire length of the cochlea, except for the helicotrema, where the scala tympani and the scala vestibuli join. Approximately 30,000 hair cells project from the neuroepithelium. When these cells are bent or distorted, sound, which has a mechanical force, is converted into electrochemical impulse. In the temporal lobe cortex, this electrical impulse is interpreted as understandable sound. By selective destruction of various areas of the cochlea in experimental animals, the cochlea has been mapped (Fig. 34–17). Thus, it is known that the high-pitched sounds stimulate the basal portion of the cochlea and low-pitched sounds stimulate the apical end. The area of the cochlea closest to the middle ear, the promontory, is stimulated by sound in the frequencies between 3,000 and 5,000 Hz, which explains why the most noise damage occurs at 4,000 Hz. The cochlea's blood supply is from the branch of the basilar artery,

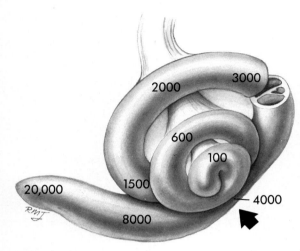

**FIG 34–17.**
Scheme showing sound localization in the cochlea. The arrow demonstrates the region of the promontory.

which is one of the terminal branches of the internal auditory artery. The internal auditory artery is an end artery, and as such, there is no collateral circulation.

The nerve impulses stimulated by movement of cochlear hair cells travel through ganglion cells, the axons that form the cochlear portion of the eighth cranial nerve. The eighth nerve leaves the posterior surface of the petrous portion of the temporal bone through the internal auditory meatus and enters the pons. From the pons, the neural stimulation passes to the superior and transverse gyrus of the temporal lobe.

### Vestibular Labyrinth

The vestibular portion of the inner ear is composed of the utricle, saccule, and three semicircular canals. Each semicircular canal is an osseous tube containing perilymph, which in turn surrounds the membranous tube carrying endolymph. The ends of each semicircular canal open into the utricle. The three semicircular canals are known as the horizontal, the superior, and the posterior semicircular canals. They are situated so that the horizontal canals on each side are in the same plane, whereas the superior canal of one side is in the same plane as the posterior canal of the opposite side. When the head is held erect, the horizontal canal is approximately 30 degrees off horizontal (Fig. 34–18). Thus the head must be inclined 30 degrees forward to bring this canal parallel to the floor. The membranous portion of the

semicircular canal is approximately a quarter of the size of the bony canal and is supported in the perilymph by minute fibrous strands (Fig. 34–19). In this way, the functioning membranous labyrinth is protected from blows or rapid movement by the perilymphatic fluid. Near the opening into the utricle, each semicircular canal, which forms approximately two thirds of a circle, is enlarged. This enlargement, known as the ampulla, contains a transverse elevation. Projecting into the ampulla is the crista, which is a projection of hair cells embedded into a thick ridge of gelatinous material called the cupula (Fig. 34–20). This projects into the ampulla like a dam and affects the flow of endolymphatic fluid.

The utricle and saccule themselves contain

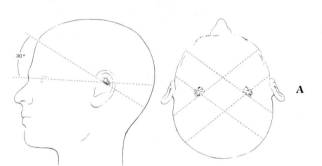

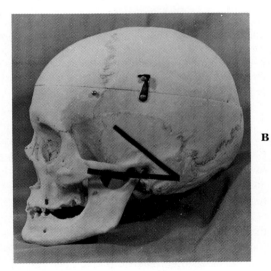

**FIG 34–18.**
**A,** relationship of the semicircular canals to the plane of the erect head and to each other. **B,** tape superimposed on skull shows the 30-degree angle between the normal erect position and the anatomic plane of the horizontal semicircular canal. The head is tipped 30 degrees down to bring the horizontal canal into a truly horizontal position.

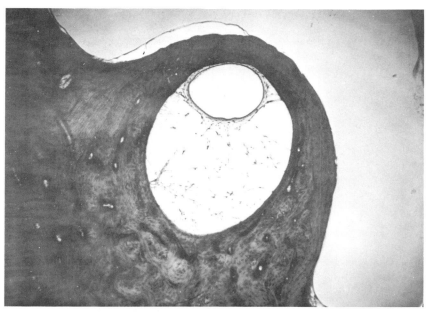

**FIG 34–19**.
Microscopic view of a cross section of the horizontal semicircular canal (monkey). Note the size of the clear endolymphatic (membranous) canal and the fine supporting stroma in the perilymphatic space. (Courtesy Dr Merle Lawrence, Ann Arbor, Mich. Used by permission.)

sensory epithelium called the macula, a broadly based mass of hair cells attached to the wall of the membranous duct. Lying on these hair cells are small granules of calcium carbonate known as otoconia, which are believed to initiate static responses owing to the effect of gravity (Fig. 34–21). Because the utricle is affected by static equilibrium, stimulation of the utricle produces compensatory eye positions, head-righting reflex, and alterations in muscle tone.

The semicircular canals are stimulated by rotation or acceleration in any direction, with inertia

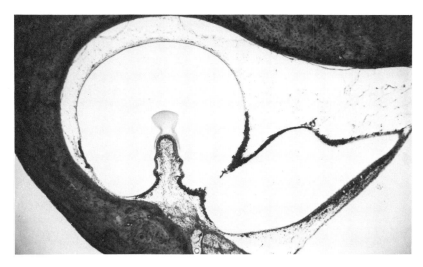

**FIG 34–20**.
Ampullated end of a semicircular canal, where it joins the utricle (guinea pig). The brushlike structure projecting into the ampulla is the crista. (Courtesy Dr Merle Lawrence, Ann Arbor, Mich.)

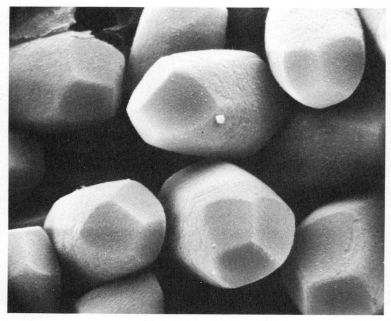

**FIG 34–21.**
Scanning electron microscope photograph shows otoconia (squirrel monkey) magnified 5,000 times. Crystals are calcium carbonate in calcite form. (Courtesy Dr David Lim, Columbus, Ohio.)

being the primary stimulus. The right and left canals always function together, except during artificial stimulation. The function of the saccule is not clearly known. The axons from the utricle and semicircular canals join to form a vestibular portion of the eighth cranial nerve, and upon reaching the brainstem, the cochlear and vestibular portions of the eighth nerve divide and terminate in their respective nuclei. Vestibular axons terminate in the medial, lateral, superior, and descending vestibular nuclei and the brainstem (Fig. 34–22). These nuclei lie on the floor of the fourth ventricle and are separated from the cochlear nuclei by the inferior cerebellar peduncle. The vestibular nuclei have connections with nuclei of the third, fourth, and sixth cranial nerves through the me-dial longitudinal bundle and with the ventral motor gray cells of the spinal cord through the vestibular spinal tract. Fibers also connect to the cerebellar cortex through the inferior cerebellar peduncle. Because the dorsal motor nucleus of the tenth nerve lies in close approximation to the vestibular nuclei in the brainstem, the vagal symptoms of nausea, vomiting, and pallor that accompany severe vestibular irritation (vertigo) suggest interconnection. The saccule, utricle, and semicircular canals receive their blood supplies from the vestibular artery, which is a terminal branch of the basilar artery.

---

**FIG 34–22.**                                                                 →
Pathways and projection areas related to vestibular system. **A,** afferent and efferent pathways, which are associated with vestibuloocular reflex, are indicated for vestibular nuclei. **B,** afferent and efferent pathways, associated with vestibulospinal reflexes, are indicated for vestibular nuclei. Vestibular connections to cerebral cortex and thalamus (ventral posterolateral and ventral posteromedial nuclei) are not shown, since pathways have not yet been clearly demonstrated. In mesencephalic nuclei: nucleus of Darkshevich and interstitial nucleus of Cajal. In motor nuclei of extraocular muscles: oculomotor nuclei including oculomotor nucleus, trochlear nucleus, and abducens nucleus. In cerebellar structures: fastigial nucleus, uvula, nodulus, and flocculus. *RF,* reticular formation. Pathways: *MLF,* medial longitudinal fasciculus: *LVST,* lateral vestibulospinal tract; *MVST,* medial vestibulospinal tract. Motoneurons: α, alpha; γ, gamma. *Arrows* in figure indicate directions of probable neural information flow.

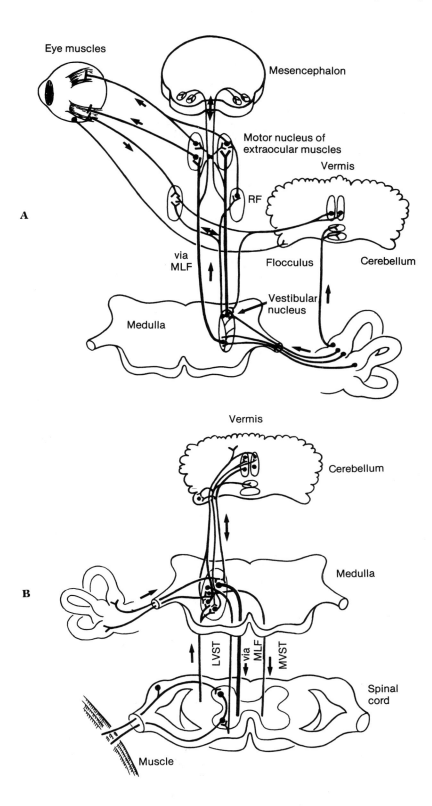

# PHYSIOLOGY OF HEARING

Before the physiology of hearing is discussed, the decibel (db), a measurement commonly used in describing hearing loss, must be mentioned. The decibel system is a logarithmic scale, because the range of human sensitivity is so great that it requires such a method. An infinitesimal movement of the hair cells in the inner ear is enough to cause faint hearing, yet a trillionfold increase in energy-producing sound pressure is still tolerable to the ear. Such an enormous increase in sound pressure is expressed as 120 db loudness. For practical purposes, the decibel system, as it is used, is shown in Table 34–1. The intensity of sound produced in various situations is shown in Table 34–2. It is important to understand that the decibel is a ratio and not an absolute value. The decibel compares the relationship between two sound intensities. Thus if we say that one sound is so many decibels, we mean that it is more intense than the reference level by that much. When hearing is tested with the audiometer and the setting is changed from a reading of 0 db to a reading of 60 db, there is an energy increase of one million times. Even so, the sound increment of 60 db above threshold is not excessively loud to the individual. Roughly, it represents the sound pressure level exerted by a moderately loud voice several feet from the ear. Percentage description of hearing loss is unsatisfactory because the pure tone signals used in audiometric tests are not all of equal importance in speech or in other common environments. Similarly, the normal ear is not equally sensitive to low and high sounds. For instance, it requires significantly more intensity to hear a 250 Hz sound than a 1,000 Hz tone, since the ear is more sensitive to the higher frequency.

Because it is desirable to have the faintest perceptible sound calibrated at 0 db, the audiometer is designed to compensate for differences in hearing sensitivity as a function of frequency. After this compensation is made, the readings may then

**TABLE 34–1.**

Relation of Decibels to Energy

| | |
|---|---|
| 10 decibels | 10 × increase in power |
| 20 decibels | 100 × increase in power |
| 30 decibels | 1,000 × increase in power |
| 60 decibels | 1,000,000 × increase in power |
| 120 decibels | 1 trillion × increase in power |

**TABLE 34–2.**

Intensity of Sound in Different Situations (Approximate)

| Decibels | Situation |
|---|---|
| 140 | Air raid siren |
| | Jet engine (pain felt in ear) |
| 130 | Tickle (sensation) |
| | Aircraft engine (close) |
| 120 | Loud shot (1 foot) |
| | Thunder |
| 110 | |
| | Aircraft engine |
| 100 | Boiler shop |
| | Discomfort for pure tones |
| | Riveting machine |
| 90 | |
| | Train |
| | Air hammer (pneumatic) |
| 80 | |
| | Heavy traffic |
| 70 | |
| | Truck (outside) |
| 60 | Average street traffic |
| 50 | Ordinary spoken voice |
| | Vacuum cleaner |
| | Automobile |
| 40 | |
| | Average office |
| 30 | Quiet room |
| | Usual home |
| 20 | Soft whisper |
| | Rural area |
| 10 | |
| 0 | Threshold of hearing |

be plotted on the chart to make an audiogram, with 0 db level reflecting the faintest sound heard.

## External Ear and Hearing

The external ear consists of the auricle and the external auditory canal. In humans, the auricle does little to increase the sensitivity of hearing. Its occasional absence in congenital or traumatic conditions is not associated with appreciable loss of hearing. On the other hand, occlusion of the external auditory meatus affects hearing seriously. Provided that the good ear is turned toward the sound source, monaural hearing is only slightly less acute than binaural hearing, but if the head is turned, hearing may be reduced by as much as 20 db in some frequencies. A more serious handicap of unilateral deafness is the patient's inability to localize the sound source. Normal individuals can determine the direction of sound because sound waves reach the two ears at slightly different times and intensities.

If the auditory canal of a person with normal hearing is occluded tightly, the resultant hearing loss is generally no greater than 40 db. This loss still permits the patient to hear a low or moderately loud voice. Earplugs and earmuffs generally protect the ear from excessive noise. The attenuation provided by these devices, however, is only partial. Uncomfortable and harmful noise can still affect the ear in some situations if the sound is loud enough. Generally, the attenuation of sound by earplugs or earmuffs is less than 30 db.

## Tympanic Membrane and Hearing

The tympanic membrane separates the external auditory meatus from the middle ear. Sound waves that strike the drumhead are partially reflected back into the ear canal and partially transmitted across the tympanic membrane. Of the transmitted waves, two routes are possible. In one, the sound enters the oval window via the chain of ossicles, and in the other, sound waves cross the tympanic membrane directly and enter the round window. In a patient with normal hearing, sound waves entering the oval window contribute a great deal more to hearing than that sound reaching the cochlea by aerial transmission across the tympanic cavity to the round window (Fig. 34–23). Interruption of the ossicle chain,

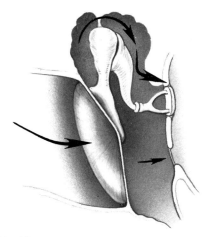

**FIG 34–23.**
Sound waves passing the ossicular chain are more effective than sound waves that enter the middle ear to the round window.

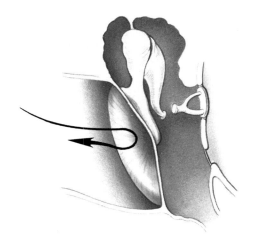

**FIG 34–24.**
Dislocation of the incus from the stapes. A 60 db hearing loss results because (1) sound waves are largely reflected and absorbed by the eardrum and ossicles and (2) sound waves that do cross the middle ear enter both windows almost simultaneously creating a cancellation effect.

for example, such as dislocation of the incus from the stapes, reduces hearing about 60 db (Fig. 34–24). However, if the tympanic membrane is absent or partially removed, hearing is improved 15 to 30 db, because sound waves are now allowed to strike the oval and round windows directly.

Perforations of the tympanic membrane exert a variable effect on hearing, depending on size and location and whether they are associated with changes in the middle ear. Small perforations may cause an almost undetectable hearing loss, and generally, uncomplicated perforations of the tympanic membrane reduce hearing by 5 to 30 db. The hearing loss extends through the entire frequency range, although it may be greater in some frequencies than others. Perforations near the attachment of the malleus are more likely to cause significant hearing loss because they contribute to loss of effective action of the ossicular chain. The condition of the ossicles, particularly freedom of motion of the stapes and the oval window, is more important to hearing than is an intact tympanic membrane. Patients with tympanic perforations and a hearing loss greater than 30 db generally have additional disturbances in the conduction mechanism of the middle ear. Examples are ossicular destruction or dislocation, stapedial fixation, and middle ear adhesions.

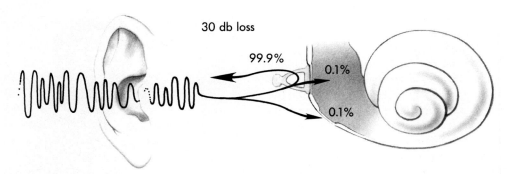

**FIG 34–25.**
Loss of energy occurring at air to liquid interface.

## Middle Ear and Hearing

The transfer of sound pressure from a gaseous medium (air) to liquid medium (endolymphatic fluid) results in a tremendous loss of energy (Fig. 34–25). In an analogy, Weaver and Lawrence point out that fishermen may talk in their boats without much likelihood of disturbing the fish, the reason being that 99.9% of sound energy is reflected from the surface of the lake back into the air, and only 0.1% enters the water. On the other hand, fishermen should be very careful not to stamp the floor of the boat or splash the water with their hands. This example illustrates clearly the task of the ear. It must transfer energy from a gaseous to a liquid medium without incurring serious loss of hearing en route. The loss of 99.9% of energy is expressed as a 30 db loss, about the level at which a person begins to complain of a hearing problem.

To help overcome this loss of energy, the middle ear acts as a mechanical transformer, and there are two devices built into the middle ear that help restore most of the sound pressure lost in the transfer.

### Lever System

Because the handle of the malleus is somewhat longer than the long process of the incus, the ear gains a small mechanical advantage. The gain is minimal, however, and restores only 3 db of the 30 db loss caused when sound pressure in the ear is transferred to a liquid media. Because of this small degree of difference, in otologic procedures the tympanic membrane can be repositioned directly on the stapes or on a straight columella to the stapes, with minimal loss of hearing.

### Hydraulic Ratio

Far more important than the lever action is the ratio between the area of the large tympanic membrane and the tiny footplate of the stapes (Fig. 34–26). This ratio, although given somewhat different values by different observers, is approximately 15:1. This ratio corresponds to approximately 23 to 25 db. Thus the transformer mechanism of the middle ear recovers about 25 to 27 of the 30 db loss when sound waves pass from air to liquid.

### Middle Ear Muscles

The stapedius muscle, supplied by the seventh nerve, and the tensor tympani muscle, supplied by the fifth nerve, have nothing to do with acuity of hearing but are protective mechanisms and react reflexively when there is a loud sound. The stapedius muscle inhibits action of the stapedial footplate, and the tensor tympani diminishes excursions of the manubrium. Sudden, sharp sounds (for example, gunshots) are too fast for the latent period of either muscle and enter the cochlea unchanged. Prolonged sounds may be diminished up to 10 db through attenuation, protecting the inner ear against intense sounds such as those over 100 db.

### Phase Relationships

In the person with normal hearing, the intact drumhead not only contributes to the very important hydraulic and lever ratio, but also shields sound from the round window. In doing so, it changes the phase relationship between the oval and round windows so that there is less likelihood of a sound wave canceling itself and entering both

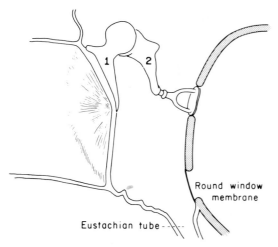

**FIG 34–26.**
Middle ear transformer system. Note that the handle of
the malleus *(1)* compared to the long crus of the incus
*(2)* adds an advantage of 1.3 to 1, allowing a gain in
sound energy of only 2.5 db. However, the areal ratio
of the tympanic membrane-footplate is much greater.
The effective ratio is 14:1 and corresponds to a 23 db
gain.

windows simultaneously. Loss of the ossicular
chain and most of the tympanic membrane may
result in an inordinate hearing loss because of the
cancellation effect—sound waves striking the stapedial footplate and the round window membrane
simultaneously and with equal intensity cause no

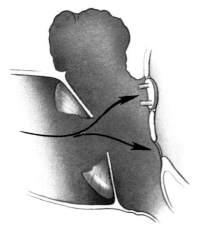

**FIG 34–27.**
Here the malleus, incus, and tympanic membrane are
destroyed—the middle ear has lost its transformer action. Additional hearing loss is caused by exposure of
both windows to approximately equal sound pressures.
Total loss is 45 to 55 db.

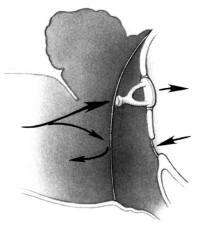

**FIG 34–28.**
Type III tympanoplasty. The negligible lever action is
lost, but the important areal ratio is restored, and there
is sound protection for the round window. There is a
free tissue graft on the stapes.

displacement of fluid. It is like placing equal pressure on two ends of an open U-shaped tube filled
with water (Fig. 34–27). In practice, when sound
waves can enter both windows, total deafness
never results, but the hearing loss may be significantly worsened. Conversely, it is possible to improve hearing in many patients without an eardrum by occluding the round window with some
substance to reflect sound waves partially. Alternatively, in an operation known as tympanoplasty, a tissue graft laid across the middle ear so
as to touch the stapes but leave an air pocket
about the round window can improve hearing.
The reason is that the sound waves are transmitted through the graft directly to the stapes and the
oval window, whereas sound waves striking the
part of the graft covering but not touching the
round window are reflected back. This sound protection of the round window is one of the two basic principles applied to restoring hearing through
tympanoplasty (Fig. 34–28).

### Sound in the Cochlea

Under normal conditions, the most effective
sound waves are those transmitted across the
drumhead and chain of ossicles to the oval window. The footplate of the stapes closing the oval
window is held in position by an anular ligament
that allows the stapes to vibrate according to the
frequency and intensity of the sound wave. Any

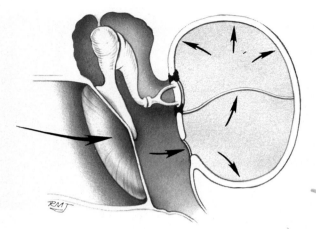

**FIG 34–29**.
Footplate otosclerosis. Very little sound can enter the cochlea. With only one window open, any sound energy from the round window is weak and spreads throughout the cochlea uniformly, so that the basilar membrane is not appreciably displaced.

disorder that affects the movement of the stapes's footplate or limits its excursion (for example, otosclerosis) adversely affects hearing (Fig. 34–29).

As the footplate of the stapes rocks in the oval window, sound pressure is transmitted directly to the perilymph of the inner ear. The perilymph acts as a protective cushion for the fragile membranous labyrinth in the cochlear duct. As the sound pressure displaces the perilymph, it results in deformation of the basilar membrane, and a

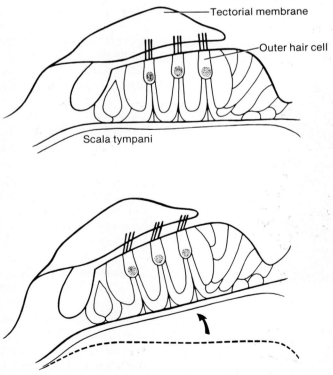

**FIG 34–30**.
Schematic drawing of radical shear of outer hair cell stereocilia resulting from displacement of cochlear partition.

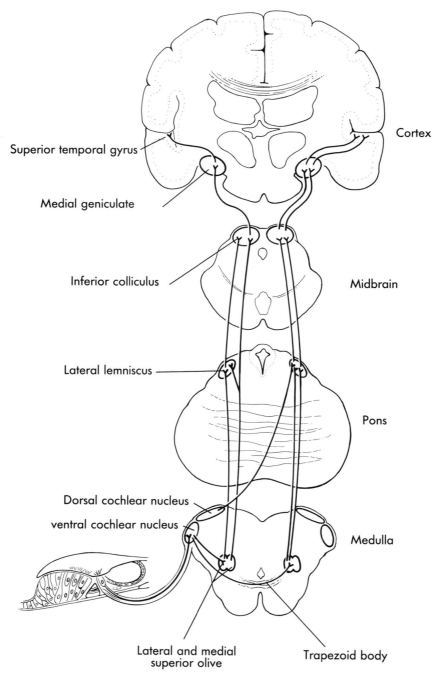

Cortex

Superior temporal gyrus

Medial geniculate

Inferior colliculus

Midbrain

Lateral lemniscus

Pons

Dorsal cochlear nucleus

ventral cochlear nucleus

Medulla

Lateral and medial
superior olive

Trapezoid body

**FIG 34–31.**
Central auditory pathways.

traveling wave is propagated from the base to the apex of the cochlea. Displacement of the basilar membrane causes movement of the organ of Corti and its hair cells, creating a shearing action between the cilia of the hair cells and the tectorial membrane, which overlies them (Fig. 34–30). This movement causes depolarization, which activates the cochlear nerve. Thus mechanical energy of the stapes's footplate motion is converted into an electrical impulse. Because the pressure wave must pass through the noncompressible liquid housed in the cochlea, there have to be compliant openings in both ends of the channel. In the person with normal hearing the round window serves chiefly as a relief outlet in the cochlea. The hair cells of the organ of Corti are susceptible to injury by oxygen deprivation, drug toxicity, and mechanical injury (usually in the form of noise and other types of trauma). There are approximately 30,000 hair cells in the human ear.

In summary, if we are to hear, hair cells must be stimulated by physical distortion and displacement. From the cochlea, the fibers of the eighth cranial nerve pass into the auditory nerve and terminate on the cells of dorsal and ventral cochlear nuclei. From there, projections eventually reach the auditory cortex, which lies in the posterior portion of the superior temporal gyrus in the sylvian fissure called Heschl's gyrus (Fig. 34–31). There are multiple synaptic pathways along the primary neural path from the cochlear nerve, and the neural input of each ear is bilaterally represented.

## Vestibular Physiology

The vestibular system is one of the triad of modalities that allows humans to maintain balance, maintain orientation in space, and respond to movement. The semicircular canals respond to angular acceleration and deceleration. Because the six semicircular canals are basically arranged in three pairs—one on each side—any rotational plane results in movement of endolymph at the ampullated ends of the semicircular canals toward the ampulla in one ear and away from the ampulla in the other. This results in deflection of the hair cells of the ampulla of the semicircular canals, which activates the vestibular nerve and its two central connections, the medial longitudinal fasciculus to the ocular system, and the vestibulospinal tracts to the lower motor neurons of the trunk and extremity. Thus in normal persons these reactions restore body position when a force of motion affects position. The semicircular canals respond to angular motion and rotation, while linear acceleration and gravity affect the macula of the utricle and saccule.

The macula of the utricle and saccule contain hair cells extending into a gelatinous mass filled with ovoid masses of calcium carbonate, called otoconia. Because the otoconia have greater density than the endolymph, they respond to changes in linear acceleration and deceleration as well as to the pull of gravity. The reactions to stimulation of the utricle or semicircular canals are nystagmus, past pointing, and falling. Other associated symptoms such as nausea, vomiting, and sweating accompany vestibular stimuli because the dorsomotor nucleus of the tenth cranial nerve is located adjacent to the vestibular nuclei in the brainstem.

Additional discussion regarding physiology of the labyrinth will be found in Chapter 43.

# 35

# Special Diagnostic Procedures in Testing for Hearing

Loss of hearing can be either partial or total. It can present in low, middle, or high frequencies or in any combination. Only when it is total or near total (more than 85 to 90 db below normal) do we speak of deafness. To say that a person with a 60 db loss of hearing is deaf leads to the erroneous assumption that nothing can be done to improve his or her hearing. Hearing loss implies a partial loss of function. Only the profoundly damaged ear is unable to respond to unamplified sound. For practical purposes, a person begins to be socially affected when hearing loss in both ears reaches or exceeds 30 db in the speech frequencies (300 to 3,000 cycles). A bilateral hearing loss of more than 30 db in these frequencies, if not medically or surgically correctable, indicates the need for amplification.

There are three types of hearing loss: sensorineural hearing loss, conductive hearing loss, and mixed hearing loss.

*Sensorineural* hearing loss (also referred to as perceptive or nerve-type hearing loss) results from disease within the cochlea, eighth cranial nerve, or brain. Causes may be infection, trauma, toxic substances, degenerative disease, or congenital abnormality. For example, purulent labyrinthitis may destroy the entire inner ear. Mumps, a common cause of severe unilateral deafness, may destroy only the hair cells of the cochlea. Intense noise destroys cochlear hair cells, and skull fracture may sever the eighth cranial nerve or injure the organ of Corti. Aminoglycosides and other drugs will cause deafness as a result of hair cell damage. Hearing loss of aging (presbycusis) may result from senile degenerative changes or loss of

central nerve pathways. Congenital nerve deafness may result from hereditary factors or intrauterine disease, for example, rubella in the pregnant woman. Multiple causes of injury to the organ of Corti produce a hair cell loss that often differs from both conductive hearing loss and hearing loss caused by nerve fiber or brain disease. To distinguish between hearing loss resulting from cochlear damage and hearing loss resulting from nerve fiber or central disease, clinicians use special audiologic examinations, which will be described.

*Conductive hearing loss,* by contrast, occurs in patients with external or middle ear disorders such as otitis media, otosclerosis, and perforated eardrum. Patients with only a conductive loss have a normal inner ear and are hard of hearing because there is a defect in the mechanism by which sound is conducted to the inner ear. Such persons can hear perfectly if the sound is amplified sufficiently; thus they can use hearing aids quite satisfactorily. By the same token, however, the hearing loss is amenable to surgical correction. Patients with sensorineural hearing loss often have more difficulty with hearing aids, although they are the more common user by far of amplification devices. In contrasting sensorineural hearing loss with conductive loss, it is worthwhile to note that disorders producing sensorineural hearing loss do not cause changes in the appearance of the tympanic membrane. On the other hand, disorders producing conductive loss, with the exception of otosclerosis and ossicle fixation, almost always cause alterations in the normal appearance of the drumhead. A mixed hearing loss involves both a conductive mechanism and the neural components.

Hearing tests commonly include the whispered or spoken voice, tuning forks, and audiometry. The best quantitative determinations are obviously made with the electrically calibrated audiometer.

## WHISPERED AND SPOKEN VOICE

The examiner who uses his or her voice to assess the patient's hearing must have had enough experience to know how well his or her own voice is heard at different distances and how to vary the intensity of his or her voice so that each patient tested is tested similarly. The intensity of sound produced by methods ranging from a soft whisper to conversational speech is listed in Table 35–1. The examiner stands 3 feet from the patient's ear and directs his or her voice toward the ear. Obviously, the whispered and spoken voice technique leaves much to be desired with regard to masking, as well as accuracy.

## TUNING FORK

Tuning fork tests for hearing acuity remain an important part of the otologic functional examination and should be common procedure in audiologic testing. The forks most useful for testing hearing are those with vibrating frequencies of 256, 512, and 1,024. The tuning fork should be stroked between the thumb and index finger or gently tapped on the knuckle. If the fork is struck too hard, overtones are produced as well as too intense a sound. Hearing tests, it must be remembered, are best performed near threshold. Because sound can be carried to a good ear when tuning forks are used for testing, masking may be necessary in the nontest ear. Two tuning fork tests, the Weber and the Rinne, are useful within certain

**TABLE 35–1.**
Relative Sound Levels at 3 Feet

| Sound | Gross Hearing Level |
|---|---|
| Faint whisper | 20 db |
| Soft whisper | 30 db |
| Loud whisper | 50 db |
| Conversational speech | 60 db |
| Shout | 80+ db |

limits in differentiating between conductive and sensorineural hearing losses and substantiating audiometric testing.

## Weber Test

In the Weber test, a tuning fork is placed on the maxillary incisors or in the midline of the skull (Fig. 35–1). The patient with conductive hearing loss hears the sound in the poor ear provided that he or she has normal hearing in the opposite ear. The reason is that ordinary room noise is always present in the usual testing situation and tends to mask the normal ear, but the ear with conductive loss, not hearing such ambient noise, has a better chance to hear the bone conduction sound. If there is sensorineural hearing loss in one ear and the opposite ear is normal, the fork is heard in the good ear. To illustrate, strike a tuning fork and place it on your skull in the midline. You will hear it in both ears. Now occlude one ear tightly with your finger; you will immediately

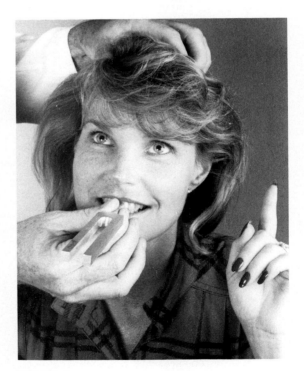

**FIG 35–1.**
Weber test. Patient indicates that sound is heard louder in the left ear. This may mean either conductive loss in the left ear or sensorineural loss in the right ear. One can hold the fork either over the maxillary teeth or forehead.

hear the sound of the fork in the plugged ear and it will be louder. You have not increased your hearing acuity, but you have limited some of the ever-present environmental sound from one ear, thus creating a temporary conductive hearing loss.

## Rinne Test

The Rinne test is performed by alternately placing a tuning fork opposite one external audi-

tory meatus and on the adjacent mastoid bone (Fig. 35–2). The normal ear hears the tuning fork twice as long by air conduction as by bone conduction. In a significant hearing loss, the air-bone relationship may be reversed so that sound of bone conduction may be heard relatively longer. A patient's Rinne test is said to be positive when he or she hears longer by air than by bone conduction and negative when the reverse is true (Table 35–2).

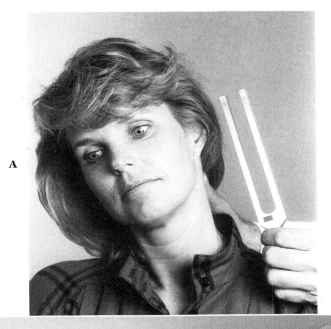

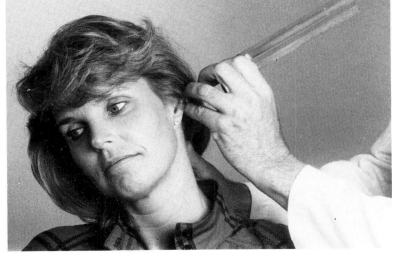

**FIG 35–2.**
Rinne test. **A,** air conduction; **B,** bone conduction.

**TABLE 35–2.**

Tuning Fork Tests for Normal Hearing, Conductive Hearing Loss, and Sensorineural Hearing Loss*

|  | Weber (bone only) | Rinne (air-bone) | Schwabach (bone only) |
|---|---|---|---|
| Normal | Not lateralized | Positive AC > BC | Equal |
| Conductive loss | Lateralized to poorer ear | Negative BC > or = AC | Patient hears longer than examiner |
| Perceptive loss | Lateralized to better ear | Positive AC > BC | Examiner hears longer than patient |

*AC, air conduction; BC, bone conduction.

## Schwabach Test

The third test, the Schwabach test, allows the examiner to compare his or her own hearing, if normal, by bone conduction with the patient's bone conduction by alternately placing the vibrating tuning fork on the patient's mastoid and the examiner's mastoid process.

## Special Considerations

The following points should be remembered in performing tuning fork tests:

1. The correct forks must be used, those with frequencies of 256, 512, and 1,024. A 256 fork is the most accurate in determining small degrees of conductive hearing loss, whereas the 512 and 1,024 forks require a greater air-bone discrepancy.
2. The forks must be applied to the proper region of the mastoid because not all parts of the mastoid are equally satisfactory for testing. Trial and error is often necessary in determining the best place to apply the fork.
3. Intermittent rather than continuous application of the forks to the bone is important.
4. The tines of the fork should be directed at the ear and not held obliquely because theoretically there would be no sound at all in this position. (For example, by holding the tuning fork to your own ear and rotating it slowly, you will note that the tone increases and diminishes in intensity depending on the position of the tines with respect to the external auditory meatus.)
5. Most inexperienced examiners strike the fork too loudly. The forks should be made to ring softly because the purpose of the test is not to determine how intense a sound the patient can tolerate, but rather at what point he or she can just hear.
6. Doubtful or conflicting results must be rechecked several times.
7. A sound-treated room is not required, but a quiet room is necessary.
8. Well-performed tuning fork tests are an important check on audiometric testing.

## AUDIOMETRY

### Pure-Tone Audiometry

Quantitative measurements of hearing are made by using a pure-tone audiometer. This device produces pure tones that can be varied according to frequency and intensity. Plotting the intensity against the frequency provides a chart such as is shown in Figure 35–3. In the audiogram demonstrated, it can be seen that there is a drop in hearing at higher frequencies and that normal hearing is preserved in the lower frequencies. Generally, in standard testing, seven frequencies from 250 cycles to 8,000 Hz are tested, first by presenting the tone loud enough for the patient to hear it distinctly and then by seeking the threshold level for frequency. Both air conduction and bone conduction measurements are recorded at threshold level.

The pure-tone audiometer is the basic instrument used in audiometry but holds many opportunities for error. The results should be checked by the tuning forks and ordinary whispered and spoken voice test. The zero reference level in the normal audiometer refers to the level obtained by testing normal human ears. Therefore, it is an average of the sound intensity that can just be de-

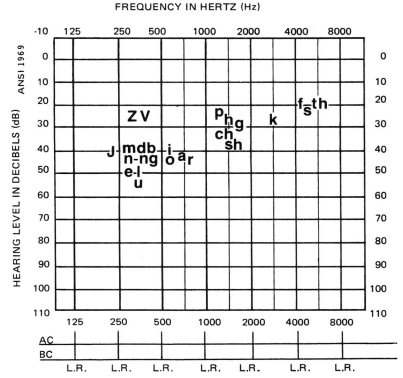

**FIG 35–3.**
This schematic audiogram demonstrated the preponderance of the vowels in the lower frequencies. Higher frequencies are dominated by the fricatives and high-pitched consonants. These higher-pitched sounds are also softer than the louder vowels. This accounts for losses of clarity and speech in high-frequency hearing loss. Note: actually the f, s, and th sounds are heard at 3,000 Hz rather than 4,000 to 6,000 Hz as shown.

tected by the average normal ear. When a person hears a given frequency at −10 db, it merely means he or she can hear that frequency better than the average person. Similarly, when the threshold of the ear is no more than 25 db above zero, the hearing is considered to be normal.

The most important range of hearing for speech is between the frequencies of 300 and 3,000 Hz. Testing is performed above and below these frequencies to thoroughly map the ability of the ear to receive sounds and to indicate minimal losses, particularly in high tones, of which the person is unaware. The optimal human ear can detect sounds from 20 to 20,000 Hz per second. The hearing in the human ear is actually most acute at about 1,000 Hz. Recent experiments with higher-frequency testing (12,000 to 18,000 Hz) are proving to be of value in early detection of cochlear damage resulting from drug toxicity. Such tests can indicate and dictate cessation of toxic drugs before significant cochlear damage oc-

curs. They may also provide early warning of damage to the eighth cranial nerve from acoustic trauma or neuroma.

### Masking

While one ear is being tested, the opposite ear must be excluded from the test. Failure to mask the good ear is a very common error and one that leads the examiner to think the patient is hearing the signal in the poorer ear that is being tested. When testing is done by air conduction, it is important to mask the better ear if the difference between the hearing level of the two ears is greater than 30 db. Masking is especially important in testing by bone conduction. The greater the discrepancy in hearing between the ears, the greater will be the need for masking in the good ear. A device used such as the Bárány noise box, placed in one ear to produce a loud noise, will effectively mask when one is testing with voice or tuning forks (Fig. 35–4). Audiometers are equipped

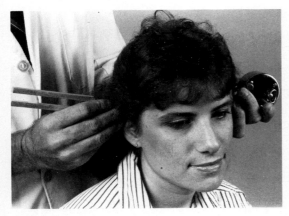

**FIG 35–4.**
Masking; the Bárány noise maker masks out all sound reaching the left ear, determining whether sound can be heard on the right.

with a masking sound that can be varied in intensity. Most important of all is simply remembering to mask. Masking seems obvious when vision is being tested (one eye is always shielded) but is very commonly disregarded when hearing is being tested.

## Speech Audiometry

Speech audiometry reproduces the spoken voice rather than pure tones. Tests include a *speech reception threshold* and *discrimination.* The *speech reception threshold* is the level at which the listener correctly repeats 50% of a specialized word list. The word list is one containing spondee (bisyllabic and equally stressed) words that are easily understood, such as *hothouse, toothbrush, horseshoe, airplane,* and *northwest.* *Discrimination* is determined by using a word list of phonetically balanced words (monosyllabic words such as *yard, cave, us, day, toe,* and *felt*). These words have been selected so as to approximate the distribution of speech sounds in ordinary conversation. Phonetically balanced words are presented at an intensity level of 40 db or more above the speech reception threshold or at a comfortable hearing level for the patient. A person with normal hearing correctly repeats 95% to 100% of these words, whereas the patient with a neurosensory or mixed hearing loss may have a much lower score. In some cases, no matter how loudly the phonetically balanced words are pre-

sented, patients may fail to understand them. In fact, in some individuals, if the intensity is increased beyond the range of comfortable loudness, the score may become worse. A person with a score less than 80% is said to have poor discrimination ability, which affects ability to understand speech.

In contrast to the patient with cochlear disease, patients with conductive hearing loss tend to score higher on this test because all that is required for them to hear well is amplification. The patient with poor discrimination ability may hear sound and realize someone is speaking but may not satisfactorily discriminate between similar words. Patients often remark, "I can hear you, but I can't understand you." Such patients have difficulty in group conversation or when listening against a background of noise. People with poor discrimination generally have a high-frequency hearing loss. They are unable to hear the high-pitched consonants and fricatives that clarify speech, though they may hear quite adequately the lower vowel sounds (Fig. 35–5). A hearing aid in such an individual may make the sound louder but may often fail to make it more intelligible, although recent developments in hearing aids are providing some improvement.

Pure-tone thresholds, speech-reception thresholds, and discrimination testing constitute the three most important audiologic tests. There are, however, several special auditory phenomena associated with hearing loss that can localize the site of pathologic conditions of the ear.

### Recruitment

*Recruitment* (defined as an abnormal increase in loudness) is exemplified by a patient who hears nothing until the sound level becomes great enough. Then a very slight increase in intensity causes the patient to find the loudness unpleasant. Often an individual with recruitment, particularly an older person, may not hear when first spoken to but, when spoken to sharply or loudly, states, "You don't have to shout at me, you know." Recruitment is a difficult problem in fitting hearing aids. These patients may have such a narrow range of tolerance between the intensity at which they are just able to hear and the intensity at which sound suddenly becomes too loud that any amplification is difficult.

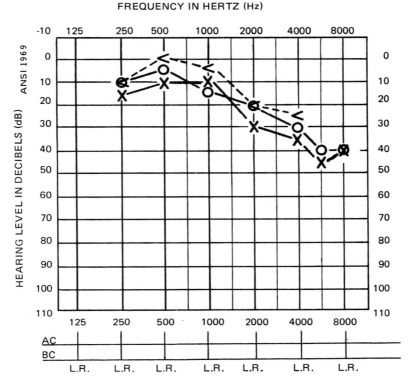

**FIG 35–5.**
Audiogram demonstrating high-frequency neurosensory hearing loss.

### *Diplacusis*

Diplacusis is a phenomenon manifested by patients with cochlear disease and (like recruitment) is produced by disorders involving the organ of Corti. With diplacusis the same sound appears to be different to the two ears. Patients with diplacusis generally may dislike music because sounds may seem discordant or instruments may seem out of tune.

## SPECIALIZED AUDIOLOGIC TESTS

Over the past few years, a variety of specialized audiologic tests have become useful in helping pinpoint the site of hearing loss and in differentiating patients with functional hearing loss from those with organic hearing loss.

### Short-Increment Sensitivity Index (SISI)

The SISI assesses the ability of an individual to detect 1 db increments in intensity. Normal individuals have difficulty detecting 1 db increments of loudness, whereas persons with cochlear injury hear most of them. Thus the SISI helps distinguish between patients with cochlear involvement and those with other types of hearing loss.

### Tone Decay

Tone decay testing is used to determine the presence of retrocochlear hearing loss. In this test, the subject is presented with a sustained pure tone at threshold. The patient signals with raised finger as long as he or she hears the tone. As the tone becomes inaudible, the intensity is increased. The procedure is continued until a single tone is heard for one entire minute. The person with normal hearing usually continues to hear the tone a full 60 seconds at levels 5 to 10 db above the threshold, but those with significant cochlear loss or with a retrocochlear abnormality may require an increase of 20 to 60 db before the tone is heard for a full minute. Some may actually be unable to hear any tone for longer than a few seconds.

## Alternate Binaural Loudness Balance (ABLB) Test

The ABLB test is a test for recruitment that generally demonstrates cochlear loss. In this test, the patient determines when a presented stimulus is equally loud in both ears. An abnormal growth in perceived loudness on the audiogram demonstrates recruitment, which is usually manifested in abnormalities associated with acoustic trauma, Ménière disease, or ototoxic drugs.

## Impedance Audiometry

Impedance audiometry uses an entirely different approach to testing hearing than does traditional audiometry. Impedance audiometry measures the compliance or its reciprocal, impedance, of the auditory system. The more compliant the system, the more sound energy that will be absorbed. The stiffer the system, the more energy turned back into the external canal. Tympanometry is a simple procedure that is easily performed in a short period and useful in children. Typically, tympanometry makes use of a specially constructed ear piece with three separate openings. One is connected to a sound source. Through this opening, a probe tone is delivered into the sealed external auditory canal. The second opening connects to the microphone and a balance meter that measures the sound pressure in the ear canal, including the sound generated by the sound source. One is able to alter the air pressure within the external canal and thus set up various conditions affecting sound transmission, which can then be compared with that transmission under normal conditions. As is true with use of a pneumatic otoscope, the acoustic compliance is greatest when the pressures are equal on both sides of the tympanic membrane. By plotting the ear's compliance on one axis and the air pressure on the other, a tympanogram is obtained (Fig. 35–6).

Some ears with disease will show more compliance (less impedance than normal), whereas in others the reverse is true (Fig. 35–7). In malleus fixation (in which the head of the malleus is fixed to the overhanging bone) the tympanogram should show greater impedance to sound transmission than in a normal ear. Some have referred to this

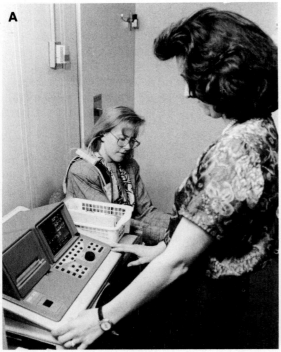
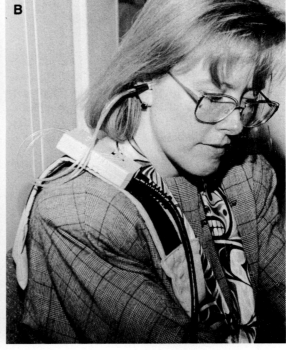

**FIG 35–6.**
Tympanometry in clinical setting.

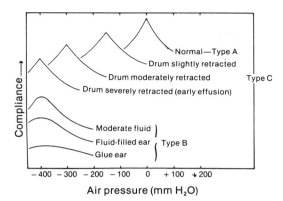

**FIG 35–7.**
Series of tympanograms illustrating various stages through which tympanogram progresses during development of acute serous otitis media. (From Jerger J, Northern J, editors: *Clinical impedance audiometry,* Action, Mass, 1980, Thieme-Stratton, Inc, in cooperation with American Electromedics Corp. Used by permission.)

as a stiff ear, and we can measure the amount of stiffness by this test. Similar findings would be encountered in serous otitis, in which there is fluid in the middle ear. In those circumstances, the system would be again stiff, with minimal motion. Impedance audiometry is of particular value in young children because voluntary responses are not required. If a normal tympanometric pattern is obtained, conductive hearing loss usually can be ruled out. However, impedance measurements do not serve as well as pure conventional audiometry to give accurate measurement of hearing acuity.

Two other tests can be performed with the use of impedance audiometry. Stapedial reflex testing demonstrates the hearing level at which the stapedius muscle will contract, altering the impedance of the middle ear. There is a significant change in compliance as the muscle contracts and pulls on the stapes. With the acoustic probe sealed in the nontest ear, a sound is delivered to the ear being tested. Bilateral contractions of the stapedius muscle should occur if the sound is loud enough—usually 70 to 80 db above threshold—and the resulting change in compliance is demonstrated on the tympanogram. Several important conditions can affect the stapedial reflex response, giving abnormal measurement. One example would be a case of recruitment, such as in Ménière's disease. In patients with recruitment, sound stimulation of the impaired ear at no more

than 40 db above threshold may result in a reflex response in the opposite (probed) ear instead of the expected 70 to 80 db level. On the other hand, retrocochlear lesions such as in acoustic neuroma may cause there to be no reflex at all, or decay phenomena may be evident (Fig. 35–8). Impedance audiometry is also useful in the case of a malingerer who complains of severe deafness in one ear. If tone presented to that ear causes a stapedial reflex in the other ear, the person obviously is not deaf in the test ear. Impedance audiometry does not replace pure-tone or speech testing or the physical examination, but in some instances it may be a valuable adjunct to conventional testing. It should never replace the pneumootoscopic examination or visualization of the tympanum.

Eustachian tube testing may also be performed in the presence of an intact tympanic membrane or with perforated tympanic membrane and myringotomy tubes. The most common test used is the swallow test, in which pressure equalization should occur with normal eustachian tube function (Fig. 35–9). When there is an intact tym-

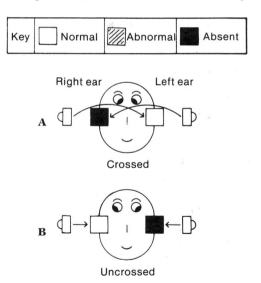

**FIG 35–8.**
Diagonal acoustic reflex pattern. **A,** When sound is delivered to the left ear, there is no reflex on the right. However, when sound is delivered to the right, there is a left reflex. **B,** When sound is delivered to the left ear, there is no reflex on the left. This pattern is consistent with left acoustic nerve (cranial nerve VII) or severe left cochlear disorder. (From Bluestone CD, Stool SE, ed: *Pediatric otolaryngology,* vol 1, Philadelphia, 1983, WB Saunders. Used by permission.)

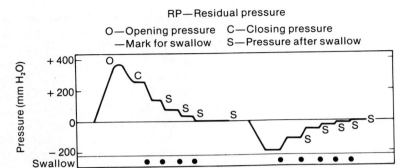

**FIG 35-9.**
Example of result of inflation-deflation ventilation studies with tympanometry that employ strip chart recorder. Normal adult with tympanic membrane perforation. This strip shows that with swallowing the negative or positive pressure is corrected, suggesting normal eustachian tube function. (From Jerger J, Northern J, editors: *Clinical impedance audiometry.* Acton, Mass., 1980, Thieme-Stratton, Inc, in cooperation with American Electromedics Corp. Used by permission.)

panic membrane, the presence of a negative-pressure tympanogram (type C) is a good indication of the presence of eustachian tube dysfunction.

*Brainstem audiometry* has become an important clinical tool in the diagnosis of ear abnormalities over the past few years. Brainstem response is similar to electroencephalographic audiometry in that it is a measure of the electrical activity in the auditory pathways. It is an accurate measure of auditory function, and it is a completely objective test that requires only that the patient remain quiet during the examination. Electrodes attached to the scalp and mastoid processes record an electrical response evoked by sound stimuli. Events are recorded during the first 10 msec following the sound stimulation. A series of rapid sounds (25+ per second) provides a stimulus. Because the potentials are small, computer averaging of these waveforms is required to extract from the background noise the response to the auditory stimulus. Measurement of latency from the stimulus to the appearance of waveforms and the appearance of characteristic waveform patterns are compared to norms. The appearance of recognizable waveforms can establish a hearing threshold (Fig. 35-10). Wave I represents activity in the cochlear nerve; wave II, activity in the cochlear nerve nucleus; wave III, activity in the neurons of the superior olivary complex; wave IV, activity in the lateral lemniscus; and wave V, activity in the inferior colliculus. Brainstem-evoked audiometry has its greatest use in testing of high-risk infants (to determine hearing loss) and in the diagnosis of retrocochlear lesions, which cause an elongation of the wave I:V ratio.

Because certain waveforms demonstrate activity in various levels of the auditory system, lesions that disturb the normal response can be localized.

Another type of electric response audiometry occasionally used is electrocochleography.

*Electrocochleography* is a measurement of potentials arising within the cochlea and the auditory nerve: the cochlear microphonics, the summating potential, and action potential of the eighth cranial nerve. In most cases, an electrode must be placed through the tympanic membrane onto the bone of the promontory to make these recordings, although ear canal recording is possible. An advantage of electrocochleographs is that they apply close proximity of the electrode to the sound generation sites, but a disadvantage is that for best recording, they require tympanic membrane penetration. Electrocochleography also does not represent auditory nerve function medial to the cochlea and thus cannot be used as an accurate test of hearing.

**Otoacoustics Emissions**

Otoacoustics emissions are low-intensity sounds produced in the cochlea and transmitted through the middle ear apparatus to the ear canal. These emissions can be detected and subtracted from the background noise in the ear canal through the use of sensitive microphone selective filtering and averaging techniques. Acoustic emissions represent the only measure of cochlear function that specifically tests the condition of the preneural components of the auditory pathways. In most cases they remain extremely stable. They

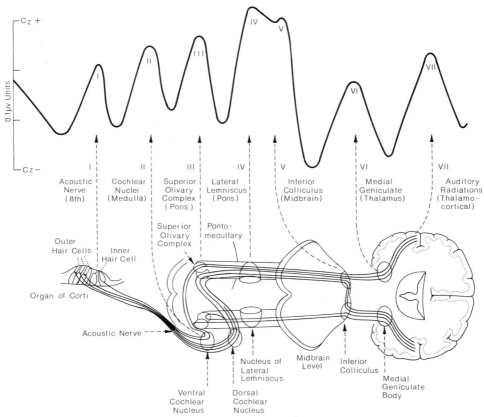

**FIG 35–10**.
Schematic tracing of brain stem evoked audiometry (BSEA), indicating the levels of the central nervous system responsible for the various wave patterns.

may eventually, therefore, be used as a long-term monitor of progressive hearing dysfunction caused by heredity, aging, or industrial noise. The test is rapid and objective. It is quite likely that otoacoustic emissions testing will be incorporated into a routine audiometric battery in the examination of hearing.

## AUDIOLOGIC METHODS IN TESTING INFANTS AND CHILDREN

Infants and young children cannot be tested by conventional methods and require a special testing battery. In infants less than 6 months of age, the startle reflex or its absence may be a clue as to whether or not the infant hears (Table 35–3). Later in the first year, the child will attempt to localize sound, and as the child becomes older, play audiometry is used in testing. Most accurate,

however, is the brainstem-evoked response (BSER), which can be used in children of any age and can obtain an approximation of hearing threshold, particularly at higher frequencies. This test remains the most reliable test for the very young child. The importance of determining, if possible, the presence of significant hearing loss in an infant or child under 18 months of age cannot be overemphasized. To learn speech, the child must hear, and if the child is hard of hearing, amplification of sound with a hearing aid is necessary early in life. Hearing aids have been successfully used by infants less than 6 months of age. If the hearing loss is profound, it is necessary to begin sensory training very early in life so the child can learn lipreading (speech reading), as well as the early simple vocal sounds. Most specialized schools for the hard of hearing or the deaf accept children for training before the age of 3 to provide the extra training necessary to compensate

**TABLE 35–3.**

Stages of Hearing Development

| Age | Characteristic |
|---|---|
| 0–4 mo | Awakens to loud noise |
| | Exhibits startle reflex to loud noise |
| | Cries with loud noise |
| 5–7 mo | Turns to sounds |
| | Follows sounds or voices |
| 8–10 mo | Makes noise in response to voice or voices |
| | Exhibits inflection in sounds—variable loudness of cry and vocalization |
| 11–14 mo | Mimics sound |
| | Makes variety of sounds |
| | Responds to voices, commands |
| 14–24 mo | Voice has inflection |
| | Vocabulary starts to develop |

for the loss of hearing. There is always an educational delay, even with children of normal or superior intelligence. The physician should never adopt the attitude of "Let's see him again in a year; he will probably outgrow it." When parents (or more frequently grandparents) who have raised a child with normal hearing are concerned enough to seek medical advice for a suspected hearing problem in an infant or a child less than the age of 1, every effort should be made to determine whether the hearing is normal or defective. If there is any suspicion of significant hearing loss, special tests, particularly BSER, may need to be repeated at intervals.

## VESTIBULAR TESTING

The neuronal connections between vestibular nuclei; the medial longitudinal vesiculus; nuclei of the third, fourth, and sixth cranial nerves; and the cerebellum are responsible for nystagmus, which occurs with vestibular stimulation. The eye movement response is the most measurable method of assessing vestibular function, and the degree of nystagmus produced is the most reliable means of estimating the qualitative and quantitative activity of the vestibular end organ.

Disturbances of the labyrinth produce a type of nystagmus known as labyrinthine nystagmus. A slow movement of the eye in one direction is followed by a rapid compensatory movement in the opposite direction. This is a rhythmic movement. The quick secondary movement is the easiest to detect, and by convention is considered the direction of the nystagmus. The severity of the nystag-

mus is expressed as first, second, or third degree. First-degree nystagmus is noted only when the one eye is looking in the direction of the rapid component. Second-degree nystagmus is noted when the eye looks straight ahead. Third-degree nystagmus is noted when the eyes look in the direction of the slow component. During tests to evaluate nystagmus, the patient is asked to follow the examiner's finger from side to side to determine the degree and the severity. Nystagmus can be observed more easily when 20+-diopter (Frenzel) glasses are placed over the eyes. They not only magnify the eyeball but also prevent the patient from fixing on any object, as fixation can suppress the nystagmus movement (Fig. 35–11).

There are other types of nystagmus, called optic or optokinetic nystagmus, that can be produced by ocular abnormalities. Such nystagmus differs from labyrinthine nystagmus in that excursions of the eyes are of equal amplitude in both directions. Also, the amplitude tends to be greater, and the motion tends to be wandering and pendulous rather than rhythmic. The most common terms used to describe nystagmus are as follows:

1. *Horizontal nystagmus*—Occurring in the horizontal plane

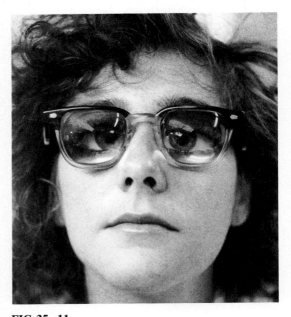

**FIG 35–11.**
Frenzel glasses. These 20+-diopter lenses are used to prevent the patient from fixing on an object, as well as allowing the examiner to note fine eye movement.

2. *Rotary nystagmus*—Occurring in the frontal plane
3. *Vertical nystagmus*—Occurring in the sagital plane
4. *Perverted nystagmus*—Any deviation from that expected
5. *Variable nystagmus*—Different direction in each eye
6. *Positional nystagmus*—Seen in a change of head position
7. *Spontaneous nystagmus*—Occurring spontaneously
8. *Induced nystagmus*—Produced by artificial stimulation

Spontaneous nystagmus indicates a disease process except when it occurs during extreme lateral gaze. Vertical nystagmus with the eyes open indicates central nervous system disease. Alteration of the expected response from artificial stimulation also indicates central nervous system disorders. Induced nystagmus caused by caloric testing is horizontal when the head is tipped 60 degrees backward and rotary when it is tipped 30 degrees forward. First-degree nystagmus and second-degree nystagmus are considered normal after artificial stimulation, but third-degree nystagmus is abnormal unless the stimulus is excessive.

A variety of tests and responses can be used for evaluation of the vestibular system.

**Test for Positional Nystagmus**

Nystagmus may be induced by changes in the position of the head. Tests are not difficult and may be performed as follows (Fig. 35–12). The patient sits on a table with his or her head turned to one side. The patient is then quickly lowered to a supine position so that the head hangs over the head of the table, 30 degrees below the horizontal. The eyes are observed for nystagmus with the use of Frenzel glasses. The patient's eyes are kept open and are watched for the appearance and duration of any nystagmus. The patient is also asked about the subjective feeling of vertigo. The test is then repeated with the head turned to the opposite side and finally with the head brought back into the hanging position. During each of these maneuvers, the examiner should assist the patient and be sure that the head and body turn together as a unit. If the head is turned independently of body motion, reflexes from the neck muscles may

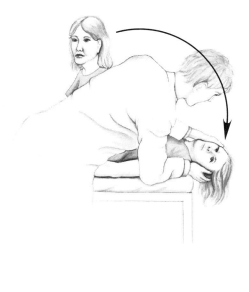
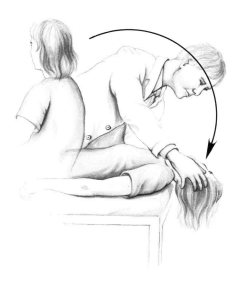

**FIG 35–12.**
Positional testing.

**TABLE 35–4.**

Positional Testing

| Localizing Features | |
|---|---|
| Peripheral | Central |
| Violent vertigo with position | Mild symptoms, "dizzy," rare vertigo |
| Lag period of a few seconds with position followed by marked nystagmus | Immediate onset of nystagmus |
| Nystagmus fatigues if position held | Nystagmus persists |
| Associated nausea common | Symptoms of nausea rare |

be initiated or compression of vascular vessels may occur that may alter the reaction. After each new position, the eyes are carefully observed for nystagmus. Any nystagmus in any position is recorded, including the direction and duration. Although positional testing has many implications, its only practical application is to separate positional vertigo of a benign peripheral type from that which is characteristic of central nervous system disease (Table 35–4).

Stimulation of the labyrinth also produces past pointing and falling as well as nystagmus. Past pointing and falling always occur in the direction of the flow of the endolymphatic fluid and are opposite the direction of the nystagmus (quick phase). The three labyrinthine findings (pass pointing, falling, and slow phase of nystagmus) occur in the same direction. However, because nystagmus is named for the fast component, nystagmus is always recorded as the opposite of falling and pass pointing. For example, nystagmus with slow motion to the left but fast to the right is called right nystagmus. It is the slow motion of the nystagmus that is the labyrinthine component—the quick motion is compensatory and a central nervous system response.

## Tests for Labyrinthine Function
### Caloric Tests

The semicircular canals can be stimulated by introducing either water or air into the external auditory canal at temperatures above or below body temperature. Water below body temperature directed against the tympanic membrane causes endolymphatic fluid to displace in a downward direction. Water above body temperature sets up convection currents in the opposite direction, causing the fluid in one or more canals to rise. This motion of the endolymphatic fluid distorts the hair cells in the cupula and produces the labyrinthine reaction. Patients vary greatly in their sensitivity to caloric stimulation. Advantages of the caloric test are that it is simple, because it requires little equipment to perform, and that it allows one to test each ear separately.

When the head is tipped 60 degrees backward, the lateral semicircular canal is vertical and therefore can be stimulated by convection currents. The results of caloric evaluation can be interpreted as normal, hyperactive, hypoactive, or absent. When no reaction is obtained from the semicircular canals, the labyrinth is said to be dead. Before and after stimulation, the patient is examined for nystagmus, past pointing, and falling (Fig. 35–13).

There are several methods of cold caloric testing. One useful technique is to direct the ice water against the eardrum, through an ear speculum, with the head tilted back 60 degrees. Twenty diopter glasses are placed over the eyes to abolish accommodation. Ice water is then directed against the eardrum from a Luer-Lok syringe through a 25-gauge needle for 10 to 12 seconds (Fig. 35–14). After a short latent period, labyrinthine reaction begins. The eyes are observed for nystagmus, and testing for past pointing and falling is performed. If no reaction occurs in response to the original stimulus, the duration of stimulus is increased—usually doubled. In the average, normal individual, 10 to 12 seconds of ice water stimulation will induce mild vertigo, definite nystagmus, and a tendency to lean or fall in one direction. Nystagmus will usually last 1 to 2 minutes. This test is known as the Kobrac caloric test and is convenient for office use. It affords minimal stimulation and can be made quantitative by varying the duration of stimulation against the eardrum. About 5 to 10 minutes should be allowed between testing the individual ears. The test is always a comparison of the two sides.

### Electronystagmography

Electronystagmography has replaced the Kobrac test as the standard for vestibular testing. This test relies on the fact that there is a difference in potential between the cornea and the retina. During nystagmus, movements of the eyes cause the

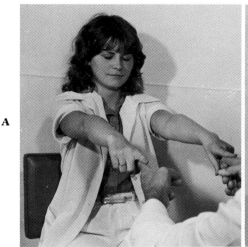 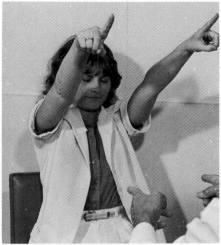

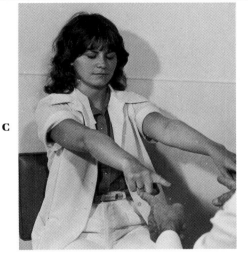

**FIG 35–13.**
Test for past pointing. Note that the eyes are closed during the test. **A,** position of hands and arms immediately after caloric stimulation. **B,** patient is raising arms vertically with elbows straight. **C,** patient has lowered arms and is past pointing to the left.

corneal retina potential to be displaced, giving rise to changes in potential that can be recorded (Fig. 35–15). Because the cornea of the eye carries a positive electrical charge and the retina a negative charge, it is possible to place electrodes near the eye and record the movements. A permanent record thus allows later study and actual calculation of the amplitude, direction, and speed of nystagmus. Obviously, this can be used to record eye tracking, spontaneous nystagmus, positional nystagmus, and gaze. In the usual test, a recording is made of the resting stage of eye movement. The direction, speed, and amplification of the

nystagmus are measured after stimulation of the labyrinth with warm and cold water or air. The temperature of the stimulating fluid is carefully controlled, generally 7 degrees above and below body temperature (Fig. 35–16). All eye motions are recorded. The test is performed in a dark room with the eyes closed to eliminate as much as possible accommodative and fixative functions of the eye that may suppress eye movements caused by the stimulus. The test supplies a permanent record that may be compared with known abnormal patterns and is used to follow the course of individual patients (Fig. 35–17). As in all tests of

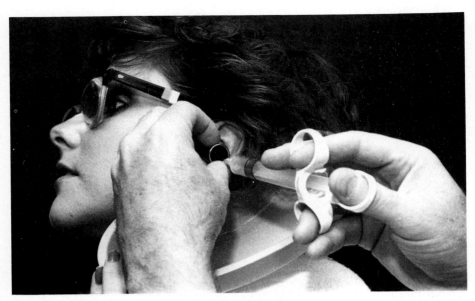

**FIG 35–14.**
Kobrac caloric stimulation. Note that the patient is wearing 20-diopter lenses and that the head is tipped backward. Ideally, at the start of the test, the head is tipped 60 degrees posteriorly.

hearing or labyrinthine reaction, the electronystagmograph (ENG) must be used only as an aid in diagnosis and integrated with other available information, including the medical history and other physical findings. The test is rarely diagnostic by itself.

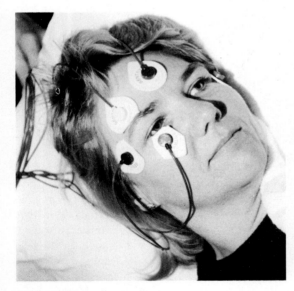

**FIG 35–15.**
Electrode placement in electronystagmography.

### Rotation Testing

Rotating testing was rarely used until recently. It was less useful in most clinical situations than was caloric testing because it stimulated both ears simultaneously (Fig. 35–18). The nystagmus produced is the result of endolymph flow occuring with both starting and cessation of rotational movement. Responses depend on the stimulation

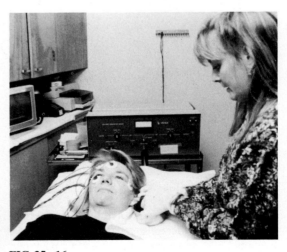

**FIG 35–16.**
Electronystagmography. Patient is undergoing caloric stimulation with recording of eye movement.

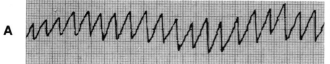

**FIG 35–17.**
"Spontaneous" nystagmus recorded from electrodes placed on patient's temples. **A**, eyes closed; **B**, eyes open, left gaze; **C**, eyes open, center gaze; **D**, eyes open, right gaze.

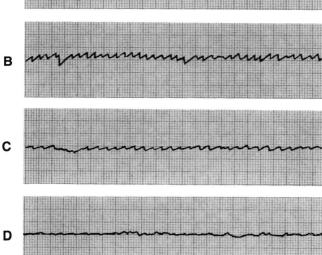

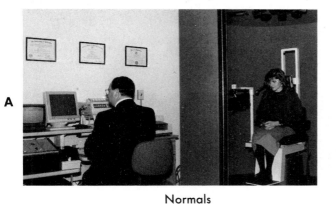

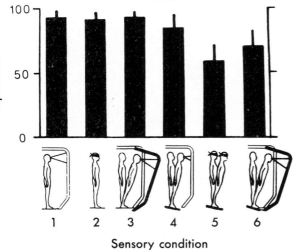

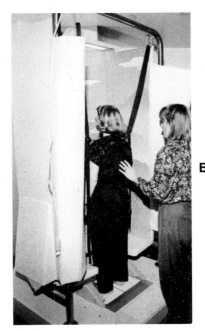

**FIG 35–18.**
**A,** computerized rotary chair system. Patient is seated in chair, which is situated in isolation enclosure. Infrared camera mounted to chair rotates with patient and allows examiner to monitor patient's head and eye position throughout test, which is conducted in total darkness (doors normally are closed during test). Slow-phase compensatory eye velocity is compared to chair velocity at a number of acceleration frequencies to determine phase, gain, and symmetry of response. **B,** NeuroCom International Equitest system shows patient standing on platform surrounded by visual scene. Pressure-sensing strain gauges beneath platform surface detect patient sway by measuring his or her vertical and horizontal forces applied to surface. Safety harness is attached to patient should loss of balance occur. The platform surface and visual surround are capable of moving independently or simultaneously. **C,** six sensory organization test conditions. A score of 100 represents no patient sway whereas a score of 0 represents maximum sway or a patient fall. (From Cummings CW, editor: *Otolaryngology-Head and Neck Surgery,* ed 2. St Louis, Mosby–Year Book, 1992. Used by permission.)

produced by the inertia of the endolymph relative to the membranous semicircular canal. More recently, computerized rotational tests with variable degrees of rotational speed have been used with the hopes of providing additional information for diagnosing of central nervous system abnormali-

ties and distinguishing them from labyrinthine disorders.

### Posturography

Recently posturography testing has been investigated with the hope of isolating those clues of

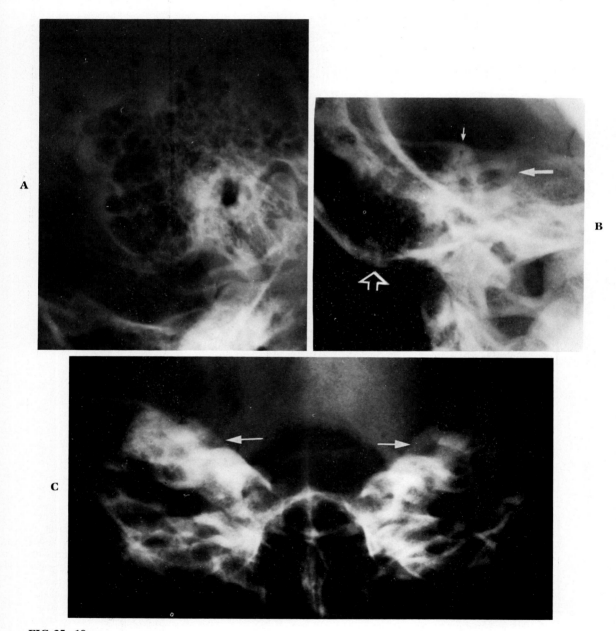

**FIG 35–19.**
**A,** lateral view of mastoid showing normal air-cell system. Note superimposition of internal and external meatus. **B,** normal Stenver's projection. *Large arrow,* internal auditory meatus (IAM); *small arrow,* superior semicircular canal: *open arrow,* mastoid tip. **C,** classic Towne projection. *Arrows* indicate IAM.

balance implicating the vestibular system. Moving platform posturography, which tests proprioceptive, visual, and vestibular activity, offers some hope for determining the cause of patient's postural instability. These tests attempt to isolate the individual components of balance by altering visual clues, joint and muscle stimuli, and vestibular stimulation. As yet, the clinical value and sensitivity of these tests is unknown.

## Drugs Affecting Vestibular Testing

Many medications exert an effect on nystagmus, and if the history, detailing the use of these drugs, is not taken, erroneous results will be obtained during vestibular tests.

### *Alcohol*

Alcohol causes positional nystagmus in the right or left ear-down position. During drunken-

ness the nystagmus beats toward the floor, and during hangover it generally beats toward the ceiling. It is stronger with the eyes closed than with the eyes open. Alcohol also causes variation in rotational testing.

### *Central Nervous System Depressants*

Central nervous system depressants suppress all types of vestibular nystagmus. This is believed to be a result of the anticholinergic or sedative effects of these drugs. It is well known that drowsiness, whether drug induced or not, suppresses nystagmus.

### *Barbiturates*

Barbiturates cause vestibular nystagmus to be stronger with eyes open than with eyes closed. This effect, known as failure of visual suppression nystagmus, is important in the interpretation of the caloric test because it may otherwise be re-

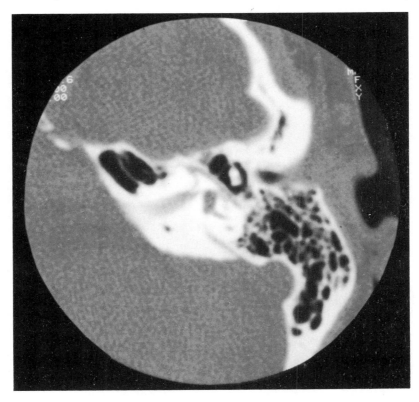

**FIG 35–20.**
**A,** normal axial CT scan of the temporal bone. *Right arrow,* ossicles with the typical "ice cream cone" appearance of the malleus and incus. *Left arrow,* the cochlea and portion of the internal auditory meatus. The labyrinthine vestibule, horizontal semicircular canal, and eustachian tube are also well demonstrated on this view. **B,** normal axial CT scan demonstrating course of seventh nerve from internal auditory meatus across middle ear *(arrow).* Note mastoid cells, external auditory canal, vestibule, and middle ear ossicles.

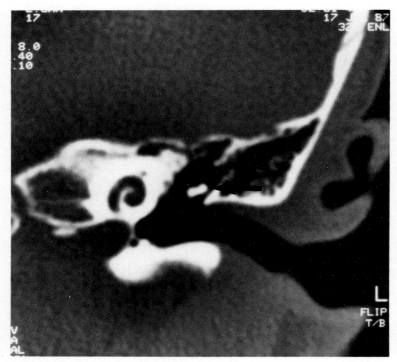

**FIG 35–21.**
Normal coronal CT scan of the temporal bone. *Arrow* demonstrates the malleus and incus. The cochlea and epitympanic region are well demonstrated.

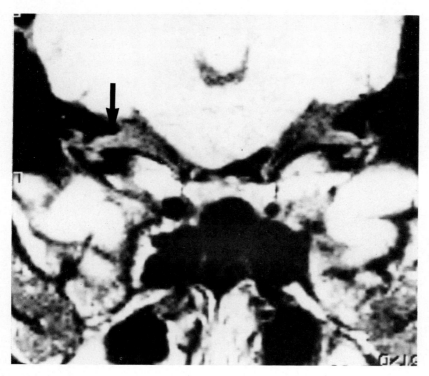

**FIG 35–22.**
Normal MRI study of the posterior fossa and internal auditory canal. Note with MRI the bony structures are radiolucent. *Large arrow* points to the eighth nerve complex lying within the internal auditory canal. *Smaller arrow* clearly defines the horizontal portion of the facial nerve as it crosses the middle ear. Structures lying within the cochlea and labyrinth are also visualized.

garded as a sign of a posterior fossa tumor. This effect is believed to be caused by selective blocking of multisynaptic vestibulocomotive motor pathways through the reticular formation.

Alcohol, barbiturates, phenytoin (Dilantin), and other central nervous system depressants can all cause degeneration of smooth pursuit movements. Higher dosage levels cause horizontal gaze nystagmus, and still higher levels can cause upbeating nystagmus during upward gaze. Clinically, it is important during vestibular testing to remember to use the same technique on all patients. Comparisons between different patients and between right and left ears of the same patients have been possible, regardless of what technique is used. The mechanics are of secondary importance. Interpretation is of primary importance. The ability to interpret results is acquired only by repeated personal experience with a given technique.

## Radiology of the Ear and Related Structures

Conventional radiology of the temporal bone and related structures has, in the past decade, been almost completely replaced by computed tomography (CT). Occasionally the Law view (lateral), Stenvors view (oblique PA view), and Towne view are taken to provide the surgeon with an idea of the cellularity of the mastoid and whether or not there is destruction (Fig. 35–19). Although other structures, such as the internal auditory canal, can be identified with these views, CT provides much improved detail.

The most valuable radiologic tool for visualization of the middle and inner ears has also been CT. Coronal and axial views are standard. With high-quality CT scans the entire course of the seventh nerve can be defined, ossicles can be visualized, and the labyrinth and cochlea can be well demonstrated. One can visualize masses, ossicular deformity, bone destruction or erosion. (Figs. 35–20 and 35–21)

While CT has given clear definition of the bony anatomy of the middle and inner ear, magnetic resonance imaging has provided increased detail of the soft tissues of the ear and related structures, especially the posterior fossa (Fig. 35–22). The seventh-eighth nerve complex, the great vessels, the brain, and brainstem structures are all clearly demonstrated. Small acoustic neuromas (as small as 1 mm) can be identified. These studies, though expensive, have greatly added to our knowledge and diagnostic skill regarding lesions of the ear and their central pathways.

# 36

# Embryology and Congenital Disorders

The auricle develops around the first branchial groove from six outgrowths of the first and second branchial arches, appearing about the sixth week of gestation. The first branchial arch contributes to the formation of the five hillocks, which form the helix, antihelix, and antitragus of the adult ear (Fig. 36–1). By the twelfth week, the auricle is formed by a fusion of these hillocks, and by the twentieth week, they have reached their adult shape. The first pharyngeal groove contributes to the formation of the external auditory canal, initially as a solid core of epithelium growing toward the middle ear. By the sixth month, the core begins to reabsorb and hollow out to form the external canal. The innermost layer of the groove, which is ectodermal, remains to become the superficial layer of the tympanic membrane. By the twenty-eighth week, the external ear canal is fully formed, although ossification is not complete until 3 years of age.

The middle ear is derived from the first pharyngeal pouch, and extension of the pouch between the first and second arches forms the eustachian tube. The close association of the first three arches is a factor in the embryologic determination of the nerve supply of the middle ear (fifth, seventh, and ninth cranial nerves). The mastoid antrum appears in the fifth month, and the tympanic membrane is formed by the twenty-eighth week. The ossicles of the middle ear initially are continuous with Meckel's cartilage of the first branchial arch and Reichert's cartilage of the second branchial arch. The head and neck of the malleus and the short process and body of the incus originate from Meckel's cartilage of the first arch mesoderm. The remainder of the middle ear ossicular chain is derived from the second arch.

At birth, all of the ossicles are of adult size and shape.

The neuroectoderm of the inner ear begins to differentiate about the third week of gestation, and by the eighth week the semicircular canals and utricle are fully formed. The cochlea is formed somewhat later, with the complete two and a half turns developed by the twelfth week. The differentiation of the neuroepithelium continues into the fourth to fifth months of gestation.

The complexity of the embryologic development of the ear contributes to a variety of congenital malformations. Abnormalities of the auricle include microtia (too-small ear), macrotia (too-large ear), and improper shape. It is rarely altogether absent. Absence or severe deformation of the auricle is often associated with atresia of the external auditory canal (Fig. 36–2). The atresia of the canal causes a conductive type of hearing loss, provided the inner ear development is unaffected. Significant malformation of the auricle implies malformation of the middle ear and seventh cranial nerve. A normal auricle with canal atresia suggests that the ossicles and middle ear are probably normal because of the later development of the external canal. Occasionally one may see an accessory auricle appearing as a tag of skin or a piece of skin or cartilage in front of the tragus. This represents remnants of the first branchial apparatus. An improper fusion of the first and second arches may result in a preauricular sinus tract, which is usually lined with epithelium generally just anterior and slightly superior to the tragus (Fig. 36–3). Treatment or removal is indicated only if these become infected or a discharge is present.

All varieties of middle ear abnormalities can

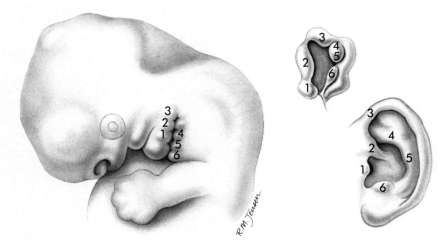

**FIG 36–1.**
External ear is formed from six hillocks—five of which form the helix and associated structures. The first hillock from the second branchial arch forms the tragus.

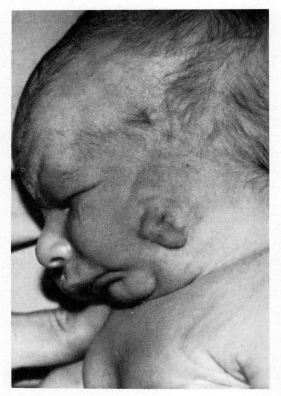

**FIG 36–2.**
Child with rudimentary displaced auricle and total atresia.

occur, including an absent stapedial tendon, persistent stapedial artery passing through the arch of the stapes, absent stapedius muscle, a dehiscence of the bone overlying the facial nerve, and congenital fixation of the malleus or stapes. These defects produce a conductive hearing loss with a normal external canal and tympanic membrane. Middle ear abnormalities are most commonly found with canal atresia.

Malformation of the auricle, external auditory canal, and ossicles occurs very often in a person with a poorly developed mandible owing to the

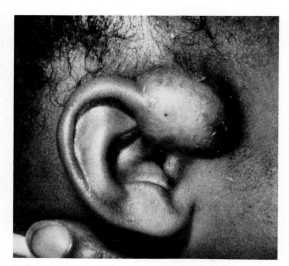

**FIG 36–3.**
Infected preauricular sinus. The pit is visible at the base of the swollen mass.

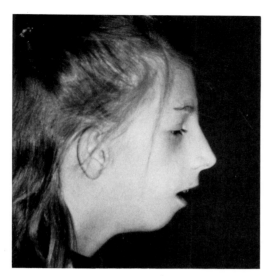

**FIG 36–4.**
Treacher Collins syndrome.

arrest of the first branchial groove and arch in the second month of fetal life. If the mandible is malformed, the patient has Treacher Collins syndrome. This is one of the more common facial deformities, consisting of antimongoloid eyes, notched lower lids, short mandible, deformed external ear, meatal atresia, and ossicular deformity (Fig. 36–4). In persons with abnormalities of the outer and middle ear, the facial nerve may have an abnormal course through the temporal bone or lie exposed in the tympanic cavity or be more lateral than is common. Because of these abnormal relationships, surgical intervention for congenital atresia is hazardous.

Unilateral canal atresia is more common, although the bilateral form is not unusual; in most cases of bilateral canal atresia, one side usually has a less marked malformation. Congenital deformities of the ear are about twice as common in males as in females.

The inner and middle ear, external canal, and pinna develop quite early, and they have been linked to simultaneous development of other organs and systems. These structures develop primarily during the first trimester of gestation. Therefore, any noxious influence operating during the first trimester may and often does affect the hearing of those infants who survive. These influences include intrauterine infections, maternal hypoxia, and fetal toxic or ototoxic drugs. In children who are born with other defects, particularly those of the central nervous system, teeth, skin, or appendages, whether genetic or exogenous, the inner ear is at significant risk. The middle ear, ossicles, and tympanic membrane share branchial origin with the pinna, external auditory canal, and other maxillofacial structures so that abnormalities of any one or more of the external visible members of the structures of the face should prompt investigation of hearing. There are a variety of genetic causes of central nervous system hearing loss, most of which entail multiple abnormalities.

# 37

# Infection and Inflammation of the Ear

## EXTERNAL EAR AND AUDITORY CANAL

Although the following are not true inflammations of the external ear and canal, they represent common problems in patient care and frequently lead to secondary infection.

## Cerumen

Cerumen or earwax is formed by special ceruminal glands in the cartilaginous ear canal. Its purposes are to lubricate the skin of the ear and to entrap foreign material entering the canal. Normally, cerumen that is produced only in small amounts dries in the ear canal and is forced out bit by bit during mastication and talking.

### Excessive Cerumen and Impacted Cerumen

Some patients have overactive glands that produce excessive accumulation of wax in the ear canal. Other patients have impacted cerumen because their ear canals are tortuous and small or abnormally narrow at one point. Still other patients have an abnormal type of cerumen often associated with dermatosis that does not dry and flake out but remains very soft and eventually fills the ear canal. If occlusion of the canal is complete, the ear feels blocked or full and the patient is hard of hearing. The hearing loss may approach 30 to 40 db. Tinnitus may be present, and occasionally there is some dizziness. Ordinarily, there is no pain unless the ear is secondarily infected. Not infrequently, patients who get water in their ears while swimming or taking showers find they have suddenly lost hearing in one ear. This may

result from increased bulk of the earwax as a result of water absorption or from the water becoming trapped behind the wax. Inspection reveals a ball of wax completely occluding the canal. Sometimes the patient has pushed the cerumen in toward the drumhead. A particularly troublesome condition results when a patient uses a cotton swab in an attempt to remove cerumen and instead impacts it medially.

Often, an ear may appear to be completely occluded, and yet the patient has no symptoms. In such an instance, there is a tiny slit where the meatus is clear, and this suffices to transmit sound and maintain normal hearing. Treatment consists of removing the wax by irrigation or with a cerumen spoon. In irrigating the canal, one need not worry that the force of the stream will injure the eardrum, provided a space is left around the syringe to allow water to escape. Ordinarily, tap water is used, but it must be at body temperature or vertigo will develop from vestibular stimulation. The canal is irrigated by pulling the ear posteriorly and superiorly, thus straightening the canal and directing the stream toward the superior quadrant of the tympanic membrane (Fig. 37–1). After irrigation, the canal should be dried by inserting a small length of cotton on a metal applicator under direct vision. Removing the wax with a cerumen spoon requires some skill. The epithelium that lines the osseous canal is exquisitely sensitive in some individuals and may bleed when touched. The eardrum itself is less likely to be injured. The cerumen spoon should be smooth edged and must be used under direct vision through an ear speculum. When possible, it is better to insert the spoon and pull the wax out-

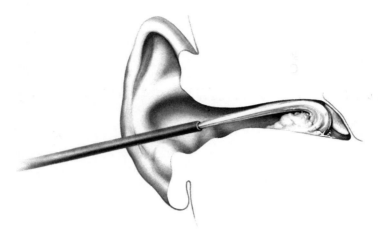

**FIG 37–1.**
Irrigation of wax or foreign body from the ear. Note that the direction of the water column is superiorly against the canal wall and tympanic membrane, as most debris and foreign material gather along the inferior sulcus.

ward in mass rather than pick it out in pieces. Usually, there is a narrow slit superiorly where the cerumen spoon can be inserted (Fig. 37–2). Occasionally, cerumen may be impacted and so dry that it cannot be removed painlessly. In such an instance, the patient is instructed to instill a few drops of hydrogen peroxide or mineral oil daily for 2 to 3 days to soften the wax. Then it can be removed easily by irrigation. The preparation Cerumenex, a proprietary drug, also can be used, but it has been noted to cause inflammatory reactions if used frequently. Occasionally, desquamated epithelium is attached to the surface of a large mass of cerumen and may look white like dead skin. In elderly men, cerumen is often mixed with long hairs, and the two form a matted obstruction of the ear canal.

### Inadequate Cerumen

Too little cerumen may be more annoying to the patient than too much because the ear canal is dry. There may be scaling, itching, and cracking of the canal in this condition. It is difficult to manage this particular problem, but it may be improved by the application of suitable ear ointments or mineral oil. Occasionally, an inadequacy of cerumen or an abnormal type of cerumen seems to be associated with dermatologic disorders such as seborrheic dermatitis.

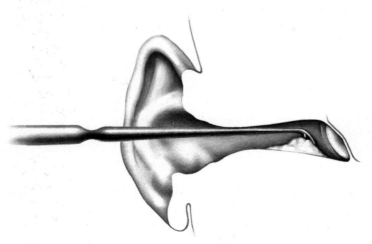

**FIG 37–2.**
Removal of wax with angled blunt curette.

## Foreign Bodies

Obstruction of the ear canal is commonly caused by an inanimate or a vegetable foreign object; this is discussed fully in Chapter 39, under Large Canal Foreign Bodies.

## External Otitis

*External otitis* is a general term used for inflammatory disease of the auricle and external auditory canal. It may be caused by either infections or dermatitis or both. Either bacteria or fungus may be the cause. Fungi produce many infections in tropical climates, whereas bacteria are the most common cause of external otitis in temperate zones. As might be expected, external otitis is much more common in summer than in winter. External otitis may be associated with infections of the face or scalp, such as an infectious eczematoid dermatitis. However, it more commonly occurs as the primary infection and is limited to the ear canal, to the auricle, or both. The normal ear canal harbors *Staphylococcus albus* and diphtheroids but generally no pathogenic organisms. The bacteria most commonly cultured from patients with acute external otitis are *Pseudomonas aeruginosa, Proteus vulgaris, Escherichia coli,* and *Staphylococcus aureus.* The *Pseudomonas* organism is especially common. External otitis is more common in people who swim frequently and thus is called swimmer's ear. These patients often have some wax in the ear that absorbs water, macerates the skin and canal, and affords a basis for infection.

The most common fungi affecting the external ear are *Candida albicans* and *Aspergillus* species, especially *Aspergillus niger,* which produces a black growth in the canal.

### Acute External Otitis

In the mild, early stages of acute external otitis, there is mild to moderate pain aggravated by movement of the auricle or tragus. There may be a low-grade fever or discharge from the ear canal that is often sticky and yellow. If the ear canal is swollen shut or obstructed by debris, there may be a partial loss of hearing and a feeling of a blocked ear, although this generally develops later. In the severe stage of external otitis, there is often intense pain and the entire side of the head aches and throbs. Some patients will not permit

aural examination because of pain. There is usually a discharge from the ear. Hearing may be diminished, and the ear feels blocked. Examination will reveal the external auditory canal to be swollen, if not entirely closed. Often the tragus and concha are swollen (Fig. 37–3). A sticky yellow or purulent discharge may ooze or pulsate from the ear canal. The temperature may be elevated, although it is usually normal or near normal. Movement of the tragus or traction on the auricle aggravates the pain because such movements are transmitted to the swollen ear. Some patients will refuse even to permit such manipulation. The increased pain caused by movement of the external ear is an important consideration in the differential diagnosis between acute external otitis and otitis media (both of which may produce ear pain and aural discharge). If an ear speculum can be inserted, the canal is usually swollen and often appears pale. Often there are desquamated epithelium and wax in the canal. Less frequently, the canal is red and may be dry. Lymphadenopathy is common, with tender nodes anterior to the tragus, behind the ear or in the upper neck. Sometimes, postauricular adenopathy or cellulitis is so great as to push the auricle forward. In such an instance, the condition must be differentiated from the subperiosteal abscess of acute mastoiditis. When the auricle itself is infected, the skin may ooze and crust. Pustules may be present, and the

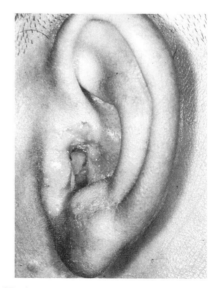

**FIG 37–3.**
Acute external otitis. Note swelling of the ear canal and lymphadenopathy anterior to the tragus.

external ear may be swollen and tender. The infection may spread to the face or the scalp. Usually, infections of the ear canal cause much greater pain than do infections of the external ear alone because the epithelium of the ear canal cannot stretch without producing pain. In acute external otitis, the eardrum often cannot be seen because of the swelling of the ear canal. When it is possible to see the eardrum, it may appear normal.

### Chronic External Otitis

In chronic external otitis, itching rather than pain is the chief complaint. Excoriation of the ear canal frequently occurs as a result of scratching. The manipulations used in cleaning the ears that patients usually find a little unpleasant or even painful under normal conditions are welcomed by most patients with chronic external otitis. Aural discharge is present in some but not all patients with chronic external otitis. Hearing is not affected unless debris accumulates and fills the ear canal. If an acute infection develops in the patient with chronic external otitis or the epithelium is broken as a result of scratching, pain may become a major symptom. The epithelium of the ear canal or auricle or both is thickened and red. Both the ear canal and the surface of the drum are remarkably insensitive to cleaning by cotton applicators. When aural discharge is present, the odor may be moderately foul, but not as foul or penetrating as with patients with certain types of middle ear disease. In contrast to acute external otitis, there is no pain when the auricle or tragus is manipulated. The tympanic membrane may appear normal or slightly thickened.

Principally, external otitis must be differentiated from otitis media. The symptoms may be very nearly the same, although the order of development is different. In severe stages, both groups of patients have pain and fever and sometimes aural discharge. Data in Table 37–1 should serve as a guide in differentiating between the two conditions.

Rarely, a bone-destroying infection called necrotizing otitis externa or malignant external otitis occurs. This is a serious infection of high mortality that occurs most frequently in elderly diabetic patients. Others predisposed to it include immunosuppressed patients and those receiving steroids. The responsible organism is *P. aeruginosa*. Generally, the disorder is characterized by progressive pain and discharge from the external canal. The findings consist of infection and granulation tissue at the junction of the osseous and cartilaginous portions of the external canal. If the infection progresses, it will extend into the soft tissue of the cartilaginous canal and through the fissures anteriorly to the parotid gland or carotid vessels, deep into the mastoid and external ear canal bone. As it progresses, it may extend medially toward the base of the skull. Pain is the major complaint throughout its course. Extensive osteomyelitis involving the base of the skull, facial palsy, and loss of hearing and vestibular function can develop. The infection is generally resistant to ordinary methods of treatment. Although local débridement is important, systemic administration of carbenicillin, gentamicin, or more recently, cephalosporins effective against *Pseudomonas* (cefoperazone, ceftazidime) are considered the treatment of choice. Ciprofloxacin and ofloxacin are also newer effective antibiotics for *Pseudomonas* and other gram negative organisms. Radical surgical resection is reserved for unresponsive cases. This disorder should always be suspected

**TABLE 37–1.**

Differential Diagnosis of Acute External Otitis and Acute Otitis Media

|  | Acute External Otitis | Acute Otitis Media |
|---|---|---|
| Season | Summer | Winter |
| Movement of tragus painful | Yes | No |
| Ear canal | Swollen | Normal |
| Eardrum | Normal (or red) | Perforated or bulging |
| Discharge | Yes | Yes—but through a perforation |
| Nodes | Frequent | Less frequent |
| Fever | Yes | Yes |
| Hearing | Normal or decreased | Always decreased |

in an elderly, diabetic patient who develops a persistent external otitis.

### Treatment of Acute and Chronic Forms

In mildly acute external otitis, topical treatment alone is all that is necessary. Local treatment begins with careful cleansing of the ear canal. In general, only bland, soothing liquid preparations with or without antibiotics and hydrocortisone should be used for the patient with acute external otitis. An important feature of any otic solution is that the pH is acidic, as most bacteria or fungi do not thrive in acidic surroundings. The ointments are not as effective and are better reserved for patients with chronic, dry external otitis. When the auricle is affected, the use of cotton or gauze compresses soaked with aluminum acetate solution (Domeboro) or the use of a saturated boric acid solution is good local treatment. In addition, systemic antibiotic medications are generally required. In mild stages, a medicated wick of cotton or packing may be inserted gently into the ear canal when the canal is partially occluded as a result of swollen epithelium. A wick should be used when one is not certain that the otic drops will effectively reach the area of inflammation. Such a wick may be moistened with a number of medications. If the ear canal is eczematous or weeping, an effective hydroscopic eardrop is Burow's solution (5% aluminum acetate). In other cases, antibiotic eardrops with or without hydrocortisone are widely available and useful. Drops containing polymyxin B, neomycin, and colistin are effective against the usual gram negative bacteria that affect the ear. In patients who have a pure staphylococcal external otitis, these medications are ineffective and antibiotics such as chloramphenicol (Chloromycetin Otic) drops or bacitracin ointment should be used. Neomycin or propylene glycol (a standard vehicle for otic drops), if used over a long period of time, may cause an allergic dermatitis. (See box and Table 37–2.)

In the mild stage of external otitis, the patient will generally not require a narcotic, and aspirin and similar analgesics will suffice. Heat may relieve discomfort. In the severe stage of external otitis when the patient's ear canal is swollen and fever and pain are present, additional treatment with systemic antibiotics such as penicillin, erythromycin, or ampicillin is advisable. These medications should be used in full dosage for 10 days. Cultures are an important guide to treatment. Pain in the severe stage of acute external otitis is severe, and aspirin alone is not sufficient. Stronger analgesics are necessary. The otic wick is generally removed in 24 to 48 hours when placed. If the canal will allow drops to reach the most medial portion of the ear canal and the eardrum, the wick can be left out. However, if the canal is still significantly swollen, the canal should be gently cleaned, the wick replaced, and the drops continued. Patients with acute external otitis may require examination and general cleaning daily or every other day until the infection subsides. Occasionally, an allergic reaction may cause or complicate external otitis. Allergic reactions may occur from the drops or from preparations such as nail polish, hair dye, hairspray, or permanent wave lotion. Dermatitis from these substances may be baffling until one thinks about their use. The condition clears rapidly when the offending agent is discontinued.

In the more chronic forms of external otitis, careful cleansing of the ear, as in acute forms, is absolutely essential as the first step in treatment. It is usually done by repeatedly wiping the canal

---

**STEPS IN TREATMENT OF EXTERNAL OTITIS**

1. Clean ear: use suction and dry swabbing (with magnification if possible).
2. Visualize the canal and tympanic membrane.
3. Swab the canal with antibiotic, antifungal, or antiseptic solution.
4. Prescribe the use of antibiotic ear drops 3–4 times/day. If the canal is so swollen that drops can't penetrate, place cotton or Merocel wick (to remain in ear 24–48 hr).
5. Use systemic antibiotics only if the nodes are increased in size, and/or fever occurs. If antibiotics are required, obtain culture.
6. Use analgesics as needed (significant narcotic medications may be needed).
7. Recheck and repeat process every 24–72 hr as necessary until the canal clears (remove and replace wick if necessary).
8. Culture if ear not improved in 48 hr or if problem is recurrent.

**TABLE 37–2.**

Commonly Used Ear Drops and Their Composition

| Preparation | Antiinfective Component | Antiinflammatory Component | Other Ingredients |
|---|---|---|---|
| Acetic acid 2% | Acetic acid | | 70% alcohol |
| Chloromycetin Otic | Chloremphenicol | | Propylene glycol |
| Ciprofloxacin Opthalmic Drops | Ciprofloxacin | | Benzethonium chloride |
| Coly-mycin S Otic | Colistin | Hydrocortisone | Thorzonium bromide |
| | Neomycin | | Acetic acid |
| | | | Thimerosal |
| | | | Polysorbate 80 |
| Cortisporin Otic Solution | Neomycin | Hydrocortisone | Cupric sulfate |
| | Polymyxin B | | Glycerin |
| | | | Propylene glycol |
| | | | Potassium metabisulfite |
| Cortisporin Otic Suspension | Neomycin | Hydrocortisone | Cetyl alcohol |
| | Polymyxin B | | Propylene glycol |
| | | | Polysorbate 80 |
| | | | Thimerosal |
| Cresylate Solution | M-cresyl acetate | | Propylene glycol |
| | | | Isopropenol |
| | | | Chlorabutanol |
| | | | Benzyl alcohol |
| | | | Castor oil |
| Diprosone Lotion | None | Betamethasone | Isopropyl alcohol |
| | | | Carbomer 934P |
| Fungizone Lotion | Amphotericin B | | Propylene glycol |
| Garamycin Ophthalmic Solution | Gentamicin | | Benzalkonium chloride |
| | | | NaCl solution |
| Lotrimin | Clotrimazole | None | Propylene glycol |
| Otic Domeboro | Acetic acid | | Aluminum acetate |
| Otic Tridesilon Solution | Acetic acid | Desonide | Propylene glycol |
| Otobiotic Otic Solution | Polymyxin B | Hydrocortisone | Propylene glycol |
| Otocort Solution | Neomycin | Hydrocortisone | Propylene glycol |
| | Polymyxin B | | Glycerin |
| | | | Potassium meta-bisulfite |
| Pyocidin-Otic Solution | Polymyxin B | Hydrocortisone | Propylene glycol |
| VōSol HC Otic Solution | Acetic acid | Hydrocortisone | Propylene glycol diacetate |
| | | | Benzethonium chloride |
| VōSol Otic Solution | Acetic acid | | Propylene glycol diacetate |

with cotton applicators, often with ointment. Special care should be given to the inferior tympanic sulcus, just external to the annulus, because discharge and debris may delay healing. When the chronic form of external otitis is caused by infection, antibiotic ointments containing neomycin, polymyxin, or colistin, with or without hydrocortisone, may be used locally three times daily for a week or sometimes longer. If the proper drops are being used, generally the ear should respond and clear within a week.

Ointments and other medications that do not contain antibiotics are also effective, particularly when the external otitis is caused by dermatosis rather than infection (Fig. 37–4). A good prescription follows.

| Rx: | Phenol | 0.9 g |
|---|---|---|
| | Salicylic acid | 0.9 g |
| | Precipitated sulfur | 0.9 g |
| | Petrolatum q.s. ad. | 30.0 g |

Sig. Apply to ear canals once or twice daily.

This ointment, a mild exfoliating agent and antipruritic, may be used for an indefinite period or until the condition clears. Sometimes, however, it is impossible to cure chronic external otitis, and the condition improves or appears to improve but

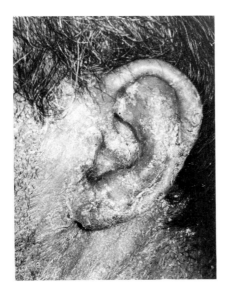

**FIG 37–4.**
Chronic scaling in external otitis associated with seborrheic dermatitis.

recurs later. Patients should be taught how to apply ear ointments or drops. Commercially prepared applicators are generally too large. The most important single treatment in chronic external otitis is meticulous removal of all debris from the ear canal.

### Fungal Infections

Fungal infections of the ear canal, common in the tropics, also occur in temperate climates. It is rare to see a pure fungal infection. One distinguishing factor between fungal and bacterial infections is that in fungal infections intense itching is the primary complaint. If the infection is mixed, pain usually accompanies the itching. Fungal infections in the external ear are usually easy to diagnose even without culture techniques, since the mycelia and hyphae of the fungal growth can be readily seen with the operating microscope under 6- to 10-power magnification.

The most common fungi affecting the ear are *A. niger*, *C. albicans*, and other yeastlike fungi. *A. niger* forms a black or grayish blotting-paper–like mass in the ear canal, and when this is removed, the underlying epithelium appears hyperemic and edematous and often denuded. Not all fungal infections of the ear canal produce symptoms, since many times the growth is sapro-

phytic. It is simply a formation found on wax or other debris in the ear and does not invade tissue. Management consists of very careful cleansing of the ear and application of an exfoliating agent such as that described in the previous section or 2% salicylic acid in alcohol. Drops of 25% mcresyl acetate, 0.5% acetic acid (Cresylate) in the ear, three times daily, are effective. Ointments and creams containing nystatin, such as Mycolog (with neomycin, gramicidin, and steroid), or Mycostatin ointment and creams are available as treatment for *Candida* organisms. Amphotericin B (Fungizone) is effective and available as a cream, ointment, or lotion. For infections not responding to nystatin, a 1% solution of thymol in ethyl alcohol can be effective. It is usually applied on a cotton wick, left in place in the ear canal several hours, and then replaced. Gentian violet (2%) in 95% alcohol is often useful. Table 37–3 lists commonly used antifungal lotions and drops. Again, frequent cleansing, every day to every other day, speeds the recovery process and allows the drops and medications to be effective. Wicks are seldom necessary in a predominantly fungal infection.

Surgical treatment is rarely indicated in chronic external otitis but can be effective in selective cases. When the patient has had external otitis for years, the ear canal can become virtually closed by swollen, fibrous epithelium. With failure by medical treatment, excision of the epithelium with application of split-thickness skin grafts are indicated. The surgeon generally enlarges the cartilaginous and bony meatus at the same time.

### Furunculosis

Furunculosis is a type of localized external otitis located in the outer half of the ear canal where there are gland and hair follicles that may become infected. Even a small furuncle causes pain until it breaks spontaneously or is incised. Symptoms and findings are similar to those of acute external otitis except that the furunculosis is more localized and the canal may not be moist or draining. Osteomas of the ear canal can sometimes be mistaken for furuncles, but osteomas are neither tender nor red. Also, they occur in the osseous rather than cartilaginous ear canal. If the furuncle is opened, the apex is incised. In some cases, gen-

**TABLE 37–3.**

Commonly Used Antifungal Drops and Lotions

| Preparation | Antifungal Component | Anti-inflammatory Component | Other Ingredients |
| --- | --- | --- | --- |
| Fungizone lotion | Amphotericin B | None | Thimerosal<br>Titanium dioxide<br>Propylene glycol<br>Cetyl alcohol |
| Lotrimin lotion | Clotrimazole | None | Sorbitan monosterate<br>Polysorbate 60<br>Cetyl alcohol |
| Lotrisone cream | Clotrimazole | Betamethasone | Mineral oil<br>White petrolatum<br>Cetearyl alcohol<br>Cetareth-30<br>Propylene glycol<br>Sodium phosphate<br>  monobasic<br>Phosphoric acid<br>Benzyl alcohol |
| Fungoid solution | Cetyl pyridinium chloride<br>Triacetin<br>Chloroxylenol | None | Oil base |
| Mycolog II | Nystatin | Triamcinolone | Aluminum hydroxide<br>Polyethylene glycol<br>  monosterate<br>Sorbic acid<br>Propylene glycol |
| Tinactin Solution | Tolnaftate | None | |
| Vioformhydrocortisone lotion | Cloquinol | Hydrocortisone | Propylene glycol<br>Polysorbate 60<br>Cetyl alcohol |
| Vioform cream | Cloquinol | None | Glycerin<br>Cetyl alcohol |
| Cresylate solution | m-Cresyl acetate | None | Propylene glycol<br>Isopropinol<br>Chlorobutanol<br>Benzyl alcohol<br>Castor oil |

eral anesthesia may be required. In early stages, ear wicks moistened with Burow's solution may be inserted to relieve pain. Local heat also affords some relief. Narcotics may be required. Antibiotics are given systemically, particularly if there is fever or cellulitis of the adjacent tissue. Because most furuncles in the ear are secondary to *Staphylococcus* infection, dicloxacillin or other antistaphylococcal agents are the antibiotics of choice.

## Perichondritis

Perichondritis of the auricle can be a serious disorder, usually secondary to *Pseudomonas* in-fection. It frequently follows external otitis, trauma, or surgery. Initially, there are redness, heat, and swelling of the auricle, which rapidly becomes painful (Fig. 37–5). There is often postauricular adenopathy. The ear may feel edematous and boggy. Rapid institution of treatment is essential, with antibiotics, including carbenicillin, ticarcillin, recent generation cephalosporins (ceftazidime), or ciprofloxacin, directed against the *Pseudomonas* organisms. If the symptoms are significant at all, the patient should be hospitalized and cultures taken. Topical treatment is generally ineffective, although if there is a weeping external otitis associated, hydroscopic solutions such as Burow's are helpful. Appearance of fluc-

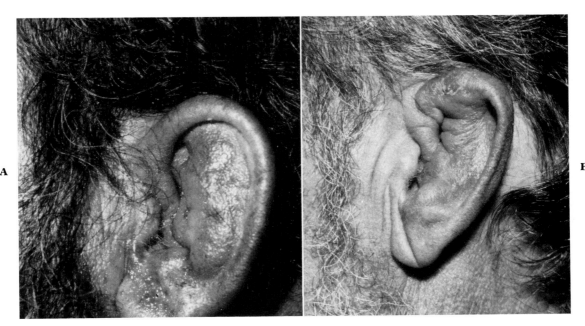

**FIG 37–5.**
**A,** acute extensive perichondritis of ear. **B,** scarring and deformity of ear secondary to perichondritis.

tuation merits incision and drainage and removal of necrotic cartilage. When necrotic cartilage is removed, the prognosis for a good cosmetic result is poor.

### Herpes Zoster Oticus

Herpes zoster oticus is a specific viral infection affecting the geniculate ganglion and nuclei of the seventh and eighth cranial nerves. It may produce vesicles in the external canal. They rupture to leave crusting in the posterior aspect of the ear canal, posterior aspect of the drumhead, or the concha and external ear. This disorder is characterized by severe ear pain; decreased lacrimation, salivation, and taste; and seventh nerve paralysis. There may, in addition, be neurosensory hearing loss and vertigo. The treatment is symptomatic at this stage, and antibiotic eardrops may relieve some discomfort.

### Aural Polyps

Aural polyps appear in the depth of the canal, are almost always covered with purulent discharge, and bleed easily. Larger polyps may be visible at the external auditory meatus (Fig. 37–6). The polyp, although it is not basically an

external ear infection, may arise from the external canal or from the middle ear and generally consists of granulation tissue. Polyps composed of granulation tissue are usually covered by squamous epithelium, but they still look redder and bleed much more easily than do mucosal polyps. In either case, polyp formation indicates chronicity of infection. The symptoms are a foul, purulent discharge and partial deafness if the polyp arises from the middle ear or obstructs the ear canal. Bleeding will frequently occur. The examiner must determine whether the polyp arises from the epithelium of the ear canal or protrudes into the canal through perforation of the tympanic membrane. The ear canal should be carefully cleaned by wiping, gentle suction, or irrigation. When the polyp can be seen more clearly, it may be moved gently with the probe to determine its relationship to the eardrum. Often the polyp fills the perforation so completely that an opening cannot be readily demonstrated. Treatment of the polyp is to remove it near its base with a small cup forcep or wire snare (Fig. 37–7). The maneuver invariably causes annoying bleeding, which may be controlled by packing or epinephrine, 1:1000, on a cotton pledget. It is best not to avulse the polyp, particularly if it comes from perforation of the posterior-superior quadrant because there is dan-

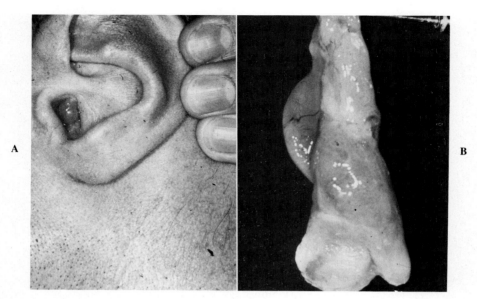

**FIG 37–6.**
**A,** an aural polyp attached to the promontory of the middle ear. There was a tympanic perforation through which the polyp hung. The polyp was bathed in foul pus. Chronic mastoiditis was also present. **B,** same polyp as shown in **A.**

ger of disturbing the stapes, facial nerve, or ossicular chain. Antibiotic eardrops are effective in reducing the associated infection. Polyps arising from the external canal heal rapidly after treatment because there is generally no underlying bone disease. Polyps arising from the middle ear are often secondary to chronic mastoiditis or chronic otitis media.

## TYMPANIC MEMBRANE

The tympanic membrane may be regarded as a translucent window through which the middle ear can be viewed (Fig. 37–8). With the exception of the fixation of the stapedial footplate and the oval window (otosclerosis) and the rare disarticulation of the middle ear ossicles, virtually all diseases of

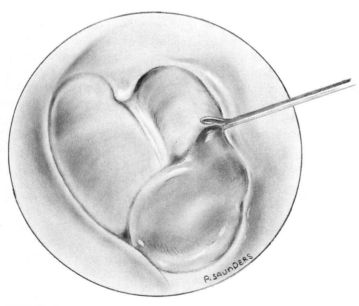

**FIG 37–7.**
Polyp being grasped with a middle ear forceps.

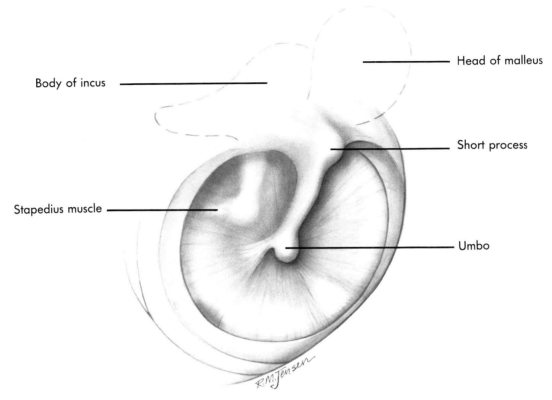

**FIG 37-8.**
Demonstration of right tympanic membrane, landmarks, and relative positions of medial structures.

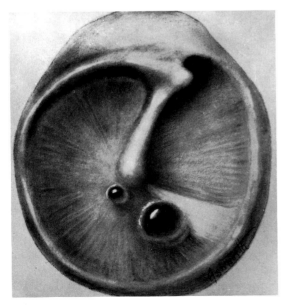

**FIG 37-9.**
Myringitis bullosa. These small vesicles are seen in viral infection at times and may also be present in herpes zoster oticus.

the middle ear reflect their presence by alterations in the position, color, and integrity of the tympanic membrane. Inflammatory change within layers of the tympanic membrane may cause vesicles to form (Fig. 37-9). Even in otosclerosis there may be a faint pink blush in the promontory that shines through the membrane. In serous otitis media, for example, the drumhead is almost always retracted and dull, often amber in color. Sometimes, an air/fluid level can be seen, or there may be bubbles of air in the middle ear fluid (Fig. 37-10). In purulent otitis media, pus under pressure pushes the drumhead outward, causing it to bulge. The usual landmarks either become faint or cannot be seen at all. Middle ear adhesions can cause irregular retraction, or the drumhead may be plastered onto the promontory medially. Cholesteatoma in the mastoid or epitympanum is often associated with tympanic perforation and a foul discharge. Rarely, a cholesteatoma can be seen through an intact drum. In that case, the tympanic membrane looks white and full but has more localized bulging than that caused by otitis

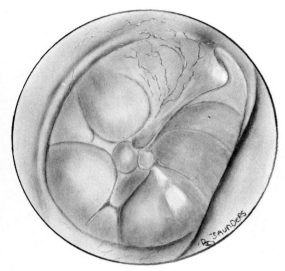

**FIG 37–10.**
Bubbles of air in serous otitis media. The bubbles move about when the examiner tilts the patient's head or exerts pressure against the drumhead with a pneumatic otoscope.

media. Also, palpation of the drumhead may elicit the sensation of probing a doughy mass, as if solid rather than liquid were filling the middle ear. Proper diagnosis of middle ear and mastoid disease depends on good visualization of the tympanic membrane, and to that end every effort should be made to clean the ear canal and the surface of the drum.

### Anesthesia

Because the outer layer of squamous epithelium is derived from skin that is not mucous membrane, customary methods of obtaining topical anesthesia for mucous membrane surfaces are useless. Solutions of cocaine, procaine, or lidocaine (Xylocaine), which afford excellent anesthesia for mucous membranes or denuded skin, are completely ineffective when applied to the intact eardrum.

Topical anesthesia to the tympanic membrane can be partially obtained by using Bonain's solution, which is a combination of phenol, cocaine, and menthol, or a saturated solution phenol. A better topical anesthetic can be obtained in the uninflamed tympanic membrane by iontophoresis using a 1:1 mixture of lidocaine and adrenaline. Anesthesia of the ear canal and tympanic mem-

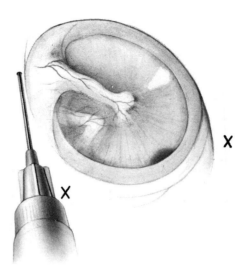

**FIG 37–11.**
Local anesthetic block of the ear canal.

brane is most effectively produced, however, by injecting a small quantity (1 to 2 cc) of local anesthetic such as lidocaine or procaine hydrochloride into the skin of the cartilaginous external canal at several points (Fig. 37–11). A fine gauged needle with short bevel is necessary.

### Features Affecting Appearance of the Tympanic Membrane

Tympanosclerosis is a disorder of the middle ear and tympanic membrane that results as the aftermath of long-standing inflammatory disease (Fig. 37–12). Long after purulent otitis media is cleared and the tympanic perforation is healed, deposits of hyaline material may be seen in the tympanic membrane. They may appear dead white or ashen grey and vary from a few indistinct flecks to large, irregular, dense plaques. Unless they are large and therefore affect the mobility of the drumhead, they have no appreciable effect on hearing. In the middle ear, however, the same deposits may seriously affect hearing, since they are prone to form around the footplate of the stapes, locking it into place. In the epitympanum, tympanosclerosis may form about the heads of the incus and malleus, fixing them. In either case, the mobility of the ossicular chain is impaired and hearing is reduced accordingly. When one is considering surgical procedures to repair a defect in the drumhead and sees a heavy white deposit of

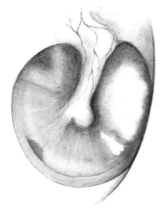

**FIG 37–12.**
Tympanosclerosis involving tympanic membrane.

tissue in the remaining portions of the drum, one should suspect that the ossicles may be similarly affected.

### Healed Perforations

Perforated tympanic membranes usually heal. Generally, healing takes place by regrowth of the inner and outer epithelial layers. Often, the fibrous layer fails to proliferate; thus the healed area is thinner, more transparent, and more flaccid than the remainder of the eardrum. The healed portion moves in and out more readily than usual when alternating positive and negative pressures are produced in the ear canal with the pneumatic otoscope. In effect, the patient acquires a second-

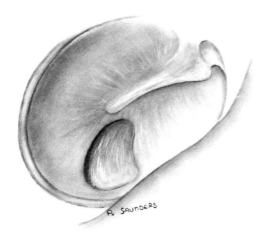

**FIG 37–13.**
Healed perforation. The healed area is often thinner, more flaccid, and more transparent than the rest of the eardrum.

ary flaccid membrane. This can be confused with a perforation by the examiner (Fig. 37–13).

### Tympanic Membrane Perforations

Tympanic membrane perforations will be discussed in the section on chronic ear diseases.

### External Otitis Involving the Tympanic Membrane

Localized infections in the ear canal such as furuncles do not affect the drumhead, but a generalized external otitis, either acute or chronic, may change its appearance. The outer layer of the eardrum is a continuation of the squamous epithelium lining the external canal. Therefore, it is subject to the same disorders. In patients with chronic external otitis, the eardrum may look dull red or even thickened or leathery. It is less sensitive than normal in these cases. Patients with chronic external otitis actually enjoy having the ear canal and drumhead cleaned, whereas normal patients or patients with acute early external otitis find this procedure unpleasant or painful.

### Granulation Tissue on the Tympanic Membrane

Granulation tissue present in the general region of the eardrum usually indicates that the tympanic membrane has been perforated and that this tissue is arising from the middle ear, protruding through the remaining membrane. Sometimes, however, granulations actually result from inflammation of the squamous epithelium of the drumhead itself. Careful examination may disclose a pinhole perforation. If the drumhead is not associated with middle ear infection, treatment consists of removal with small forceps. The base is cauterized with silver nitrate, and antibiotic eardrops are instilled. Treatment is usually successful in these circumstances.

## Myringotomy

Incision of tympanic membrane is called myringotomy. Draining fluid from the middle ear, whether by incision or needle aspiration, is called paracentesis. Instruments needed for myringotomy are a very sharp knife and an aural speculum. Myringotomy is best performed posteriorly and inferiorly where the drumhead can be readily seen and where there are no ossicles to be injured (Fig. 37–14). The membrane should not be excised above the line connecting the 9 and 3 o'clock positions (Fig. 37–15). If the incision is too deep, the mucosal covering of the promontory may be cut. Although pain and bleeding ensue, the mistake is not serious. In extremely rare instances, there may be a high-lying jugular bulb that could be injured by the myringotomy. Before the advent of antibiotics, it was common practice to open the tympanic membrane as widely as possible, often sweeping through a wide arc from back to front. Today, in most patients with suppurative otitis media, a generous incision is unnecessary because antibiotics are usually given concomitantly and greatly reduce the amount and duration of discharge. Nevertheless, in patients in whom a myringotomy is done for purulent otitis, an incision larger than mere needle puncture should be made. A smaller opening is sufficient when serous or mucoid material is aspirated from the middle ear in patients with serous otitis. Needle paracentesis in such cases can be performed with a short-bevel, 20-gauge needle and a 2-mm syringe.

## INFECTIONS AND DISEASE OF THE MIDDLE EAR AND MASTOID

One should realize that almost all inflammation and infection of the middle ear and mastoid are an extension of infection from the nose and nasopharynx. Exceptions are those secondary to trauma and tumor. Almost all ear disease is the result of poor or inadequate eustachian tube function. Any management of ear disease is thus dependent primarily on improving eustachian tube function. The most common causes of eustachian tube obstruction are:

1. Acute upper respiratory infection
2. Allergy
3. Enlarged adenoids
4. Chronic sinusitis
5. Failure of physiologic opening in the eustachian tube with palatal maldevelopment (for example, submucous cleft of the palate, neurologic disease)
6. Tumor
7. Recurrent suppurative otitis or chronic suppurative otitis media

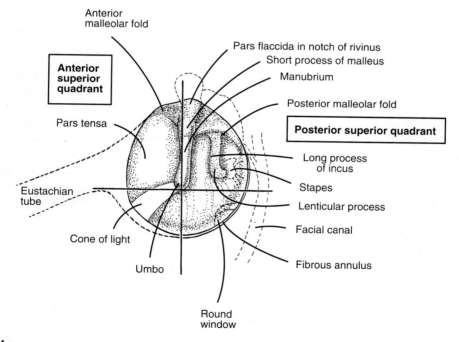

**FIG 37–14.**
Relationships of important middle ear structures to be considered in myringotomy. Often the incudostapedial joint can be seen dimly through the intact tympanic membrane. (Drawing is of left ear.) (From Saunders WH, Paparella MM: *Atlas of ear surgery,* ed 2, St Louis, 1971, Mosby–Year Book. Used by permission.)

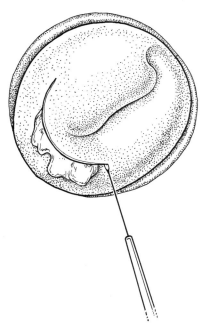

**FIG 37–15.**
Technique of myringotomy (right ear).

8. Systemic factors (for example, hypothyroidism, diabetes)
9. Ethnic factors (probably anatomic)

Eustachian tube obstruction results in the middle ear air being absorbed into the middle ear–capillary complex, thus creating a relative negative pressure compared with the atmospheric pressure on the outside of the drum. The eardrum then becomes retracted. A condition called aerotitis occurs in some people when the eustachian tube fails to open during descent of an airplane. Generally, symptoms of eustachian tube blockage are mild intermittent pain, mild hearing loss, and fullness in the ear. Examination generally would reveal a retracted tympanic membrane, although its color would be normal in the absence of any infection. Any treatment of acute eustachian tube blockage is directed toward forcing air up the eustachian tube and into the middle ear. Inflation of the eustachian tube by the Valsalva maneuver or by blowing against pressure or swallowing may help. However, the tube should never be inflated while the nasopharynx is infected because of the danger of causing otitis media. In the case of aerotitis, however, a myringotomy is often necessary because of pain.

## Acute Suppurative Otitis Media

Acute otitis media is one of the most common infections of childhood. Careful statistical studies have shown that 60% to 70% of children have at least one episode of otitis media before their third birthday. Approximately one third of all children in the United States have had three or more such infections by the age of 3. The frequency of infection is much higher in children with cleft palates. Acute otitis generally accompanies any upper respiratory tract infection. It frequently is a complication of viral infections, such as the common cold, measles, or influenza.

### Symptoms
Initially, there may be a slight decrease in hearing or fullness in the ear. This is rapidly followed by mild pain and increasing pressure. Later, severe deep throbbing pain of the ear is a cardinal symptom, usually accompanied by an elevation in temperature as high as 104° or 105° F, particularly in infants and children. The pain is described as steady and boring. Infants and children tend not to sleep, and they cry and pull at their ears. There may be vomiting and diarrhea in young children. In adults, there may be complaints of vertigo. There are usually associated symptoms related to the upper respiratory infection. Examination will show a markedly infected tympanic membrane or a bulging tympanic membrane if the pressure is increased in the middle ear space. The landmarks are generally indistinct (Fig. 37–16). If the eardrum has ruptured, the pain and pressure will be relieved and examina-

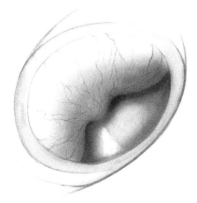

**FIG 37–16.**
Acute otitis media (right ear).

tion will show discharge in the canal. This is initially a bloody, serous fluid, but after a few hours it may become frankly purulent. The discharge may be pulsating. Hearing is reduced, and there may be pain to pressure over the mastoid antrum.

Various organisms have been reported to be involved in acute otitis media. It is believed that 50% to 75% of acute otitis is on a viral basis, at least initially. Bacteria usually found are *Haemophilus influenzae, Streptococcus pneumoniae,* β *Streptococcus,* and, infrequently, *S. aureus.* Until recently, it was thought that involvement with *Haemophilus* was infrequent above the age of 5, but changing bacterial patterns have demonstrated that *Haemophilus* is now the primary acute bacterial infection in children under the age of 10. In newborns and infants, *E. coli* is a predominant causative organism. Rarely, *Klebsiella, E. coli,* and *Bacteroides* species can produce an otitis media in children and adults.

### *Treatment*
Prompt antibiotic therapy hastens resolution of the infection. Amoxicillin or ampicillin is now considered the drug of choice for acute otitis media, particularly in children under the age of 10. If patients are allergic, secondary drugs include erythromycin, sulfonamides, and cephalosporin. Treatment with antibiotics should be for a full 10-day course and should be closely monitored by the physician. Resistant strains of *Haemophilus* are becoming common in some locales, and cultures may be necessary if response is not prompt.

Pain medication and decongestants may be used initially in the treatment of otitis media, but persistence of pain or fever for more than 24 to 48 hours suggests a complication or an unresolved infection and the patient should be reevaluated. Should the tympanic membrane rupture, clean cotton should be kept in the outer ear to prevent extension of the discharge. Ear drops are generally of no value. Ordinarily, the ear will drain purulent material for 2 to 3 days, and then the discharge will become scant and mucoid. It eventually should cease by the seventh day. When the eardrum ruptures, pain usually resolves within a few minutes. Reevaluation of the patient following the completion of therapy is critical in the long-term management of recurrent otitis media. Myringotomy, which was the primary mode of treatment for acute otitis media before the avail-

ability of antibiotics, is still indicated under the following circumstances:

1. Extreme toxicity or history of febrile convulsions
2. An immunologically compromised child
3. Failure of antibiotic therapy
4. Severe pain in a cooperative patient
5. Complications of acute otitis media

Myringotomy is usually performed to drain pus from the ear. The only instrument required is a myringotomy knife with a small pointed blade and long handle. A good light source is necessary, and this is used under magnification. The procedure may be performed with the use of general anesthesia, local anesthesia, or no anesthesia at all. An inflamed eardrum is generally more painful than a normal eardrum and does require some type of anesthesia. A small piece of cotton moistened with Bonain's solution against the tympanic membrane and left in place approximately 5 minutes will give some anesthesia. Iontophoresis using lidocaine and epinephrine is useful in anesthesia of the tympanic membrane, but it is less effective in the acutely inflamed ear. General anesthesia may be used in adult patients or in older children who require myringotomy; however, local block with lidocaine is generally preferred.

There are generally two types of myringotomy: circumferential and radial. Circumferential myringotomy allows wide drainage and is used to remove fluid or pus under pressure and acute infections (Fig. 37–17). The incision is begun by placing the knife against the eardrum, posteriorly and superiorly below the malleolus. One should be careful to avoid injury to the medial wall and middle ear. The knife is swept downward and forward with the blade 2 to 3 mm away from the drum margin. It ends in an anterior-inferior position. A cotton pledget will absorb the blood and fluid that is released. A radial myringotomy uses a smaller, stab type of incision but is sufficient to release serum from the middle ear and is most useful for noninfected ears.

## Complications of Acute Otitis Media
### *Secretory Otitis Media (Serous Otitis Media)*
Secretory otitis media is one of the main causes of hearing loss in children and may follow

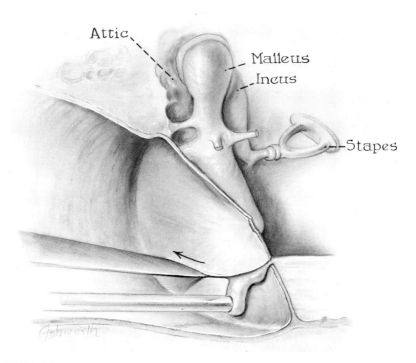

**FIG 37–17**.
Type of myringotomy used for acute suppurative otitis media. (See also Fig. 37-15).

acute otitis media, although not necessarily. It may be secondary to such conditions as allergy, infection, barotrauma, and adenoid enlargement. In fact, any cause of eustachian tube dysfunction is a factor in the development of serous otitis. Diagnosis is made on the basis of history and examination. History is relatively noncontributory, except if there is antecedent infection trauma or hearing loss. This may not be brought to the attention of the parents in young children. Examination will reveal one of several changes in the eardrum.

**Retraction of the Tympanic Membrane.** Tympanic membrane retraction is best observed as foreshortening of the malleus on otoscopy and the fact that the short process appears much more prominent. The tympanic membrane appears to be tented over the short process of the malleus (Fig. 37–18).

**Discoloration of the Tympanic Membrane.** The entire drum may be amber colored or a dull gray. In fact, almost any color or appearance can be represented in serous otitis. Occasionally, the lower half of the drum may be amber colored and the upper half normal, suggesting the presence of a transudate in the middle ear. Occasionally, a meniscus may be seen, indicative of fluid level. If blood is present in the middle ear (which occasionally occurs), the eardrum will appear blue or black. Air bubbles can be seen through the drum, giving it a ground-glass appearance.

**Immobility of the Tympanic Membrane.** The tympanic membrane is relatively immobile. This is perhaps the most reliable of all the physical findings and demonstrates the presence of negative pressure in the middle ear along with the fluid. Hearing testing will demonstrate a conductive loss (Fig. 37–19). The Weber test will lateralize to the side of the lesion (conductive loss), and the Rinne test will be negative (bone conduction greater than air conduction). Audiometric studies may demonstrate a conductive hearing loss if the child is old enough to perform the test. It is with possible serous otitis media in the very young that tympanometry is of value. The response most likely in serous otitis would be a type B tympanogram or occasionally a type C

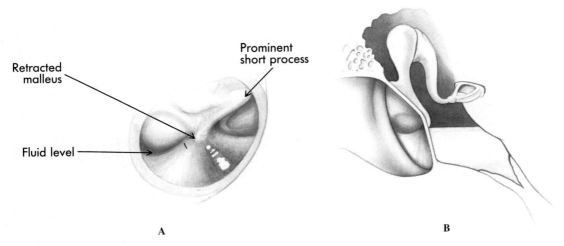

A                                                      B

**FIG 37–18.**
**A,** several features of serous otitis media are demonstrated: (1) marked prominence of the short process of the malleus with tympanic membrane retraction: (2) foreshortening of the malleus; (3) discoloration of tympanic membrane and fluid level. **B,** fluid level demonstrated. The tympanic membrane would not move on pneumootoscopy.

tympanogram in which the ear demonstrates a significant negative pressure. Although tympanometry does not replace pneumootoscopy as a diagnostic tool, it is useful, particularly in small infants and young children, in that it is a simple procedure, is atraumatic, and can be accomplished in a brief period of time. The hearing loss in children with secretory otitis is often mild enough to go undetected until routine testing is done when the child enters school at the age of 5

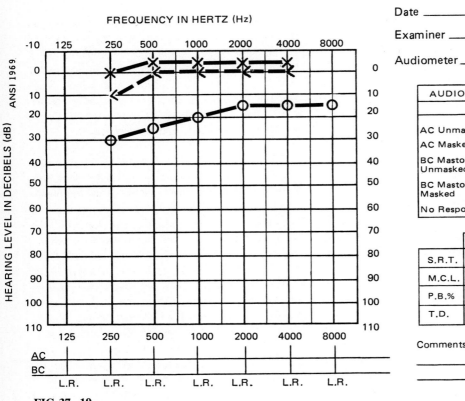

**FIG 37–19.**
Unilateral right-sided serous otitis.

or 6. Studies of acute infections have demonstrated that 70% of children will retain a middle ear effusion for at least 2 weeks following an acute ear infection. Forty percent will still have effusion after 1 month, and 20% for longer than 2 months. In some cases, the fluid contains antibiotic-resistant bacteria. For this reason, careful follow-up is indicated for any child or adult who has persistent serous otitis.

### Recurrent Otitis Media of Infancy

One of the most difficult problems in the treatment of otitis media is the child who develops recurrent episodes five or six times a year. This is particularly a problem in the infant or the child under the age of 1. Again, in these circumstances the causes of eustachian tube dysfunction must be carefully investigated. One must always consider the possibility of recurrent sinusitis in youngsters with this condition. Careful evaluation for palatal insufficiency must be undertaken. A youngster with a cleft uvula or a submucous cleft is at high risk for recurrent infections. The history is usually one of recurrent episodes, one following another, starting in the fall and extending through the spring. The child may never develop a normal-appearing tympanic membrane during this period. When a child with multiple occurrences is seen, treatment should be directed at managing the underlying infection. A course of antibiotics should be extended to 14 to 21 days in an acute episode. Nasal decongestants can be given with each upper respiratory infection. Certain precautions in feeding must be emphasized, particularly in the infant. Children should never be fed bottles while they are lying supine but should always be propped up. Some people have advocated stopping milk products and substituting soybean products because of the high incidence of milk allergies, particularly in youngsters who have been breast-fed. If these more conservative means of management do not break the cycle of recurrent infections, the use of prophylactic antibiotics is indicated. Studies have demonstrated that the use of low-dose sulfisoxazole (Gantrisin) or amoxicillin reduces the number of acute infections to one fourth the previous rate of infection. These drugs are usually given for 2 to 3 months continuously at one quarter to one half of the usual daily dose. If the child persists with recurrent infections or

breaks through the prophylactic therapy, myringotomy with a ventilation tube is the final choice of therapy. It must be remembered that placement of a ventilation tube is not done to allow drainage but to allow equalization of pressure between the middle ear space and the atmosphere and thus substitute for the nonfunctional or poorly functioning eustachian tube.

### Chronic Serous Otitis Media

Chronic serous effusion of the middle ear presents a serious threat to hearing if untreated. Although chronic serous otitis media has been recognized for many years, the incidence has markedly increased in the past 40 years. It is generally secondary to factors previously mentioned, including overgrowth of lymphoid tissue in the nasopharynx, chronic sinus infections, and allergy of the nose and nasopharynx. Lowered resistance to infection from a variety of causes may contribute to middle ear effusion. However, inadequate treatment of acute or subacute suppurative otitis media is an important factor in the increasing incidence of chronic serous otitis media. Treatment of acute otitis media with antibiotics for only 24 to 48 hours may create a low-grade, smoldering infection that may occur repeatedly until a thick mucoid effusion remains in the middle ear for weeks or months. In addition, recent studies indicate that children in day care have approximately a 10 times greater rate of recurrent otitis media or serous otitis media than children cared for at home. This may help explain the increased incidence of these disorders over the past 15 years.

The symptoms of chronic secretory otitis media are generally minimal. Hearing loss is characterized by fluctuation, generally down, with acute respiratory infection. Patients may complain of fullness or heaviness in the head, and certain sounds may be distorted. There is no pain, no fever, and no discharge from the ear. Examination of the ear in long-standing serous otitis may be deceiving. Minimal changes occur in the tympanic membrane. The drum may be pearly-gray in color, with only minimal dullness of the appearance on minimal retraction. Limitation of motion on tympanometry and pneumootoscopy is the most useful physical finding. Audiometric studies are generally diagnostic, showing conductive hearing loss. A history of fluctuating hearing loss suspected in a child by a parent or teacher should immediately make the physician think of middle ear effusion. This calls for an audiogram, even though the eardrum may appear normal. The surgical treatment of serous otitis media is discussed in Chapter 40.

Complications related to persistent chronic serous otitis media or secretory otitis media include development of cholesteatoma, perforation, fibrosis of the middle ear space, and tympanosclerosis, all of which may create a permanent hearing loss. For that reason, follow-up of patients with acute or chronic secretory otitis media is imperative.

Finally, the physician must remember that chronic serous otitis media in an adult may be caused by carcinoma of the nasopharynx. When unilateral effusion occurs in an adult, nasopharyngeal carcinoma should always be suspected and every possible diagnostic procedure used to prove or disprove its presence.

## Abnormal Patency of the Eustachian Tube

An abnormally patent eustachian tube may mimic symptoms of serous otitis. This occurs when there is loss of tissue about the eustachian tube orifice. One cause is recent severe loss of weight. The symptoms are otophony and fullness in the ear, which are relieved when the patient lies down. Patients can even hear themselves breathe and the too-free exchange of air along the tube is annoying. Insufflation of a four-to-one mixture of boric acid and salycilic acid powder into the tubal orifice is a useful diagnostic test, as well as temporary treatment. The use of SSKI will also cause hypertrophy of the secretory glands around the orifice of the eustachian tube and temporarily improve the patient's symptoms.

The method that produces a more lasting result is injection of polytetraflorylethylene paste into the anterior wall of the eustachian tube orifice. Although not always successful, it works well enough to be used for the occasional patient with persistent marked symptoms.

## Acute Mastoiditis

Acute mastoiditis was a common complication of acute otitis media before the advent of antibiotics. It is still seen in patients in whom otitis media has not been treated or has been inadequately treated. It occurs when infection has persisted in the middle ear or has been treated with an incorrect antibiotic. Classically, symptoms develop 10 to 14 days after an acute infection. They are manifested by a slowly increasing, thick, purulent discharge from the ear, usually recurrent after it had pretty well ceased. There is a dull, aching postauricular pain, most severe at night, and a low-grade fever of 99 to 100° F.

When acute mastoiditis is uncomplicated, examination demonstrates a copious, thick, foul-smelling, purulent discharge filling the external auditory canal. After the canal has been cleaned, the eardrum may appear dull, edematous, and thick, sometimes with a pulsatile discharge. Occasionally, the tympanic membrane may be intact when the mastoid infection has loculated itself from the middle ear. Pressure over the mastoid process produces a deep, dull bone tenderness. Firm pressure is generally necessary to demonstrate tenderness, in contrast to the light pressure required in acute external otitis. There may be sagging of the soft tissue of the auditory canal lateral to the drum and the ear may be pushed outward and downward (Fig. 37–20). Computed tomography of the temporal bone will confirm the diagnosis. Characteristic radiographic findings are clouding of the mastoid cells and decalcification of the bony walls between the cells with the breakdown of cellular structures (Fig. 37–21). Before the use of antibiotics, treatment almost always required an operation. Today, if only clouding of the mastoid air cells and early decalcification of bone are visible, high-dose antibiotics plus wide myringotomy may clear the disease. If destruction of bone has occurred, an operation will be necessary.

The operation for acute mastoiditis is a simple (complete) mastoidectomy and can be performed through either a postauricular or an end-aural incision (Fig. 37–22). Both incisions give large exposure over the mastoid cortex. The inner table of bone over the dura is left intact, and the middle ear is not disturbed. A myringotomy is performed to drain the middle ear. Antibiotics are continued postoperatively. The usual organism involved in acute mastoiditis is *S. pneumoniae*. Less frequently, acute mastoiditis is caused by *H. influenzae*. The relative rarity of *H. influenzae* as a cause of acute mastoiditis suggests that the disease secondary to *Haemophilus* infection is more mucosal

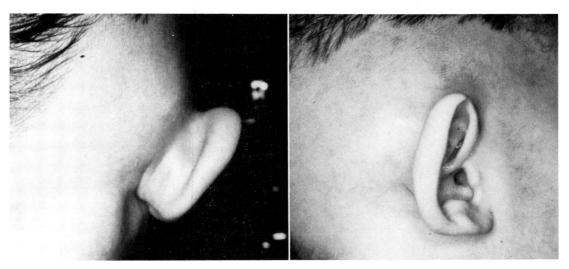

**FIG 37-20.**
Acute mastoiditis demonstrating the ear being pushed downward and forward by the subperiosteal abscess.

and less prone to develop bone destruction. The difficulty with diagnosis of acute mastoiditis occurs in patients without classic symptoms who have only a pulsating, dull discharge with minimal pain and systemic symptoms. In these cases, the patient has usually received some form of treatment, but the discharge is not completely resolved. Symptoms may recur several times over a period of months, and the bone destruction may not become clearly evident until 3 to 4 months after the acute infection. In these cases, a confirm-

ing CT scan is imperative. Generally, after the operation complete healing occurs in 7 to 10 days, and hearing is unaffected after resolution.

Complications of acute mastoiditis are caused by extension of infection from the mastoid to the contiguous structures. The complications take the following forms.

### Facial Nerve Injury

There may be erosion of the bone protecting the facial nerve in the middle ear space or mas-

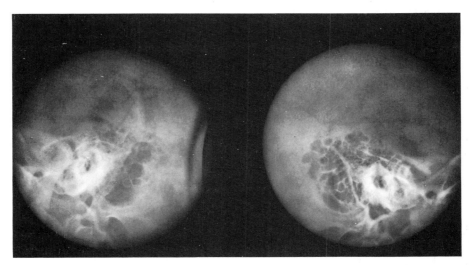

**FIG 37-21.**
Comparative study of the right and left mastoids. The x-ray film on the right shows normal cells. In the film on the left the cells are indistinct and clouded, and some intercellular walls have disappeared. This is typical of acute mastoiditis.

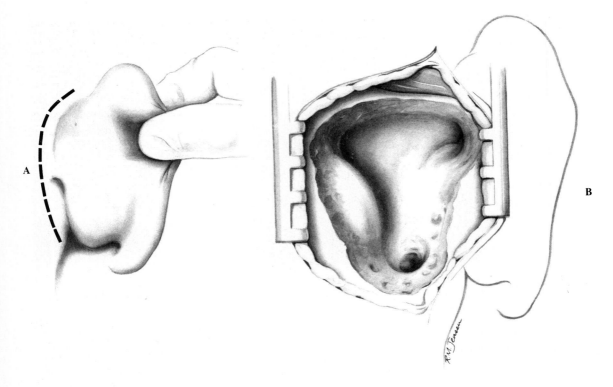

**FIG 37–22.**
**A,** postauricular mastoid incision. **B,** the cortex of the mastoid has been removed, demonstrating the posterior external canal wall, the sigmoid sinus curving posteriorly and the middle fossa superiorly. The ossicular chain and tympanum are unaffected by this procedure.

toid. Inflammation of the nerve then produces paralysis of the facial muscles. Differential diagnosis and management of facial paralysis are discussed in Chapter 43.

### Meningitis

Eighty percent of meningitis is secondary to otologic disease. It occurs by extension of infection, either blood borne or indirectly, through the inner table of the cortex into either the posterior fossa or middle cranial fossa through the tegmen. Symptoms and treatment of meningitis are the same as for meningitis from any other cause. The management of the ear abnormality follows treatment for meningitis.

### Brain Abscess

An extension of infection through the inner table may also cause an epidural or brain abscess involving the temporal bone or cerebellum. The diagnosis of epidural abscess is more difficult to establish than diagnosis of meningitis. Usually,

only a dull, persistent headache, recurring mild fever, and minor changes in sensorium are the symptoms. An abscess of the temporal lobe of the brain causes slowly increasing signs of an expanding intracranial lesion following a brief period of meningeal irritation. Papilledema is usually slight, and gross neurologic signs are infrequent, since the temporal lobe is a relatively silent neurologic area of the brain. By contrast, abscess of the cerebellum may produce ataxia, and papilledema is often severe. Coma may occur abruptly. When any of these symptoms or signs are associated with otitis media or previous otitis media or mastoiditis, neurosurgical consultation is imperative.

### Thrombosis of the Sigmoid Sinus

Thrombosis of the sigmoid sinus occurs when the infection spreads through the dura over the posterior fossa. An infected thrombus forms inside the sigmoid sinus. The thrombus may extend in retrograde fashion through the transverse sinus or distal to the jugular bulb. Such a thrombus is accompanied by a severe septicemia, with temperature spikes to 104 or 105° F being characteristic. There may be tenderness over the jugular vein in the neck and on the involved side. Treatment demands immediate hospitalization with intravenous antibiotics. Mastoidectomy and removal of the infected thrombus from the sigmoid sinus may be required. This is accomplished by removal of the inner table of the mastoid, incision of the outer dural layer of the sinus, and removal of the thrombus until free venous bleeding is obtained from both the superior and inferior cavities of the sinus. Often, to prevent embolism, the jugular vein has to be ligated, particularly if the thrombus has extended beyond the jugular bulb.

### Suppurative Labyrinthitis

Invasion of the internal ear by infection produces suppurative labyrinthitis. It is manifested by severe, whirling vertigo with nystagmus, nausea, vomiting, tinnitus, and sensorineural hearing loss. The symptoms persist for days to weeks. If the infection is untreated or neglected, it may extend through the labyrinth and cause meningitis. Treatment again consists of hospitalization, administration of high-dose antibiotics, and occasionally drainage of the labyrinth through the mastoid. Following a suppurative labyrinthitis, there is usually a total hearing loss and a nonfunctional labyrinth.

### Subperiosteal Abscess

When infection of the mastoid causes erosion to the outer cortex, a subperiosteal abscess is produced. This is often manifested in acute mastoiditis and is associated with temperature elevation and deep fluctuation of the soft tissue behind the ear. It generally forms slightly above the mastoid process. Rarely, erosion occurs through the medial aspect of the mastoid tip, causing abscess formation deep to the attachment of the sternocleidomastoid and digastric muscles and producing pain, swelling, and tenderness under the mastoid or between the mastoid tip and the mandible. This uncommon type of subperiosteal abscess is known as Bezold's abscess.

### Chronic Suppurative Otitis Media

The term *chronic suppurative otitis media* implies permanent perforation of the eardrum. Recurrent episodes of infection, even though frequent and occurring intermittently for years, are not considered to be chronic suppurative otitis media unless there is a permanent perforation of the eardrum.

Chronic infection of the middle ear is much more common in persons who have had ear disease in early childhood. Disease of the ear in infancy and early childhood may arrest the normal pneumatization of the mastoid (Fig. 37–23). It is possible that the same process alters the mucosa of the middle ear, making it more susceptible to recurrent infection than the normal ear. Most patients with chronic suppurative otitis media have small, undeveloped, and acellular mastoids that can be demonstrated on x-ray film (Fig. 37–24).

Many different bacteria may be associated with chronic suppurative otitis media. Some are virulent and others are common saprophytes. The appearance and odor of the discharge may be helpful in identifying certain bacteria. *P. aeruginosa* is a common invader and causes a greenish dis-

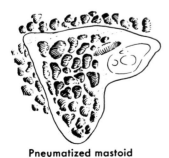
**Pneumatized mastoid**

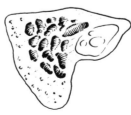
**Partially pneumatized mastoid**

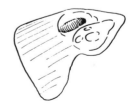
**Contracted (infantile or sclerotic) mastoid**

**FIG 37–23.**
Types of mastoid pneumatization. Otitis media in infancy or early childhood can arrest normal pneumatization at any stage.

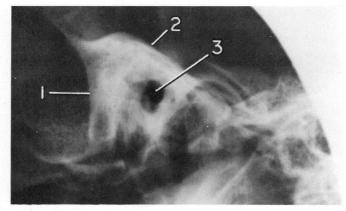

**FIG 37–24.**
X-ray film of an infantile type of temporal bone with no pneumatized cells. *1,* anterior wall of the sigmoid sinus. *2,* tegmen between the mastoid and the middle fossa. *3,* external auditory canal. (Compare with Fig. 37–21).

charge. *E. coli* may be introduced by finger contamination and has the characteristic odor of coliform bacilli. The *Proteus* bacilli cause a foul or fetid odor. Culture of the discharge is important. *Staphylococcus, Streptococcus,* gram-negative bacilli, and *Pneumococcus,* as well as diphtheroids, are commonly present. Most often a culture grows several different bacteria, and thus sensitivity studies should be performed. It should be recalled that antibiotics that are effective in vitro are not always effective in vivo, and repeat cultures may be necessary when the response to treatment is inadequate. When cholesteatoma is present, there is not totally satisfactory treatment for the discharge, and surgical treatment is mandatory.

Any otitis media that is virulent enough to destroy part of the eardrum or ossicles damages the middle ear to such an extent that chronic disease may follow. Scarlet fever and measles were common offenders before the use of antibiotics. This result is now much less frequent. Neglected otitis media or serous otitis media is the most common cause of chronic changes in the middle ear and tympanic membrane. Rare is the individual with good eustachian tube function who develops chronic suppurative otitis media.

In chronic otitis media, there are three basic types of perforations (Fig. 37–25). When the perforation does not involve the margin of the drum, it is considered to be a *central* perforation. The term *central* means that some eardrum remains at all points around the circumference of the perforation. When the anulus or the margin of the drum is destroyed, the perforation is called *marginal.* The distinction between central and marginal perforation and prognosis cannot be overemphasized. Central perforation generally indicates a more benign disease process than marginal perforation. Cholestea-

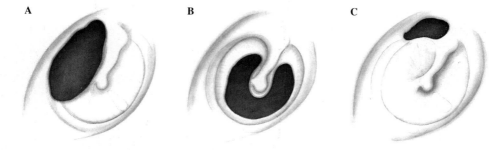

**FIG 37–25.**
Three common tympanic perforations. **A,** Posteriomarginal-perforation (hearing maybe poor). **B,** large central perforation around the handle of the malleus (hearing is usually poor). **C,** Attic perforation of Shrapnell's membrane (hearing is usually good). Cholesteatomas commonly occur in patients with a marginal perforation and are always present with attic perforation.

toma is much less likely to occur when there is only a central perforation, although this is not always the case in children. Marginal perforations usually occur in the posterior-superior quadrant. These perforations result most commonly from acute otitis media. Another type of marginal perforation is called an *attic perforation* or pars flaccida perforation. These perforations can lead into the epitympanum through the pars flaccida. Several theories as to the pathogenesis of these perforations include:

1. Eustachian tube obstruction or retraction, developing a pocket that eventually creates a perforation
2. Hyperactivity of the basal cell layer of the epidermis from negative pressure and long-standing inflammation that result in a secondary cholesteatoma
3. Possibility of primordial dermal arrest, which causes primary cholesteatoma

Exacerbations of chronic suppurative otitis media can occur secondary to eustachian tube dysfunction and the migration of microorganisms into the middle ear by way of the obstructed tube during upper respiratory infections and by way of the external auditory canal when water has gained access to the middle ear.

### Cholesteatoma

Cholesteatoma occurs most frequently when there is a marginal perforation of the eardrum or a pars flaccida perforation that allows squamous epithelium from the external auditory canal to grow to the middle ear (Fig. 37–26). As this epithelium grows, it desquamates, and the keratin cellular debris collects inside the middle ear (see Fig. 37–27). Gradual enlargement of the cholesteatoma leads to expansion into the mastoid antrum and epitympanum. After a number of years, bony destruction may cause erosion of important adjacent structures.

Pathologically, cholesteatomas are identical to epidermoid inclusion cysts. They occur in other parts of the skull when other inclusions have been left beneath the bony surface. They are more common in the ear, however, and more dangerous because of the contiguous structures they damage. Cholesteatomas tend to be recurrently infected, are characterized by foul, draining discharge, and produce white masses of debris. These can be seen in the middle ear, often associated with granulation tissue or polyps. As cholesteatomas tend to destroy ossicular bones, hearing loss may be severe.

The most common symptom of chronic suppurative otitis media with or without cholesteatoma is a painless discharge from the ear that may be foul smelling. There may be periods of days or weeks with no discharge, but discharge always recurs. It is frequently made worse by upper respiratory tract infection or by water in the ear. When discharge from an ear begins during an upper respiratory disorder and is unaccompanied by pain in

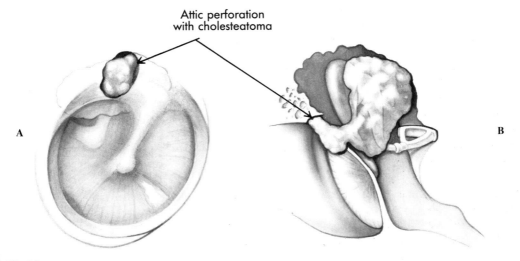

Attic perforation
with cholesteatoma

**A**

**B**

**FIG 37–26.**
**A,** lateral view of attic perforation and cholesteatoma extending around incus and epitympanum. **B,** attic perforation with visible cholesteatoma.

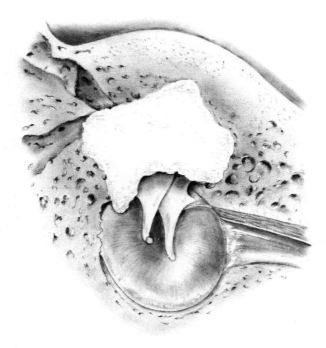

**FIG 37–27.**
Cholesteatoma viewed from the medial side of the left eardrum. Usually the surrounding bone is less pneumatized.

the ear, it can be assumed there is a permanent perforation of the drum. Occasionally, there is slight discomfort in the ear, but significant pain in the ear in patients with chronic suppurative otitis is a dangerous sign indicating possible complications. Hearing loss is almost always present, varying from a minimal loss when the perforation is small to as much as 50 to 60 db when the ossicles are destroyed or fixed by tympanosclerosis. The loss is usually of a conductive type, but in some patients one may expect a cochlear sensorineural component producing a mixed type of loss. The cochlear involvement is probably the result of the toxic effect of recurrent purulent material on the permeable round window membrane, causing a chemical change and end-organ disease. It is somewhat surprising that not all patients with chronic or even acute suppurative otitis media suffer cochlear damage.

Pain or vertigo is not expected to be present in uncomplicated chronic suppurative otitis media. The presence of either symptom may indicate an impending complication. Deep, persistent pain may indicate the presence of purulent pus under pressure. It may also indicate irritation of the dura or a brain abscess. Vertigo indicates irritation of

labyrinth or erosion of the bone on the labyrinth. Either symptom may be an indication for operative involvement.

In patients with cholesteatoma, particular types of vertigo merit discussion. Patients often become dizzy when the ear is cleaned or when pressure is placed against the canal. Most often, the vertigo in these patients is momentary, but it may be so extreme that the patient falls. Nausea and vomiting generally do not occur. Such a patient probably has a fistula of the horizontal semicircular canal. The fistula can be present through the bony labyrinth, exposing membranous labyrinth, but the patient does not have continuous vertigo. An easy examination that demonstrates such a fistula is compression of the ear of the external auditory canal, usually by inserting the tip of a Politzer bag into the external meatus and compressing a rubber bulb. Alternatively, a pneumatic otoscope may be used, or thumb pressure may be exerted on the external canal. When a fistula is present, compression of the ear causes an immediate conjugate deviation of the eyes toward the opposite side, a sudden feeling of whirling or propulsion, and a tendency to fall. This is called a positive fistula test. While performing the test, the physician should be careful not to let the patient fall out of the chair. A positive fistula test is an indication for surgery.

Many pathologic changes may occur in chronic suppurative disease of the middle ear. Perforations may vary from small, clean holes to complete destruction of the eardrum. Sometimes only the handle of the malleus remains. Granulation tissue or polyps may be present in the middle ear. Polyps may obscure the eardrum when it extrudes into the external auditory canal through the perforation. Cholesteatoma is generally seen as a shiny, white, or opalescent mass with squamous debris. The drum and its perforation may be obscured by purulent matter or crusted discharge. To adequately evaluate patients with chronic suppurative disease, the physician must carefully remove all pus and foreign matter by wiping or suctioning before examining the ear.

The discharge from chronic suppurative otitis media is variable but occasionally can be diagnostic if the drainage is secondary to eustachian tube obstruction with an anterior central perforation. In this case, the discharge is usually mucoid. It can occasionally be secondarily infected and is usually exacerbated by acute respiratory infections. The mucosa appears to be generally weepy and shiny. By contrast, if the discharge is secondary to a large central perforation without an attic or mastoid disease, usually mucopurulent exacerbations occur secondary to water contamination.

Discharge may be purulent but is usually odorless, and responds rapidly to treatment. If the discharge is secondary to cholesteatoma, it has a foul odor, suggesting tissue or bone necrosis. The purulent discharge is usually associated with granulation tissue or polyp formation.

To recapitulate, diagnosis of chronic suppurative otitis media is made on the basis of the history, which is demonstrated by a painless otorrhea and hearing loss. The development of pain, vertigo, or symptoms of the seventh cranial nerve suggests complication. The otologic examination demonstrates perforation with variable qualities of discharge and odor. The eustachian tube function is generally abnormal, and hearing is reduced.

Radiologic examination of the temporal bone of patients with chronic suppurative otitis media usually shows the mastoid to be small, without air cells. Sclerosis of bone evidenced by increased calcification is almost always present. Any areas of bone destruction demonstrate that the pathologic process has extended beyond the middle ear. Such areas of obstruction may be variable in size and extent. Their presence suggests an operation is necessary. If the cholesteatoma has extended into the mastoid, the radiologic studies will often show a sharp, defined, round area of radiolucency surrounded by sclerotic bone (Fig. 37–28). Temporal bone computed tomography (the study of choice) will demonstrate bone erosion, ossicular loss, and a soft tissue mass (Fig. 37–29). Blunt-

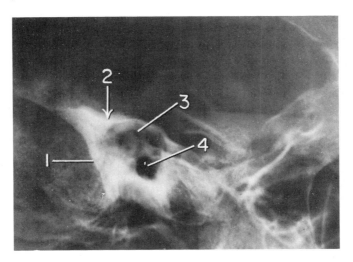

**FIG 37–28.**
X-ray film of the right temporal bone. The rounded radiolucency above and behind the external canal is destruction caused by a cholesteatoma. *1,* anterior margin of the sigmoid sinus. *2,* floor of the middle fossa. *3,* destruction by cholesteatoma. *4,* external auditory canal. The lumen of the superior semicircular canal can also be seen.

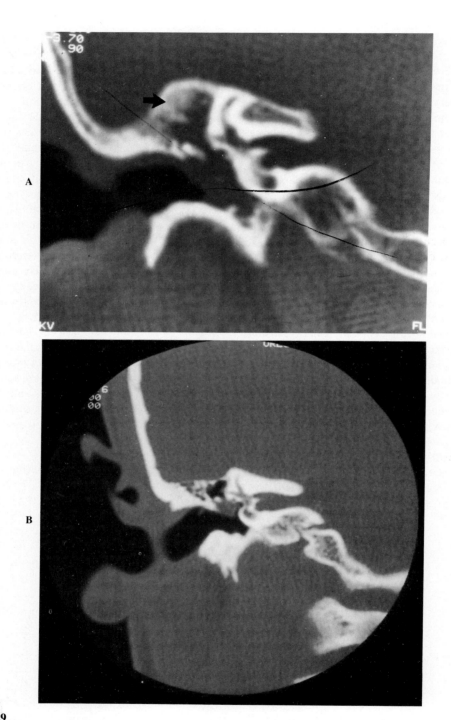

**FIG 37–29**.

**A,** extensive cholesteatoma involving the middle ear and mastoid. The *upper small arrow* delineates the margin of erosion of the mastoid air cells. The *lower arrow* demonstrates the mass within the middle ear space. Also demonstrated on this CT scan are the superior and horizontal canals with the neural pathways to the internal auditory meatus. **B,** coronal CT scan demonstrating cholesteatoma invading middle ear. Note erosion of scutum. This scan demonstrates the horizontal and superior canals and the seventh cranial nerve well.

ing of the scutum in the absence of previous surgery is indicative of cholesteatoma.

### Medical Treatment

Medical treatment of chronic suppurative otitis media consists of the use of local medications in the ear and eradication of any contributing factors creating a poorly functioning eustachian tube and infection in the middle ear. Careful removal of granulation tissue, polyps, and visible cholesteatoma will allow local medication to reach areas of infection more adequately. Aural irrigation using sterile saline solution at body temperature will do much to clean up disease in the middle ear and epitympanum. Sterile saline irrigations may be done twice daily in reliable individuals. The ear is dried as carefully as possible, and antibiotic drops are instilled. The usual organisms involved in the discharge of chronic suppurative otitis media are *Pseudomonas aeruginosa, P. vulgaris, Aerobacter, E. coli, S. aureus,* and *Bacteroides fragilis.* The gram negative organisms are generally susceptible to neomycin, colistin, polymyxin B, and an acidified vehicle. However, *Staphylococcus* and *Bacteroides* infections are not sensitive to these drugs and must be treated with either acidified solutions or chloramphenicol drops. The medications listed in the section on acute external otitis are useful in treating chronic suppurative ear disease. In addition to the ear drops listed, 2% acetic acid drops can be used. Almost all eardrops should be given as four drops, four times daily. Instillation of the ear medication is important, particularly in children. The involved ear should be up for 2 minutes after the placement of the eardrops to allow effective contact of the medication. Children may complain of burning or refuse the acidified ear preparations. In those cases, garamycin ophthalmic or ciprofloxacin ophthalmic drops can be given as they contain no acid and are less irritating. Occasionally, some patients with draining ear or perforation respond poorly to treatment with drops. This may be related to maceration caused by the drops or an allergy to the vehicle, particularly propylene glycol. In these patients, various powders may be useful.

Examples of powders used are as follows:

1. Sulfanilamide powder
   Sulfathiazole powder     Equal parts
   Zinc peroxide powder
   Sig. Blow powder in each ear 3 times daily.

2. Iodine                        0.3 g
   Solvent ether            4.0 ml
   Boric acid powder      30.0 g
   Dissolve iodine in ether. Mix with boric acid powder until dry. Sig. Blow in ear with powder blower 3 or 4 times daily.

3. Chloramphenicol powder
   Sig. Use powder from 20 capsules of chloramphenicol. Blow small quantity in the ear 3 times daily.

Systemic antibiotics have not proved helpful in chronic suppurative otitis media except when there is a superimposed acute process. When there is an acute exacerbation in a chronically infected ear, systemic antibiotics are essential. In the absence of pain or signs of complication, local treatment may be necessary for months or years.

### Surgical Treatment

Surgical treatment of chronic suppurative otitis media is based on the following two objectives: total removal of the disease, and reconstruction of hearing. A variety of surgical techniques have been devised and are possible, depending on the degree and extent of the disease.

**Tympanoplasty.** In patients with central perforations without cholesteatoma, tympanoplasty or reconstruction of the tympanic membrane and ossicular chain is the procedure of choice. The objective is to restore a sound-transmitting mechanism and a closed perforation. Tympanoplasty and attendant procedures involving hearing loss will be discussed in Chapter 40. In patients with extensive mucosal disease or cholesteatoma, a modified radical or radical mastoidectomy may be required.

**Modified Radical Mastoidectomy.** Modified radical mastoidectomy is a procedure that removes the attic and mastoid ear disease but preserves and reconstructs the middle ear space. The operation differs from radical mastoidectomy in that the middle ear structures and the eardrum are preserved. The skin of the eardrum and the external auditory canal is used to seal the middle ear from the mastoid cavity. After a modified radical mastoidectomy, the ear should have serviceable hearing. Modified radical mastoidectomy is of

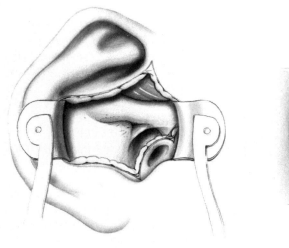 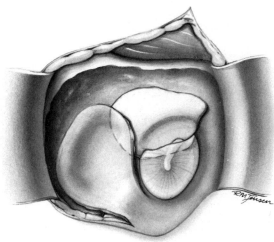

A

B

**FIG 37–30.**
Modified radical mastoidectomy. **A,** endaural incision with exposure of the mastoid. **B,** the tympanic membrane perforation has been repaired by an underlay of fascia graft, while the canal skin has been rotated over the graft into the mastoid bowl. The tympanic membrane and middle ear space are preserved.

particular value when the perforation is small or high on the posterior margin of the drum and when the disease involves the epitympanum but not the middle ear. The middle ear may be normal in such cases except for changes in the attic, a common situation when cholesteatoma is present. Modified radical mastoidectomy is usually done in conjunction with various tympanoplasty techniques (Fig. 37–30).

**Radical Mastoidectomy.** Radical mastoidectomy is rarely performed. It is considered necessary when the cholesteatoma extends deep into the eustachian tube and cannot be completely removed. In a radical mastoidectomy performed through a postaural incision, all mastoid air cells, granulation, and purulent matter are removed. The posterior wall of the external auditory canal is removed, as are the remnants of the eardrum, ossicles, and all mucosa of the middle ear are removed. Finally, the tensor tympani muscle is removed, and the eustachian tube is cleaned of all infected mucosa. The resulting cavity heals by an ingrowth of the epithelium from the skin of the external canal (Fig. 37–31). In some instances, the cavity formed by the removal of the mastoid cells, if excessive in size, can be filled with muscle. A flap is fashioned from the temporalis muscles superiorly, leaving a pedicle for blood

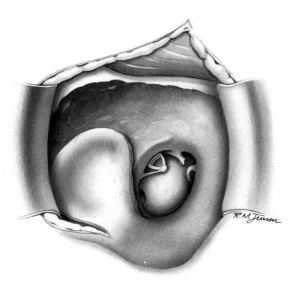

**FIG 37–31.**
Radical mastoidectomy. The mastoid cells and their mucosa, the tympanic membrane with the malleus and incus as well as middle ear mucosa have been removed. The canal skin has been rotated to help obliterate the inferior portion of the mastoid. The tensor tympani muscle is tucked into the eustachian tube to seal it from the nasopharynx. The cavity will heal by epithelialization.

supply, and is turned into the mastoid cavity. The cavity thus created is smaller than usual and requires minimal postoperative care. However, such a flap should not be used unless all infected material has been removed (see Fig. 37–31).

After either radical mastoidectomy or modified radical mastoidectomy, the epithelium-lined cavity is opened to the outside through an enlarged external meatus and thus can be cleaned from time to time. Both procedures are designed to cure infection and provide the patient with a safe ear. With modern otologic techniques, the need for radical mastoidectomy is rare, and variations of tympanoplasty, modified radical mastoidectomy, and tympanoplasty with mastoidectomy have been devised to treat the chronically infected ear.

Occasionally, an ear that is chronically infected can be made dry and safe by medical treatment rather than surgery. A spontaneous cessation of chronic discharge may occur, although there may still be an open perforation of the drum, a partially eroded ossicle, or adhesive bands that impede the normal ability of the eardrum and the ossicles. In the absence of cholesteatoma, the ear can be considered safe in those instances, although hearing is diminished. Patients may not desire any further treatment, although reconstructive procedures are generally advised. Each case must be considered individually, and the decision as to the exact method of reconstruction or repair must be made in the operating room after the middle ear has been exposed and the extent of the mechanical disarrangement and disease has been observed. The necessary tissues for repair of the ear are generally obtained from nearby tissues, such as the fascia of the temporalis muscle or the perichondrium from the tragus.

### Complications
Complications of chronic suppurative otitis media are the same as those occurring in acute mastoiditis—for example, meningitis, epidural abscess, brain abscess, sigmoid sinus thrombosis, and paralysis of the seventh cranial nerve.

# 38

# Trauma to the External Ear

The ear can be cut or torn from the head during fights, in automobile accidents, or on the playing field. Because the blood supply to the ear is extremely good, such wounds generally heal well. The physician should be careful not to discard any torn or free tissue unnecessarily. Often auricular tissue that looks nonvital recovers, and even if torn completely from the head, an ear can sometimes be reattached successfully if it is kept in a cool physiologic solution and if anticoagulants are given after surgery. Strict aseptic technique is important in handling and cleaning the tissue of the ear.

Lacerations of the auricle, which extend through the skin, cartilage, and perichondrium, are resutured in layers; the technique includes careful closure of the skin, subcutaneous tissue, and perichondrium (Fig. 38–1). The cartilage should not be sutured because of risk of perichondritis. Gauze or cotton should be placed behind the ear before ear dressings are applied so that the ear is not crushed painfully against the skull. A gentle pressure dressing is generally placed over the ear.

## HEMATOMA

Subperichondrial hematoma may result from trauma to the pinna, most frequently seen in wrestlers. It generally occurs on the anterior surface of the auricle and represents bleeding between the cartilage and perichondrium (Fig. 38–2). The ear has a reddish purple, shapeless elevation. The risk of damage from hematoma is mainly to the cartilage because the perichondrium carries the blood supply to the cartilage. Avascular necrosis of the cartilage may result from untreated hematoma and deformity of the ear may result from organizing blood clots. Hematomas also are a common site for infection, making the final result worse. Should there be extensive scarring or a loss of cartilage, a cauliflower ear is the result. This most frequently occurs after repeated injuries to the ear. When a hematoma is seen soon after injury, the blood should be aspirated with sterile technique and a needle. A pressure dressing that molds itself to the curves of the ear should be carefully applied. If the hematoma reforms (and it should be checked within 12 to 24 hours), it should be incised and either a drain or suction drainage applied. It is important to hold the perichondrium tightly against the cartilage by means of a molded splint and well-padded pressure dressing. Incisions in the auricle for the hematoma should be made along the curves of the helix or under the antihelical folds so that the scar will not be visible after the injury (Fig. 38–3). All head trauma must be strictly avoided during the period of healing.

## FROSTBITE OF THE AURICLE

Frostbite of the auricle is difficult to treat. Different techniques have been used over the past 15 years, but present authorities suggest slow warming at body temperature with minimal trauma to the ear. Avoidance of extreme hot or cold temperature and removal of blebs as they develop are advised. The use of steroids is not recommended.

Massaging with snow should be avoided, as should any manipulation. No dressings should be used because they further compromise circulation,

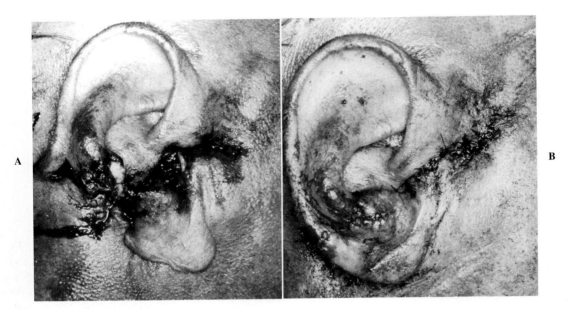

**FIG 38–1**.
**A,** severe laceration of external ear with almost total evulsion of the inferior third. **B,** preservation of soft tissue with meticulous closure of perichondrium and skin.

particularly venous return. In severe or prolonged exposure with severe frostbite, the use of heparin to prevent venous sludging and intravascular clotting is sometimes recommended, though still controversial. Antibiotics are indicated only in the development of secondary infection.

## HEMATOMA OF THE EXTERNAL CANAL

Hematoma of the epithelium lining the osseous part of the external canal is easy to produce inadvertently by wiping too hard with cotton applica-

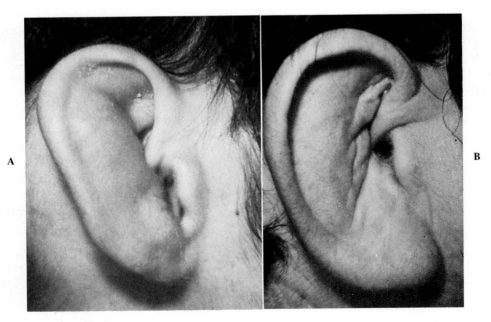

**FIG 38–2**.
**A,** hematoma of external ear. **B,** deformity of auricle following a hematoma.

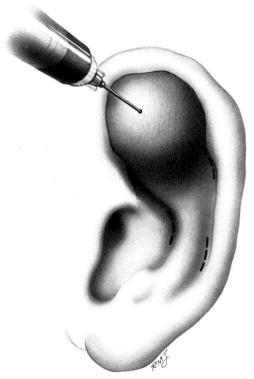

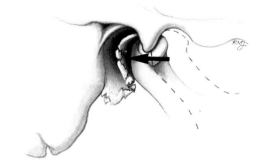

**FIG 38–4.**
Posterior displacement of the anterior bony ear canal by blow to the mandible.

**FIG 38–3.**
Hematoma of auricle. The hematoma can either be aspirated and firm packing placed against the ear or incisions made either in the helical fold or under the antihelical curl.

tors or other instruments. This can often be caused by the patient trying to clean the ear. This epithelium is so delicate that sometimes even the slightest trauma produces a hematoma. On the other hand, the epithelium lining the cartilaginous or external half of the ear canal is thick and not as sensitive. Generally, no treatment is required unless there is significant pain, under which circumstances the hematoma can be aspirated and a wick placed.

## FRACTURES OF THE EXTERNAL CANAL

Generally, the external ear canal is fractured only in severe skull fractures; occasionally, however, displacement of the mandibular condyles posteriorly by a blow to the jaw will fracture the anterior bony wall of the external canal, compressing it posteriorly (Fig. 38–4). Treatment of these cases is based on recognizing the damage initially and differentiating between occluding external ear infection and a macerated posteriorly displaced anterior canal wall. Treatment consists of local anesthesia and replacement of the fragments of the canal wall with the use of a thin nasal speculum or similar instrument. Early treatment is required because displaced fragments may cause stenosis of the external canal. After reestablishment of the canal, a wick or stent is placed to hold the canal open.

## TYMPANIC MEMBRANE AND MIDDLE EAR TRAUMA

The incidence of traumatic perforation has always been high. Trauma to the tympanic membrane may have many causes.

### Picking the Ear

The tympanic membrane is not as delicate as is usually thought. The warning "Never clean the ear with anything smaller than the elbow" may be good advice, but actually the eardrum is less likely to be injured than is the very delicate epithelium covering the osseous canal. The fibrous layer between the two epithelial layers makes the eardrum a substantial structure. Many patients who pick their ears to remove wax or stop itching cause bleeding or pain. However, examination almost invariably reveals that the injury was actually to the ear canal near the drumhead, rather than to the drumhead itself.

## Concussion

An explosion or hard slap on the ear can easily tear the tympanic membrane, often resulting in severe pain and partial deafness. Particularly common are water-skiing injuries or diving accidents. Tinnitus or vertigo may also be present. The middle ear may become infected. Occasionally, there is dislocation of the ossicles. The ruptured tympanic membrane is treated by keeping sterile cotton in the meatus and changing it as necessary. No irrigation, insufflation, or manipulative treatment is advisable unless the tear is extremely stellate and cannot be approximated. In those cases, under local anesthesia and sterile technique, the drum can be approximated over a piece of sterile Gelfoam placed in the middle ear. Ninety percent of traumatic perforations heal spontaneously in several days to weeks. If the drum does not heal, a tympanoplasty may be required.

## Barotrauma

Barotrauma, which may be caused by too rapid descent during air travel, for example, is a common cause of injury to the tympanic membrane. Ordinarily, the eardrum is not perforated, but sometimes there is marked ecchymosis of the drum. Bleeding into the tympanic cavity, another rather common result of barotrauma, produces a blue drumhead.

## Skull Fracture

Fractures through the base of the skull can tear the tympanic membrane. If the fracture line passes through the tympanic sulcus, there may be a steplike effect to the annulus when healing occurs.

## Hot Slag

Welders sometimes have a red-hot piece of slag fly into the ear. There is pain, followed almost invariably by an infection that is difficult to clear. The patient is left with a perforation of the tympanic membrane caused by the hot metal burning its way through the drumhead. Frequently, tympanoplasties or even mastoidectomy with tympanoplasty may be required to clear the infection and repair the defect of the tympanic membrane. Surgical results with slag burns are not consistently successful, in contrast to other types of trauma. This may be because of the thermal burn and scarring or retained foreign body.

## Middle Ear Trauma

Perforations of the tympanic membrane are generally associated with dislocations or fractures of the ossicular chain. Incus disarticulation at the incudostapedial joint is the most common traumatic injury. The second most common is subluxation of the stapes or fracture of the stapes into the vestibule, which is usually associated with vertigo and sensorineural hearing loss. When the ossicular chain is disrupted, the tympanic membranes usually heal spontaneously, and secondary surgery to explore the ossicular chain is necessary. Results of repair of traumatic abnormalitiues are generally excellent in the absence of sensorineural damage.

## Traumatic Noise-Induced Hearing Loss

Frequently, in addition to tearing the tympanic membrane, explosive blasts or injuries can produce a severe sensorineural hearing loss that may be total in some instances. These losses are generally nonreversible, although there may be some improvement in the weeks following blast-type injury. Noise-induced hearing loss is further discussed in Chapter 40.

## TEMPORAL BONE FRACTURE

Fractures of the skull may involve the temporal bone. Eighty percent of temporal bone fractures are longitudinal, that is, in the longitudinal plane of the petrous pyramid. Twenty percent are considered transverse, in that the fracture line extends across the cochlea and vestibule (Fig. 38–5).

The associated pathologic condition with longitudinal fractures is less severe than that with transverse fractures. Only a third of longitudinal fractures will cause significant sensorineural hearing loss, although a much higher percentage have conductive loss. Facial nerve injury is much less

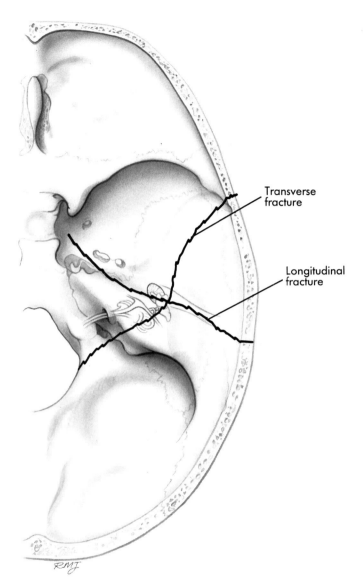

**FIG 38–5.**
Temporal bone fracture.

common in longitudinal fractures than in transverse. Longitudinal fractures generally tear the tympanic membrane and cause bleeding into the middle ear space. Frequently there are leaks from the subarachnoid space into the middle ear, creating a leak of cerebrospinal fluid. A sign of longitudinal temporal bone fracture is ecchymosis of the postauricular area. This usually develops within the first day and is called Battle's sign.

Transverse fractures are usually associated with profound neurosensory hearing loss and 50% are associated with facial nerve injury. Transverse fractures usually destroy the vestibular mechanism, resulting in severe vertigo (Table 38–1). Initial treatment generally involves careful observation. Because of the risk of cerebrospinal fluid leak, the ear should be treated under sterile conditions and care of the external canal should be aseptic. Prophylactic antibiotics are used for 7 to 10 days following the injury. Generally, the dural

**TABLE 38–1.**

Temporal Bone Fracture

|  | Longitudinal | Transverse |
|---|---|---|
| Incidence | 80% | 20% |
| Tympanic membrane | Perforation with tear—superior canal | Usually intact |
| Hearing | Mild to moderate high-frequency loss, frequent conductive loss | Significant neurosensory loss—may be total |
| Vertigo | Rare | Frequent |
| Seventh nerve paralysis | 10%-15% | 50% |

tears and cerebrospinal fluid leak will seal spontaneously.

Surgery is generally reserved for two circumstances: persistent hearing loss following injury in which there is good cochlear reserve and those cases of injury to the facial nerve in which there is thought to be traumatic disruption of the nerve or bony fragment penetration into the nerve (see Chapter 12). Generally, reconstruction of the disrupted ossicular chain following injury is very successful. Sensorineural hearing loss and vestibular abnormalities after traumatic injury are generally persistent.

# 39

# Tumors

## EXTERNAL EAR

Tumors of the external ear are quite common. Occasionally there appears about the ear a tag of skin, or skin and cartilage, that is an accessory auricle inside and in front of the tragus. This represents remnants of the first brachial apparatus (Fig. 39–1,A) There may be a sinus tract or dimple just anterior to and above the tragus. This requires no treatment unless it is recurrently infected. Lop ear, or outstanding auricle, is a fairly common abnormality of the external ear, readily corrected by plastic surgery. It is necessary to cut and re-form the conchal cartilage. Mere excision of the skin behind the ear does not hold the auricle back permanently. The procedure is generally performed at the age of 6 or 7 years (Fig. 39–1,B).

### Benign Tumors of the External Ear
#### Sebaceous Cysts
Sebaceous cysts often appear just behind the lobule of the ear or in the meatus of the canal (Fig. 39–2). The content of the cyst is sebum, a soft, cheeselike material. If the cyst becomes infected, enlarges rapidly, and is painful, treatment in the acute stage consists of antibiotics, incision, and drainage and the use of hot compresses. Some advise excision of the cyst in the acute phase. If the cyst is recurrent, all of the lining should be excised surgically.

#### Keloids
Keloids, which are massive overgrowths of reparative (scar) tissue, form predominantly in blacks but are also seen in whites. About the ear

they are most commonly attached to the lobule as a result of the ears having been pierced for earrings, but they may occur after any type of trauma to the auricle (Fig. 39–3). The best treatment is excision, followed by repeated injections of long-acting steroids, such as methylprednisolone acetate (Depo-Medrol) or triamcinolone acetonide (Kenalog), into the suture line area or developing keloid.

### Chondrodermatitis Nodularis Chronica Helicus (Painful Nodule)

Painful nodule is the name given to small indurated areas of chrondritis along the superior rim of the auricle (Fig. 39–4). The condition is quite painful, and the cause is unknown. Treatment is injection of long-lasting steroids or excision. Chondromas, lipomas, and fibromas of the external ear tend to be extremely rare and are a pathologic diagnosis.

### Relapsing Polychondritis

Relapsing polychondritis is a rare disorder characterized by episodic inflammation of cartilage, particularly the ear. Symptoms consist of a red, tender, edematous pinna with sparing of the external canal, thus differentiating the condition from external otitis. Diagnosis is primarily clinical. Laboratory findings include an elevated erythrocyte sedimentation rate, anemia, and positive rheumatoid factor. The disease can involve other cartilaginous structures, including those of the nose, trachea, and larynx.

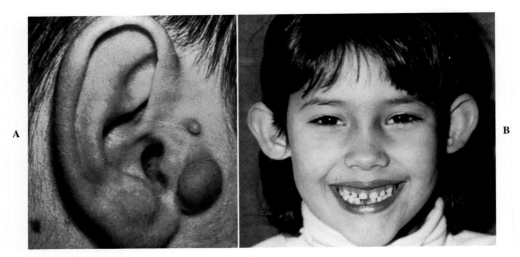

**FIG 39–1.**
**A,** two accessory auricles. This pretragal position is common. **B,** protruding auricle, or lop ear.

## Malignant Tumors of the External Ear

Carcinoma of the auricle is common. The cancer may be either a basal cell or squamous cell carcinoma (Figs. 39–5 and 39–6). Carcinoma of the external ear accounts for approximately 4% to 8% of all skin cancers. Approximately 80% to 85% of carcinomas occur on the external ear, and 10% to 15% of them are seen in the external ear canal. Squamous cell carcinoma is much more common on the auricle than is basal cell carcinoma. Squamous cell carcinoma usually occurs in older men on the posterior or superior portion of the pinna and usually in individuals with extensive sun exposure. Basal cell carcinomas are more common on the face than squamous cell carcinomas and less common in the auricle. They generally occur later in life than do squamous cell carcinomas. Squamous cell carcinoma tends to be more exophytic, whereas basal cell carcinoma is more endophytic and indurated and tends to bur-

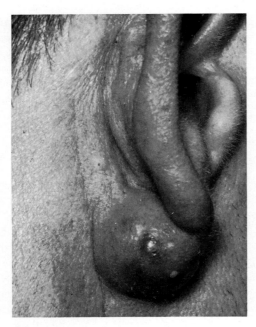

**FIG 39–2.**
Large sebaceous cyst in a characteristic location.

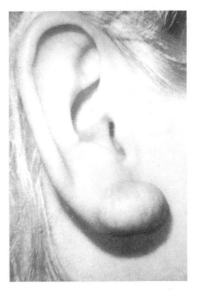

**FIG 39–3.**
Keloid involving lobule from perforated earlobe.

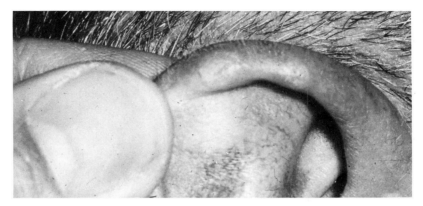

**FIG 39–4.**
Painful nodules of the auricle.

row subcutaneously beyond the visible limits of the tumor.

The first consideration in the treatment of malignant neoplasms of the auricle is adequate removal. The cosmetic result is secondary. Generally, wide local excision of the tumor is satisfactory. Tumors of the external ear should be reviewed histologically for persistent tumor at the time of excision. Sometimes the entire auricle must be excised and bare bone of the skull exposed. Radiation therapy for both basal and squamous cell carcinoma of the external ear is effective. However, when there is involvement of cartilage or bone, irradiation is less effective than surgery. When regional lymph nodes are involved, extensive local excision associated with block neck dissection and possible parotidectomy is necessary. Important in both basal and squamous cell carcinoma is early identification. If identified early, 95% of these tumors can be cured.

When carcinoma of the external ear invades the bony ear canal or the mastoid, the prognosis is much worse than when the cancer is limited to soft tissues. Such cases may require extensive excision, not only of the entire ear, but also of the temporal bone, to control the tumor.

### Malignant Melanoma

Fortunately, malignant melanoma of the external ear is uncommon. Because of the frequency of nevi upon the ear, it must be considered. Gen-

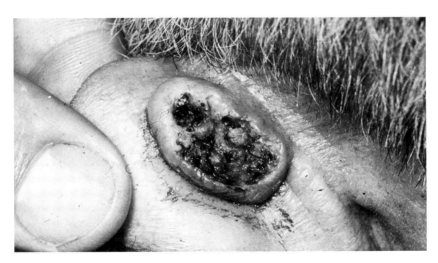

**FIG 39–5.**
Basal cell carcinoma on the posterior surface of the auricle. Note the rolled borders. The lesion's margin is not as it appears, and treatment required excision of the majority of the auricle.

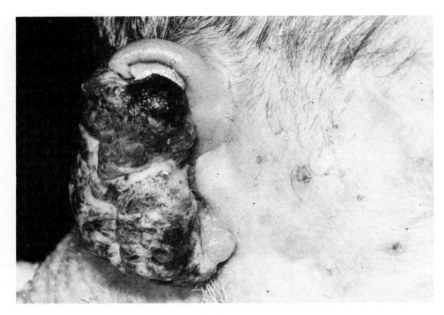

**FIG 39–6**.
Squamous cell carcinoma of the ear. Treatment should include wide local excision, parondectomy, and radial neck dissection to remove lymphatic drainage.

erally, extensive local excision with regional node removal is the treatment required. Prognosis is directly related to the extensiveness of the lesion and depth of involvement.

### Benign Tumors of the External Ear Canal
#### Exostosis and Chondromas

Exostoses in the ear canal arise near the tympanic membrane, where they attach to the osseous canal. They are small, broad-based, bony, hard lumps covered with normal epithelium. Often, they are multiple and usually they are bilateral (Fig. 39–7). Some authorities believe that exostoses form because of periosteal irritation resulting from swimming in cold water. Others believe that they result from embryologic maldevelopment. Exostoses are usually not large enough to hide all the eardrum from view and are usually asymptomatic. Treatment is usually unnecessary. Rarely, however, they may cause obstruction and require removal. If removal is indicated because of size, the operation may be performed directly through the meatus or through an endaural incision such as that used for mastoidectomy. Exostoses usually arise from the posterior wall of the ear canal, where their bases are in close relationship to the facial nerve.

Chondromas arise at a location more external to the drumhead than do exostoses, since chondromas spring from the cartilaginous ear canal. They are quite rare. Like the more common exostoses, they are asymptomatic unless very large.

#### Keratosis Obturans

Keratosis obturans is an example of cholesteatoma of the external auditory meatus. The cause is undetermined. This is a rather unusual condition, in which the cholesteatomatous mass is found on the floor of the osseous portion of the ear canal. The symptoms are pain, usually mild, and sometimes discharge when the ear is secondarily infected. Treatment consists of removing the squamous epithelium and debris and enlarging the external canal.

#### Ceruminoma

A ceruminoma is an adenoma of sweat gland origin. This uncommon tumor presents as a smooth, introverted polypoid swelling in the outer end of the external canal. The presenting symptom is usually a blocked feeling within the ear, and there is no history of otorrhea or previous ear trouble. A diagnosis is made on histologic examination.

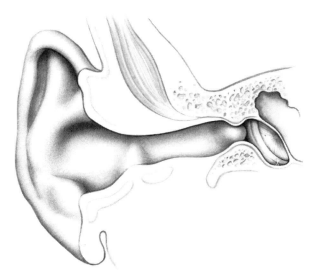 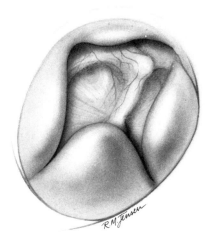

**FIG 39–7.**
Exostosis of the ear.

### Osteomas

Unlike exostoses, osteomas are relatively rare in the external canal, and their appearance is more that of a single foreign body or cyst. Generally, they are solitary, bony, hard enlargements of the canal of varying size.

### Adenomas

Adenomas are less common tumors found within the external canal.

### Aural Polyps

Aural polyps appear in the ear canal and are almost always actively draining infected material. They bleed with the slightest trauma. Besides representing chronic ear disease, their major significance is their differentiation from malignant tumors; consequently, a biopsy should always be done.

### Large Canal Foreign Bodies

Obstruction of the ear canal is commonly caused by inanimate and vegetable foreign bodies placed in the ear by young children. These may be confused with tumors if allowed to remain in place for long periods. Cotton is the most common foreign body in the ear canal of adults. Such objects as small stones, pieces of wood, peas, beans, and paper are fairly commonly found in the ear canals of children (Fig. 39–8). Sometimes there are no symptoms. The physician often finds the foreign body during routine examination. At other times, there may be pain or pus may drain from the ear. Occasionally, an insect will fly or crawl into the ear canal and cause great distress by beating its wings and crawling about. When an insect is in the canal, an oily substance such as mineral oil or olive oil should first be dropped into the ear to immobilize and smother the insect. It can then be removed by gentle irrigation or forceps.

The external auditory canal is very sensitive to touch, and the skin over the bony canal is thin, bleeds easily, and forms subepithelial hematomas from minor trauma. Therefore, the removal of solid foreign bodies (for example, beads, BB shot, or pieces of wood) carries a definite risk of additional trauma to the ear if the patient is not completely cooperative or if removal is difficult. Whenever the removal is painful enough that the patient cannot remain quiet (which often proves to be the case when the patient is a child), further attempts without anesthesia should not be made. The foreign body is removed with the patient under light general anesthesia. If a difficult removal is attempted without anesthesia, the foreign body may be forced through the eardrum into the middle ear, resulting in subsequent hearing loss or chronic infection. Trauma to the ear canal, if significant, also causes stenosis of the external canal, which may require operative correction and grafting to obtain patency.

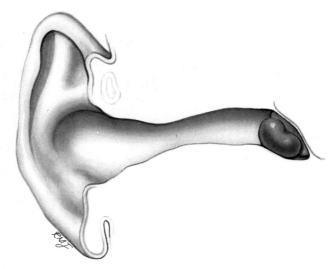

**FIG 39–8.**
Bean lying medial to the isthmus of the bony canal against the tympanic membrane.

## Malignant Tumors of the External Ear Canal
### *Basal Cell, Squamous Cell, and Adenoid Cystic Carcinomas*

Basal cell, squamous cell, and adenocystic carcinomas are found in the external auditory meatus. Basal cell carcinomas are found much less commonly in the external auditory canal than on the auricle and generally invade the meatus and ear canal from the external ear. Squamous cell carcinomas, on the other hand, constitute 70% of malignancies of the external canal (Fig. 39–9). They may come from the skin of the auricle or arise in the epithelium of the ear canal, middle ear, or mastoid. Symptoms of tumors of the external ear include drainage from the ear; a deep, boring pain; hearing loss; and in later stages a peripheral type of facial paralysis. After pus is cleared from the ear canal, examination reveals a granular, readily bleeding tumor. The diagnosis must be differentiated from that of an aural polyp or granulation tissue. The diagnosis is usually not difficult when the lesion is extensive but may be overlooked if the tumor is visible only in the depths of the canal. For this reason, all granula-

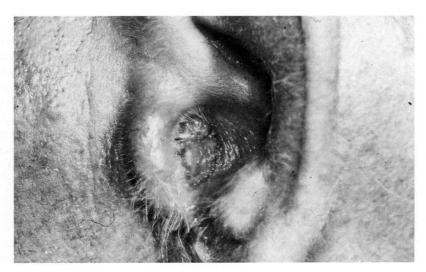

**FIG 39–9.**
Carcinoma of the external auditory meatus. This lesion extended into the mastoid, was friable, drained purulent material, and bled easily.

tion tissue in the middle ear should be retained for pathologic examination. Repeat biopsy is indicated when tumor is suspected and initial biopsy is negative. A squamous cell carcinoma commonly develops in chronically infected and draining ears.

The prognosis for carcinoma of the ear canal is reasonably good as long as the tumor is confined in the cartilaginous canal. Wide local excision and skin grafting may result in a cure. However, if the osseous canal is invaded, treatment is compromised and the cure rate is greatly reduced. Radical mastoidectomy followed by radiation therapy is required to control the tumor if the bony canal is involved. In advanced cases, when judgment indicates a poor prognosis even with the combination of radical mastoidectomy and radiation therapy, the entire temporal bone can be removed surgically. This operation, usually performed by a neurosurgeon and the otolaryngologist working as a team, is a last-resort, life-saving procedure that carries a high operative mortality rate (15%). Even when it is successfully accomplished, the cure rate is quite low.

### Adenocystic Carcinoma (Cylindroma)

Adenocystic carcinoma (cylindroma) is a particularly vicious tumor. Short-term survival rates are good, but long-term rates are very poor. Extremely wide surgical excision is needed for good result. The tumor is noted by its skiplike behavior, slow relentless growth, and neural invasion.

### Rhabdomyosarcoma

The most common malignant tumor involving the external canal or middle ear in children is embryonal rhabdomyosarcoma. Though extremely rare, this tumor occurs almost exclusively in children and is associated with chronic ear drainage, ear pain, and hearing loss. Diagnosis is by biopsy of a hemorrhagic mass, and treatment consists of chemotherapy and irradiation. Recently, with the combination of a variety of chemotherapeutic agents and radiation therapy, a significant rate of cure (60%) has been reported.

## TUMORS OF THE MIDDLE EAR

Tumors of the middle ear are rare. The three most common types are neurofibroma of the facial nerve (discussed in Chapter 44), squamous cell carcinoma, and glomus jugulare tumor.

### Squamous Cell Carcinoma

Squamous cell carcinoma of the middle ear generally occurs after long-standing chronic suppurative otitis media, although it also can occur spontaneously. Discharge from the ear, often blood-tinged, is the only early symptom. Eventually, there is hearing loss on the affected side. In the advanced stage, pain and facial paralysis are common. Diagnosis is made by biopsy of tissue removed from an ulcerating, fungating mass seen through the ear speculum.

Treatment must be radical. Irradiation alone has been unsuccessful in effecting a cure. Rarely, a thorough radical mastoidectomy preceded or followed by irradiation may eradicate all tumor cells. However, a complete resection of the temporal bone is usually necessary to prevent recurrence. The prognosis for squamous cell carcinoma in the middle ear is therefore poor, regardless of treatment.

### Glomus Jugulare Tumor

A glomus jugulare tumor arises from the glomus bodies located in the adventitia of the dome of the jugular bulb. It may also be found on the medial wall of the middle ear, attached to a tiny arteriole. In this case, the tumor is called a glomus tympanicum. Such tumors ordinarily are small and much less serious than glomus jugulare tumors. The carotid body tumor looks the same microscopically as the glomus tumor, and similar tumors have been found in numerous other parts of the head and neck, where they are sometimes called chemodectoma or nonchromaffin paraganglioma. These tumors grow slowly and may remain unnoticed for years. In reported series, the average length of time from appearance of the original symptoms to diagnosis was 7 to 8 years.

Early symptoms may be tinnitus, slight hearing loss, or a throbbing, pulsating discomfort. Later, pain, dizziness, total unilateral deafness, and multiple cranial nerve paralysis are seen. The striking feature of this tumor is its tendency to bleed profusely when manipulated. Spontaneous hemorrhage is rare but does occur. Any episode of profuse bleeding following manipulation of a mass in the external canal, or in the middle ear, should

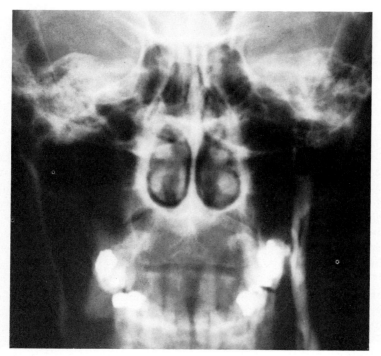

**FIG 39–10.**
Venous phase of an angiogram demonstrating the extension of a glomus tumor into the internal jugular vein. Arrow points to the base of this radiolucency lying within the jugular vessel.

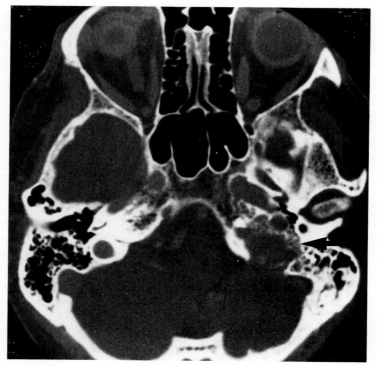

**FIG 39–11.**
CT scan demonstrating glomus jugulare. The arrow points to the extensive destruction of the mastoid air cells and petrous bone by this large vascular tumor. The cartoid artery is surrounded on its posterior aspect by this tumor mass.

make the physician suspect a glomus jugulare tumor. Clinically, the erroneous diagnosis of granulation tissue polyp is often made. Only a biopsy will establish the correct diagnosis. When neglected, a glomus jugulare tumor expands slowly and causes extensive destruction of the mastoid and internal ear. It may also extend intracranially. A carotid angiogram, as well as retrograde venogram of the internal jugular vein, is often essential in diagnosing and determining the extent of the tumor (Fig. 39–10). Aneurysms of the internal carotid may mimic a glomus tumor in symptoms and appearance. Contrast-enhanced computed tomography (CT) is frequently useful in demonstrating size and position of the tumor but has not replaced the angiogram (Fig. 39–11).

Treatment is generally surgical, except in cases of extensive tumor involving the entire skull base. In the case of glomus tympanicum, often all that is needed is to reflect the drumhead, as one would do for a stapedectomy, and excise the small red tumor on the promontory. In those cases the diagnosis is generally made on observation of a pulsa-

tile tumor behind the intact tympanic membrane. In the case of glomus jugulare or large glomus typanicum, surgery may be formidable, and complete surgical removal is not always possible. Recently, newer surgical approaches exposing the skull base have allowed more extensive removal of the large or recurrent glomus jugulare or recurrent glomus tumor. Radiation therapy, although it does not destroy the tumor, sometimes prevents progression and regrowth and is used when the tumor cannot be resected safely.

### Tumors of the Facial Nerve

Tumors of the facial nerve occasionally present as middle ear tumors. Most have been reported as benign neuromas (schwannomas) or neurofibromas. Most of them arise within the fallopian (facial) canal. The tumor originates from the displacement of meningeal tissue laterally during embryologic development and grows attached to the facial nerve sheath. Prognosis is generally based on the slow development of facial paraly-

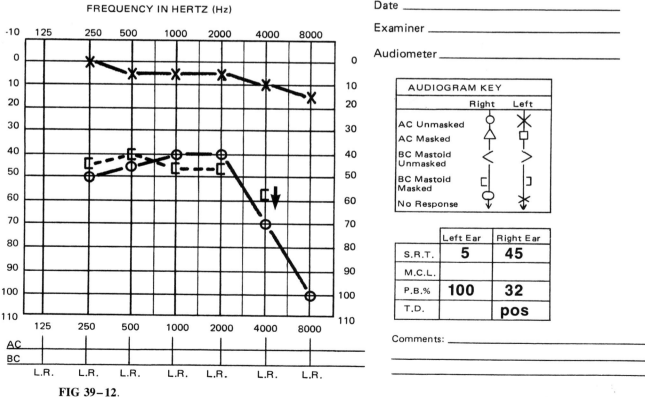

**FIG 39–12**.
Acoustic neuroma. Note the extremely poor discrimination and the positive tone decay in unilateral hearing loss.

sis. Computed tomography is used for diagnosis, demonstrating evidence of bone destruction. Treatment demands adequate surgical excision of the tumor with end-to-end anastomosis or nerve grafting (see also Chapter 44).

### Histiocytosis X

Although not a true tumor, histiocytosis X (or reticuloendotheliosis) produces a tumorlike condition not infrequently involving the temporal bone. The three types of clinical syndromes are Letterer-Siwe disease, Hand-Schüller-Christian disease, and eosinophilic granuloma. Occasionally, the first two types are seen as a draining ear. Treatment is irradiation, but mortality is high. Eosinophilic granuloma is seen in young adults and children and demonstrates an osteolytic lesion involving the temporal bone and/or skull. Symptoms may include otorrhea, deafness, and facial paralysis. Treatment consists of surgical excision or curettage with radiotherapy for more extensive lesions. Prognosis is generally good for adequately treated eosinophilic granuloma.

### Tumors of the Internal Ear

Acoustic neuromas account for 80% of cerebellopontine angle tumors and deserve special attention because of their great importance to otologists. Acoustic neuroma is a benign tumor arising from the neurilemmal sheath of the eighth cranial nerve. The vestibular portion of the nerve is more frequently involved than the auditory portion. The

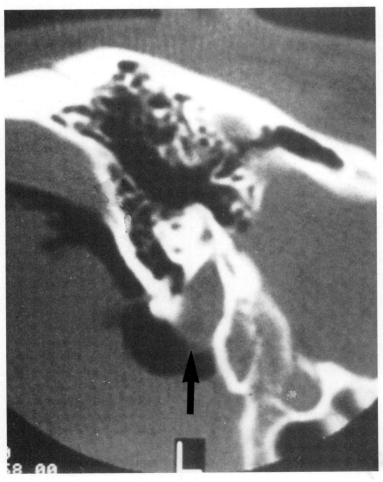

**FIG 39–13.**
Air-contrast CT scan demonstrating intracannulicular acoustic neuroma. Note widening of the internal auditory meatus and the margin of the tumor just at the opening of the canal.

importance of the disease is based on its complex of symptoms, which tend to mimic a variety of other ear abnormalities. Usually, the first symptom is tinnitus, with the onset of hearing loss, which may be delayed for months or years. The hearing loss may be of any degree but generally is characterized by a high-frequency or flat type of loss. In about 10% of cases, there may be a sudden neurosensory loss. Early diagnosis of acoustic neuroma is made on the basis of suspicion in a patient with unilateral sensorineural hearing loss or tinnitus. When the tumor is large, there generally is unsteadiness of a constant, though usually mild, degree. True vertigo is unusual, although it may occur. Finally, facial paralysis may occur as the seventh and eighth cranial nerves are compressed in the internal auditory canal. Tumors that grow large enough to expand into the cerebellar pontine angle produce the symptoms of intracranial space-occupying lesions.

Special hearing tests may pinpoint the site of the lesion and thus differentiate between a cochlear and a neural hearing loss. One common finding is that the patient's discrimination score is unduly poor in comparison with his or her ability to hear pure tones (Fig. 39–12). In this condition, special auditory tests (for example, reflex decay and tone decay) are positive. Tomograms of the internal auditory meatus may show widening of the internal auditory meatus. Computed tomography scans with contrast usually will light up small acoustic neuromas (Fig. 39–13). Magnetic resonance imaging will detect very early tumors within the internal auditory canal and is the most accurate diagnostic study (Fig. 39–14). Vestibular examination generally demonstrates a reduced or absent caloric response on electronystagmography. Early diagnosis is important because preservation of hearing and facial nerve function is directly related to the size of the tumor.

Treatment is usually by surgical removal. Small tumors can be resected through the middle cranial fossa. Medium-size tumors are generally removed through a translabyrinthine approach, which, though it destroys hearing in the involved ear, provides good access to the tumor and allows preservation of the seventh cranial nerve. Tumors greater than 3 cm in diameter are probably best approached through the suboccipital approach. Occasionally small tumors in older patients can be observed and followed by sequential magnetic resonance imaging. Recently, radiosurgery has

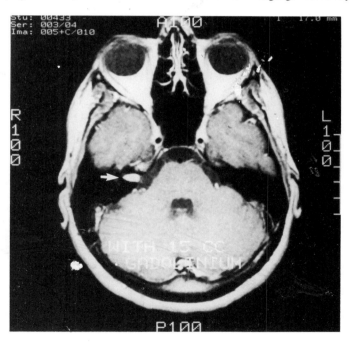

**FIG 39–14.**
MRI of posterior fossa showing a small intracannulicular acoustic neuroma. This study demonstrates the clarity with which small acoustic neuromas can be identified within the lateral portion of the internal auditory canal. The "lighting up" of this area is diagnostic. The tumor is just over 1 cm in size.

been used to selectively irradiate acoustic tumors (gamma knife). However, this technique, which precisely concentrates a high level of radiation to the tumor, is reserved for unusual cases and circumstances.

Meningioma is the second most common posterior fossa tumor. Generally, other cranial nerves are involved in developing meningiomas, which tend not to arise within the internal auditory canal. Radiographic studies may show hyperostosis and calcification within the tumor. The diagnosis is developed similarly to that of acoustic neuromas, although frequently the tumor is seen to be more medial to the internal auditory meatus.

# 40

# Hearing Loss

Communicative disorders account for the greatest number of handicapping disabilities in the United States. Studies by the National Center for Health Statistics and Centers for Disease Control indicate that more people suffer from hearing, speech, and language impairment than from heart disease, venereal disease, paralysis, epilepsy, blindness, tuberculosis, cerebral palsy, muscular dystrophy, and multiple sclerosis combined. According to the Department of Health and Human Services, the yearly loss of earnings caused by communicative disorders is a staggering $2 billion. By a conservative estimate, hearing loss affects 30 million Americans significantly. Of these, 3 million are school-age children. Hearing loss, however, is most common among the elderly. Almost half of those needing assistance are more than 65 years of age. Reliable statistics indicate that more than 12 million persons in this over-65 age group have hearing disorders. More than 11.5 million Americans suffer from a significant uncorrected hearing handicap. Studies by family practice physicians indicate that inflammation of the middle ear in children is the second most prevalent disorder seen by the family physician, the first being the common cold.

The incidence of hearing loss in children is between 2% and 4%, and in almost one third of hard-of-hearing children the problem can be traced to something that happened before or during birth. These include rubella (German measles) contracted by the mother in the first trimester of pregnancy, influenza, shingles, other viral diseases, and drugs.

Hearing loss has major socioeconomic implications, with a direct cost of approximately $750 million for the education, management, and compensation of those with problems.

Hearing losses fall into two broad categories: conductive and sensorineural. Each has a variety of independent causes.

## SENSORINEURAL HEARING LOSS

Sensorineural hearing loss occurs when the cochlea or eighth cranial nerve is damaged. This damage may take place before birth, during delivery, or later in life. *Hereditary deafness* may be defined as a defect of cochlear development secondary to a genetic defect. This may be present at birth, being called *congenital,* or developed later in life, being called *acquired.* In hereditary deafness, there is usually more than one child in a family involved, although, in most cases, there are usually family members with no hearing loss whatsoever. In a marriage between persons with hereditary deafness, genetic counseling is imperative, since the likelihood of having deaf offspring is greatly increased. Although many types of hereditary deafness are recognized, the easiest grouping to remember is one based on associated abnormalities.

Most types of hereditary, congenital hearing loss are associated with other abnormalities and involve a wide variety of systems (see the box on page 454). The list of congenital and hereditary causes of hearing loss associated with physical defects increases yearly as we learn more about genetic transmission and development.

Types not associated with other abnormalities include dominant types of congenital severe deafness, unilateral deafness, low-frequency hearing loss, and mid-frequency hearing loss. Recessive forms may occur in all these types. There are also acquired forms of hereditary deafness that mani-

CONGENITAL HEREDITARY HEARING LOSS
ASSOCIATED WITH SKELETAL DEFORMITY
- Treacher Collins syndrome (congenital)—abnormal ear, microstomia, micrognathia, mixed hearing loss
- Crouzon's disease (congenital)—craniostenosis, midface hypoplasia, exophthalmos, mixed hearing loss
- van der Hoeve's syndrome (acquired congenital)—fixed stapes, blue sclerae, fragile bones, conductive hearing loss
- Paget's disease (congenital)—micrognathia, glossoptosis, ear deformity, mixed hearing loss
- Klippel-Feil syndrome (congenital)—short neck, spina bifida, canal atresia, mixed hearing loss

ASSOCIATED WITH OCULAR ABNORMALITY
- Usher's syndrome (acquired congenital)—retinitis pigmentosa, sensorineural hearing loss (progressive)
- Cockayne's syndrome (acquired congenital)—mental retardation, premature senility, visual loss, sensorineural hearing loss

ASSOCIATED WITH RENAL DISEASE
- Alport's syndrome (acquired congenital)—progressive nephritis, sensorineural hearing loss (progressive)

ASSOCIATED WITH METABOLIC DISORDERS
- Pendred's syndrome (acquired congenital)—goiter, sensorineural hearing loss
- Richards-Rundle syndrome (acquired congenital)—hypogonadism, ataxia, sensorineural hearing loss

ASSOCIATED WITH CARDIAC DISORDERS
- Trisomy 13-15 (congenital)—micrognathia, cleft lip, congenital heart disease, sensorineural hearing loss
- Trisomy 16-18 (congenital)—cardiac abnormality, low-set ears, atresia

good discrimination. The progressive development of hearing disability is premature.

## NONHEREDITARY CONGENITAL DEAFNESS

The three main nonhereditary causes of congenital deafness are viral infection, birth trauma, and kernicterus (see box below). When a pregnant woman contracts German measles during the first trimester of pregnancy, there is a 5% to 10% chance the child will be born deaf or profoundly hard of hearing. Of those children who develop the rubella syndrome (including cataracts, cardiovascular abnormalities, mental retardation, retinitis, and hearing loss) 70% present with some degree of deafness. Pathologic damage generally occurs at the level of the organ of Corti.

The probability of other viruses affecting hearing when they occur in the first trimester of pregnancy is quite high, though not clearly defined.

Prolonged anoxia in a newborn infant may damage the cochlea and produce hearing loss. This is often associated with cerebral palsy. Occasionally there is intracranial hemorrhage and damage to the cochlear nerve.

Kernicterus or erythroblastosis fetalis often damages the cochlea, cochlear nuclei, and brainstem (superior and inferior colliculus). Twenty percent of patients with kernicterus have severe deafness. This is directly related to the bilirubin level and its duration of elevation.

Congenital deafness can also be caused by toxic reaction to medications. Drugs such as quinine and streptomycin may damage the cochlea of the fetus. Certain tranquilizers and central nervous system depressants have been implicated as possibly causing congenital neurosensory hearing loss.

Although less frequent, congenital syphilis must always be considered as the cause of other-

fest themselves later in life, such as progressive nerve deafness. For example, one type of hearing disability that manifests in middle age is associated with a flat hearing loss at all frequencies and

NONHEREDITARY CONGENITAL DEAFNESS
- Measles—first trimester
- Kernicterus
- Birth trauma
- Drug toxicity
- Congenital syphilis

wise unexplained neurosensory congenital hearing loss. The onset may be from birth, or hearing loss may actually develop in adolescence or adult life. One or both ears may be affected. The hearing loss is usually fluctuating and often associated with vertigo. It may be indistinguishable from other forms of vestibular cochlear disorders, for instance, Ménière disease, in the adult population. The hearing loss and vertigo are rapidly progressive. The patient may or may not have been treated for syphilis. Other signs of congenital syphilis are helpful, but serologic confirmation is mandatory for diagnosis. Treatment is with penicillin and steroids.

## NONHEREDITARY HEARING LOSS

Nonhereditary forms of hearing loss constitute, by far, the largest group of hearing loss patients (see boxes on pages 454 and 455). These include

---

> **NONHEREDITARY ACQUIRED SENSO-RINEURAL HEARING LOSS**
> - Presbycusis
> - Occupational or noise-induced hearing loss
> - Head trauma
> - Drug toxicity
> - Sudden sensorineural hearing loss
> - Endolymphatic hydrops
> - Perilymphatic leak
> - Tumor

presbycusis, noise-induced or occupational hearing loss, trauma, toxicity, metabolic causes, endolymphatic hydrops, sudden neurosensory hearing loss, tumor, and perilymphatic leak.

### Presbycusis

*Presbycusis* is a term given to hearing loss associated with aging, which in many cases is a re-

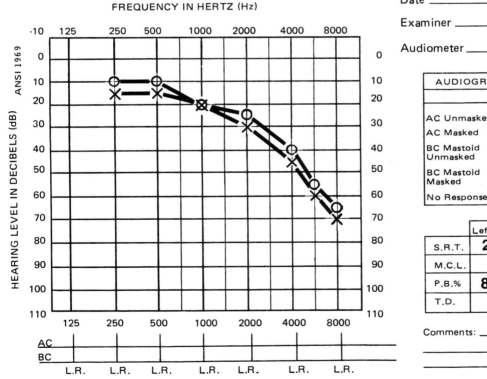

**FIG 40–1.**
Classical-appearing pure-tone audiogram of a mild to moderate neurosensory loss with aging. The high-frequency loss will evidence itself by inability to hear the high-pitched fricatives and consonants, creating difficulty with discrimination, especially in noise. The relatively good discrimination scores in quiet environments are deceiving in most elderly patients.

sult of atrophy of the ganglion cells in the cochlea or changes in the basilar membrane. The degenerative changes produced in this type of hearing loss parallel those which occur in other tissues of the body. Presbycusis is characterized by a bilateral, gradual loss of hearing, particularly of high frequencies, which slowly progresses to involve lower and middle tones (Fig. 40–1). It accounts for the majority of neurosensory hearing loss in the elderly. Because the hearing loss is initially in the higher frequencies, patients will initially complain of loss of the ability to discriminate. They will complain that people are mumbling to them but will deny any other type of hearing loss. With progression, the hearing loss will involve all frequencies and amplification will be a major factor.

Characteristics of presbycusis are:

1. Gradual, progressive development
2. Loss of higher frequencies, manifested by loss of discrimination in noise
3. Often a narrow range of tolerance to sound intensity

As patients' hearing falls below 30 to 35 db, they should be involved in amplification programs. The earlier the patient with presbycusis begins to use amplification, the better he or she will do as the hearing loss progresses.

### Noise-Induced or Occupational Hearing Loss

Hearing loss caused by loud noise is the most common and most important type of occupational hearing loss. Exposure to industrial noise levels greater than 85 to 95 db over a period of months or years causes cochlear damage. In earlier stages there is a loss of hearing at or near the frequency of 4,000 cycles per second (Fig. 40–2). As time passes, the damage will extend to both higher and lower tones, the lower tones being affected the least initially. Considerable damage occurs before individuals are aware of the hearing loss because speech reception is not altered seriously until the hearing loss is greater than 30 db in speech frequencies. Noise-induced hearing loss has two phases; the first is known as temporary threshold

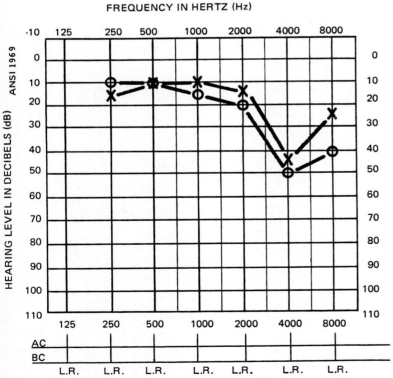

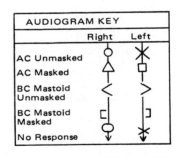

Date _____

Examiner _____

Audiometer _____

| AUDIOGRAM KEY | | |
|---|---|---|
| | Right | Left |
| AC Unmasked | ○ | ✕ |
| AC Masked | △ | □ |
| BC Mastoid Unmasked | < | > |
| BC Mastoid Masked | □ | □ |
| No Response | ○↓ | ✕↓ |

| | Left Ear | Right Ear |
|---|---|---|
| S.R.T. | 10 | 15 |
| M.C.L. | | |
| P.B.% | 88 | 92 |
| T.D. | | |

Comments: **Noise induced**

**FIG 40–2.**
Classical noise-induced hearing loss with notch at 4,000 Hz.

shift. This means that the human ear, when exposed to loud sound, will show a loss of sensitivity, that is, a rise in the threshold for sound. If the hearing returns to its previous level after the noise has been removed, the shift was temporary and no permanent damage has occurred. On the other hand, if the hearing loss does not return to its previous level, permanent hearing loss has occurred. Such a permanent threshold shift is the second phase of damage. Temporary threshold shift can be superimposed on permanent damage. The ears of some people are more easily affected by noise than are those of others. Again, as with presbycusis (perhaps even more so), patients complain that they are unable to discriminate words, particularly in circumstances in which there is competing noise (for example, restaurants, picnics, buses, cars).

Hearing loss caused by noise has become a serious economic problem. Lawsuits totaling millions of dollars against industry, insurance carriers, and state industrial accident commissions are now in the courts. The laws in many states now make the last employer responsible for all previous noise-induced hearing loss. For this reason, and because conservation of hearing is important, many industries require preemployment audiometric examinations. In individuals who work where

**TABLE 40–1.**

Permissible Exposures for Continuous Noise*

| Level in dbA | Maximum Exposure Duration (hr) |
|---|---|
| 90 | 8 |
| 95 | 4 |
| 100 | 2 |
| 105 | 1 |
| 110 | 0.5 |
| 115 | 0.25 |

*Based on a 90 db TWA for an 8-hour workday, using the 5 db exchange rule.

the sound intensity level is greater than 85 db, periodic hearing tests are required so that cochlear impairment can be detected early. In many circumstances, however, it is impossible for a person to avoid a high noise level (Table 40–1). The use of ear protectors such as earplugs, muffs, and sound shields is necessary (Fig. 40–3). Earplugs reduce the noise reaching the middle ear by 10 to 30 db but must seal the ear canal firmly to be effective. Cotton is unsatisfactory as an ear protector. Some protectors can be custom fitted to the individual ear. In those industries in which loud noise exposures cannot be avoided, earplugs alone are not satisfactory and earmuffs must be used in addition. Occasionally, shields over the

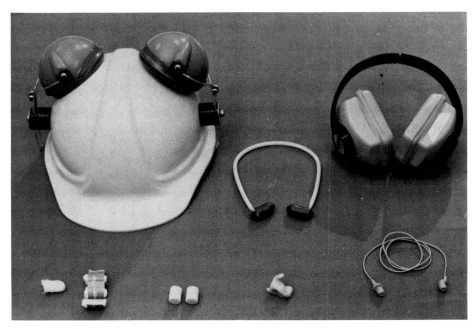

**FIG 40–3.**
Typical industrial ear defenders. *Above, left* and *right*, earmuffs. *Below* and *center*, earplugs.

entire head may be used to protect the individual from noise damage. Most important, however, is the periodic evaluation of the patient's hearing and removal from the source of noise when any evidence of loss occurs.

Noise-induced hearing loss can be associated with the use of firearms, including guns used in sport. The loss generally tends to be greater in the left ear of right-handed persons because the right ear is protected from the sound impulse by resting closer to the stock of the rifle. By contrast, with revolvers the hearing loss is symmetric. Patients should be warned that if firing guns causes tinnitus or a sensation of fullness in the ears, they have had a temporary hearing loss and probably should avoid that type of exposure or wear more suitable ear protection. In recent years, it has been clearly observed that high-intensity popular music can produce hearing loss. Sound-pressure levels of 110 to 140 db have occurred near loudspeakers. A typical reading of 110 db sound pressure level 30 feet from a loudspeaker will produce a severe temporary threshold shift in 16% of listeners.

The widespread use of personal stereos with earphones is also of concern. Studies have shown that the sound output of tape recorders such as Walkmans often exceeds standards of safety. The average output of a Walkman in the 5/10 setting is near 94 db, an exposure that over a prolonged period of time is capable of producing significant hearing loss. The sound settings that are generally used by younger people while listening to these devices are generally considerably higher, since they are often exposed to competing sound at the same time.

Patients with noise-induced hearing loss often complain more of tinnitus than hearing loss, and this tends to be a warning that they are developing some significant, irreversible threshold shift. When hearing has been affected by noise, it is important that the worker avoid noise exposure for several weeks before final hearing evaluations are made. This avoids complicating any compensation reward for permanent loss, since in some patients the hearing may not revert to the final hearing level for several weeks.

Occasionally, hearing loss can occur from injuries such as explosive blasts or explosions around the head. The results of these injuries may vary widely but include significant damage to both the tympanic membrane and the inner ear. This might even include rupture of the tympanic membrane. The inner ear itself may be severely damaged or destroyed owing to the concussion injury and hemorrhage and tearing of soft tissues in the cochlear vestibule.

In 1970 the U.S. Congress passed the Occupational Safety and Health Act. The act has the following specific provisions regarding occupational hearing loss:

1. Sets maximal permissible noise levels and exposures
2. Demands protection against the effects of noise when certain specified noise levels are exceeded.
3. Differentiates intermittent and continuous noise, the latter being defined as noise with intervals between maximal peaks of 1 second or less
4. Requires industry to use *feasible* administrative and/or engineering controls to protect against excessive noise exposure
5. Demands the provision of personal protective equipment if other controls (as noted in provision 4) are ineffective
6. Requires a "continuing, effective hearing conservation program" to be administered in all cases in which sound levels exceed the values stated in the act.

The Hearing Conservation Amendments of 1981 and 1983 further specify noise exposure criteria. They establish standards for maximum permissible noise exposure, as well as procedures for reducing noise levels and monitoring employees' hearing.

Because no medical therapy has any effect on the hearing loss caused by noise and because this problem, once established, is irreversible, much effort is required to warn about the risks of high-level noise at work and in sport. Further loss can be prevented by ear protection with muffs and earplugs in all those exposed to loud noise or gunfire.

## Head Trauma

The diagnosis of cochlear damage is usually clearly indicated from the history of head injury. If the ear has bled, there is strong suspicion of a

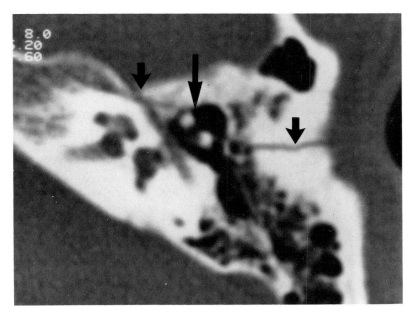

**FIG 40–4**.
CT scan demonstrating longitudinal temporal bone fracture. The *arrow on the right* clearly denotes the fracture line. The *center arrow* identifies separation of the malleus and incus demonstrating ossicular disruption, and the *arrow to the left* demonstrates the fracture extending into the area of the geniculate ganglion and internal genu of the facial nerve. Facial paralysis was present in this particular patient.

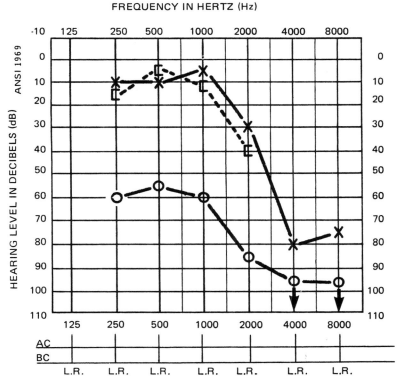

**FIG 40–5**.
Audiogram in acute traumatic head injury demonstrating a high-frequency sensorineural hearing loss in addition to a low-frequency conductive loss in the right ear. This would suggest a longitudinal fracture with ossicular discontinuity on the right.

temporal bone fracture, which is a diagnosis supported by concomitant facial weakness, vertigo, or confirmatory x-ray films. As a rule, hearing loss from head injury or trauma is permanent if the cochlea is damaged; however, if a temporal bone fracture has not occurred, the injury may be of a more concussive nature and some improvement can be expected with time. Temporal bone fractures are usually accompanied by a period of unconsciousness. These fractures can either be longitudinal along the petrous ridge, in which the hearing loss is generally conductive, or horizontal, in which the loss is neurosensory. With longitudinal temporal bone fracture there is almost always a marked high-frequency hearing loss. With horizontal fractures there is very frequently concomitant seventh nerve injury and profound cochlear damage (Figs. 40–4 and 40–5).

Other forms of trauma that can cause hearing loss are postsurgical, such as occur during operations of the temporal bone or intracranially.

## Drug Toxicity

Drug toxicity is an increasingly important cause of sensorineural hearing loss. The drugs most well known for this are the aminoglycoside antibiotics, salicylates, quinine, and related antimalarials. The ototoxicity resulting from all the aminoglycosides is quite similar and best understood. Aminoglycoside-induced ototoxicity is complicated by factors related to the absorption and elimination of the drug. Although the aminoglycosides are generally poorly absorbed in the gastrointestinal tract, oral administration can result in ototoxic responses. The same is true when these drugs are used to irrigate a wound, as the amount of absorption may be sufficient to cause hearing loss. The sole mechanism for elimination of aminoglycosides is renal excretion. Thus, any abnormality of the renal system will affect the concentration in the inner ear. The pathologic site of the destruction is the sensory hair cells. As is true with most ototoxic drugs, the basal turn of the cochlea is most affected and high-frequency loss is the earliest to develop and the most permanent (Fig. 40–6). Another unique feature of ototoxicity, not just true of aminoglycosides, is that ototoxic effects might not be detected during drug administration but can occur days to weeks after therapy has been terminated. Ototoxicity can also be unilateral. In addition to aminoglycosides, an-

**DRUGS KNOWN TO PRODUCE COCHLEAR AND VESTIBULAR TOXICITY OR TO PRODUCE SYMPTOMS (HEARING LOSS, DIZZINESS, TINNITUS) RELATED TO THE INNER EAR**

- Toxic to cochlea and/or labyrinth
  - Amikacin
  - Chloramphenicol (topically)
  - Chloroquine
  - Cisplatin
  - Dibekacin
  - Dihydrostreptomycin
  - Ethacrynic acid
  - Furosemide (Lasix)
  - Gentamicin
  - Kanamycin
  - Neomycin
  - Netilmicin
  - Nitrogen mustard
  - Quinidine
  - Quinine
  - Salicylates
  - Streptomycin
  - Tobramycin
  - Vancomycin
  - Viomycin
- Causing dizziness
  - Antihypertensives
  - Barbiturates
  - Central nervous system depressants
  - Estrogens
  - Oral contraceptives
  - Phenothiazines
  - Phenylbutazone

tibiotics have been shown to interact with loop-inhibiting diuretics, such as ethacrynic acid, and this interrelation can result in an enhanced neurosensory hearing loss.

Nonsteroidal antiinflammatory drugs such as aspirin produce a temporary hearing loss and tinnitus in patients receiving large doses (Fig. 40–7). In most cases, however, both the hearing loss and the tinnitus disappear when the drugs are terminated. Although there are a few cases in which permanent ototoxicity resulted from aspirin, the data are not convincing. Other drugs more recently reported as ototoxic are quinine, quinidine, and the antineoplastic drugs cisplatin and nitrogen mustard, viomycin, vancomycin, and 6-aminonicotinamide. Erythromycin in large

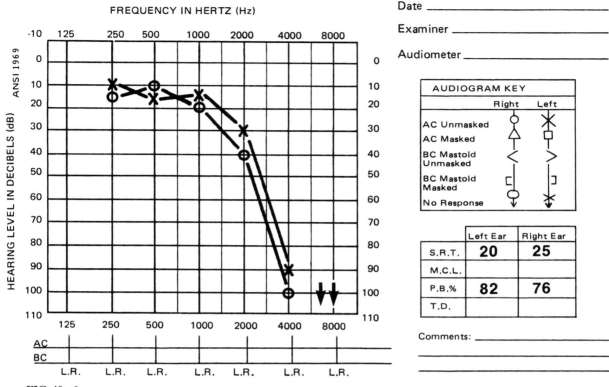

**FIG 40–6.**
Profound high-frequency loss typical of neomycin ototoxicity. Note that discrimnation scores with this hearing loss are relatively good in a quiet environment. However, in noise these scores would be in the 40% to 50% range.

doses has also recently been reported to produce a temporary hearing loss.

## Metabolic Causes of Neurosensory Hearing Loss

Whether congenital or acquired, hypothyroidism causes recognizable changes in the ear, and deafness is the principal symptom. In cretins the hearing loss is severe and sensorineural in type. Hearing loss in hypothyroid adults is usually not profound and generally reversible. The actual pathologic change is unknown, but proper replacement of circulating thyroxin, as for any hypothyroid state, will arrest or correct the hearing loss.

## Sudden Sensorineural Hearing Loss

Sudden deafness may appear instantaneously in a person who has had no previous hearing loss. The hearing loss is usually profound. Some pa-

tients describe a clicking or buzzing in one ear, then realize they are deaf. Some go to bed and wake up deaf in one ear and are uncertain when their deafness occurred. Occasionally, this is associated with dizziness. Subsequently, over a period of days or weeks, this profound loss may lessen and, in some cases, completely recover (Fig. 40–8). Tinnitus may be present. This clinical entity of sudden, profound sensorineural hearing loss has long been considered to have a vascular basis, but more recently, viral factors have been recognized as a possible cause. It has been long known, for example, that mumps causes the most profound unilateral hearing loss in children. This virus is probably just one of many capable of affecting the cochlea. Sudden, unilateral, sensorineural hearing loss unrelated to otitis media or trauma may therefore be the result of any of many etiologic agents. Among the suspected causes of sudden, sensorineural hearing loss are

1. Change in physical environment, for example, surgery, stress, travel

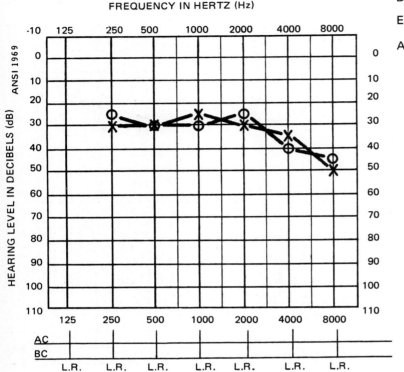

**FIG 40–7.**
Flat neurosurgery hearing loss seen in aspirin toxicity. This patient had a normal pure-tone average of better than 10 db. This is usually the case with aspirin. The patient also had marked tinnitus. The hearing returned to normal after stopping aspirin.

2. Viral illnesses—25% of patients have had a predisposing viral illness
3. Vascular vasospasm—sludging embolism
4. Fistula, usually related to straining stressful physical activity (e.g., scuba diving)
5. Tumor—a small percentage of neuromas will cause sudden loss, probably secondary to vascular drug ototoxicity
6. Immunologic disorders

The treatment of sudden deafness has included vasodilators, steroids, and antihistamines, but it has not been clearly defined which drugs are helpful. There is some evidence that high-dose steroids (60 mg prednisone/day) associated with intermittent carbogen (5% carbon dioxide and 95% oxygen) have been helpful in restoring hearing compared to no treatment. One of the most effective treatments has been rest and avoidance of stress. Large studies have suggested that almost all patients with sudden hearing loss are experiencing stressful conditions. If the patient is seen within 48 to 72 hours after onset of hearing loss, bed rest, even hospitalization, and sedation should be advised.

**Perilymphatic Leak**

Sudden perilymphatic leaks, secondary to rupture of either the oval or round window as a result of severe barotrauma or sudden exertion, are sometimes suspected. However, such causes are infrequent and usually related to some severe episode of trauma. This cause, however, is the one type of sudden neurosensory hearing loss for which the course may be altered by early surgical intervention, that is, sealing of the perilymphatic leak. These leaks can occur from either the oval or round window.

**Endolymphatic Hydrops**

Endolymphatic hydrops (Ménière disease) causes a fluctuating sensorineural hearing loss,

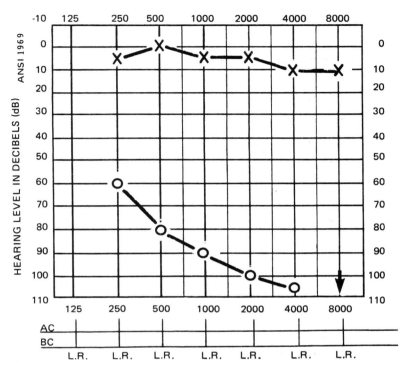

**FIG 40–8**.
Pure-tone audiogram of sudden sensorineural hearing loss. Sudden hearing loss may take the form of either low- or high-frequency damage, although high-frequency loss is most common. In a case such as this, the discrimination score might be 0% to 20%. The majority of such losses will improve over the weeks following the insult.

initially of the low tones (Fig. 40–9). As the disease progresses, the loss may become greater, involving all frequencies, and may become total. Usually it is unilateral, although in 20% to 25% of patients symptoms develop in the second ear. Hearing loss with Ménière disease is often accompanied by intermittent tinnitus, initially low pitched but later of high frequency. In addition, episodes of fullness, pressure and vertigo are part of the disorder. Ménière disease is discussed in detail in Chapter 43, Dizziness and Vertigo.

Other causes of sensorineural hearing loss include multiple sclerosis and cochlear otosclerosis. Otosclerosis usually causes a classic conductive hearing loss, but occasionally it can involve the cochlea itself, causing a progressive neurosensory loss.

## Treatment of Severe Sensorineural Hearing Loss

See Chapter 41, Rehabilitation of Nonsurgical Hearing Loss.

## Conductive Hearing Loss

Conductive hearing loss appears when sound cannot reach the cochlea. The blockage may result from abnormality of the canal, eardrum, or ossicles, including the footplate of the stapes. Lesions central to the footplate produce a sensorineural hearing loss. The box on page 464 lists the causes of conductive hearing loss.

The external auditory canal can be obstructed by impacted cerumen, foreign bodies in the canal, tumors, and swellings during infection of the external ear. The most common cause is impacted cerumen. Still another cause is atresia of the ex-

---

**CAUSES OF CONGENITAL CONDUCTIVE HEARING LOSS**
- Atresia of the external canal
- Congenital stapes fixation
- Congenital malleus fixation
- Ossicular discontinuity or maldevelopment
- Primary cholesteatoma

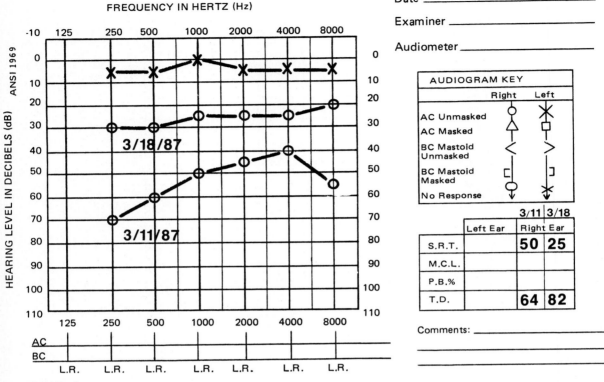

FREQUENCY IN HERTZ (Hz)

**FIG 40–9.**
Low-frequency sensorineural hearing loss from Ménière's disease showing the marked fluctuation from one test to another. Note also the marked difference in discrimination.

ternal auditory canal, a congenital condition in which the external auditory canal fails to develop normally. It is sometimes associated with mandibular deformities or an underdeveloped pinna. There may be bony occlusion of the canal with a normal pinna or complete absence of the canal and entire external ear (Fig. 40–10). A syndrome related to maldevelopment of the external ear known as Treacher Collins syndrome (mandibulo-

**CAUSES OF ACQUIRED CONDUCTIVE HEARING LOSS**
- Obstruction of the external ear canal
- Tympanic membrane perforation
- Serous otitis media
- Adhesive otitis
- Ossicular discontinuity—trauma, infection, cholesteatoma
- Tympanosclerosis
- Otosclerosis
- Ossicular fixation

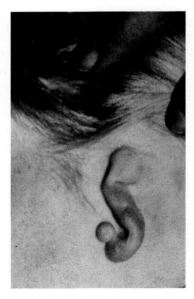

**FIG 40–10.**
External canal deformity with atresia.

facial dysostosis) is characterized, in addition to abnormalities of the external and middle ear, by agenesis of the mandible, abnormally developed eyelashes (medial part of the lower lid), and hypoplasia of the malar bones. There is a marked hereditary tendency in this condition. The hearing loss may be the result of both external and middle ear deformities.

The eardrum may be affected as the result of thickening (as in tympanosclerosis), scarring, perforation, or retraction. Hearing loss in the middle ear may be caused by liquid (pus, serum, or blood), absence or increased mobility of the ossicles (tympanosclerosis or otosclerosis), adhesions, tumors, or dislocated or absent ossicles (congenital or acquired). Almost all hearing loss secondary to damage to the eardrum or middle ear can be corrected by modern microsurgical techniques.

## Treatment of Conductive Hearing Loss

In most patients with conductive hearing loss, the condition can be treated, and normal hearing can be restored.

### *Hearing Loss Resulting From Cerumen Obstruction*

There are three methods of cleaning the ear canal. Often the simplest way to remove particulate manner is with a cerumen spoon working under direct vision through the ear speculum. The second method of cleaning the ear canal is by irrigation. The third method is by using a small, angulated sucker tip to aspirate the soft wax or any other liquid material from the ear canal. This is more useful when removing purulent matter from the ear canal but can be used when cleaning very soft wax. For discussion of wax and foreign body removal, see Chapter 39.

### *Hearing Loss Resulting From Serous Otitis Media*

Removal of thick mucoid secretion from the middle ear is necessary in many patients with serous otitis media. A myringotomy is performed. The incision in the tympanic membrane is made in a radial direction, and the liquid is removed by suction. Tenacious mucoid material occasionally must be removed by using both suction and small middle ear forceps. Both types of fluids may be forced out

of the eustachian tube by gentle inflation of the eustachian tube if it is patent. In adults the myringotomy is generally made in the anterior-inferior quadrant. A variety of tube prostheses are available. In adults myringotomy through the normal eardrum can be performed with iontophoresis or a local anesthetic block (Fig. 40–11). In children a short-duration anesthetic may be necessary. If there are no other contributing factors, hearing often returns to normal after removal of the fluid.

Patients with chronic recurrent serous otitis media often require myringotomy. Frequently it is necessary to insert a tube through the eardrum (Fig. 40–12). The tube allows aeration of the middle ear and hastens resolution of the eustachian tube obstruction, which has helped to create the negative pressure in the middle ear. The myringotomy site heals around the tube after a few hours. Tubes may be left in place until they are extruded spontaneously. Generally, a tube will remain in position for an average of 6 months. In patients who have had repetitive myringotomy and tubal placement, longer-acting tubes with a larger flange can be used. In children, serous otitis media can be associated with large or recurrent adenoids or chronic sinusitis. If adenoid hypertrophy is a major factor in causing blockage of the eustachian tube and affecting respirations, an adenoidectomy is indicated. The lymphoid tissue behind the eustachian tube orifice (Rosenmüller's fossa) must be removed under direct vision for best results.

### *Hearing Loss Resulting From Congenital Atresia*

In almost all patients with canal atresia and a normal pinna the cochlea is normal; therefore, a bone conduction hearing aid can be worn to restore hearing loss. Restoration of useful hearing is also possible by surgery. The steps of the procedure are as follows:

1. Through an endaural incision, the area of the bony meatus is identified.
2. An oval area of cortex is removed above and behind the site of the atresia, just posterior to the temporomandibular joint and exposing the tegmen (floor of the middle fossa).
3. Dissection is carried inward, enlarging the opening until the attic or antrum is ex-

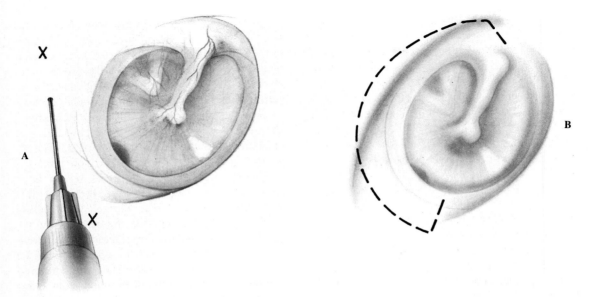

**FIG 40–11.**
**A,** sites of injection for local anesthesia of the ear include superior, posterior, and inferior sites along the bony cartilaginous junction. Some infiltration can descend medially along the canal. **B,** outline of the incision for tympanomeatal approach to middle ear.

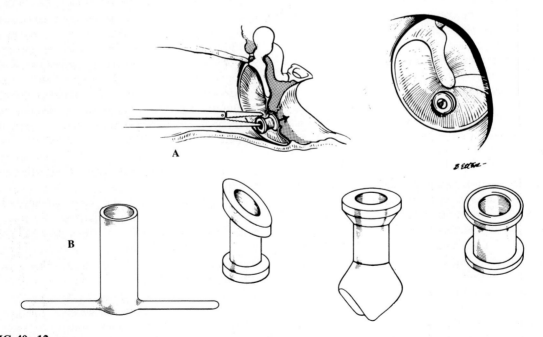

**FIG 40–12.**
**A,** plastic tubular buttons in place through the tympanic membrane. **B,** various types of plastic tubes and buttons used in serous otitis media. The tube on the left is a Goode tube with the larger flange. This tube is used for long-term placement of ventilation.

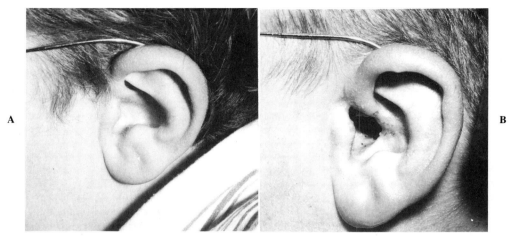

**FIG 40–13.**
**A,** congenital atresia of the external auditory canal. The pinna is well formed in the patient shown. However, it may be small, distorted, or absent entirely. **B,** postoperative skin-lined cavity as kept open by acrylic mold. This is not always necessary. (From DeWeese, DD: *Portland Clin Bull* 8:63, 1954. Used by permission.)

posed, demonstrating the head of the malleus and/or incus.

4. Once the middle ear is located, the bony plate representing the tympanic membrane is removed, sparing the ossicles.
5. If the malleus and incus are fused and fixed, they are removed, leaving the stapes intact. If the malleus and incus are normal or mobile, they are left in place.
6. The middle ear is then covered with fascia, and the cavity is lined with split-thickness skin. The external canal is enlarged (Fig 40–13).

In some cases, a simple mastoidectomy is performed through a postauricular incision, thus exposing the ossicles from behind. The risk in surgical repair of atresia is the possibility of unusual placement of the facial nerve, which can be inadvertently damaged. Therefore, the surgical dissection is meticulous.

The operation is generally not recommended if the atresia is unilateral and the uninvolved ear has normal hearing. Neither is it advised in bilateral congenital atresia before the age of 6 years.

### Hearing Loss Resulting From Other Congenital Defects

Sometimes patients with a conductive hearing loss (but not otosclerosis) have a normal or nearly normal tympanic membrane and a history of deafness since early life. See the box on page 463 for a list of causes of congenital conductive hearing loss. The diagnosis is not readily apparent, and it may be necessary to explore the middle ear to ascertain the cause of hearing loss and to correct it, if possible, during the same operative procedure. A transcanal approach is used and a flap is turned similar to the one used for stapedectomy (see Fig. 40–16). Once the drumhead is reflected, the middle ear can be inspected. One may find, for example, a missing long crus of the incus or a missing lenticular process of the incus. In the former case, the remaining part of the incus may be pulled out from the epitympanum and repositioned on the head of the stapes, or between the stapes and malleus. If only the lenticular process is absent, a piece of cartilage from the tragus or a small piece of bone may be wedged between the head of the stapes and the long crus of the incus. Sometimes the bodies of the incus and malleus are fused in the epitympanum and must be removed to free the ossicular chain. If the superstructure of the stapes is missing and the body of the incus still remains, it is possible to establish a connection between the malleus and the stapedial footplate by removing and remodeling the incus and carefully interposing it. A prosthetic incus may be used to connect the malleus to the footplate. There are thus a great many variations in

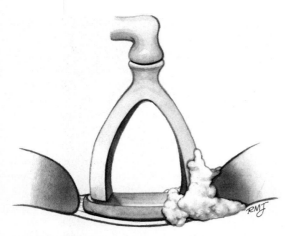

**FIG 40–14.**
Otosclerotic focus on anterior margin of the stapes.

middle ear anatomy that must be anticipated with congenital ear problems. Most of them are amenable to surgery, but usually exploratory tympanotomy is necessary before one can be certain of what technique will be required.

### Hearing Loss Resulting From Otosclerosis

Otosclerosis is the most common cause of conductive hearing loss in people between the ages of 15 and 50 years. It is a hereditary defect of unknown cause. According to postmortem studies, 10% of the white population have otosclerosis. It is not common in blacks. Women are more affected than men.

In otosclerosis, dystrophy occurs in the bony labyrinth (otic capsule). Normal bone is absorbed and replaced by otosclerotic bone, which is highly vascular and tends to overgrow the normal bony labyrinth. When the otosclerotic bony focus advances posteriorly from its usual site of origin (immediately anterior to the oval window), it causes a progressive fixation of the footplate of the stapes, which is manifested by a slowly progressive conductive hearing loss (Figs. 40–14 and 40–15). In women it may progress more rapidly during or immediately after pregnancy, but no definite causal relationship has been established. The eardrum usually appears normal, although occasionally a faint pink blush can be seen

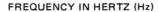

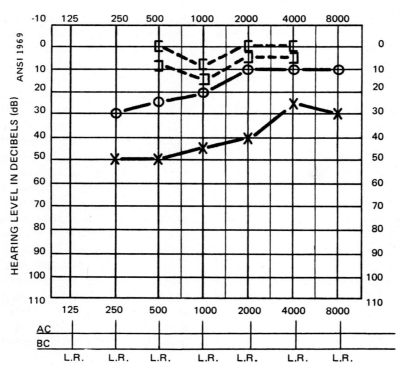

**FIG 40–15.**
Bilateral otosclerosis. This is a predominantly low-frequency conductive hearing loss. Discrimination scores in conductive losses will generally be excellent. This patient is a surgical candidate for left stapes surgery.

through the eardrum. This coloration is called Schwartz's sign and represents the vascularity of the active otosclerotic bony focus.

Hearing loss is usually first noticed in the late teens or early twenties. Both ears are usually affected but not always. Although otosclerosis characteristically produces more conductive hearing loss, it can involve neural elements and cause mixed hearing loss or sensorineural hearing loss. If cochlear function is normal or near normal, the hearing loss produced by otosclerosis can be improved by surgical means.

The evolution of surgery for otosclerosis since 1950 has been a triumph of microsurgical techniques. Initially the procedure consisted of fenestration, in which a new window was created in the horizontal semicircular canal after a mastoid cavity was made. This procedure is rarely used now and is generally of historical interest only, since it has been supplanted by stapedectomy. Because the middle ear lost its mechanical advantage, the hearing loss persisting after the fenestration procedure was 20 to 30 db and therefore normal hearing was never approximated.

In 1952, with improved lighting and magnification, the stapes mobilization procedure became popular. This consisted of mobilization of the fixed stapes. It was found, however, that only 30% of patients had persistent closure of the air-bone gap, with refixation of the stapes occurring either by new otosclerotic bone or by healing of the fractured footplate margin. Thus the stapes

mobilization procedure was replaced by partial or total stapedectomy.

In 1957 Shea first reported successful removal of the stapes with its footplate and replacement of it with a prosthetic stapes made of polyethylene tubing. Since then numerous modifications have been devised. More recent procedures have somewhat less risk to sensorineural hearing reserve and better long-term results. In properly selected patients who retain normal or nearly normal bone conduction, usable and often normal hearing can be restored 90% to 95% of the time. Some patients do not improve despite careful stapedectomy and prosthetic replacement. This risk of damage to the cochlea and partial or total hearing loss is reported to be as high as 6% following the procedure. There is a 1% to 2% risk of total loss. This potential risk must always be considered before a decision is made to perform a stapedectomy. There are also some patients who have initial good results but later show cochlear damage.

The two procedures most commonly used at present are (1) a total stapedectomy with replacement with a prosthesis and (2) a stapedotomy (a small hole placed in the stapes's footplate through which a wire and piston are inserted). The procedure consists of the following steps:

1. A local injection about the ear (see Fig. 40–11)
2. The elevation of a canal tympanic membrane flap, called the tympanomeatal flap,

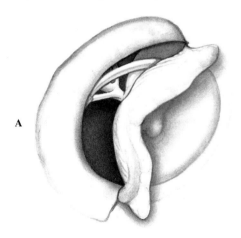 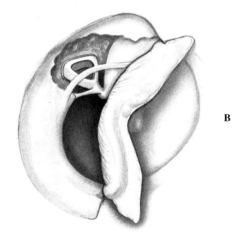

**FIG 40–16.**
**A,** elevation of the tympanomeatal flap demonstrating the incus, stapes, and chorda tympani crossing the incus. **B,** removal of additional posterior-superior canal wall bone demonstrating course of the facial nerve and the oval window niche with the anterior and posterior crura.

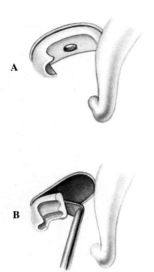

**FIG 40–17.**
**A,** after fracture and removal of the superstructure of the stapes, a small hole or fenestra is made in the oval window. **B,** if a small fenestra is not possible, the entire stapes footplate should be removed.

with elevation anteriorly exposing the ossicular chain (Fig. 40–16)
3. Separation of the incudostapedial joint
4. Division of the stapedius muscle
5. Removal of the superstructure of the stapes from the footplate
6. Creation of a small fenestra into the stapes or total removal of the stapes's footplate with fine microsurgical instruments (Fig. 40–17).
7. Placement of a prosthesis. In the small fenestra technique, the piston is placed in the fenestra. In total stapedectomy, a perichondrium, or fascia "boat," is placed over the oval window and the prosthesis is positioned on it (Fig. 40–18).

Several different prosthetic devices are used (Fig. 40–19).

Good hearing may be maintained for many years following stapes procedures; however, a high percentage of patients develop a slowly progressive high-frequency cochlear loss. For this reason, many feel it best to delay performing a stapedectomy on the opposite ear of the same patient until several years after the first operation. One advantage of the small fenestra stapedotomy has been the lessened risk of high-frequency hearing loss developing over time, a feature which may make this the procedure of choice of the future.

In some instances, after a stapedectomy has been performed, there is incomplete closure of the oval window. Perilymph may then leak about the prosthesis and into the middle ear. If such a leak continues, the hearing level that has been improved by the operation may fluctuate widely or may suddenly diminish. Such changes may also be accompanied by tinnitus or mild to very sudden, intense vertigo. Whenever a patient who has undergone stapedectomy complains of fluctuating hearing, increasing tinnitus, or recurrent or abrupt vertigo, a perilymph leak should be suspected. Often the operation must be repeated and the leak repaired to preserve the hearing improvement and, in some cases, to prevent serious, irreversible loss of hearing.

**Medical Treatment.** In addition to the several surgical procedures devised for correction of hearing loss caused by otosclerosis, sodium fluoride is said to promote recalcification and inactivation of the actively expanding demineralized focus of otospongiosis. This results in stabilization of a progressive sensorineural hearing loss. Thus,

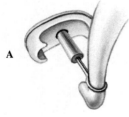
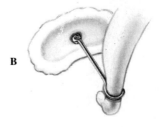

**FIG 40–18.**
**A,** placement of the wire piston firmly crimped about the incus. **B,** total stapedectomy after placement of perichondrium over the oval window. A wire loop prosthesis is crimped and placed against the oval window membrane.

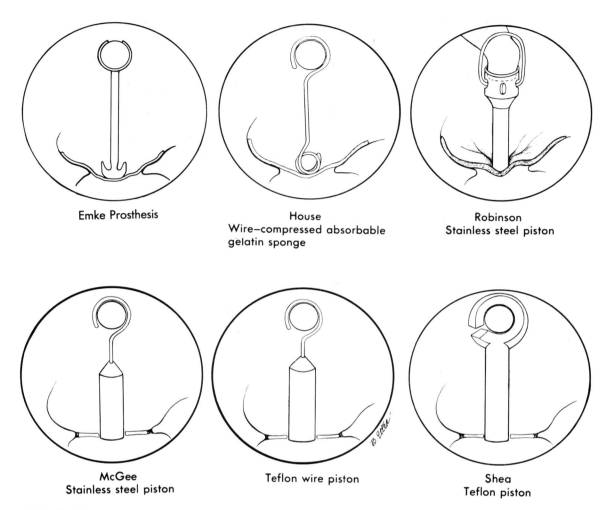

Emke Prosthesis

House
Wire–compressed absorbable
gelatin sponge

Robinson
Stainless steel piston

McGee
Stainless steel piston

Teflon wire piston

Shea
Teflon piston

**FIG 40–19.**
Stapedectomy prostheses. Top three diagrams show various prostheses used after footplate has been removed. Bottom three diagrams indicate that the footplate has been "drilled" to precisely accept a prefabricated piston. (Adapted from Saunders WH, Paparella MM, Miglets AW: *Atlas of ear surgery,* ed 3, St Louis, 1980, Mosby–Year Book. Used by permission.)

the drug is used not to correct the element of conductive loss that has already taken place, but to prevent the superimposed sensorineural loss that sometimes occurs. There is still active controversy concerning the effectiveness of this treatment. The various doses recommended include 25 to 40 mg of sodium fluoride taken with calcium and vitamin D daily for up to 2 years.

### Hearing Loss Resulting From Chronic Suppurative Otitis Media

The aim of temporal bone surgery is eradication of infection. A radical or modified radical mastoidectomy requires removal of part or all of the eardrum, the mucosa of the middle ear, the malleus, and the incus. Such an operation is still necessary to control infection in some patients with extensive chronic suppurative otitis media. As a separate procedure, radical mastoidectomy is very infrequently performed (see Chapter 37).

**Tympanoplasty.** Over the years there have been numerous definitions and classifications of tympanoplasty, which is defined as reconstructive surgery of the tympanic membrane. Tympanoplasty has been facilitated by the development of

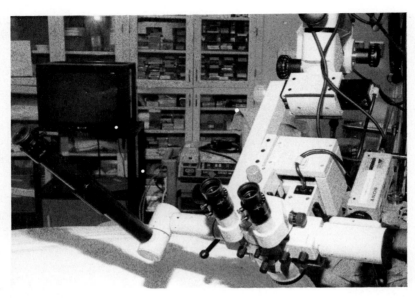

**FIG 40–20.**
Operating microscope used during middle ear and mastoid surgery. The lens system allows a change from 6 to 40 magnification.

the operating microscope (Fig. 40–20). The normal ear provides a great mechanical advantage to sound pressure by means of the transformer action. This is made possible in small part by the lever action of the ossicles and in greater part by the tympanic membrane-to-footplate ratio. This mechanical advantage afforded by the middle ear explains its chief purpose. It must regain as much as possible of the sound pressure that is lost when sound is transferred from air to a liquid medium. The transformer action of the middle ear is effective in recovering some 25 to 27 of the 30 db lost. Also important in the normal scheme of hearing is the sound protection afforded to the round window by the presence of an intact tympanic membrane. In the normal ear, the round window acts as a relief mode for sound pressure driven into the cochlea across the ossicular chain. If it were not for round window protection, sound waves could reach both the oval and round windows simultaneously and cause a cancellation effect. In chronic otitis media, in which the tympanic membrane and often the malleus and incus are partially or completely absent, sound waves can enter both windows with approximately equal intensity. Therefore, there is a chance for partial cancellation. More important, with loss of the eardrum, the area ratio is lost or reduced. Thus tympanoplasty improves hearing by reestablishing

two important middle ear functions: (1) it restores the area ratio, which is the chief component of the transformer action, and (2) it creates sound protection for the round window.

More recent classifications for surgery of chronic ear infection are as follows:

1. **Myringoplasty,** an operation in which the tympanic membrane perforation is closed without modification of the ossicular chain
2. **Tympanoplasty with ossiculoplasty, without mastoidectomy,** an operative procedure in which the middle ear conductive mechanism and tympanic membrane are repaired without involving the mastoid cavity
3. **Tympanoplasty with ossiculoplasty, with mastoidectomy,** an operation that eradicates disease in both the mastoid and middle ear cavity with reconstruction of the tympanic membrane and ossicular chain. Various types of reconstructive procedures are possible within this classification but have to be described. Therefore, when the tympanic cavity is restored and the ossicular chain is corrected in some fashion, one would expect hearing levels to approach the normal bone conduction level.

***Indications.*** Tympanoplasty with ossiculoplasty is indicated when chronic suppurative otitis
media produces a significant conductive loss. The
patients must have good nerve function (cochlear
reserve) if hearing is to be improved. The greater
the difference between the air and bone measurements, the greater the chances for improvement.
It must be noted that tympanoplasty may at times
be performed for reasons other than improvement
of hearing. For example, there are patients with
perforation of the tympanic membrane who have
essentially normal hearing but who still need the
perforation closed to prevent intermittent discharge. Others, who may have chronic suppurative otitis media but a sensorineural rather than a
conductive hearing loss, still require tympanoplasty as part of an operative procedure to help
clear infection, even though hearing improvement
is not possible. Ossiculoplasty may also be used
in patients with no perforation, such as those with
traumatic effects (dislocation of the incus), those
with congenital middle ear problems, and those in
whom tympanosclerosis has fused the malleus to
the incus or fixed the malleus to the bone of the
epitympanum. Here the problems are ossicular
and may involve the use of metal or plastic prostheses, otogenous material (especially in incus
transposition,) or homograft ossicles. In these
cases, the results are often surprisingly good,
since there is no concomitant infection.

***Contraindications.*** Tympanoplasty with ossiculoplasty is contraindicated in patients whose
cochlear reserve is poor, as tested by bone conduction. The procedure should be delayed in patients with active infection.

***Techniques.*** Many approaches and techniques are used. Some surgeons use a postauricular approach, whereas others use an endaural approach. The use of full-thickness or split-thickness skin graft, which was the original grafting
material, has been abandoned. A sliding skin
graft fashioned from the inner part of the ear canal can be used successfully, but most surgeons
now use fascia or perichondrium. Tympanoplasty
may be performed even in the presence of mastoid or middle ear disease, such as infection or
cholesteatoma, although the results are not as
good.

Many surgeons prefer, in extensively diseased

ears, to perform the operation in stages. When a
tympanoplasty is performed to correct defects
caused by chronic suppurative otitis media, the
results are better if the suppurative disease is
cleared first. Then all that remains to be accomplished is the mechanical correction of the deficient sound-transmitting system. The operation
can be combined, however, with mastoidectomy
in patients with active suppurative disease. In
fact, inspection of the mastoid is advised as part
of tympanoplasty whenever there appears any
likelihood of such disease. Sometimes good results are obtained when the posterior wall of the
ear canal is left standing rather than being removed, as occurs in a radical or modified radical
mastoidectomy.

Most important in any surgery is eustachian
tube function. The eustachian tube must be patent
for good middle ear function. An air-filled middle
ear is necessary if there is to be an air pocket between the graft and the round window. If the
middle ear mucosa is in good condition, it is left
undisturbed. However, if it has been replaced by
squamous epithelium growing in from the ear canal through a perforation or absent drumhead, it
must be removed. Then care is taken to interpose
nonadherent sheeting of Silastic or similar material between the denuded promontory and the new
drumhead. Otherwise, the fascia would adhere to
the promontory and obliterate the middle ear
space. In addition, Gelfoam (an absorbable substance) frequently is placed in the middle ear
space to support the new graft temporarily. As the
Gelfoam is absorbed, the eustachian tube begins
to ventilate the ear. The fascia or perichondrial
graft picks up its blood supply from the margins
of the tympanic membrane.

In *myringoplasty* (also known as Type I tympanoplasty) there are two general techniques: an
underlay method and an onlay technique. In the
onlay method the graft material used (fascia) is
placed lateral to the tympanic membrane remnant.
In this technique, all squamous epithelium on the
tympanic membrane must be removed to prevent
burying squamous epithelium. In the underlay
method the margins of the perforation are denuded and the graft is placed medial to the perforation supported by Gelfoam (Fig. 40–21). Usually the ear has been approached with a canal
flap, and the graft can be tucked under the posterior canal skin. In some cases, the loss of the

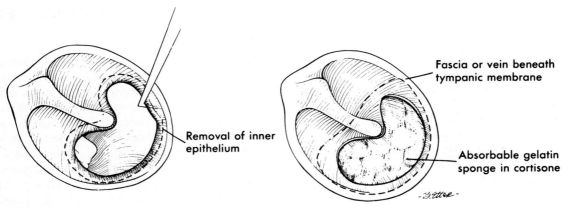

**FIG 40–21.**
Type I tympanoplasty (myringoplasty) performed by placing the graft against the medial surface of the drumhead. Epithelium is removed from the rim of the perforation, and the fascia or vein is placed beneath the tympanic membrane. Absorbable gelatin sponge must first be placed in the middle ear to support the graft against the undersurface of the drumhead. (From Saunders WH, Paparella MM: *Atlas of ear surgery,* ed 2, St Louis, 1971, Mosby–Year Book. Used by permission.)

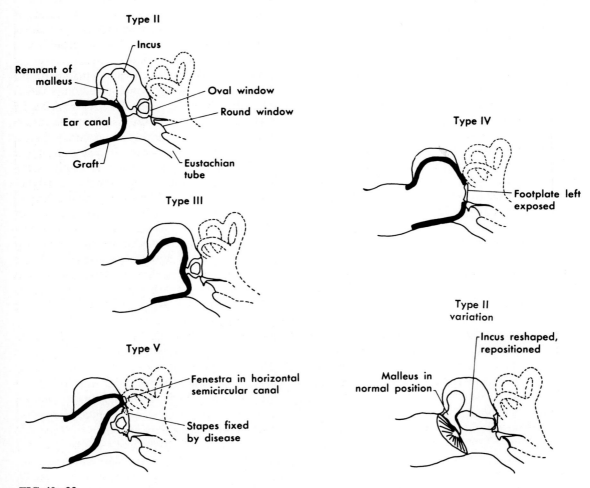

**FIG 40–22.**
Different types of tympanoplasty. In each diagram a graft (fascia, perichondrium) is indicated by the heavy line. The diagram of type V illustrates fenestration, and the diagram of type II shows correction of an ossicular defect without a tympanic membrane perforation. Note that in all types there is round window protection.

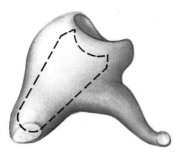

**FIG 40–23.**
Creation of a bony ossicular strut from an incus.

tympanic membrane may be near total. In those cases, homograft tympanic membranes obtained from cadavers have been used with a high success rate to replace the components of the normal tympanic membrane.

**Ossicular Reconstruction.** With ossicular deformity, a variety of surgical techniques have been devised and a variety of materials used to reconstruct the ossicular chain. The multiple possibilities of repair are represented in Figure 40–22.

An *incus interposition* is probably the most common procedure done in tympanoplasty, as the most frequent ossicular deformity is loss of connection between the malleus and the head of the stapes. There are a variety of methods of incus in-

terposition. If the body and short process of the incus are still present and unaffected by chronic ear disease, the incus can be detached from the malleus. The incus is then remodeled so that the short process fits on the head of the stapes, and the body is notched to fit under the malleus. This procedure is frequently performed when there is no active suppurative disease—for example, in healed chronic otitis media in which the tympanic membrane is present so that the fascia graft is not needed. In general, the use of either autogenous or homogeneous incus interposed between a mobile stapes and an intact tympanic membrane or fascia graft gives very good hearing. Best results are obtained if the interposed bone is drilled and shaped in such a fashion that there is a secure fit between the head of the stapes and the handle of the malleus (Figs. 40–23 and 40–24). Good results demand meticulous surgical dissection and a secure fit of all the interposed parts.

A variety of anatomic defects may face the otologic surgeon, including absence of the superstructure of the stapes, as well as the long process of the incus. In these cases the prosthesis must bridge the interval between the footplate of the stapes and the undersurface of the malleus or tympanic membrane. A variety of materials have been used for this prosthesis, including homograft ossicles, cartilage, and synthetic grafts, including

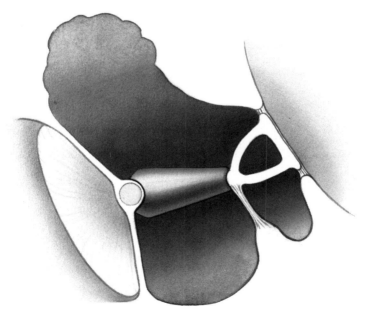

**FIG 40–24.**
Placement of an incus strut notched to fit the head of the stapes and placed under the handle of the malleus.

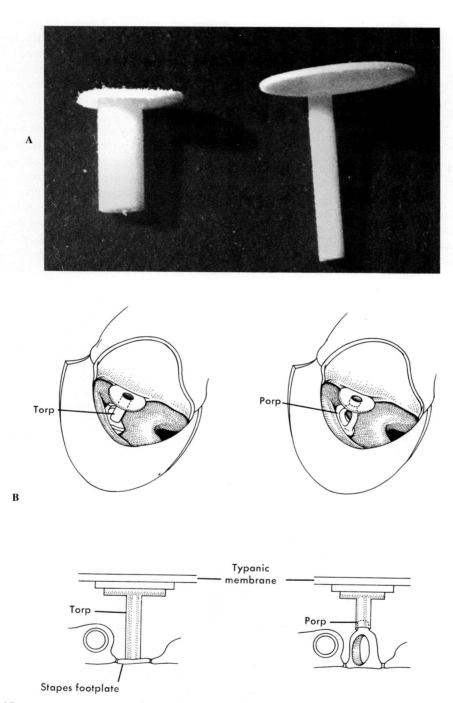

**FIG 40–25.**
**A,** *Left,* partial ossicular replacement prosthesis (PORP). *Right,* total ossicular replacement prosthesis (TORP). The PORP fits between the eardrum and the head of the stapes. The longer TORP fits between the eardrum and the footplate of the stapes. **B,** the left-hand figures *(above* and *below)* show total absence of the superstructure of the stapes. A TORP prosthesis is required. This may bridge from the footplate to the undersurface of a fascial graft, or it may bridge to the medial surface of the residual handle of the malleus. The right-hand figures *(above* and *below)* show the placement of the shorter PORP when most of the stapes still remains. Note the placement of the cartilage overlying the TORP or PORP deep to tympanic membrane. This is placed to prevent extrusion of the prosthesis through the graft or tympanic membrane.

ceramic and various Teflon prostheses. Modifications and innovations of replacements for middle ear structures continue to be devised. An example is the partial ossicular replacement prosthesis shown in Figure 40–25. Similarly, a total ossicular replacement prosthesis can be substituted for the entire chain if the footplate of the stapes is intact. Best results still appear to be obtained, however, by either the patient's own material or homograft ossicular material if it can be fashioned properly to reconstruct the ossicular chain.

Results of tympanoplastic procedures are not perfect, but patients generally will get some improvement. Improvement to the level of socially adequate hearing (greater than 30 db) will be gained in 95% of cases with straightforward myringoplasty. Generally, an 80% to 90% success rate to socially adequate hearing can be expected with incus interposition and a 60% to 80% success rate with more involved procedures. Very often revision procedures greatly improve the initial surgical results. Results are affected by active infection, eustachian tube dysfunction, and patient noncompliance.

# 41

# Rehabilitation of Nonsurgical Hearing Loss

Although many patients with hearing loss receive benefit from surgical treatment, there are many others whose hearing cannot be improved by these means. Although figures vary, over 20 million people will need help for hearing problems at some time during their lives. As many as half of these will have a hearing loss great enough to handicap them. For this segment of the population, help must come from amplification of sound (hearing aids), other assistive devices, or speech (lip) reading. The physician remains as the logical counselor to the patients with a hearing loss problem. The physician must advise the patients as to suitable rehabilitation. In no field of medicine is rehabilitation more important than in hearing loss. Under the guidance of otologists and with the assistance of audiologists, speech therapists, speech teachers, and educators of the deaf, rehabilitative programs must be outlined for each individual with hearing disability.

## HEARING AIDS

Generally, a hearing aid is nothing more than an audioamplification system, more modified by its necessary size than by any other factor. It has the following parts: (1) a microphone that converts sound waves into electrical energy; (2) an amplifier; (3) a receiver that converts this electrical energy back to sound waves; and (4) a power source, batteries or transistors, that provides the power to run the system. In recent years, the hearing aid industry has made tremendous strides in the miniaturization of hearing aids. Also, hear-

ing aids are now capable of amplifying over a much greater range of sound. Formerly, they would amplify only up to 2,000 Hz, but now aids are capable of amplification to 4,000 Hz or higher, an advance providing added assistance at higher frequencies. Hearing aids have also become more frequency specific. In other words, they can amplify certain frequencies to the exclusion of others, usually increasing the higher tones. Finally, with modern hearing aids, it is much easier to control the output, to limit the loudness, and to compress the range of sound intensity to a narrow band.

There are many types of hearing aids (see box) including ear-level aids, body aids, bone conduction aids, and contralateral routing of offside signals (CROS) aids. There are four main ear-level aids: (1) behind-the-ear, (2) in-the-ear, (3) canal, and (4) in glasses or other devices (Fig. 41–1). Each of these devices has both advantages and disadvantages. The advantage of the behind-the-ear aid is a stronger battery source and, hence, more output. It is also less likely to cause feedback because the microphone is separate from the amplifier. The in-the-ear and canal aids have the advantage of improved cosmetic appearance and good fidelity, but the disadvantage, because of their smaller size, is slightly decreased output or volume gain (Fig. 41–2). The eyeglass hearing aid has the advantage of concealed appearance and is frequently used as a CROS aid but has the disadvantage of being removed frequently, depending on how often the individual takes off his or her glasses.

Bone conduction aids are still used for severe

## TYPES OF HEARING AIDS

- Ear level aids
  - Behind-the-ear aid
  - In-the-ear aid
  - Canal aid
  - Eyeglass aid
- Body aids
- Bone conduction aids
- CROS aids
- Cochlear implant

conductive losses in children, especially those with atresia. Body aids are rarely used, except with patients with profound hearing loss. The advantage of body aids is that they have the greatest gain (power) of all the hearing aids and do not have feedback. However, they are less acceptable to patients unless there is a profound hearing loss.

The CROS hearing aid is a modified ear-level aid that can be either in eyeglasses or behind the ear. It was especially designed to reduce the listening problems encountered by patients with hearing loss in only one ear. In the CROS aid, the signals are picked up by the microphone placed near the poor ear and routed across to an ear phone mounted beside the good ear. The amplified signals are directed into the good ear either by placing a plastic tube in the ear canal or by using a special nonoccluded ear piece that holds the tube firmly in the canal. Some newer aids use a frequency modulated (FM) transmission system that negates the need for wire connections. Such an arrangement does not block the normal reception of sound in the good ear. Modifications of the CROS aid (Bi-CROS and IROS) are also useful because they separate the microphone from the ear phone, thus avoiding the feedback that may result when both elements are close together on one side of the head. The Bi-CROS is an aid in which signals from the right ear are transferred to the left and those from the left ear are transferred to the right.

Conventional hearing aids amplify sound through conventional analog amplifiers. However, digital technology is slowly being added to hearing aids so that some of today's analog amplifiers are being controlled with digital electronics. These are called hybrid systems. The use of hybrid systems and all digital techniques allows for additional useful features, including noise reduction and memory (development of several sets of adjustment patterns in the hearing aids and the remote control). These new advancements will mean significant improvements in amplification for the hard of hearing.

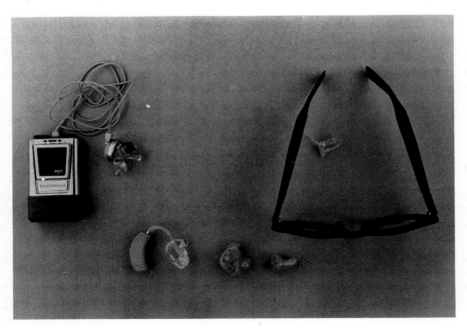

**FIG 41–1**.
Hearing aid types. *Left to right, front row:* behind-the-ear, in-the-ear, canal type. *Back row:* body-style, eyeglass.

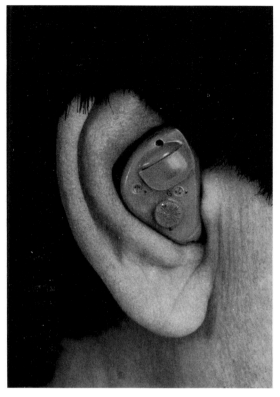

A

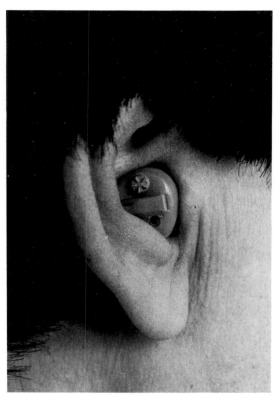

B

**FIG 41–2.**
**A,** custom in-the-ear hearing aid. **B,** canal type of hearing aid. Smaller canal aids are now available.

Four features contribute to the poor acceptance of hearing aids: (1) cosmetics; (2) cost; (3) problems with use, particularly in noise; and (4) poor instruction in hearing aid use.

Vanity plays a major role in hearing aid rejection; however, recent improvement of ear models and the acceptance of hearing aids by major public and entertainment personalities has done much to change this attitude.

The cost of hearing aids is a major deterrent, especially since they are rarely paid for by insurance. Hearing aids may cost $250 to $800 or more each.

Problems with noise and feedback continue to plague the industry as the major complaint of hearing aid users.

Finally, too few patients are counseled as to what hearing aids are capable of providing and what they are unable to do. Too many individuals have false hopes or are not knowledgeable concerning the capabilities of their hearing instrument.

The patient who benefits most from the use of hearing aids is the one who has a major conductive hearing loss. However, this is also the patient in whom surgery is most successful. There are several reasons for the good results of the hearing aid in conductive hearing loss: (1) in conductive loss all tones are more likely to be affected to nearly the same degree. This so-called flat type of hearing loss is easily altered by straight amplification. (2) In the true conductive loss, there are no problems with discrimination. If sound is loud enough, the patient can understand what he hears. (3) Recruitment is usually not present. Therefore, the patient with conductive hearing impairment can receive sound over a wide range of intensities without discomfort.

The patient with a mixed or sensorineural hearing loss has more difficulty using a hearing aid. Sensorineural hearing losses, in most instances, involve the high tones or the high and middle tones, leaving the low frequencies nearly normal. Compensation for the high-tone loss can be built into the electrical circuitry of the hearing aid, but for patients who have major differences in sensitivity between the high and low frequencies, sound specificity may not be sufficient. In spite of these difficulties, almost all patients with sensori-neural hearing loss can wear a hearing aid effectively and can improve speech. Even profoundly deaf patients with a loss of 85 to 90 db obtain benefit from hearing aids. This is true even if the patient is unable to discriminate words clearly. The perception of tonal differences helps understanding and lip reading.

In the selection of a satisfactory hearing aid, speech and pure tone audiograms are useful, not only in determining whether the patient will benefit from amplification but also in selecting the most suitable type of amplification. Pure tone thresholds indicate the severity and frequency of hearing loss. The comfort level and maximal tolerance level are also important in hearing aid selection, since the patient needs to be comfortable listening without noise intolerance. This is often difficult to achieve when the range between comfort level and tolerance level may be as little as 10 to 20 db, which requires immense compression of speech sounds into a very narrow range of loudness, a factor difficult to achieve without distortion. Patients who have damaged cochlear hair cells and exhibit recruitment are the most difficult to fit with a hearing aid. They will hear soft sounds poorly or not at all, and loud sounds will cause distortion and even pain. The tolerance of such patients to minute increases in volume and the narrow range between comfortable loudness and uncomfortable loudness create problems that sometimes cannot be resolved. Differences in the ear molds are also important in achieving good results with hearing aids. Better discrimination can often be achieved by using an open mold with an air vent, which creates only partial occlusion. These vented aids make it possible to selectively amplify at higher frequencies without equally amplifying the lower frequencies and allow lower tones, usually better heard, to reach the ear through the vent.

In considering the use of hearing aids, the following features are of great importance: (1) Most patients with sensorineural hearing loss can be aided and thus should not be ignored because of the nature of their loss. It is impossible to prejudge whether a patient will or will not be assisted by an aid. (2) Hearing aids should not be used only for those with moderate-to-profound hearing loss, but for those whose hearing is better and thus require lesser hearing gain. Not only do patients get accustomed to hearing amplified sound, but management of hearing aid controls becomes automatic. Thus, as they become older, they are able to avoid a learning process. (3) It must be made clear to the patient that a hearing aid does not give normal hearing. Almost all hearing aids will cause some problem in noise because they amplify all sounds. In a restaurant, for instance, the hearing aid user may complain bitterly about hearing the conversation at the tables around him as loudly as that at his or her table. This continues to be the most difficult adjustment to using a hearing aid. (4) In fitting a hearing aid, the patient and physician must repeatedly try to improve the function and use of the aid. Making sounds louder is not enough for most patients, and efforts should continue to develop better clarity of speech perception. (5) Hearing aids can be and are of value in the unilateral losses. Many patients who are business people, teachers, automobile drivers, and so on will all benefit from a hearing aid in a poor hearing ear. (6) Even if patients complain that with the hearing aid they hear louder but not clearer, it is important that they be encouraged to continue the use of the aid, particularly for the sake of their family and friends. The value of not having to shout at an individual is critical in families maintaining social contact with a hearing-impaired relative or friend. Federal regulation requires that before the sale of a hearing aid the patient have a trial period of use; it is important that this trial period never be cut short. The potential of the instrument must be demonstrated clearly to the individual.

## COCHLEAR IMPLANTS

Cochlear implant technology has expanded rapidly over the past several years. The cochlear implant is an attempt to replace the nonfunctional inner ear with a direct electrical stimulus to the auditory nerve. There are a variety of implant designs, but all have similar components, including: (1) a microphone that receives the sound and sends it to a speech processor; (2) a processor that transforms the acoustic energy into an electrical signal that is passed to (3) an electrode implanted near the auditory nerve. This electrode stimulates

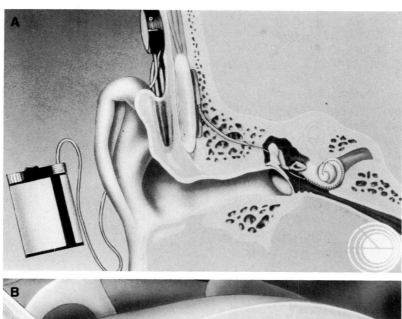

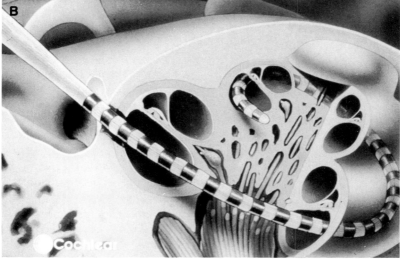

**FIG 41–3.**
**A,** schematic representation of cochlear implant showing receiver processor and probe passing through mastoid into middle ear and through round window. **B,** twenty-two channel electrode placed into scala tympani and passed around basal turn of cochlea.

the remaining auditory nerve fibers (Fig. 41–3).

Patients who have acquired language before losing their hearing attain the most benefit from the cochlear implants. The implants thus far have been used only on patients who had profound hearing loss and who obtained no usable hearing with the use of the most powerful hearing aids. Congenitally deaf patients are not able to process information delivered by implants as effectively and have not done as well. The surgical procedure involves standard approaches to the middle ear through a facial recess approach and exposure

of the round window. The majority of the implants involve placement of an electrode within the cochlea through the round window. It is becoming apparent that, although results are variable, some patients are able to use the information and understand some speech. Almost all patients are able to detect sound as faint as 25 to 30 db, which in the profoundly deaf provides significant auditory improvement. Perhaps the greatest value of the cochlear implant has been its ability to provide sound clues to patients who have heard no sounds for years. This aids in their lipreading ability, helps modulate their speaking tones, and gives a greater sense of safety and well-being. As yet, however, the majority of patients do not hear speech as a normal person hears it, but rather hear a tonal sound of various description. For the patient who has no hearing, this is an immense event. Significant research is continuing in a variety of centers with a number of devices.

There are many other aspects of a hearing rehabilitation program (see box below). A number of these areas will be discussed.

## LIPREADING

The ability to understand speech through the observance of lip and tongue movement and facial expression is known as lipreading. Some persons have a natural ability to read lips and practice it as a matter of habit. Others, even after long training, never learn to read lips well. Lipreading is an additional aid to anyone with a hearing impairment. Although some patients learn by themselves, help from a teacher gives more satisfactory results. The combination of a well-fitted aid and good lipreading ability is the ultimate in hear-

---

**FEATURES OF AURAL REHABILITATION PROGRAM**
- Use of hearing aids
- Possibility of cochlear implant
- Assistive communication
  - Speech reading
  - Auditory training
  - Cued speech
  - Finger spelling
  - Signing
  - Telephone devices
  - Telecommunication devices for the deaf (TDDs)
  - Computer technology
  - Hearing dogs
- Assistive listening devices, including FM systems, induction loops, and infrared systems
- Special sensory devices
  - Caption television
  - Gongs and bells
  - Vibrators
  - Lights

---

ing rehabilitation. The sounds most frequently lost are, fortunately, the sounds most easily lipread (e.g., consonants and fricatives).

## TELEPHONE DEVICES

A multitude of devices to help improve telephone communication are available. None of these devices, however, extend the frequency response, improve the signal-to-noise ratio, or reduce distortion. Their main action is simple amplification. These devices include two groups: (1) volume control and (2) couplers for use with telecoil loops incorporated into individual hearing aids. With volume control, a wheel or button on the handset will amplify the signal up to approximately 30 db.

## TTY-TDD

Devices are available to allow a deaf individual to have phone communication by using teletypewriters. In using teletypewriters (TTY) and telecommunication devices for the deaf (TDDs), the patient dials a phone number, places the handset on the acoustic coupler of the TDD, and types a message. The electrical signals are converted into auditory signals, and the receiving TDD then converts the signals from the receiving telephone into electrical impulses that are directed to a screen, printer, or storage device (Fig. 41–4). Basically, what is typed in one machine is printed out on the other. Technology has significantly advanced in this area, making these devices smaller, more portable, and less expensive. Operation of the system requires low-level typing ability and ability to read.

## ASSISTIVE LISTENING DEVICES

Assistive listening devices are readily accessible and bring the listener closer to the source of sound, eliminating undesirable background noise and providing greater intelligibility. They are designed to amplify the source of the desired sound, thereby improving signal-to-noise ratios and enhancing intelligibility. The simplest assistive listening devices are ear phones or ear molds connected directly to an immobile amplified source.

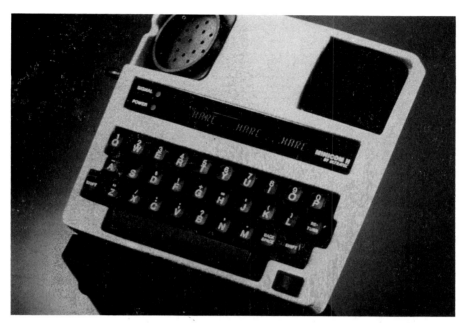

**FIG 41–4.**
Portable TDD. (Courtesy of HARC Mercantile Ltd.)

This source may be a television set, a microphone amplifier, a radio, or the like. These systems are frequently used by individuals with mild-to-moderate hearing loss who have difficulty understanding television or radio. These devices are also excellent for one-to-one communication in patient interviews, counseling sessions, and so on. There are a variety of pocket microphones and receivers available.

Another assistive device is the infrared system, which uses a new technology for transmission of the audio signal based on invisible modulated infrared radiation. Infrared, gallium arsonide, luminescent diodes are used to generate the modulated signals. A photosensitive diode, coupled with a lens to concentrate the incident radiation, is used as a receiver. Areas up to 5,000 square feet, which will typically accomodate 400 to 500 people, can be illuminated. For instance, 12 transmitter emitters are used in the New York Metropolitan Opera House to serve the 4,265-seat auditorium. The receiver decodes the signal into intelligible high-quality audio signals, and these signals are then transmitted to the listener through a stethoscope-type headset or through the individual's own hearing aids (Fig. 41–5). These systems offer excellent fidelity without noise interference. Indoor use of infrared systems is ex-

cellent in rooms such as TV areas, theaters, auditoriums, and churches.

Another advance has been the development of FM systems consisting of an FM transmitter and one or more receivers. The transmitter microphone is placed near the sound source, and the signals are sent to the receiver. The receiver picks up the signal, amplifies it, and sends it to the listener by way of either ear phones or hearing aids (Fig. 41–6). These systems allow the listener freedom of motion within the range of transmission, which varies depending on the device. Some will have ranges up to 600 feet. The one disadvantage is that there is no assurance of privacy, as anyone with a receiver may hear the signal. FM is the technology most commonly used in classroom teaching for hearing disabled children.

There are a variety of rehabilitation amplification devices available. These devices are relatively inexpensive and must be considered in the overall rehabilitation program for the hearing impaired.

## SPECIAL EDUCATION

The deaf or profoundly hearing-impaired child presents critical educational problems. Early rec-

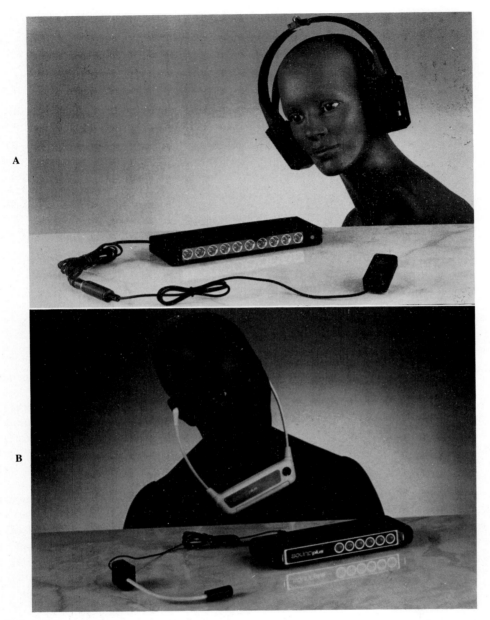

**FIG 41–5.**
Infrared personal ALD system with **A,** earphones, and **B,** cushions. (Courtesy of HARC Mercantile Ltd.)

ognition of the hearing loss is essential for good results. One of the most cogent principles concerning communicative disorders is the importance of starting communication in the first year of life. At 1 year of age, the deaf child cannot be distinguished from the hearing child by many observers, but the differences between the deaf and the hearing child in development become marked thereafter. A large proportion of so-called deaf children have sufficient residual hearing to enable them to respond and to recognize the majority of sounds in their environment by wearing a hearing aid. Few, if any, children who are considered deaf really have absent residual hearing. Use of the child's residual hearing is markedly improved through the use of an aid. Deaf children will tolerate hearing aids even under a year of age. Delay of hearing aid placement for more than 1 to 1½

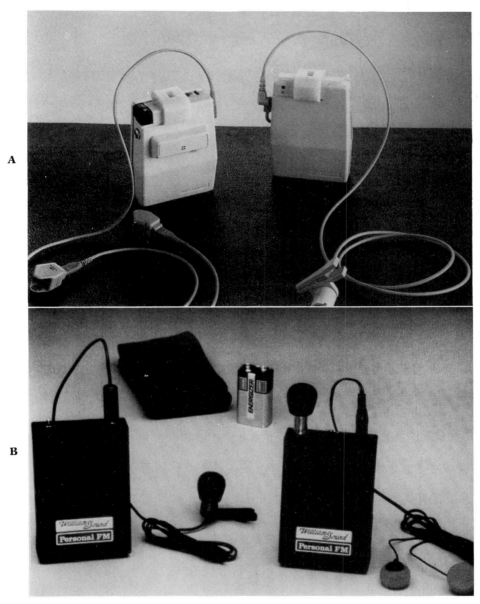

**FIG 41–6.**
FM portable assistive listening systems. **A,** Phonic Ear. **B,** Williams Sound. (Courtesy of HARC Mercantile Ltd.)

years after birth severely impairs the development of acquired language skills and causes delays in development that are almost impossible to recoup. Constant auditory and environmental training is actually most critical in language development in the first 3 years of age. Therefore, special training of the deaf child should occur at the time of identification, which should be before the age of 1. Early training in sense perception, attention to the face and lips of the parents, and visual associa-

tions are important foundations for later education. Preschool training is critical, starting as early as 12 months of age. This is important, as most special education programs start around the age of 3 to 4. Fortunately, facilities for education of people who are profoundly hard of hearing are available in every state. There are state schools for the deaf, special municipal schools in the larger cities, and private schools. In general, early educational efforts are directed toward teaching awareness of sound and speech and attempts to elicit early speech sounds from the child. In addition, there are hearing and speech clinics located in many cities throughout the country and in many hospitals and universities. These clinics offer audiometric tests of all types, advice in fitting of hearing aids, lipreading classes for adults and children, preschool classes for deaf children, classes for the parents of children who are hearing

impaired or deaf, speech diagnosis and therapy, and recreational activities. The American Academy of Otolaryngology/Head and Neck Surgery provides information on rehabilitation facilities to any physician. Information can be obtained by contacting American Academy of Otolaryngology/Head and Neck Surgery, 1101 Vermont Ave N.W., Suite 302, Washington DC 20005.

# 42

# Tinnitus

Tinnitus is defined as a noise or ringing in the ear. It is usually subjective and audible only to the patient. Occasionally it is objective and audible to the examining physician who uses certain techniques. When tinnitus is slight, it may be annoying only at night or when the usual environment noise is low. During most of the day, and especially when busy at work, the patient does not notice the ringing. When tinnitus is continuous and loud, it may actually interfere with hearing and be so annoying that a neurosis develops. In rare instances of extremely loud tinnitus a patient may consider suicide.

Tinnitus is often a sign of disease of the ear, and it may be the first or only sign of such disease. Thorough aural and general systemic examinations must be made. In many instances the cause cannot be determined. Sometimes, when there are no other signs or symptoms, the cause can only be suspected.

## SUBJECTIVE TINNITUS

Subjective tinnitus may arise from a disturbance of the external ear, tympanic membrane, ossicles, cochlea, eighth cranial nerve, brainstem, or cortex. The character of the tinnitus does not aid in determining the site of the disturbance. However, certain conditions are known to give rise to one type of tinnitus more often than to another (Table 42–1).

Cerumen in the external canal, perforation of the tympanic membrane, or fluid in the middle ear may cause subjective tinnitus. This type of tinnitus most often causes a muffling of other sounds and a change in the patient's voice. The patient may describe his or her voice as sounding hollow. The tinnitus is usually low pitched, and it may be intermittent.

At some time in its course, otosclerosis is almost always accompanied by tinnitus, which may last for months or years and then disappear as the disease progresses. The tinnitus associated with otosclerosis is variable. There may be ringing, roaring, or whistling sounds. Several sounds may occur together. When present, the tinnitus is constant. It does not fluctuate widely.

Inflammation of the middle ear may be accompanied by tinnitus that is often pulsating in character. The tinnitus subsides with the inflammation. Chronic infection of the middle ear is rarely accompanied by tinnitus.

In presbycusis and after acoustic trauma, tinnitus is usually high pitched and ringing in character. In these conditions the pitch of the tinnitus is usually near the frequency at which the hearing loss is greatest.

When tinnitus follows exposure to accustomed acoustic trauma, such as that produced by the firing of a high-powered rifle, it frequently is associated with temporary hearing loss. Patients should be told that tinnitus serves as a warning: if they continue to expose their ears to excessive noise, they may lose their hearing permanently. Anyone with tinnitus after exposure to loud noise should be careful to protect the ears against the noise.

Certain drugs cause tinnitus (Table 42–2). The same drugs are known to damage the cochlea or eighth cranial nerve. Such tinnitus is usually high pitched and may continue after the drug has been stopped. Quinine and salicylates commonly produce tinnitus when used over a prolonged period

**TABLE 42–1.**

Causes of Subjective Tinnitus

Otologic
  Presbycusis
  Noise-induced hearing loss
  Ménière disease
  Otosclerosis
  Chronic suppurative otitis

Metabolic
  Hypothyroidism
  Hyperthyroidism
  Hyperlipidemia
  Zinc deficiency/vitamin deficiency

Neurologic
  Skull fracture/closed head trauma
  Whiplash injury
  Multiple sclerosis
  Following meningitis

Pharmacologic
  Aspirin compounds
  Nonsteroidal antiinflammatory drugs
  Aminoglycosides
  Heavy metals

Dental
  Temporomandibular joint syndrome

Psychologic
  Depression
  Anxiety

**TABLE 42–2.**

Drugs That May Cause Tinnitus

| Aspirin-Containing Products | |
|---|---|
| Acetidine | Empirin Compound |
| Alka-Seltzer | Excedrin |
| Anacin | Florinal |
| Anahist | 4-Way Cold Tablets |
| APC | Inhiston |
| Aspirin | Liquiprin |
| Aspergum | Midol |
| Bromo Quinine | Pepto-Bismol |
| Bromo-Seltzer | Persistin |
| Bufferin | Saccharin |
| Coricidin | Sal-Sayne |
| Darvon Compound | Stanback |
| Dristan | Theracin |
| Ecotrin | Trigesic |
| Edrisal | |
| Aminoglycoside Antibiotics | |
| Amikacin | Neomycin |
| Gentamicin | Streptomycin |
| Kanamycin | Tobramycin |
| Nonsteroidal Antiinflammatory Drugs | |
| Fenoprofen | Naproxen |
| Ibuprofen | Phenylbutazone |
| Indomethacin | Sulindac |
| Ketoprofen | Tolmetin |
| Heterocycline Antidepressants | |
| Amitriptyline | Protriptyline |
| Amoxapine | Trazodone |
| Desipramine | Trimipramine |
| Doxepin | |
| Imipramine | |
| Nortriptyline | |

of time. In some patients only a small, single dose causes the ears to ring. Streptomycin, dihydrostreptomycin, neomycin, kanamycin, gentamicin, and similar, chemically related drugs may cause both tinnitus and hearing loss. Heavy metals, such as arsenic used in the treatment of syphilis, may cause the same damage. Often, the onset of tinnitus is a warning that the drug should be discontinued before irreversible hearing loss occurs.

Vascular changes in the central nervous system associated with arteriosclerosis and hypertension commonly cause a high-pitched tinnitus. In hypertension, the tinnitus will often fluctuate with the blood pressure.

Tumors of the posterior fossa, particularly in the cerebellopontine angle, produce tinnitus early in their course. Continuous high-pitched or low-pitched tinnitus may be the first symptom of an acoustic neuroma and may precede loss of hearing or disturbance of equilibrium by several years.

Tinnitus is one of the triad of symptoms characterizing labyrinthine hydrops (Ménière disease). The characteristic sound is low pitched and, although continuous, fluctuates in intensity. It may become quite loud immediately before an acute attack of vertigo, and it may almost disappear after the attack. When the disease is under control, the tinnitus partially subsides but usually does not disappear. Distortion of sounds and diplacusis also accompany Ménière disease and, along with the annoying tinnitus, make the patient's hearing even worse than it seems to be on the pure-tone audiogram.

Anemia and low blood pressure may produce a variable tinnitus of mild intensity. The tinnitus usually clears when the anemia is controlled or the blood pressure is normal.

Syphilis of the central nervous system may produce tinnitus, usually high pitched and continuous. Attacks of epilepsy and migraine may be preceded by tinnitus.

Some patients hear certain vascular sounds that are interpreted as tinnitus. Perhaps *head noise* would be a better term for these sounds produced during venous congestion or when plaques are present in the walls of the carotid arteries (pulsating, or "swishing," tinnitus synchronous with the heartbeat may be heard). Pressure over the common carotid artery may abolish this tinnitus temporarily. Some loud cardiac murmurs are transmitted to the skull and are heard as a pulsating tinnitus. Vascular tinnitus is usually low pitched.

Finally, some types of tinnitus are neurogenic or functional in origin. They have no characteristic sound. Examination of the ear and central nervous system reveals no cause for the tinnitus. Often the tinnitus increases during emotional stress. This type of tinnitus is worse toward the end of the day than it is in the morning. Any type of tinnitus seems louder when the patient is fatigued.

Certain muscular sounds in the head and neck may be heard by patients and disturb them. Chewing, stretching of the neck, tight closing of the eyes, and tight clenching of the jaws produce subjective sounds that any of us can hear. When a conductive hearing loss is present, all such sounds are accentuated because the masking effect of ambient noise is lost. Also, when a conductive hearing loss is present, motion of the eardrum and contraction of the muscles of the middle ear may become audible intermittently.

If persons hear organized sounds (such as voices or music) when no such sound is present, they are said to have auditory hallucinations. Central nervous system dysfunction is certain. Auditory hallucinations may occur in the psychotic person, but they may also be caused by localized or diffuse encephalitis of the temporal lobe of the brain.

## OBJECTIVE (AUDIBLE) TINNITUS

When a patient's tinnitus can also be heard by the physician, certain definite conditions are suggested (Table 42–3). Audible tinnitus should be suspected when the tinnitus is blowing in character and coincides with respiration; when it is pulsating, biphasic, and rough in character; or when there is a rapid succession of clicking sounds. For audible tinnitus to be heard, the physician must place his or her ear against the patient's ear or use a stethoscope against the patient's external auditory canal.

**TABLE 42–3.**

Causes of Objective Tinnitus

Vascular abnormalities
  Arteriovenous shunts
    Congenital arteriovenous malformations
    Acquired arteriovenous shunt
      Glomus jugulare
      Glomus tympanicum
  Arterial bruits
    High-riding carotid artery
    Carotid stenosis
    Vascular loop (internal auditory canal)
    Persistent stapedial artery
  Venous hums
    Dehiscent jugular bulb
    Hypertension
Mechanical abnormalities
  Patulous eustachian tube
  Palatomyoclonus
  Idiopathic stapedial muscle spasm

A blowing tinnitus that coincides with inspiration, expiration, or both usually indicates an abnormally patent eustachian tube. This type of tinnitus is extremely distressing to the patient. It may appear after extreme weight loss in debilitated patients. Fortunately, most such instances of tinnitus are of short duration. Some relief can be obtained by repeating the Valsalva maneuver (swallowing with the mouth and nose obstructed to produce negative pressure in the nasopharynx).

Rarely, a patient will have tinnitus characterized by a series of sharp, regular clicks heard for several seconds or minutes at a time. This type of tinnitus is almost always intermittent, although it may occur many times during the day. The cause is not definitely known, but the mechanism is understood. It is produced by tetanic contractions of the muscles of the soft palate, and the palate can be seen to contract spasmodically when the tinnitus is audible. The contractions are very small and rapid, approximately 175 to 200 a minute. Occasionally, several injections of procaine hydrochloride (Novocain) or lidocaine (Xylocaine) into the palatal muscles on the involved side will break the reflex activity. Anticonvulsant medications are also used when this disorder occurs.

Audible tinnitus that is pulsating and synchronous with the heartbeat almost always indicates an arteriovenous aneurysm somewhere in the head or neck. Rarely, a carotid bruit is audible. The most common sites of arteriovenous aneurysms causing audible tinnitus are intracranial or are in the vessels immediately in front of the ear (anterior auricular artery). Arteriograms help locate the aneurysm. Resection of the aneurysm and ligation of the involved vessels may be indicated.

## TREATMENT

Tinnitus caused by changes in the external canal and middle ear can usually be relieved. The type accompanying acute or subacute middle ear disease disappears when the inflammation subsides. The tinnitus that accompanies otosclerosis cannot be treated except by surgical correction of the hearing loss. In most patients who have an operation for otosclerosis, the tinnitus diminishes when the operation is successful but remains if hearing is not improved (Fig 42–1).

Tinnitus caused by disturbances in the cochlea, eighth cranial nerve, and central nervous system cannot be treated specifically unless it is associated with a known disease and disappears with control of that disease.

Patients with specific medical disorders merit directed therapy. The majority of patients have some otologic disease in which complaints are mild and can only be treated symptomatically.

Treatment modalities include the following: (1) nonspecific medical management, (2) masking, (3) biofeedback, (4) drug therapy, (5) electrical stimulation, and (6) surgery.

### Nonspecific Management

If symptoms are mild, the following general rules should be observed:

1. The physician should discuss with the patient all etiologic factors regarding the complaint and reassure him or her at the completion of the evaluation as to the unlikelihood of tumor or life-endangering disease. The patient should also be told that the symptoms improve significantly or go away in approximately 25% of patients and decrease over a period of months in 50%. Only 25% of patients will have persistent symptoms, and in only a small proportion will the symptoms increase.
2. Patients should totally avoid loud noise and, if exposed for any duration, should use noise protection. Almost invariably, patients with hearing loss will find their

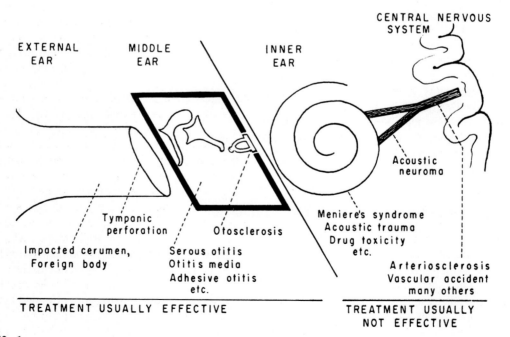

**FIG 42–1.**
Possible areas giving rise to tinnitus. The great majority of patients with tinnitus have the symptom from inner ear or central causes, not external or middle ear disorders.

tinnitus accentuated by loud noise exposure whether it be from music, athletic events, or work.

3. All caffeinated beverages or medications with stimulants must be avoided. Coffee, tea, cola, and chocolate must be excluded or at least reduced to increase the possibility of a reduction in symptoms. It is important to understand that decaffeinated beverages are not caffeine-free. In fact, many decaffeinated coffees have only a 50% reduction in caffeine.

4. Patients should stop smoking. More than 50% of patients with mild tinnitus note a significant reduction in their complaint with avoidance of caffeine and nicotine.

5. All medications must be reevaluated, and specific avoidance of aspirin-containing compounds and nonsteroidal antiinflammatory drugs should be attempted. Other medications can be substituted; if not, dosages can be lowered. Other drugs or combinations of medicines that might be implicated as causal should be altered in an attempt to alleviate symptoms.

6. A variety of home masking techniques should be tried, including music or placing the radio dial between frequency-modulated stations at a loudness level that masks out the tinnitus. A bedside masker can also be recommended. Generally, the sounds required to mask the tinnitus are quite soft and not necessarily disturbing to the patient or other family members. These techniques are particularly useful in patients who have difficulty getting to sleep.

7. In patients with depression or anxiety, psychologic testing and evaluation are advisable. This allows the physician to review the patient's emotional status before further treatment and to intelligently advise medications if necessary.

These general rules usually prove successful in managing the typical patient with tinnitus. In fact, 80% of patients will have sufficient relief and will not require further treatment. However, in some patients the cause cannot be reversed and general treatment is insufficient. More specific therapy regimens can be outlined for patients with this unresolved symptom. These regimens include (1) masking instruments, (2) stress management, (3) medications, (4) electrical stimulation, and (5) surgery.

## Specific Management

Specific medical treatment of tinnitus remains of uncertain value. In the past 10 years, lidocaine, carbamazepine (Tegretol), primidone (Mysoline), phenytoin (Dilantin), and tocainide (oral lidocaine) have been tried in controlled series of patients. These drugs have proved of little value for tinnitus, although occasionally a patient may improve on one of them. The use of alprazolam (Xanax) (0.5 mg bid) has helped a number of severely afflicted patients. No drugs are specific for tinnitus, but they offer future hope of tinnitus control in some patients. Because the causes of tinnitus are undoubtedly several rather than one, it is probable that control of tinnitus must wait for more precise localization of its origins.

When drug toxicity is the cause of tinnitus, withdrawal of the drug may stop it. If cochlear damage has already occurred, the tinnitus may continue.

It is interesting to note that even sectioning of the eighth cranial nerve, which has been performed many times for Ménière disease and for acoustic neuroma, often fails to stop tinnitus. This raises the suspicion that central nervous system tinnitus is more common than is usually thought. It may also indicate that tinnitus represents autonomic dysfunction rather than a disturbance of the cochlea or eighth cranial nerve.

Biofeedback, in conjunction with learned techniques of relaxation, has been used for control of tinnitus with variable success. Results are difficult to evaluate, but biofeedback may offer future help for the tinnitus sufferer.

When the loudness of a patient's tinnitus is matched by a similar sound from the audiometer presented to the unaffected ear, it is surprising how weak a signal is needed to match the tinnitus. The average is about a 10 db intensity, and often 5 db in the left ear, for example, will match with the tinnitus in the right ear. A matching of 20 db is unusual.

It has been known for a long time that mild tinnitus is frequently masked by everyday sounds. Such tinnitus is unnoticed when the afflicted person is in ordinary room noise or outside in the

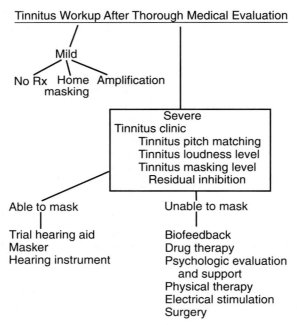

Tinnitus Workup After Thorough Medical Evaluation

**FIG 42–2.**
Tinnitus workup after a thorough medical evaluation.

traffic noise. Only in quiet surroundings, as at bedtime, is the tinnitus annoying. Even rather loud tinnitus is diminished by surrounding noise. Studies of this natural modifying of tinnitus have led to the development of electronic masking devices worn by the patient. In many cases these devices can reduce the intensity of the tinnitus or mask it completely. Sometimes a hearing aid alone, since it amplifies external sound, not only improves hearing but also diminishes or stops the tinnitus while it is worn. A masking instrument can be used alone if tinnitus without hearing loss is the problem. The masking unit can also be incorporated with a hearing aid to relieve both hearing loss and tinnitus in some patients. This type of management is now widely used in the United States. Improvements in the instrument and further research will undoubtedly refine the technique in the future.

From the use of masking, phenomenon known as residual inhibition has been studied. Certain people have found that, if a masking device is used even for a short period of time, the tinnitus may be markedly diminished or absent for some

time after the masking sound is removed. A few persons have been free of tinnitus for hours or longer after using a masking device for several hours. Residual inhibition is incompletely understood and will require further work to determine whether, or in what circumstances, it can be of practical value.

There is also evidence suggesting that certain psychologic states (specifically depression) can accentuate tinnitus. Antidepressant medications have been used with some success in many tinnitus sufferers. It is never clear, however, whether the depression causes tinnitus or the reverse is true. Therefore it is imperative that all other means of diagnosing and treating tinnitus are considered before embarking on antidepressant therapy.

In the control of tinnitus the physician must remember that tinnitus is only a symptom and that a specific cause must be sought and eliminated if possible. Only when no treatable cause can be found should the symptom alone be treated. Tinnitus is sometimes a warning of other serious disease (Fig 42–2).

# 43

# Dizziness and Vertigo

Dizziness indicates a disturbed sense of relationship to space. It is a subjective sensation that rises to the level of consciousness, alarming the patient, who is often unable to describe exactly what he or she is feeling. The sensation may be one of turning or whirling, or it may be a less well-defined symptom of giddiness, weakness, confusion, blankness, or unsteadiness.

Subjective orientation of the body in space is controlled by a complicated system that includes all of the following:

1. Eyes and eye muscles
2. Proprioceptive system
3. Labyrinth (semicircular canals) and utricle
4. Eighth cranial nerve
5. Vestibular nuclei and brainstem
6. Neural pathways from the vestibular nuclei to the midbrain and to the temporal lobe (medial longitudinal fasciculus)
7. Central coordination mechanisms in the cerebellum
8. Vestibulospinal tract (posterior columns)
9. Afferent fibers coming from muscles and joints via the vestibulospinal tract

The end organ of equilibrium (semicircular canals and utricle), the vestibular division of the eighth cranial nerve, and the vestibular nuclei are commonly referred to as the statokinetic system (Fig 43–1). Whirling or spinning sensations or a subjective feeling of propulsion or tilting directs attention to the statokinetic system, whereas the other less specific complaints of dizziness may be caused by a disturbance in any part of the body.

The interrelationship between the labyrinth,

eyes, and proprioceptive system is the important mechanism. Loss or disturbances of function of any one of these structures will upset normal equilibrium. When loss of function of one occurs, the other two may gradually compensate so that equilibrium or locomotion is almost normal. However, loss of function of any two results in incapacitation. For example, a patient with tabes dorsalis, whose vestibulospinal tracts are damaged, may be able to walk when he can see but be unable to maintain his balance when in the dark. Similarly, a blind person becomes very disoriented under water when normal proprioceptive information is lost. An underwater scuba diver who has severe vestibular stimulation may, because of lack of proprioceptive and visual input, swim toward the bottom. Causes of death in deep-water divers are often believed to be secondary to this multiple-system disturbance.

A sensation of true whirling or turning means disturbed function in the semicircular canals, eighth cranial nerve, or vestibular nuclei. Various other sensations that patients may describe as dizziness indicate the presence of lesions at higher levels or regions farther away.

Of all the symptoms a patient presents to a physician, dizziness is one of the most common and one of the most confusing. Within certain limits, it is possible to classify dizziness according to recognizable entities. By doing so, the physician not only clarifies his or her confusion, but establishes some basis for rational therapy. The statements "within certain limits" and "clarifies his or her confusion" are used advisedly because, regardless of classification, there will always remain certain patients whose dizziness is never ex-

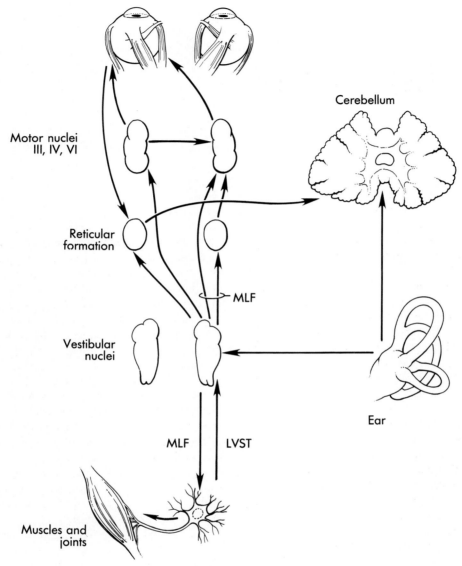

**FIG 43–1**.
Schematic representation of coordinated vestibular ocular and proprioceptive function determining balance.

actly understood and whose treatment must be a regimen of trial and error. This does not imply that classification so far as is possible is of no value. Just the opposite is true. The physician must have a certain established complex of symptoms in mind, which, when all of the criteria of each are met, points to a specific diagnosis and leads to a specific treatment.

Symptoms of true whirling or sensation of motion can be called vertigo. Nonmotion-related symptoms may be classified as nonsystematized dizziness. The classification in the box is based on this premise.

## HISTORY

Before the history and examination of patients with the complaint of dizziness are discussed, it should be made clear that the work-up of a dizzy

| NONSYSTEMATIZED DIZZINESS | VERTIGO |
|---|---|
| I. Eyes | I. Ear |
|   A. Muscle imbalance |   A. External ear |
|   B. Refractive errors |     1. Wax or foreign bodies |
|   C. Simple glaucoma |   B. Middle ear |
| II. Proprioceptive system |     1. Retracted tympanic membrane |
|   A. Pellagra |     2. Acute disease |
|   B. Chronic alcoholism |       a. Acute suppurative otitis media |
|   C. Pernicious anemia |       b. Otitis media with effusion |
|   D. Tabes dorsalis |     3. Chronic disease |
| III. Central nervous system |       a. Labyrinthitis |
|   A. Mild cerebral anoxia |       b. Cholesteatoma (fistula reaction) |
|     1. Arteriosclerosis |     4. Injury with hemorrhage |
|     2. Hypertensive cardiovascular disease |   C. Internal ear |
|     3. Chronic hypertension |     1. Acute toxic labyrinthitis |
|     4. Anemia |     2. Vascular episodes |
|     5. Paroxysmal auricular fibrillation |     3. Trauma |
|     6. Aortic stenosis with insufficiency |     4. Allergy |
|     7. Heart block |     5. Hydrops of the labyrinth (Ménière disease) |
|     8. Carotid sinus syndrome |     6. Motion sickness |
|     9. Simple syncope |     7. Postural vertigo |
|     10. Postural hypotension | II. Eighth nerve |
|   B. Infection |   A. Infection |
|     1. Meningitis |     1. Acute meningitis |
|     2. Encephalitis |     2. Tuberculous meningitis |
|     3. Brain abscess |     3. Basilar syphilitic meningitis |
|     4. Syphilis |   B. Trauma |
|   C. Trauma |   C. Tumors |
|   D. Tumors | III. Brain stem (nuclei) |
|   E. Migraine |   A. Infections |
|   F. Petit mal epilepsy |     1. Encephalitis |
|   G. Endocrine conditions |     2. Meningitis |
|     1. Menstrual-pregnancy-menopause pattern |     3. Brain abscess |
|     2. Hypoparathyroidism with tetany |   B. Trauma |
|     3. Hypothyroidism |   C. Hemorrhage |
|     4. Paroxysmal hypertension associated with adrenal medullary tumor |   D. Thrombosis of posteroinferior cerebellar artery |
|     5. Hypoglycemia |   E. Tumors |
|   H. Psychoneurosis |   F. Multiple sclerosis |

patient cannot be accomplished in a limited amount of time. Therefore, a routine must be established that allows the physician the opportunity to work with a dizzy patient over a series of visits. Otherwise, the patient with these complaints will have an abbreviated and inadequate evaluation, and the physician will dread the chief complaint "I am dizzy."

The evaluation of dizziness must begin with the history. It is the most important part of the examination because certain diseases or syndromes present a characteristic history. In many patients with vestibular disorders the physical examination, x-ray films, and laboratory tests are normal and the probable diagnosis must be suspected from history alone.

In taking the history, the examiner should ask six basic questions.

1. *Does the patient experience true whirling?* The direction and character of the motion are not important. The fact that there either is or is not a real sense of motion is important. With eyes open, the patient feels that objects are moving around him or her, but with eyes closed, the patient feels that he or she is in motion. Both indicate true vertigo and narrow the field of investigation to the statokinetic system. If it is not possible to elicit a history of sense of motion, the entire body becomes field for investigation.
2. *What is the pattern of dizziness?* A history of paroxysmal attacks with intervals of complete relief between attacks may indicate certain diseases. The onset, course, severity, and duration all may suggest specific disorders. The time of day and any relationship to menstrual periods, occupation, and trauma may be important.
3. *What are the associated symptoms?* Nausea and vomiting accompanying vertigo are, in the absence of central nervous system disease, usually caused by labyrinthine disease. Less severe dizziness without demonstrable pattern may arise from disease in any part of the body.
4. *Is there hearing loss or tinnitus?* Any associated hearing loss or tinnitus accompanying dizziness helps localize the disorder.
5. *Is there a history of motion sickness or vestibular sensitivity?* Patients with no history of previous motion sickness or vestibular difficulty who experience true whirling vertigo have significant vestibular abnormalities. By contrast, patients who have a long history of motion sensitivity (for example, inability to ride in the backseat of a car, inability to ride a merry-go-round, or a history of airsickness) require a less severe degree of ocular, proprioceptive, or vestibular abnormality to elicit their symptoms.
6. *What is the drug history?* In the initial evaluation, history of drug intake is critical. Almost any classification of drugs can cause the symptom of dizziness. It is im-

---

**CLASSES OF DRUGS CAUSING VERTIGO**
- Antibiotics
- Anticonvulsants
- Antihistamines
- Antihypertensives
- Antiinflammatory
- Diuretics
- Muscle relaxants
- Sedatives
- Tranquilizers

---

portant to consider drugs primarily in the management of any patient with this complaint. Drug classifications generally thought to elicit symptoms of dizziness on certain occasions are listed in the box.

Those who have treated many dizzy patients through the years believe that the history alone can provide 90% of the diagnosis. Therefore, it is extremely important that the physician spend the time with the patient to elicit a clear description and evaluation of his or her complaint.

**Examination**

General physical examination may be indicated by the history. A full ear, nose, and throat examination is always necessary, including blood pressure recordings with the patient sitting and standing. An audiogram should always be taken. If it is normal, further hearing tests are generally unnecessary. If it is abnormal, it is imperative to determine definitely whether the hearing loss is conductive or sensorineural in nature. Care must be taken in determining bone conduction. The opposite ear should be masked to ensure accuracy, and the audiometric findings should be rechecked with tuning forks (see discussion of hearing tests in Ch 40). However, an abnormal audiogram does not always indicate that the statokinetic system is responsible for the dizziness. It may be an incidental finding unrelated to the symptom being investigated.

The function of the labyrinth can be tested in several ways (see discussion of labyrinthine tests in Ch 40). Regardless of the technique used and assuming that it is constant from patient to patient, the interpretation of the reaction produced by stimulation is of primary importance. The patient should be questioned about the intensity of the subjective sensation and asked before the test begins to compare the sensation produced with the dizziness he or she usually experiences. If the response produced by labyrinthine testing (caloric examination) is described by the patient as being much more severe than the symptom being investigated, one can be sure that the patient is not suffering from an end-organ lesion of any significance. If the response is similar to or less severe than the patient's spontaneous dizziness, disease in the statokinetic system should be suspected. If there is definite hyperactivity of the subjective response without a coincident hyperactivity of the observed labyrinthine reactions, a neurosis should be suspected. True hyperactive responses can be anticipated from the history. A history of swing sickness, carsickness, or seasickness suggests that the labyrinths are hypersensitive. If no reaction can be produced, one can safely consider that labyrinthine function is absent, that is, that the labyrinth is dead. Perverted nystagmus, such as vertical, oblique, variable, third-degree, or greatly exaggerated nystagmus, is suggestive of central nervous system disease. One must guard against placing too much emphasis on caloric reactions or electronystagmographic interpretation in attempting to emphasize minute deviations. Often one can be sure only of normalcy, hyperactivity, hypoactivity, or complete loss of function.

Attempts to elicit positional nystagmus should be repeated several times if postural vertigo is a possibility. Positional nystagmus cannot be reproduced every time a given change of position is assumed. When positional nystagmus can be demonstrated, the direction of the nystagmus must be noted. If the nystagmus elicited changes direction with different head positions, it is most likely caused by a central disorder. If the direction of the nystagmus produced by position change is constant, either central or peripheral disease may be indicated (see Fig 35–12).

Correlation of the history, physical examination, and special testing is necessary to arrive at the correct diagnosis. One must not make the error of dumping into a general "wastebasket" cases bearing such labels as "pseudo-Ménière disease," "Ménière-like syndrome," or "functional dizziness." Such diagnoses, without careful examination, increase the probability of error in exact di-

agnosis and lead to trial-and-error management, which is often unsuccessful. If the dizziness is disturbing enough to make the patient seek medical advice, it may require as complete an investigation as fever of unknown origin or other obscure symptoms with few confirmatory signs.

When the symptom of dizziness is obscure, whether or not the sensation is one of motion, discovery of the cause may be difficult. Often the combined talents of the otolaryngologist, neurologist, ophthalmologist, and internist are required to determine the underlying cause. Unless the cause is apparent or the symptom self-limited, close cooperation among several physicians offers the best chance for successful diagnosis. In spite of all efforts, there will still be patients in whom the cause of dizziness cannot be determined and in whom treatment must be on an empiric symptomatic basis. It is important in developing the differential diagnosis of the dizzy patient that one systematically exclude the common entities responsible for dizziness. The following will be a brief review of the differential diagnosis, history, and physical examination of causes of nonsystematized dizziness and vertigo.

## NONSYSTEMATIZED DIZZINESS— DIFFERENTIAL DIAGNOSIS

### Eyes

*Abnormal vision* will make it difficult to maintain a normal relationship of the body to the environment. The blind person has lost one of the three senses that maintain equilibrium and must rely on the labyrinth and the proprioceptive system. Therefore a disturbance of vision may produce dizziness when all other systems of the body are normal.

*Ocular muscle imbalance* is an occasional cause of dizziness. The dizziness is not severe, nor is it whirling in nature. Muscle imbalance should be suspected as a causative factor when the patient has mild dizziness that is difficult to describe and is annoying but not incapacitating. The patient may describe transient diplopia or the sensation of objects appearing to move slightly as he or she sits still.

*Errors of refraction* may produce the same subjective complaint. They are more easily suspected, since there is more likely to be an actual complaint of visual difficulty. Errors of refraction should be suspected if the patient complaining of dizziness has had a new prescription for glasses at the time of or shortly before the onset of dizziness. Errors of refraction should also be suspected when there is a history of frequent correction or if the patient has newly acquired bifocal or trifocal lenses. Often these patients will have difficulty when looking up and down rows of stacked items, as occurs in a grocery store.

*Glaucoma* may also produce a sensation of dizziness through visual disturbance. There is certainly good evidence to suggest that some patients are more dependent on ocular function for their balance and sensation relationship space than others. Some of these individuals can be trained to overcome their increased sensitivity by ocular exercises such as following a moving ball or a moving object with the head stable.

## Proprioceptive System

Disorders of the proprioceptive system or of the spinal tracts carrying proprioceptive sensation to the central nervous system may be accompanied by dizziness. Advanced stages of these diseases are also associated with a disturbed sense of position and therefore may produce ataxia. An ataxic or staggering gait also can occur as part of the disturbance involving the statokinetic system or the cerebellum; thus ataxia is nondiagnostic.

*Pellagra* and other vitamin deficiencies still exist in many areas. These may produce dizziness, ataxia, or both.

*Chronic alcoholism* produces peripheral changes in the vestibulospinal pathways. It may also be a factor in the reduced absorption of vitamins from the gastrointestinal tract, producing symptoms. Patients with this type of proprioceptive abnormality complain of difficulty walking in the dark or over uneven ground, where there is significant stimulation to the proprioceptive system and ocular compensation is difficult.

*Pernicious anemia,* though rarely seen, frequently causes unsteadiness. When it is advanced, dizziness may be accompanied by ataxia, loss of motion or position sense, and loss of vibratory sensation in the lower extremities.

*Tabes dorsalis* may produce symptoms identical to those produced by the preceding three entities, since the disease process commonly involves the posterior and lateral columns of the spinal cord. Again, these individuals have difficulty functioning in the dark, over uneven ground, up and down steps, or with any rapid motion.

## Central Nervous System Disease

Any disease of the central nervous system may irritate or partially inhibit pathways that influence equilibrium. Certain conditions are more likely to produce dizziness as a single presenting complaint.

### Cerebral Anoxia

Mild cerebral anoxia is produced by a variety of conditions and may be of variable duration. Frequently, the underlying condition will give rise to a sensation of dizziness that lasts only a few moments and occurs at any time of the day or night. In none of these conditions is tinnitus or hearing loss found as part of the picture. Although tinnitus and hearing loss may be present in patients with cerebral anoxia, they are not part of the symptomatology. Usually, other evidence of cerebral flow or brainstem anoxia is present.

*Arteriosclerosis, hypertension,* and *chronic hypotension* may all produce the picture described. The patient will complain of feeling imbalanced or insecure and has great difficulty describing the symptoms. Dizziness is not constantly present and does not usually occur while the individual is sitting or lying down. It may occur several times a day for brief periods and with varying intensity. It may be influenced by fatigue, emotional upset, or overwork. It is generally described as a light-headed feeling.

*Anemia* may produce cerebral anoxia. Any condition that causes low hemoglobin, from simple iron deficiency to leukemia, may be an underlying cause of dizziness.

*Paroxysmal auricular fibrillation, aortic stenosis with insufficiency and regurgitation, heart blocks of various nature,* and *carotid sinus syndrome* are important causes of dizziness. The dizziness is sudden and paroxysmal, separated by variable intervals during which there are no symptoms. Because of the paroxysmal nature of these symptoms, the underlying condition may be misinterpreted as Ménière disease, unless care is taken with the history and examination. In heart block and carotid sinus syndrome, the onset of symptoms may be so sudden that the patient falls to the ground without chance to seek support. The patient generally does not describe true vertigo but rather a fainting sensation. The onset of symptoms is usually more abrupt than with Ménière disease, and the duration is measured in seconds. Simple syncope also may cause lightheadedness or dizziness and, of course, loss of consciousness. Vestibular disorders do not cause loss of consciousness. Transient ischemic episodes may cause sudden lightheadedness, vertigo, or drop attacks. Duration is for seconds and may result in a fall. There are secondary symptoms of dysarthria, diplopia, and other evidence of motor weakness that help make the diagnosis.

*Postural hypotension* is found in many patients who, particularly in the latter decades of life, complain of dizziness when they arise from bed or from a sitting position. The dizziness lasts only a few moments and is rarely severe enough to cause falling. It is followed by complete recovery until the next sudden change of posture. Such dizziness can also occur with a sudden change of position or rapid turning in a standing position. It is usually caused by failure of the blood pressure to rise in response to assuming the standing or changed position and is commonly referred to as postural hypotension. Recordings of blood pressure while the patient is in the recumbent position and immediately after he or she arises will usually demonstrate that the blood pressure falls abruptly. Treatment consists of educating the patient to make a habit of rising slowly. The hypotension may also be caused by antihypertensive drugs or the many other medications that affect a patient's response to change in position. Obviously, any combination of medications given to the elderly must be investigated.

### Infection

Infection or septicemia may be an underlying cause of dizziness.

*Meningitis, encephalitis,* and *brain abscess* are frequently accompanied by dizziness. The dizziness is not violent or paroxysmal but is usually slowly progressive. Spontaneous nystagmus may be present, postural vertigo should be expected, and perversion of caloric responses from the labyrinths may occur. Encephalitis may involve the cochlear or vestibular nuclei and may be associated with hearing loss. The diagnosis is established from such signs as fever or disturbance of other cranial nerves, increased intracranial pressure, papilledema, or seizures.

*Syphilis* has been known for centuries as the great imitator. In many areas of the central nervous system it can cause changes that will produce dizziness, nystagmus, or both. There is nothing characteristic about the dizziness produced by syphilis. It can mimic any vestibular disorder.

### Trauma

*Trauma* to the central nervous system is a frequent cause of dizziness. Dizziness without whirling occurs frequently. Fortunately, this form of dizziness is mild, recedes slowly (in 6 to 8 months), and usually does not recur. The sensation is one of unsteadiness, giddiness, or weakness. It is often made worse by change of position or exertion and frequently is accompanied by near blackouts. Other symptoms such as headache, fatigue, and difficulty in concentration are common but not diagnostic. The location of the exact pathologic site producing this dizziness is unknown. It may be caused by multiple small hemorrhages of the central nervous system or by concussion alone, as well as by disturbance of the normal neuronal pathways from the inner ear. The ultimate prognosis is good, and reassurance should be given to the patient to prevent the development of a neurosis on the basis of fear from continued insecurity.

### Tumors

Brain tumors may cause dizziness. When they arise in or near the statokinetic system, they may produce whirling (systematized) vertigo. When they originate in other areas of the central nervous system, they produce nonspecific dizziness. Dizziness of this type is neither characteristic nor diagnostic. Generally, the rapid progression of brain tumors makes the diagnosis clear over a very brief period. Other evidence of a brain tumor is necessary before the diagnosis can be established. Acoustic neuroma and meningioma, common tumors of the eighth nerve, will be discussed under Vertigo.

## Migraine

Migraine may be preceded by an aura of dizziness, or it may be accompanied by dizziness. The typical pattern is a unilateral headache associated with scotoma, nausea, and vomiting for 1 to 4 days and vertigo. In some persons, dizziness is an outstanding symptom, and the headache is secondary. When dizziness predominates, it is often referred to as a migraine equivalent.

## Petit Mal Epilepsy

Petit mal epilepsy may cause dizziness. It is not uncommon in children. A careful history will help to establish that such dizziness is actually a sudden, momentary loss of consciousness. No nystagmus, tinnitus, or hearing loss accompanies this condition.

## Metabolic Conditions

Endocrine dysfunctions can give rise to dizziness. The mechanism by which this is produced is unknown. Clinical observation reveals many instances in which dizziness is part of the menopausal pattern or is associated with pregnancy, the menstrual cycle, or the administration of estrogens. In obscure cases of dizziness, the patient's case history should be carefully taken and evaluated in an effort to determine whether there is a relationship between the dizziness and the menstrual-pregnancy-menopausal pattern. The widespread use of hormone therapy must be considered as a possible cause of the symptom.

*Hypoglycemia* should be suspected when there is a definite time relationship between the dizziness and ingestion of food. The dizziness resulting from low blood glucose comes on gradually over a period of 15 to 30 minutes and lasts from 1 to 2 hours (or until food is ingested or the level of blood glucose rises again). It is usually accompanied by a feeling of fatigue. The symptoms may progress to apprehension, overexcitability, shakiness, and convulsive movements such as those seen in a diabetic patient who has an overdose of insulin. Hypoglycemia can be proved by a blood sugar drawn at the time of symptoms or a glucose tolerance curve. The possible diagnosis of islet cell tumor of the pancreas must be considered.

*Hypothyroidism* with or without tetany, hyperthyroidism, or paroxysmal hypertension associated with an adrenal medullary tumor may also cause dizziness. Usually other systemic systems are quite apparent in these patients.

## Psychoneurosis

Psychoneurosis undoubtedly accounts for many instances of nonsystematized dizziness. There is nothing characteristic about this type of dizziness. In the absence of disease of the ear, it is not accompanied by tinnitus and hearing loss. Tinnitus may have a functional basis, but its association with dizziness on this basis is probably coincidental. In these cases, the physician can make no definite rules except to be aware of the possibility and to exclude all other possibilities. The practice of labeling any set of symptoms the physician cannot explain as functional not only dulls the investigative powers of the physician, but also may lead to errors in diagnosis or to neglect of organic disease. The physician should form the habit of searching for organic causes first; furthermore, even when organic disease cannot be demonstrated, the diagnosis of functional dizziness should be made only when that diagnosis is supported by other symptoms and signs of psychoneuroses.

## VERTIGO—DIFFERENTIAL DIAGNOSIS

The characteristic of dizziness caused by the disturbance of the statokinetic system is a sense of motion. The sense of direction or character of the sense of motion is not as important as the fact that there is a feeling of whirling or propulsion. The patient's feeling of turning, which occurs with the eyes closed, is of no more significance than the feeling that the environment is turning around him or her, which occurs with the eyes open. Any sensation of movement, even if it be up and down movement or oblique movement, suggests involvement of the statokinetic system. Vertigo is frequently accompanied by nausea or vomiting. It is often accompanied by loss of hearing, tinnitus, or both. Spontaneous nystagmus is frequently present with whirling vertigo. It may be present only at times of severe vertigo, or it may not be seen because the patient consults the physician between attacks. However, when spontaneous nystagmus is seen, it is indicative of disease, and in most cases the disease is in the statokinetic vestibular system.

## External Ear and Middle Ear

Vertigo may be caused by disease of the external ear and middle ear.

*Wax* and *foreign bodies* in the external ear may produce the sensation of vertigo. The symptom is usually quite mild and is most commonly caused by wax firmly impacted against the tympanic membrane. Foreign bodies or a hair resting against the tympanic membrane may also cause the sensation of vertigo or a vague sense of imbalance.

*Negative pressure in the middle ear* from eustachian tube blockage of any type may cause vertigo. The vertigo may be constant or paroxysmal but is generally mild.

*Acute suppurative otitis media* and its complications can cause vertigo. The vertigo is mild when it accompanies uncomplicated otitis media. It is whirling when it is associated with mastoiditis complicated by labyrinthitis. Purulent invasion of the labyrinth usually causes severe loss of hearing in the involved ear and almost always results in a dead labyrinth. Vertigo associated with suppurative middle ear disease is always a danger signal. When it occurs secondary to suppurative infection and destruction of the labyrinth, symptoms are significant for 3 to 6 weeks.

Destruction of the inner table of the mastoid, which produces an epidural abscess on the anterior face of the cerebellum, can give all the signs of labyrinthitis. These complications are rare today because of antibiotics, but they still occur in patients who have been undertreated or untreated.

*Otitis media with effusion* is often accompanied by dizziness. The dizziness is often a feeling of imbalance rather than a whirling sensation and is usually more noticeable when the patient changes position. It is not as severe as postural vertigo, but the dizziness occurs during changes of position.

*Chronic suppurative otitis media* and its complications may cause vertigo. Acute exacerabations of chronic disease may produce a labyrinthitis identical to that seen with acute mastoiditis.

*Cholesteatoma* causes erosion and enlargement of the attic of the middle ear, erosion of the mastoid antrum, and the horizontal semicircular canal. If erosion of the labyrinth occurs, patients may experience sudden, severe vertigo that throws them to the floor. Typically, the onset is so rapid that patients cannot protect themselves. However, the vertigo is over in a few moments, and there are no after symptoms. There may be history of such episodes immediately following sneezing or blowing of the nose. An attack may occur if the patient puts a finger into the ear canal to scratch or cleans the ear with an applicator or an irrtigating solution. This history is pathognomonic of a fistula of the labyrinth and can be confirmed by the fistula test (see the discussion of tests for labyrinthine reaction).

*Trauma* to the middle ear can produce vertigo. Blows over the ear with the open hand may rupture the eardrum and dislocate the ossicles, particularly the stapes, which can be subluxated into the vestibule. This may cause temporary or permanent vertigo. Fractures through the middle ear produce vertigo and may be accompanied by bleeding or leaking of cerebrospinal fluid from the middle ear.

## Internal Ear

Many conditions of the middle ear can give rise to vertigo.

### Acute Toxic Labyrinthitis

*Acute toxic labyrinthitis* is probably the most dramatic cause of whirling vertigo the physician sees. Typically, there is a gradual onset of whirling vertigo that reaches its maximum within 24 hours. At its height, the vertigo is accompanied by nausea and vomiting, then the patient gradually regresses to normal over 3 to 6 weeks. *Tinnitus and hearing loss do not occur.*

The patient suffering from acute toxic labyrinthitis is frequently incapacitated for 3 to 5 days, during which time any motion of the head brings on symptoms. The supine position is sought. During recovery, a less severe sensation of whirling occurs when the head is turned suddenly in any direction. This syndrome may accompany acute febrile illnesses such as pneumonia, cholecystitis, and influenza. In many patients it follows the ingestion of drugs, overindulgence of alcohol, food or drug allergy, or extreme fatigue. Reassurance of recovery is important in management.

Vestibular examination may demonstrate any degree of hypoactivity of a single labyrinth. The exact area of irritation of the statokinetic system that gives rise to acute toxic labyrinthitis is generally unknown. The use of the word *toxic* is in itself an admission of ignorance and should be recognized as such. In most cases, it means that the physician is assuming the presence of a toxic irritation from some source without having any proof that such is true. Nevertheless, the syndrome is common and characteristic, and the name given to it is descriptive.

### Vestibular Neuronitis

Vestibular neuronitis, first described by Dix and Hallpike in 1952, is a form of acute labyrinthitis that occurs in epidemic proportions, usually as a result of some respiratory virus. It is believed that the virus affects the vestibular nuclei. Characteristically, it may occur in minor epidemics related to an upper respiratory infection. Individuals have a sudden loss of vestibular function accompanied by severe vertigo, nausea, vomiting, and spontaneous nystagmus. The symptoms, as in acute toxic labyrinthitis, generally peak rapidly, and recovery generally takes 1 to 3 weeks. Again, tinnitus and hearing loss do not occur. There is, however, marked suppression of vestibular function on one side, which may be permanent.

Treatment of acute toxic labyrinthitis and vestibular neuronitis consists of bed rest, sedation, and administration of antivertiginous medications. Generally, patients are advised against rapid movement, which tends to accentuate their symptoms. With vestibular neuronitis, there is generally no permanent disability. Individuals with unilaterally suppressed vestibular function, as occurs with this disorder, have a tendency toward later developing positional vertigo or nystagmus.

### Vascular Episodes

Vascular episodes of several types can disturb the physiology of the internal ear and produce vertigo. Arterial spasm may reduce the blood supply to the labyrinth and produce transient whirling vertigo with nystagmus. It is most frequently seen in hypertensive cardiovascular disease. Rupture of a vein or artery with hemorrhage into the labyrinth or arterial occlusion may produce a sudden, dramatic, incapacitating vertigo. This is accompanied by a loud tinnitus and a sudden loss of hearing. Complete loss of hearing and caloric response is evident early in these disorders and is permanent. In 3 to 4 weeks, even after total loss of unilateral labyrinthine function, equilibrium is reestablished and nearly normal physical activity can be resumed. Some instability remains with rapid motion.

### Trauma

Trauma of the internal ear may result from fracture through the internal ear, concussion, or sudden loud noise. Fracture through the cochlea and vestibule may give a picture exactly like that of hemorrhage into the internal ear. The seventh cranial nerve will frequently be injured, and facial paralysis occurs in 50% of transverse temporal bone fractures and 15% of longitudinal fractures.

*Whiplash injury* is a common cause of dizziness following injury. Generally, the onset of dizziness is delayed until 7 to 10 days following the accident, at which time the patient will begin to complain of some dizziness with head movement, generally toward the side of the injury. In many cases, there is no objective evidence of the disorder. Occasionally, benign positional vertigo or electronystagmographic evidence of spontaneous or positional nystagmus with the head turned in the direction of the whiplash may develop. Audiometric studies are generally normal, unless there is other significant head trauma. The physician is often asked to estimate the duration of probable incapacity or to evaluate the extent of disability as a basis for determining unemployment compensation. The prognosis as to the duration of the disability should always be guarded in traumatic injuries, and the patient should be followed at intervals to determine at what time a return to work will be safe. Such a patient should be warned about the dangers of working in high places and driving a car if symptoms persist. Patients may also have complaints of unsteadiness with motion. They may display a variety of eye complaints from blurring to intolerance of moving visual images (for example, TV).

Malingering, or compensation neurosis, must constantly be borne in mind when one is evaluating the condition of patients with evidence of trauma to the internal ear. In the absence of evidence of a neurosis when malingering is suspected, the patient should be given the benefit of doubt until further observations are made.

### Motion Sickness

*Motion sickness* is the term applied to the disturbance of equilibrium caused by repeated motion, such as the movement of a ship.

During stimulation, the patient has almost continuous dizziness, nausea, and frequent vomiting. These symptoms last until some hours after the stimulation ceases, although they generally are not as severe. A large number of persons who are otherwise normal experience motion sickness when they are on a merry-go-round, on a swing, or riding for any distance in the rear seat of an automobile. Some people find even riding for a few blocks in a car impossible. Both visual input and proprioceptive input, obviously, play a factor in creation of these symptoms. A variety of medications have been utilized. The most successful are dimenhydrinate (Dramamine), scopolamine, or central nervous suppressants such as diazepam (Valium). See Table 43–1 and box on page 506 for listing of useful medications.

### Endolymphatic Hydrops (Ménière disease)

Endolymphatic hydrops, which is usually called Ménière disease, is a common cause of paroxysmal, whirling vertigo. In this condition, a triad of symptoms is seen: (1) attacks of whirling vertigo, (2) tinnitus, and (3) fluctuating sensori-

**TABLE 43–1.**

Medications for Control of Acute Vertigo

| Hospital Setting | Dose |
| --- | --- |
| Atropine | 0.2–0.4 mg (IV) |
| Droperidol | 1.5–2.5 mg (IV slowly) |
| Diazepam (Valium) | 5–10 mg (IV slowly) |
| Promethazine | 12.5–25 mg (IV slowly) |
| Diphenhydramine hydrochloride | 50 mg (IV slowly) |

| Outpatient Setting | Dose |
| --- | --- |
| Meclizine (Antivert) | 25–100 mg q.i.d. (oral) |
| Dimenhydrinate (Dramamine) | 50 mg q 4–6 h (oral) |
| Promethazine (Phenergan) | 12.5–25 mg q 4-6 h (oral) |
| Transderm Sc&op (Scopolamine) | 1 patch 0.5 q 3 d (dermal) |
| Dephenidol (Vontrol) | 25–50 mg tid (oral) |
| Diphenhydramine hydrochloride (Benadryl) | 25–50 mg q 4–6 h (oral); 50 mg/10 ml solution (IV) |

neural hearing loss. Early in the disease, one or two of the symptoms may occur without the third. In two thirds of patients, vertigo is the primary symptom. Final diagnosis of endolymphatic hydrops should not be made, however, until all three symptoms are present. In most patients, the vertigo, tinnitus, and hearing loss exhibit certain patterns that are characteristic of endolymphatic hydrops. It is most common in adults between the ages of 30 and 50.

Isolated attacks of severe, whirling vertigo with no dizziness, or instability between attacks is the most characteristic symptom of early Ménière disease. Each attack begins abruptly, but not so suddenly that the patient falls. In the typical attack, the vertigo increases for 10 minutes to an hour, persists for 20 minutes to several hours, and subsides. It is important to remember that the vertigo lasts hours, not days or weeks. *Continuous vertigo for several days is not typical of endolymphatic hydrops.*

The attacks may be several weeks or months apart. Initially, they may be years apart. If the patient is not treated, the attacks may become more frequent and more severe, until they occur as often as every few days. Rarely, in the most severe cases, they occur daily, but they remain paroxysmal and there are periods of complete relief between attacks. Late in the disease or during a particular flare of symptoms, the patient may complain of some unsteadiness between episodes. Most instances of severe vertigo are associated with nausea and vomiting for several hours. Nausea without vomiting may be seen in milder attacks.

The hearing loss associated with Ménière disease is typically a sensorineural loss of low tones. It is present initially in only one ear. Bilateral hydrops occurs in about 25% to 40% of patients and usually develops within the first 3 years of the disease. The loss of hearing tends to fluctuate abruptly, and between episodes the patient's hearing tends to return toward normal. Eventually the hearing loss progresses slowly to severe cochlear damage. A sense of fullness or pressure in the involved ear is a frequent complaint when the hearing is impaired. Distortion of words and diplacusis are common.

The typical audiogram of patients with endolymphatic hydrops reveals a low-frequency hearing loss in contrast to other types of sensorineural hearing loss. Recruitment of loudness to some degree is almost always present. The condition may be suspected when the patient complains that loud, sharp sounds are annoying or painful in the ear that has poor hearing.

The tinnitus that accompanies endolymphatic hydrops is typically a low, buzzing sound initially, later fluctuating. It is frequently louder preceding or during the attack of vertigo. Both hearing loss and tinnitus remain between attacks of vertigo. Late in the disease, the tinnitus may develop a high-pitched component.

One may see patients with attacks of vertigo that are without hearing loss or tinnitus but are otherwise typical of endolymphatic hydrops. In these patients the diagnosis should not be made until hearing loss or tinnitus appears, and a toxic or allergic cause should be sought. Similarly, there are patients who have a fluctuating, neurosensory, low-frequency hearing loss typical of the hearing loss associated with hydrops, but again, the diagnosis of Ménière disease should not be made until the hearing loss or tinnitus appears. Rather, these episodes should be considered as *cochlear* hydrops.

The predominant pathologic feature is dilatation of the endolymph-containing structures. There is gross distention of the endolymphatic system, particularly the scala media, and consequent degeneration of the neural end organs of both the labyrinth and the cochlea. The cause is as yet unknown, although there has been extensive speculation in the 120 years since the disorder was first described. It has been attributed to many things, including adrenal cortical dysfunction, disturbances in the control of salt and water balance, allergy, vasospasm, toxicity, and metabolic abnormalities in the inner ear. It is possible that each of these conditions may play a part in producing the disorder.

Too often, Ménière disease has been another "wastebasket" into which unclassified cases of vertigo are carelessly thrown. Regardless of its cause, the syndrome presents a clear-cut history and functional changes in the ears. All elements of the disease should be rigidly demanded before paroxysmal vertigo is labeled Ménière disease. Endolymphatic hydrops that occurs secondary to ear disease or trauma is often called Ménière syndrome to differentiate it from the idiopathic disorder that is called Ménière disease. The symptoms may be identical.

Physical examination, including neurologic and otolaryngologic examination, is generally normal in Ménière disease, except for the vestibular and auditory tests. Caloric stimulation of the involved ear may produce normal responses, but more often the reaction is one of hypoactivity. Hyperactive response to caloric stimulation should make one doubt the presence of endolymphatic hydrops. The glycerol test has become a prominent diagnostic tool that can be used to confirm the historical diagnosis of Ménière disease. Glycerin (1.2 mg/kg) is given by mouth with an equal volume of grapefruit juice. There is generally improvement in the hearing threshold and the speech discrimination scores 1 to 3 hours after ingestion. This improvement is transient, but if the patient is having frequent episodes of vertigo, the test can occasionally break a series of spells. The response to glycerin is believed to reflect acute dehydration of the inner ear secondary to its osmotic effect.

**Medical Treatment of Vertigo.**    All patients should be strongly reassured that the attacks ultimately stop of their own accord or that they can be stopped. Control of the anxiety and fear caused by the violence of the vertigo and retching will make any other treatment more effective. It is important that the attending physician have a thorough knowledge of both the diagnosis and treatment of the disorder and provide understanding as well as confidence to the patient.

Acute spells of Ménière disease can be treated effectively with the use of anticholinergics, vasodilators, or sedatives (see box).

---

**MEDICAL TREATMENT OF MÉNIÈRE DISEASE**
  I. Low-salt diet
 II. Drug therapy
    a. Diuretics: Dyazide, hydrochlorothiazide
    b. Peripheral vestibular suppressants: meclizine, diphenhydramine
    c. Central nervous system vestibular suppressants: diazepam
    d. Antiemetics: promethazine
    e. Anticholinergics: scopolamine

1. Atropine, given subcutaneously, often will stop an attack within 20 to 30 minutes. Dose is generally 0.6 mg intramuscularly.
2. Diphenhydramine hydrochloride (Benadryl) is effective when given intravenously. The dosage is up to 100 mg given slowly in full strength as supplied for intravenous use (10 cc) or added to 250 ml of 5% dextrose and water.
3. Diazepam (Valium) has a strong sedative effect on the central nervous system and is used intravenously to control an acute episode. Intravenous doses of 5 to 15 mg titrated to the patient's response are usually sufficient to stop acute attacks. This must be done under medical supervision. Larger doses are occasionally necessary.
4. In a hospital situation, intravenous droperidol (a narcoleptic agent) may be used. Dosage is 2.5 to 5.0 mg every 12 hours. This agent is very effective is lessening the effects of an acute episode.

The long-term management of vertigo and hearing loss in Ménière disease is more difficult. A low-salt diet remains the basis of management. A diet of approximately 1.5 g has widest acceptance. On this diet patients are advised not to salt food, either while cooking or at the table. Salt substitutes may be used. The patient is told to avoid any salt-containing foods such as potato chips, peanuts, nuts, beer, and canned soups. It is imperative that patients eliminate or curtail cigarette smoking because of its known effects on the vascular system. Similarly, many physicians restrict caffeine intake.

Diuretics remain a basis of medical treatment. Chlorothiazide (Diuril), 500 mg every day, or hydrochlorothiazide (HydroDIURIL), 25 mg twice a day, are commonly used. Chlorothalidone (Hygroton), 100 mg once a day, or triamterene with hydrochlorothiazide (Dyazide), 1 tablet per day, are used by some with reported good response. Potassium supplementation must be used with certain diuretics. Generally, most patients on this regimen, provided the vertigo does not recur, may reduce or stop the diuretic after 3 to 4 months. However, the patient must continue the salt restriction.

Although vasodilators have been used for many years in the treatment of Ménière disease, there is no clear evidence that cerebral flow is improved with the standard drugs used. Other vasodilating regimens have included histamine or carbogen, which is a commercially prepared mixture of 5% carbon dioxide and 95% oxygen.

Methantheline bromide (Banthine) has been effective when used either alone or in conjunction with salt restriction and vasodilators or both. In some instances it has had a dramatic beneficial effect on tinnitus and hearing loss. The initial dose may be either 50 or 100 mg every 6 hours. If 100 mg are used, the dosage should be dropped to 50 mg every 6 hours after a therapeutic effect has been achieved. Propantheline bromide (Pro-Banthine) in doses of 15 mg every 6 hours, will occasionally give the same results.

Meclizine (Antivert), 12.5 to 25 mg three times a day, is an antihistamine that suppresses peripheral labyrinthine function and in many patients has been given long term with beneficial results. In any patient who gives a history of episodes of allergic reactions, the antihistamine drugs may be beneficial and may be occasionally all that is necessary for control. However, in only 5% of patients with Ménière disease is there an allergic cause identified. Dimenhydrinate raises the threshold of labyrinthine irritability and therefore may be successfully used without other treatment in patients with mild vertigo.

Dimenhydrinate (Dramamine) in the ordinary doses of 50 to 100 mg every 4 to 6 hours has been used in the management of Ménière disease with varying degrees of success. If patients are free of symptoms for several months, the antihistamine medications can be discontinued.

Many patients benefit from long-term mild sedation to allay anxiety. Diazepam is often used in low doses. Occasionally doses as low as 2.5 mg three times a day can be effective in controlling symptoms, particularly those of mild unsteadiness in the patient with long-standing Ménière disease. However, because diazepam tends to suppress central pathways, large doses of it in a vestibularly debilitated patient can increase symptoms.

In recent years, the scopolamine patch (Transderm-Sc&o) has been used for patients with frequent, recurrent episodes of Ménière disease. These patches, placed behind the ear, are effective transdermally over a 3-day period. Generally, in full dosage, side effects of dry mouth and blurred vision are quite disturbing. It is useful in the severely affected patient.

**Surgical Treatment.** Failure of medical therapy to adequately relieve the severe vertiginous spells is primary indication for surgical therapy. Less than 10% of patients with Ménière disease ever require surgery. These are generally the patients in whom the attacks continue to cause disability (despite medical management), those whose occupation makes it imperative that they take no chance in having an attack, or those for whom it is impossible to follow medical management. Almost all patients chosen for operative intervention have failed to respond to any type of medical care. The disease in these patients is progressive, with the hearing in the affected ear rapidly diminishing.

The variety of surgical procedures available emphasizes the lack of any one "perfect" surgical therapy for Ménière disease. The procedures can be divided into conservative or destructive procedures (see box). Conservative procedures include endolymphatic shunt, endolymphatic decompression, tack procedure, vestibular nerve section,

SURGERY FOR ENDOLYMPHATIC HYDROPS
I. Endolymphatic sac procedures
   1. Endolymphatic sac decompression
   2. Endolymphatic shunt
II. Vestibular nerve procedures
   1. Middle fossa vestibular nerve section
   2. Retrolabyrinthine vestibular nerve section
III. Destructive procedures of vestibular apparatus
   1. Transtympanic labyrinthotomy
   2. Labyrinthectomy
   3. Translabyrinthine vestibular nerve section

cryotherapy, or ultrasound. Destructive procedures include transtympanic labyrinthotomy or transmastoid labyrinthectomy.

The endolymphatic shunt operation opens the endolymphatic sac, theoretically releasing perilymph into either the subarachnoid or mastoid space. In this procedure, the endolymphatic sac is exposed over the posterior fossa by a mastoidectomy approach (Fig 43–2). A tube is then placed

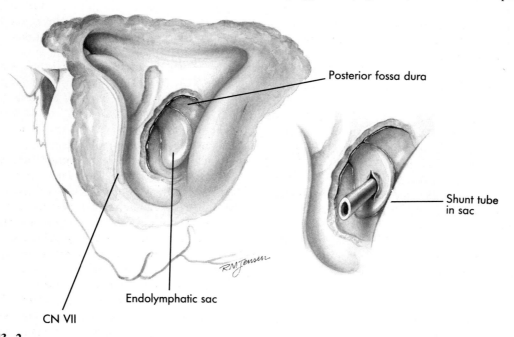

**FIG 43–2.**
Endolymphatic mastoid shunt demonstrating simple mastoidectomy to expose the posterior fossa dura and endolymphatic sac posterior to the posterior semicircular canal. Inset demonstrates the shunt tube placed through an incision in the lateral wall of the endolymphatic sac and brought out into the mastoid cavity.

into the endolymphatic sac, which is usually easily identified, and brought laterally into the mastoid cavity or placed medially into the subarachnoid space. Because surgical results of both procedures appear similar, the endolymphatic mastoid shunt is preferable because there is decreased risk of meningitis and cerebrospinal fluid leak. Long-term results suggest a 60% to 70% control of vertigo and a 50% to 60% stabilization of hearing. The risk to existing hearing with this procedure is 3% to 4%, and the hospitalization is generally less than a day. Some physicians are satisfied with exteriorizing the endolymphatic sac by uncovering the bone over it, believing that the increased vascularity with healing and decompression of the sac are adequate treatment. A small percentage of patients continue to have symptoms of such severity that a more involved procedure is necessary.

The tack procedure, popularized by Cody, is less frequently done. It consists of placing a tack (a 3 mm pin) through the stapes's footplate under direct vision. The theory is that the hydropic saccule will swell against the tack and rupture, eventually developing a permanent endolymph-perilymph fistula. The control over vertigo with this procedure seems similar to that with the shunt procedure, but the hearing loss appears more progressive. Thus the procedure is often reserved for elderly patients who are at risk for more extensive procedures and have poor hearing.

Recently there has been increased interest in vestibular nerve section in uncontrolled Ménière disease. In this procedure, done either via the middle fossa surgical approach or by a retrolabyrinthine approach, the superior and inferior vestibular nerves are sectioned, preserving the cochlear and seventh nerves (Fig 43–3). The advantage of the procedure is the better than 95% control of vertiginous attacks. One disadvantage is the increased risk to the seventh nerve and cochlea, compared with the shunt procedure. About 10% of patients will develop a significant increased loss of hearing, which is a considerable risk in those who have serviceable hearing. In addition, the operative procedure is more difficult and the hospitalization significantly longer than with the shunt procedures. Therefore, it is a better secondary procedure for those who have good hearing.

Cryotherapy and ultrasound to the horizontal or posterior canal through a mastoidectomy approach have been used. These procedures are not as widely accepted, however.

A small percentage of patients continue to have symptoms following previous surgical procedures or have so little function in the affected ear that the function is considered worthless. In those individuals, labyrinthine destruction is indicated. Control of vertigo is 100%, but the hearing loss is similarly total. The morbidity from the operation is generally low. The procedure consists initially of a simple mastoidectomy. When enough mastoid cells are removed to uncover the three semicircular canals, these canals are then widely opened, including the vestibule, and the membranous labyrinth is removed (Fig 43–4).

A second destructive procedure is accomplished by reflecting the tympanic membrane, as is done in operations on the stapes, removing the stapes, and destroying the labyrinth through the oval window. Further destruction of the cochlea has been advocated in the hope of stopping tinnitus, but this approach has not always been successful.

Streptomycin, administered systemically and carefully controlled by serial audiometry and electronystagmographic testing, has been used to decrease labyrinthine activity and prevent attacks of vertigo caused by hydrops in patients with bilateral disease. Because such treatment has a risk of causing a toxic effect in both ears, it is reserved for those individuals in whom the disease is bilateral and no other treatment can be considered.

## Other Peripheral Labyrinthine Disorders
### Cogan's Syndrome

In 1945 Cogan described a condition of nonsyphilitic interstitial keratitis with symptoms of a vestibuloauditory disorder, including tinnitus, vertigo, and hearing loss. They were essentially the triad of Ménière disease, plus interstitial keratitis. Other bodily findings were negative. It is now apparent that Cogan's syndrome is only part of a larger immunologic complex. If the patient is seen early, large doses of steroids might be expected to halt the rapidly progressive hearing loss, tinnitus, and vertigo. Although treatment has been unsuccessful in the long term, a temporary response can be obtained with the use of steroids.

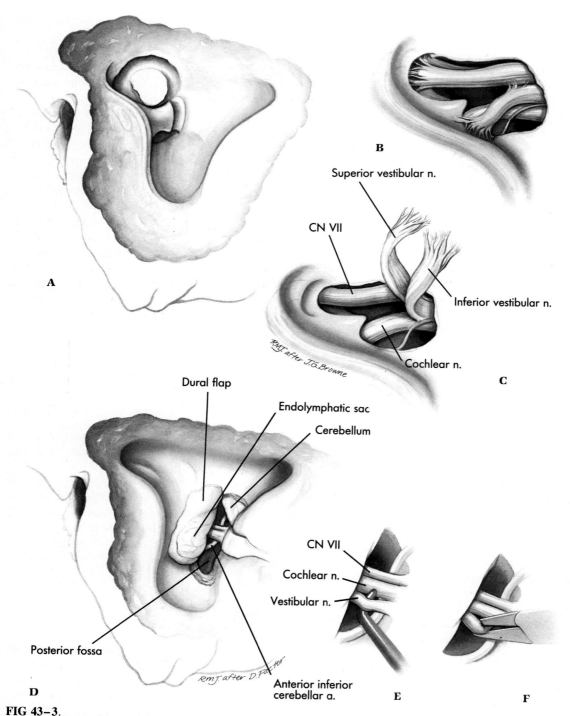

**Superior vestibular n.**

**CN VII**

**Inferior vestibular n.**

**Cochlear n.**

RMJ after J.G.Browne

**A**

**B**

**C**

**Dural flap**

**Endolymphatic sac**

**Cerebellum**

**CN VII**

**Cochlear n.**

**Vestibular n.**

**Posterior fossa**

RMJ after D. Factor

**Anterior inferior
cerebellar a.**

**D**

**E**

**F**

**FIG 43–3**.

Translabyrinthine vestibular nerve section. **A,** completion of labyrinthectomy with isolation of horizontal, superior, posterior semicircular canals. **B,** further dissection medial to the facial nerve and vestibule demonstrating the internal auditory meatus. Visualized are the superior vestibular nerve overlying the facial nerve and the inferior vestibular nerve lateral to the cochlear nerve. **C,** section of the superior and inferior vestibular nerves demonstrating the remnant of cranial nerve VII and the cochlear division of cranial nerve VIII. **D,** retrolabyrinthine approach demonstrating cochlear vestibular complex in the posterior fossa. Note the endolymphatic sac and dura flap are turned forward, clearly exposing the nerves to be sectioned. Insets (**E** and **F**) show the separation of the vestibular nerve from the cochlear division and sectioning with microscissors. (**C** redrawn from Nelson, A: *Temporal bone surgical dissection manual,* Los Angeles, 1982, House Ear Institute. Used by permission.)

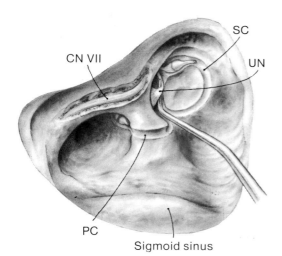

**FIG 43-4.**
Transmastoid labyrinthectomy (surgical position). Delineation of vertical and tympanic segments of the facial nerve (cranial nerve VII) permits wide exposure of vestibule by removal of bony semicircular canals. Hook may then be used to extract utricular nerve *(UN)* and ampullary nerves. *(SC),* Superior semicircular canal; *PC,* posterior semicircular canal.

### Benign Positional Vertigo

Benign positional vertigo produces a sudden sensation of severe whirling, lasting from 5 to 30 seconds, that can occur when a person changes position when standing but is more frequent when lying down or turning over. It is accompanied by nystagmus, occasionally by nausea, and rarely by vomiting. It does not occur every time the person assumes the inciting position. It should be noted that this sensation is true vertigo (that is, whirling) and should not be confused with postural hypotension, which produces a feeling of lightheadedness or mild syncope. Benign positional vertigo occurs rarely in persons with central nervous system disease, and for the most part, the lesion is peripheral. It is common, although often overlooked. Usually it is self-limited, and no specific cause can be demonstrated. Generally, the duration of symptoms is less than 6 months, but recurrence is common. This disorder is thought to be caused by a deposit (probably of otolith debris or degenerative matter from the macula) lodging against the cupula of the posterior semicircular canal. This theory is supported by histologic evidence in temporal bones. When positional vertigo is observed, it is necessary to investigate both ears and the central nervous system. It is often

seen after head injuries. Tests for positional nystagmus, when positive, help establish the diagnosis (see discussion of labyrinthine tests).

### Perilymphatic Fistula

Occasionally, fistulas from the oval or round window will cause fluctuating episodes of vertigo, usually associated with some hearing loss and tinnitus. Most frequently, the patient will give a history of previous head trauma or excessive exertion immediately preceding the onset of symptoms. The diagnosis of perilymphatic fistula is exceedingly difficult and generally only surgically verified. If the intermittent vertigo is stimulated by pressure to the ear by straining, coughing, or sneezing, treatment may relieve the vestibular symptoms. Rarely is hearing improved.

### Vertebral Basilar Artery Insufficiency

Vertebral basilar artery insufficiency is caused by decreased blood flow of the posterior and/or anterior inferior cerebellar artery. It is associated with drop attacks, generally precipitated by head motion. It is accompanied by dizziness in about 50% of individuals. Associated symptoms include visual disturbances, dysarthria, headache, and loss of consciousness.

## Eighth Nerve Causes of Vertigo

Irritation or destruction of the eighth nerve pathways to the brainstem may cause dizziness that is often accompanied by some disturbance in hearing. Frequently, the damage to the hearing is total.

### Inflammation

*Infection,* such as meningitis, may cause irritation to the nerve during the active stage and produce dizziness, tinnitus, and hearing loss. Permanent damage to the nerve with residual permanent reduction in hearing acuity may result, but dizziness occurs only during the irritative phase. The dizziness so produced is frequently accompanied by spontaneous nystagmus.

### Trauma

*Trauma* to the eighth cranial nerve occurs as a result of basilar skull fracture, usually through the petrous apex. Such trauma may produce severe or total hearing loss that does not recover. The dizziness produced is whirling in nature, but it lasts only during the period immediately following the damage. If total section of the nerve or destruction of the labyrinth is the result, the immediate symptoms last 3 to 6 weeks, during which time the opposite labyrinth assumes control, as in hemorrhage of the internal ear or suppurative labyrinthitis. Frequently, the sixth and seventh cranial nerves are damaged at the same time because of their close anatomic relationship to the eighth nerve. Therefore, facial paralysis and lateral rectus palsy are frequently seen with trauma to the eighth nerve.

### Tumors

*Tumors* of the posterior fossa or cerebellopontine angle can produce systematized vertigo that is often accompanied by spontaneous nystagmus. In patients with cerebellar tumors, the symptoms are most likely to be slowly progressive dizziness, ataxia, uncoordination, and headache. In those with tumors of the cerebellopontine angle, for example, acoustic neuroma or meningioma, dizziness is similar but accompanied by hearing loss. Acoustic neuroma usually produces cochlear symptoms first, and these symptoms precede the onset of dizziness. The hearing loss is sensorineural and progressive. Response to vestibular stimulation becomes more hypoactive and is finally lost. As such tumors enlarge, other cranial nerves are involved. After the eighth nerve, the fifth nerve is most commonly involved. The earliest and most common sign is partial or complete corneal anesthesia of the involved side. It takes but a moment to test the corneal reflex, and it should never be overlooked in the routine examination. When tumors are very large, the seventh nerve may be involved. Treatment is surgical removal by a transmastoid or occipital approach. Hearing is generally lost, but seventh nerve function is preserved.

## Brainstem (Nuclei) Causes of Dizziness

Involvement of the brainstem in the region of the vestibular nuclei, regardless of origin, may produce whirling vertigo. When the lesion is small, vertigo occurs without hearing loss or tinnitus. Larger lesions cannot affect the vestibular nuclei alone because of the close proximity of the nuclei to other cranial nerves. Therefore, lesions of the brainstem producing vertigo and hearing loss together are accompanied by signs of dysfunction of adjacent cranial nerves. Treatment is usually symptomatic. Diagnosis is often made on CT or MRI.

### Inflammations and Trauma

*Inflammations* such as encephalitis, meningitis, and brain abscess or trauma may cause damage to the brainstem directly or through pressure.

### Hemorrhage

Bleeding into the brainstem cannot cause dizziness alone because of the close proximity of other nuclei. Small petechial hemorrhage might conceivably do so, but this theory is unproved and unlikely.

### Thrombosis of the Posteroinferior Cerebellar Artery

*Thrombosis of the posteroinferior cerebellar artery* produces sudden vertigo associated with other signs. The onset is typically sudden. In addition to vertigo and nystagmus, examination shows dysphagia, weakness of the palate, impairment of sensation of pain and sensation of temperature on the face, Horner syndrome, and cerebellar signs in the arm and leg on the same side of the body as the lesion. Impairment of sensation of pain and temperature on the opposite side of the body accompanies these signs.

### Tumors

*Tumors* of the brainstem produce symptoms and signs similar to those of other brainstem damage, but progression is less rapid. Diagnosis depends on careful neurologic examination, CT or MRI.

### Multiple Sclerosis

Multiple sclerosis may cause vertigo, which can be the only complaint. Here the picture is similar to that described as acute toxic labyrinthitis. A maximum of vertigo is reached in hours or a day. The dizziness may then last several days or even several weeks, after which it gradually subsides. Tinnitus and hearing loss are usually not associated. The only assistance one may gain from the history is that most patients who have acute toxic labyrinthitis relate that they were well on the way to recovery in 10 days. The symptoms from multiple sclerosis are more prolonged.

When there is suspicion of multiple sclerosis, a detailed history should be taken with regard to any past neurologic episodes, such as a sudden blurring of vision followed by recovery. Tempo-ral pallor of the optic disks is characteristic but may not appear until later. Abnormalities of opto-kinetic and ocular function can be identified on electronystagmogram in a small percentage of patients with multiple sclerosis. Diagnosis is aided with magnetic resonance imaging and a spinal tap demonstrating abnormal proteins.

# 44

# The Facial Nerve

## ANATOMY AND PHYSIOLOGY

### Facial Nerve

The facial, or seventh cranial nerve, leaves the pons, travels a short distance, and enters the internal auditory meatus together with the eighth cranial nerve. This close relationship of the seventh and eighth nerves is maintained throughout the petrous portion of the temporal bone. Leaving the eighth nerve, which is distributed to the cochlea and labyrinth, the seventh nerve, with the chorda tympani, continues laterally and emerges on the anterior and superior aspect of the medial wall of the middle ear. Here the nerve turns sharply, posteriorly and inferiorly, to make a bend known as the genu of the facial nerve and traverses the medial wall of the middle ear, superior to the oval window and the stapes (*intratympanic* portion). The geniculate ganglion is located 2 to 3 mm proximal to the genu of the facial nerve.

At the stapes, the seventh nerve makes an arch posteriorly and passes inferiorly to the prominence of the horizontal semicircular canal (*pyramidal* portion), bringing the nerve deep into the bone of the external auditory canal. It continues vertically downward (*vertical* portion) and emerges from the skull through the stylomastoid foramen (Fig 44–1).

On leaving the stylomastoid foramen, the facial nerve turns forward, passes immediately lateral to the base of the styloid process, crosses the posterior belly of the digastric muscle (*cervical* portion), and enters the parotid gland. In the parotid gland it travels between the superficial and deep lobes and divides into three trunks that fan out between the lobes (Fig 44–2). The point of division is called the *pes anserinus,* or goose's foot. After traversing the gland, the branches of the facial nerve emerge from the anterior and superior borders of the gland to supply the muscles of facial expression. The cervical branch of the facial nerve is in close relationship with the posterior facial vein (Fig 44–3).

### Surgical Landmarks

The facial nerve can be easily located in the temporal bone because of its constant relationship to the oval window, horizontal semicircular canal, and stylomastoid foramen (see Figs. 44–1 and 44–3). In its cervical portion, it can be located by its relationship to the styloid process and digastric muscle. The facial nerve can also be located by its lateral relationship to the posterior facial vein.

### Function

The facial nerve supplies motor fibers (Fig 44–4) to the muscles of facial expression, that is, those of the lips, nose, cheeks, eyelids, and forehead. Motor fibers from branches of the facial nerve go to the stapedius, extrinsic auricular, stylohyoid, and platysma muscles, as well as to the posterior belly of the digastric muscle.

The facial nerve also has sensory fibers. Exact sensory pathways have not been proved. A portion of the outer one third of the external auditory canal and a portion of the concha of the external ear receive cutaneous branches from the facial nerve. These sensory branches have connections with the trigeminal, glossopharyngeal, and vagus nerves. Sense of taste to the anterior two thirds of the tongue and secretory fibers to the sublingual and submaxillary salivary glands are carried by the chorda tympani (Fig 44–5).

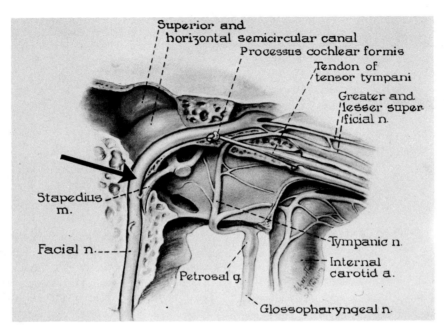

**FIG 44–1.**
Medial wall of the middle ear showing the facial nerve and other structures. Arrow points to the most common site of injury during an operation on the temporal bone.

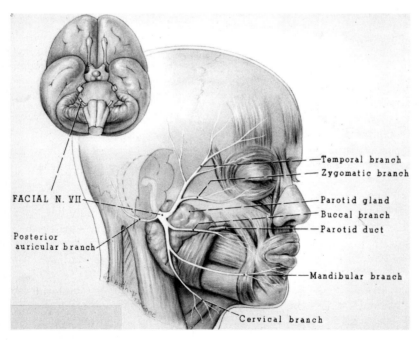

**FIG 44–2.**
Distribution of the facial nerve after its exit from the stylomastoid foramen. (From Jacob SW, Francone CA: *Structure and function in man*, Philadelphia, 1978, WB Saunders. Used by permission.)

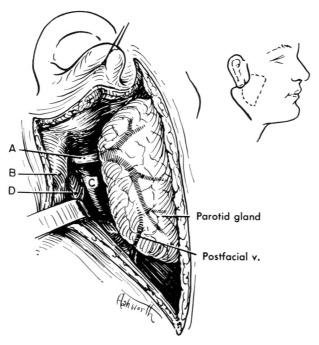

**FIG 44–3.**
Relationships of the facial nerve at the stylomastoid foramen. **A,** main trunk of the facial nerve. **B,** mastoid tip. **C,** styloid process. **D,** posterior belly of the digastric muscle. Note the relationship of the posterior facial vein. *Inset,* incision to expose gland and facial nerve.

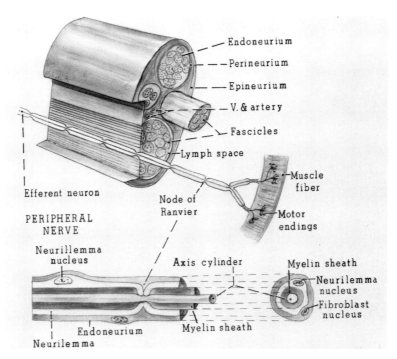

**FIG 44–4.**
Peripheral motor nerve, such as the seventh nerve. (From Jacob SW, Francone CA: *Structure and function in man,* Philadelphia, 1978, WB Saunders. Used by permission.)

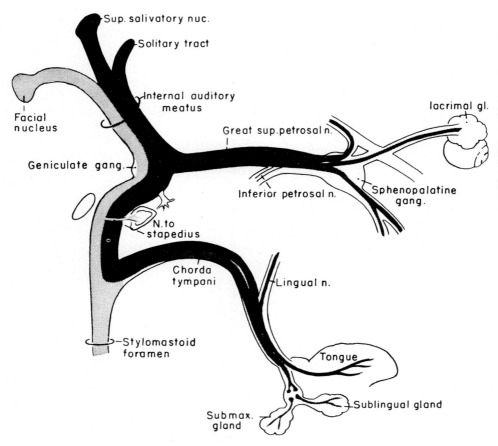

**FIG 44–5.**
Components of the facial nerve. (Adapted from Mielhke A: *Die Chirurgie des Nervus facialis,* Berlin, 1960, Urban & Schwarzenberg. Used by permission.)

### *Chorda Tympani Nerve*

The chorda tympani (special visceral efferent) nerve accompanies the facial nerve to a point just below the horizontal semicircular canal. Here the two nerves separate. The chorda tympani leaves the facial (fallopian) canal through a small foramen (iter chordae posterius) and then crosses the tympanic membrane between the fibrous and mucous layers of the eardrum at the level of the malleolar folds and between the incus and the neck of the malleus. Leaving the ear through a small foramen (itér chordae anterius), the chorda tympani joins the lingual nerve medial to the mandible and is distributed to the tongue and to the sublingual and submaxillary salivary glands.

### Sensory Disturbances

Disturbance of the sensory function of the facial nerve may produce pain in and around the ear. It may also impair the sense of taste in the anterior two thirds of the tongue. Two conditions incident to disturbed sensory function of the facial nerve are herpes zoster oticus and geniculate ganglion neuralgia.

### *Herpes Zoster Oticus (Ramsay Hunt Syndrome)*

Some otolaryngologists believe that herpes zoster oticus (Fig 44–6) results from inflammation of the geniculate ganglion. It produces severe pain in the ear, vesicles in the external auditory canal, and facial paralysis. The pain and vesiculation may be present without paralysis. The cutaneous area involved is supplied by fibers from the fifth, ninth, and tenth cranial nerves, as well as by fibers from the facial nerve. It also receives fibers from the cervical plexus. Consequently, it is impossible to establish which nerve is responsible for the inflammation. Further discussion of herpes

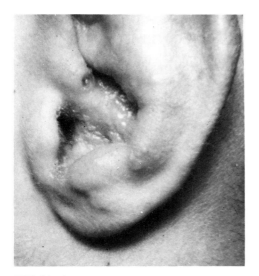

**FIG 44–6.**
Herpes zoster oticus. Note vesicles.

zoster is in the section on motor disturbances of the facial nerve.

### Geniculate Ganglion Neuralgia

In patients with geniculate ganglion neuralgia, the primary site of pain is deep in the ear. The

pain occurs in paroxysms, is sharp and shooting in nature, and its severity is comparable to that of tic douloureux. It may radiate to the jaw, face, and neck. Treatment initially consists of drug therapy. The drug of choice is carbamazepine (Tegretol), 200 mg, three or more times daily. This drug must be closely monitored for side effects. Other drugs used are phenytoin (Dilantin) and, more recently, baclofen (Lioresal). Prolonged and intractable pain can be completely relieved by intracranial section of the *nervus intermedius*.

## Motor Disturbances of the Facial Nerve

Because of the well-defined anatomic mapping of the seventh nerve, localization as to site of lesion or blockage can be clearly defined (Fig 44–7). Localization can be summarized as follows:

1. Facial nerve paralysis, presence of taste, lacrimation, and stapedial reflex; lesion peripheral to stylomastoid foramen
2. Facial nerve paralysis, loss of taste and submaxillary salivary flow, presence of

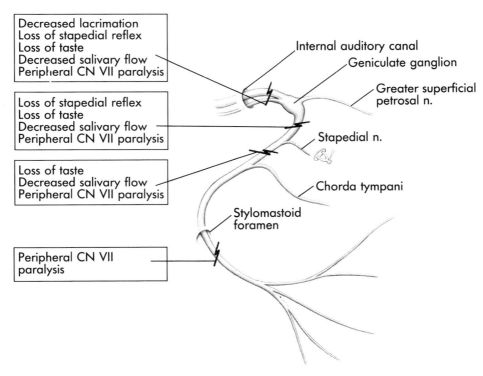

**FIG 44–7.**
Symptoms related to site of facial injury.

lacrimation and stapedial muscle reflex; lesion distal to take-off of chorda tympani nerve

3. Facial nerve paralysis, loss of stapedial reflex and taste; presence of lacrimation; lesion peripheral to the geniculate but proximal to the nerve to the stapedius muscle

4. Facial nerve paralysis, loss of lacrimation, loss of stapedial reflex, loss of taste; lesion proximal to geniculate ganglion

5. Seventh nerve paralysis with the exception of presence of bilateral forehead motion; lesion superior to the nucleus of the seventh nerve

Irritation to, or injury of, the motor portion of the facial nerve produces twitching, spasm, weakness, or paralysis of the facial muscles. Paralysis is the most important. If paralysis is uncorrected, the resulting deformity of the face not only is disfiguring but also may be accompanied by serious psychologic trauma, particularly in women.

On the involved side of the face, the buccinator and other muscles are completely paralyzed in total facial paralysis so that there is a total lack of motion. Consequently, on the involved side of the face mastication of food is difficult. Saliva may drool from the corner of the mouth. Irritation of the lids and cornea occurs. Foreign bodies may easily enter the eye, since the lids will not close to protect the cornea. Smiling, laughing, and frowning on the uninvolved side of the face produce a one-sided grimace (Fig 44–8).

Neurophysiologists have described three degrees of damage that can occur when a nerve is injured.

1. *An injury that causes no degeneration of the nerve distal to the injured side.* There may be, however, some interruption of the continuity of the myelin sheath at the site of injury. This slightest of the three degrees of damage is known as *neuropraxia.* Recovery from this type of injury is usually rapid and complete.

2. *An injury that causes division of the axon with degeneration of both the axon and the myelin sheath peripheral to the injury with no degeneration proximal or toward the nerve cell.* Some changes do take place in the nerve cell, but the cell does not degenerate. The other components of the nerve (the neurilemma and endoneurium) remain

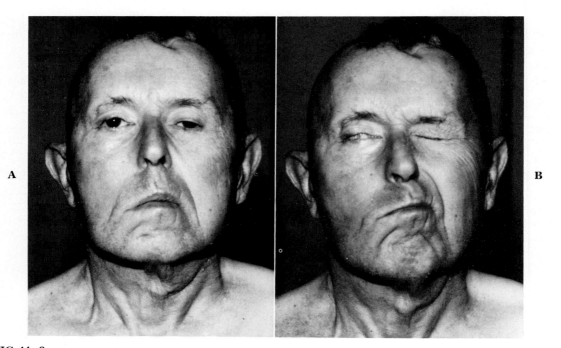

**FIG 44–8.**
**A,** total facial paralysis. Note flattening of facial creases on the right and pulling of the mouth to the left even at rest. **B,** this is markedly accentuated with attempts at grimacing. The eye does not close.

normal. A person who has this degree of injury may also recover without serious sequelae; however, the recovery is slow, since the myelin sheath and axon must re-form and grow out to the nerve end. This degree of injury is called *axonotmesis*.

3. *An injury that completely disrupts all the essential elements of the nerve with subsequent degeneration of the axon and myelin sheath and sometimes the parent cell itself.* When this degree of damage has occurred, the new sheath and axon must grow from the cell body (provided that it has not degenerated) and traverse the entire length of the nerve. This type of injury results in the most severe degree of damage, which is known as *neurotmesis*. The term does not necessarily imply physical severance of the nerve, but regeneration in this situation carries some hazards. The axons and sheath cells may not regrow into the same channels from which they originated. They may grow part of the way to the extremity of the nerve, or they may grow out of the sheath if an aperture is present through which they can travel.

All three degrees of injury can and do occur in Bell's palsy. Some of the nerve fibrils may show a minor degree of injury and others a severe degree. There is no specific method of determining the type of degeneration that has occurred in a patient with Bell's palsy. It is ascertained only by evaluating the amount and rapidity of recovery. The term *injury* as related to Bell's palsy is used here in its broadest sense. Traumatic injury is not implied.

### Tests of Facial Nerve Function

A variety of tests (see box) are available in the otolaryngologic examination, including electrical tests to determine the site of lesion and the degree of nerve damage. The most commonly used electrical tests are the nerve excitability test and the electromyographic muscle test.

**Nerve Excitability Test.** Several electrical tests are used to stimulate the nerve following facial nerve paralysis. In the nerve excitability test, an active electrode stimulates the individual branches of the facial nerve, and a comparison is

---

**TESTS OF SEVENTH NERVE FUNCTION**
ELECTRICAL STIMULATION TESTS
- Nerve excitability test (NET)
- Maximal stimulation test
- Conduction latency testing
- Strength-duration curves
- Electroneuronography
- Electromyography (EMG)
TESTS FOR LOCALIZATION
- Shirmer test
- Stapedial reflex
- Salivary flow
- Taste
- Hyperacusis

---

made between the amount of electrical stimulus required to cause facial movement. The normal side is used as a control. If the paralyzed side requires only slightly more current, the prognosis is good. If it requires a much larger amount of current (greater than 3.5 mA), there is evidence of degeneration. No response to stimulation on the paralyzed side indicates the nerve has already degenerated. This test has no clinical value in partial paralysis or within 3 days of total paralysis, as changes generally take 3 to 5 days to occur even if the nerve is severed. With the nerve excitability test, day-to-day changes in neural function can be followed. In general, if the face requires less and less current to produce a contraction, the prognosis is good. If, however, there is a sudden change that requires more current or the function is lost on the paralyzed side, there is indication of continuing damage.

Variations of the nerve excitability test have been devised. One is called the maximal stimulation test, in which the stimulus is carried to maximal facial contraction. The normal side is compared with the paralyzed side. Some authors believe that this is a better means of detecting abnormality and shortens the delay in detecting denervation of the nerve. Other authors are strong proponents of electroneuronography, which is an electrodiagnostic test that measures the compound action potential of facial muscles.

**Electromyographic (EMG) Muscle Test.** The electromyographic muscle test determines the activity of the muscle itself. An electrode is inserted into the muscle and recordings are made during rest and during voluntary contraction. Normally, in striated muscle there is no electrical activity at rest, but with voluntary contraction one can record voluntary action potentials. One is looking for the development of fibrillation potentials, which are an electrical fibrillation that occurs in denervated muscle. The absence of fibrillation potentials indicates that the nerve is incompletely degenerated, and the presence of active motor unit potentials or voluntary action potentials indicates that the nerve is still intact and has some function. Although there is significant information to be gained from electromyographic studies, abnormality does not occur until 14 to 21 days after the development of the facial paralysis. Again, electromyography is of no particular value in partial facial loss.

**Schirmer Test.** The Schirmer test is used to aid in localization of nerve damage and possibly to aid in prognosis (Fig 44–9). In this test a piece of dry litmus paper is lightly placed on each lower eyelid. The amount of moistening of the litmus paper is observed over 5 minutes. Wetting of the paper for a distance of at least 1.5 cm is considered to be normal. Less than 1.5 cm indicates the probability that edema, compression, or injury is present at or proximal to the geniculate ganglion. A marked diminution of tearing or a marked dry eye indicates poor prognosis.

**Stapedius Reflex.** A further test of facial function is the stapedius reflex. Because the sta-

pedius muscle is innervated by the seventh nerve, it will contract when stimulated by a short, sharp sound. It can be motivated by the sound being produced in the opposite ear, since there are bilateral, crossing neural connections. The reflex will not be initiated if the facial nerve is not functioning properly at the level of the branch to the stapedius muscle (pyramidal portion of the nerve).

**Submaxillary Salivary Flow.** The test for submaxillary salivary flow is based on measurement of flow of saliva from the submaxillary gland. Preganglionic parasympathetic nerve fibers are on the outside of the seventh nerve bundle, and it has been assumed that these fibers are injured before motor fibers. When there is ischemia of the facial nerve, there is also some impairment of function of the chorda tympani. This impairment results in a decrease of salivary flow to the involved side.

### Congenital Facial Paralysis

Facial paralysis may be present at birth. When it is caused by a disorder of embryologic development or by intracranial hemorrhage before birth, the prognosis for recovery is poor. Associated with this type of facial paralysis may be paralysis of the abducens, oculomotor, trigeminal, glossopharyngeal, and hypoglossal nerves. Paralysis may also be caused by pressure from obstetric forceps and other trauma during delivery. In these instances, the prognosis is generally good. Al-

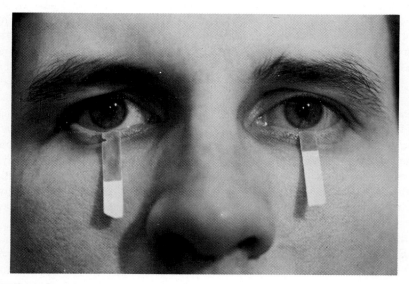

**FIG 44–9.**
Schirmer test. Note the diminution of wetting from the left eye (the involved side).

though these points should be carefully evaluated, there is generally no treatment.

### Central Facial Paralysis

The frontalis muscles receive a bilateral supranuclear innervation. When there is a lesion superior to the nucleus of the seventh nerve, usually a brain tumor or abscess, the lower half of the face on the contralateral side is paralyzed. Forehead motions (frowning and raising of the eyebrows) are retained. Awareness of this aids in localization of the cortical lesion.

Thalamic lesions influence involuntary motions such as laughing and crying. When a lesion of this type is present, the face is paralyzed or weak during involuntary acts but moves normally when voluntary movement is attempted. Remember, in peripheral paralysis the face does not move at all on the involved side. The involuntary emotional motions are retained in central lesions not involving the thalamus.

### Hemifacial Spasm

Hemifacial spasm is manifested by twitching of one or more muscles supplied by the facial nerve. Although not painful, it is extremely annoying and difficult to manage. It does not progress to paralysis of the nerve, although prolonged contraction can cause some grimacing. Blocking of individual branches of the nerve with alcohol may give relief but is usually not suggested. Decompression of the facial nerve has been successful but only for short periods. Surgeons, in the past, have selectively lysed fibers of the nerve to the eye, nose, and mouth, which prevents the spasm but does not produce complete facial paralysis. More recently, this problem has been linked to increased pressure of a loop of the anterior-inferior cerebellar artery resting on or compressing the facial nerve near the internal auditory canal. Decompression of this area and placement of a muscle or synthetic sponge between the vessel and nerve, has yielded excellent relief of symptoms. Hemifacial spasm is highly associated with lesions of the cerebellopontine angle, so all patients with these symptoms should undergo a thorough neuro-otologic evaluation.

### Bell's Palsy

Spontaneous facial paralysis without evidence of other disease or injury is known as idiopathic Bell's palsy. It affects all ages, with peak incidence between the ages of 20 and 40 years. Bell's palsy is not rare: the overall annual incidence is between 10 to 20 per 100,000 population. The incidence in pregnant women is a little more than three times the general incidence. The reason for this is unknown.

Paralysis occurs suddenly or gradually over a period of 24 to 48 hours. Symptoms of disturbance of the chorda tympani (impaired taste and dryness of the mouth) may or may not occur simultaneously and can precede the paralysis by 2 to 7 days. Pain behind the ipsilateral ear occurs in more than 20% of Bell's palsy sufferers, and numbness of the face occurs in about 20%, both often preceding the paralysis. Although the specific cause of Bell's palsy is unknown, it is recognized that swelling of the facial nerve (whether traumatic or idiopathic) causes ischemia, which in turn leads to more swelling and more ischemia. The edema produced may seriously compress the nerve, which has a long course through the temporal bone in a rigid bone canal. There is some evidence that the original insult in Bell's palsy is viral in origin. Between 30% and 50% of patients with Bell's palsy have a prodrome of viral nature, and a study has suggested that two thirds of Bell's palsy victims have other cranial nerve symptoms, including evidence of dysfunction of the fifth, ninth, and tenth nerves. This would suggest a polyneuropathy. However, the viral origin is as yet unproved. A thorough history and physical examination are critical in the evaluation of any facial paralysis, particularly Bell's palsy. Any evidence of chronic ear disease makes that disorder suspect as the cause of the facial paralysis. Slow, progressive onset of facial paralysis would suggest tumor enlargement as the cause of the paralysis. All too often a referring physician assumes the facial paralysis is the result of Bell's palsy and fails to examine the ear or the remainder of the neurologic system.

Every patient with facial paralysis should have pure-tone air and bone conduction audiograms, with masking of the opposite ear and speech discrimination. A unilateral hearing loss on the side of the facial paralysis suggests a possible posterior fossa lesion. In Bell's palsy, the vestibular nerve is not involved. X-ray evaluation should be considered in all cases of idiopathic facial paralysis. Although plain films may rule out the presence of an intracanalicular lesion in the internal acoustic canal, they are of less value in tracing the course of the facial nerve. Polytomography of the temporal bone has been replaced by computed tomography. This is of particular use in determining lesions of the cerebellopontine angle, but more recent advances have allowed CT to trace the course of the facial nerve accurately through the temporal bone. It should be used in all cases of slowly developing seventh nerve paralysis.

There is general agreement that the immediate treatment of Bell's palsy should be medical. Many medical regimens have been recommended through the years. Currently the use of steroids is regarded as useful. The recommended treatment is a course of oral steroids in high doses over 8 to 10 days. One recommended regimen is 60 mg of prednisone for 3 days, 40 mg for 3 days, then 20 mg for 3 days. Although this does not necessarily cause regression of the palsy, there is some evidence that it may reduce the number of patients in whom the condition progresses to complete nerve degeneration. It does cause resolution of pain in those patients who are affected. Some recent studies suggest that the herpes virus may be an etiologic factor, and acyclovir may be useful in treatment.

While resolution of the facial paralysis is awaited, care of the eye must be continued. A dry eye frequently leads to corneal ulceration, and consequently the use of Lacri-Lube or other eyedrops is indicated in most patients, particularly those who are unable to close the eye sufficiently to moisten the cornea.

Under conservative treatment (or with no treatment at all), 80% to 85% of patients suffering from Bell's palsy will recover completely or with so little residual weakness that no further management is required. Most of the remaining patients recover only partially. A few do not recover at all. The problem that has faced otologists through the years has been to determine what, if anything, can be done for the 15% to 20% of patients who are to recover only partially or not at all.

Surgical management for idiopathic Bell's palsy has been an area of intense controversy for years and is as yet unresolved. Some neurologists and otologists believe that idiopathic seventh nerve paralysis should not be treated by surgical means. It is their feeling that the recovery is unaffected by the surgical decompression. Other prominent physicians recommend that in patients with total seventh nerve paralysis any difference in the neuroexcitability testing of 3.5 mA or greater between the normal and abnormal side merits decompression of the seventh nerve in its horizontal and descending course. Some advocate immediate decompression of any total seventh nerve paralysis associated with pain, as this is generally considered a poor prognostic sign. Other neurologists believe that the seventh nerve should not be decompressed until the EMG demonstrates reaction of degeneration. There is also major controversy concerning the type and extent of surgery required. Some otologists believe that the entire bony course of the seventh nerve must be uncovered from the internal auditory meatus to the stylomastoid foramen. Their reasoning is that the narrowest point in the seventh nerve's course is medial to the geniculate ganglion, and that this area is most likely to be the source of compression. Failure to expose this area of the seventh nerve accounts for the inability to clearly demonstrate alteration of the course of facial improvement after surgery.

The attractiveness of seventh nerve decompression remains because all otolaryngologists with experience in seventh nerve decompression have seen rapid (over 1 or 2 days) return of facial motion after decompression, a circumstance that does not occur with medical treatment alone. Likewise, the seventh nerve in patients with Bell's palsy is markedly edematous and fairly "explodes" when the nerve sheath is divided, whereas similar findings do not occur with the seventh nerve exposed for other causes.

There are several indications for seventh nerve decompression, although even these have their detractors. These indications are: (1) patients who develop a trace of return of function after 1 to 2 weeks and then do not improve beyond that point, (2) recurrence of seventh nerve paralysis multiple times on the same side, (3) indication of a possible tumor, however slight, and (4) cases that show conductive block initially on EMG and then gradually start to develop evidence of denervation. In those instances, at the minimum the vertical and horizontal course of the seventh nerve must be uncovered, and preferably the entire course of the seventh nerve must be exposed.

Decompressions and facial nerve surgery must be done skillfully and with minimal trauma to the nerve. The occasional operator is not at home in this particular procedure, and poor technique can only add insult to injury.

The problem with determining the 10% to 20% of patients who can expect incomplete or poor return remains an enigma. The sequelae of even partial return of function can be quite distressing to the patient. Synkinesis, or mass motion of the face, is particularly distressing and common. This consists of grimacing when the eye attempts to blink or closing the eye on the involved side with smiling. Synkinesis is thought to be a result of innervation by nerve fibers of widely scattered muscle segments or, in other words, regrowth of the nerve fiber to the wrong muscle bundle.

At this point, the pathology, etiology, and treatment of idiopathic Bell's palsy are still unresolved.

### Herpes Zoster Oticus (Ramsay Hunt Syndrome)

Herpes zoster oticus is a manifestation of multicranial nerve involvement with the herpes zoster virus. Typically, the patient manifests a rather sudden facial paralysis associated with vesicles involving the ear canal and ear. Paralysis is thought to be secondary to edema of the facial nerve and involvement of either the facial nerve nucleus or the geniculate ganglion with the virus. Occasionally, the eighth cranial nerve is involved, presenting as a neurosensory hearing loss and vertigo. Treatment follows the same course as for idiopathic facial paralysis. Recent studies suggest that the antiviral drug Acyclovir (Zirovax) in a dose of 400 mg to 800 mg, 5 times a day for 5 days, may be beneficial in alleviating symptoms (e.g. vesicular eruption, pain, and paralysis).

### Paralysis Associated With Acute and Chronic Infections of the Ear

Commonly seen in children is a paralysis associated with acute otitis media and occasionally with mastoiditis. Generally, this represents an inflammatory involvement of the facial nerve, and treatment is directed at the primary infection. Seldom is any treatment required for the facial nerve, which, in almost every case, returns to normal after control of the infection.

Facial nerve paralysis associated with chronic ear disease is occasionally seen with cholesteatoma. Characteristically, the cholesteatoma matrix erodes the horizontal portion of the facial nerve, particularly at its posterior genu. Pressure and superimposed infection, therefore, affect the facial nerve function. Surgical management is necessary.

### Melkersson's Syndrome

Melkersson's syndrome is rare. It produces unilateral facial edema (supposedly lymphedema) and is often accompanied by facial paralysis. The cause is unknown. Usually the paralysis clears, although the edema may persist. Episodes are often recurrent.

### Tumors of the Facial Nerve

Tumors of the facial nerve are rare. The majority that have been reported are benign neuronomas (schwannomas), neurofibromas, or angiomas. Most arise within the fallopian (facial) canal. Very rarely, a meningioma may occur. This tumor originates from displacement of meningeal tissue laterally during early embryonic development. The tissue grows attached to the sheath of the facial nerve, and may compress the nerve or invade it. In these locations (either the vertical or horizontal portion of the nerve), the only symptom of a tumor is a slowly progressive facial paralysis. If the tumor arises distal to the stylomastoid foramen, it can be palpated in the neck. The tumor in this location does not produce facial paralysis until quite late. Because benign tumors in the ear grow slowly, it may take several months to years until there is clinical evidence of a tumor or before erosion occurs in the bony external auditory canal. Diagnosis of tumors of the facial nerve has been aided by improved x-ray studies and computed tomography. Sometimes this may be the only way to distinguish between idiopathic Bell's palsy and tumors of the nerve.

Treatment demands adequate surgical excision of the tumor, with end-to-end anastomosis of the nerve when possible. When anastomosis is not possible, grafting must be done to replace the resected segment of nerve.

### Injury to the Facial Nerve

The facial nerve may be compressed or severed either intracranially or in the petrous portion of the temporal bone by (1) brainstem tumors, (2) acoustic neuromas, or (3) fractures of the base of the skull. Repair of the nerve in the petrous portion of the temporal bone after skull fracture is

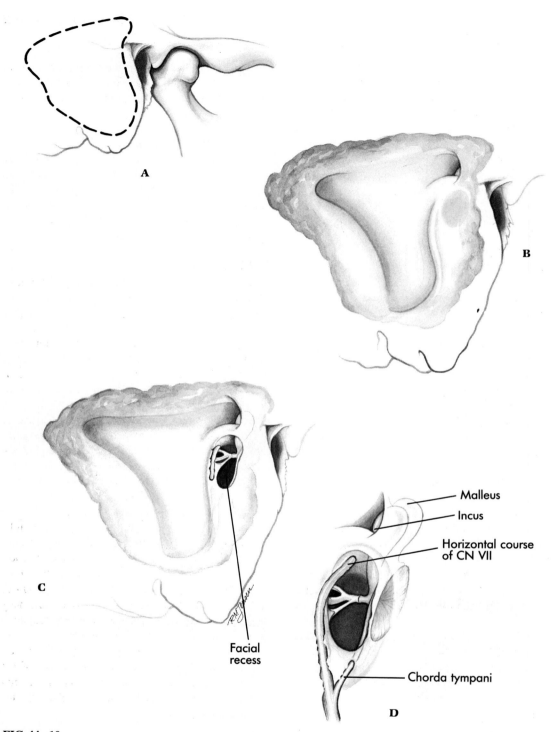

**FIG 44–10.**
**A,** site of bone removal for mastoidectomy. **B,** simple mastoidectomy completed with skeletonization of the sigmoid sinus and facial nerve. The bone is being thinned over the facial recess. **C,** a window is made through the posterior canal wall exposing the incus and stapes in the middle ear space. Facial nerve is uncovered in this particular section and the chorda tympani nerve is identified. **D,** representation of the uncovered facial nerve through its descending and horizontal course to the geniculate ganglion. Visualization of the nerve is satisfactory through this posterior approach.

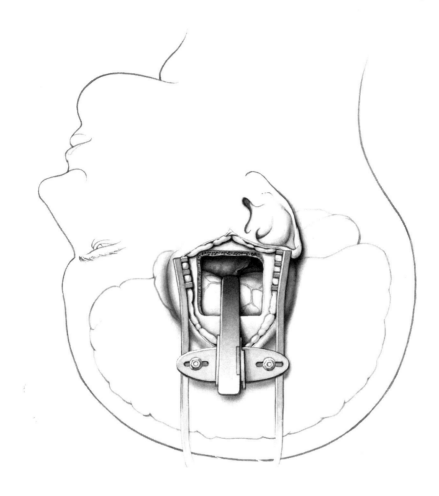

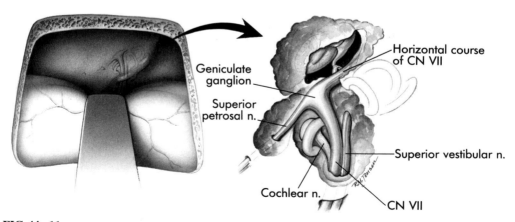

**FIG 44–11.**
Middle fossa decompression demonstrating course of the facial nerve medial to the geniculate ganglion.

possible. The repair is accomplished by way of a combined mastoid and middle fossa approach to the superior portion of the temporal bone, location of the injury, and decompression or suture of the nerve as indicated by the extent of the injury.

Most often, the facial nerve is damaged in the middle ear or in its descending vertical portion. Injuries in these areas occur either during operations on the mastoid or from external trauma. Damage to the facial nerve outside the skull is most frequently caused by trauma such as gunshot or automobile injuries. Another source of injury is resection of the nerve during partial or total parotidectomy. Invasion of the nerve by malignant tumor of the parotid gland also causes paralysis. A benign tumor of the parotid gland rarely causes a facial paralysis.

When facial paralysis is caused by a parotid tumor, the tumor must be considered malignant until proven otherwise. Frozen sections of such tumors at the time of operation, when indicated, will determine whether they can be removed safely without sacrificing the nerve. Safe removal can be accomplished when the tumor is benign. If pathology frozen section reveals squamous cell carcinoma, high-grade mucoepidermoid cancer, or adenocarcinoma, the nerve must be sacrificed and removed with the tumor. One or several grafts (usually from the anterior femoral cutaneous nerve or greater auricular) can be sutured in place during the same operation to give the best chance for return of facial tone and function.

## Repair of the Facial Nerve

The facial nerve has remarkable powers of regeneration. Even after complete section, which causes, as in other nerves, wallerian degeneration to the nucleus, recovery can and does take place if the tunnel back to the muscle end plates is not compressed.

Electrical tests of the nerve and facial muscles aid in determining whether repair can be performed successfully or should not be attempted. If the facial muscles still react to a faradic current applied to the skin over the nerve trunk, there is no actual interruption of continuity. In this event, surgical measures are delayed. When the nerve will not react to faradic stimulation but the muscles will still respond to galvanic current, continuity of the nerve has been interrupted. Attempt at surgical repair is then the procedure of choice. If the muscles fail to respond to a galvanic stimulus at all, nerve repair is generally useless.

### Decompression

When there is pressure on the nerve from edema, tumor, or depressed bone causing paralysis, decompression of the facial nerve is indicated. Decompression can be performed from the petrous portion to and including the internal auditory canal (Figs. 44–10 and 44–11). It is accomplished by careful uncapping of the nerve in its bony canal in the temporal bone. At the end of the dissection, the nerve is no longer encased in a solid bony tunnel but lies in a trough of bone with three sides uncovered. The sheath of the nerve can then be slit to remove all pressure. Decompression allows the return of normal blood supply, reduces edema, and provides an unobstructed pathway through which regenerating nerve fibers can grow.

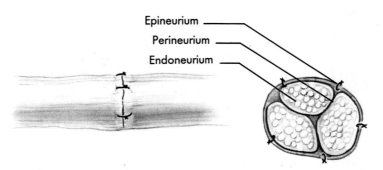

Epineurium
Perineurium
Endoneurium

**FIG 44–12.**
End-to-end anastomosis of facial nerve with fine sutures of 9-0 suture to the epineurium.

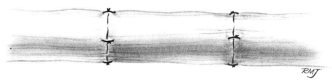

**FIG 44–13.**
Cable graft of facial nerve. Generally, the postauricular or the sural nerve is used for this graft.

### End-to-End Anastomosis

When the nerve has been severed, the best results are obtained by an end-to-end anastomosis. This provides only one juncture over which the nerve must regrow. The procedure must be performed with care so that the approximation of the severed nerve ends is firm but not too tight. Careful suturing of the epineurium with two or three 9–0 silk sutures around the edges of the nerve gives optimal results (Fig 44–12). Some authors feel that a single 6–0 suture through the nerve itself, including the epineurium, is less traumatic.

### Nerve Grafts

When it is not possible to accomplish end-to-end anastomosis, nerve grafts are used. The greater auricular nerve or the femoral cutaneous nerve is used most often. Either can be dissected to give a single- or a multiple-branched graft. Both are about the size of the facial nerve. Grafts can be both intratemporal or extratemporal. Successful grafting can be performed between the main trunk and all branches after extensive removal of the nerve during an operation on the parotid gland (Fig 44–13).

### Substitution Anastomosis

When the facial nerve is damaged so that it cannot be repaired, or the ends of the nerve cannot be found, substitution anastomosis may be performed. Either the spinal accessory or the hypoglossal nerve is used. When the spinal accessory nerve is sacrificed for anastomosis to the facial nerve, the resulting shoulder drop and atrophy of muscles create an undesirable deformity. For this reason, it is rarely done today. Most surgeons prefer to use the hypoglossal nerve. Use of this nerve causes some loss of motion and some atrophy of the tongue on the side of anastomosis, but the resulting disability is less than when the spinal accessory nerve is used as the donor.

Sometimes only one half of the nerve is used for the anastomosis. Substitution anastomosis gives less satisfactory results than end-to-end anastomosis or grafting, but it improves muscle tone and allows some motion, which is far more desirable than permanent total paralysis.

### Plastic Procedures

In recent years, numerous facial plastic procedures have been used to improve the appearance of total facial paralysis. When the facial muscles have so atrophied that they no longer respond to stimulation of any kind, none of the previously mentioned procedures is of value. Some cosmetic improvement can be gained by fascial slings or by a face-lift, which is accomplished by the use of fascia lata to support the facial tissues from the zygoma or temporalis muscle. Portions of the masseter muscle can be used as well. The temporalis muscle can be dissected from the skull and turned down into the cheek to increase bulk and supply the appearance of tone and slight motion. This is considered an "active fascial sling." Slight motion can be learned by clenching the teeth when either the masseter or the temporalis muscle is used. These muscles have their motor nerve supply from the fifth cranial nerve.

With the advent of microsurgery, muscles from other parts of the body can also be used. These types of muscle-nerve-vessel transplants require meticulous anastomosis of arteries, veins, and nerves under high magnification and have not been particularly successful.

When facial distortion is significant, it may be advisable to combine the aforementioned procedures with blepharoplasty, tarsorrhaphy, face-lift, brow lift, or lip transplantation to obtain the best cosmetic result. Although these procedures may improve the appearance of the face at rest and correct sagging of the soft tissues, no motion of the face occurs.

# PART IX
# Face

# 45

# Anatomy

The facial bones provide the rigid support and framework of all facial structures. They are attached to and suspended from the cranium. The facial bones include the malar bone, which provides the cheek prominences; the maxilla, which provides the contour of the upper jaw and support of the midface; the nasal bones; and the mandible (Fig 45–1). The zygomatic arch is actually a combination of the zygomatic process of the temporal bone posteriorly, which joins with the zygomatic process of the malar bone anteriorly. The relationship of the facial bones to each other has been extensively studied by a variety of disciplines. This data base provides the mechanism for defining normal relationships based on cephalometric measurements. It is possible to evaluate facial bones radiographically and to define the specific deviations from these standard measurements. Although information about these bony relationships has been available for a long time, only recently has there been considerable interest in the surgical change in these bony relationships.

Numerous muscles cover the facial bones. There are two sphincters. The orbicularis oculi is located within the upper and lower eyelids and suspended from the facial bones by the medial and lateral canthal ligaments. The orbicularis oris is the circular muscle incorporated within the upper and lower lips. The mimetic muscles are a group located throughout the mid and lower portions of the face; they provide the mechanism for facial expression (Fig 45–2). The mimetic muscles are individually named, but that extent of anatomic detail is not necessary for the clinician's comprehension. The muscles of mastication are located in the lateral facial area around the temporal, zygomatic, and lateral mandibular region.

The temporalis and masseter muscles contribute to the surface anatomy of the lateral facial area and are involved with closing the mandible (Fig 45–3). The medial pterygoid muscle is located on the medial side of the vertical ramus of the mandible and is also involved with closing the mandible. The lateral pterygoid muscle is located in a similar position but is involved with protruding the mandible (Fig 45–4).

The facial area is rich in vascularity. This creates a surgical challenge because extensive blood loss is an ongoing possibility with any facial surgery. However, the rich blood supply often is advantageous because it permits aggressive approaches to transposing tissue. It is important to recognize that the internal carotid artery runs medial to the vertical ramus and posterior to the maxilla to enter the carotid canal en route to the brain. It is imperative that the clinician understand the anatomic proximity of these structures. The facial soft tissue is supplied primarily by the branches of the external carotid artery. The facial artery courses over the midmandibular body to extend superiorly as it further branches to support the soft tissue of the lips. The superficial temporal and occipital branches also provide blood to the more superiorly located facial soft tissues. The venous blood supply is usually associated with the arteries and drains primarily into the internal jugular system. However, there is some drainage to the external and anterior jugular veins.

The motor innervation of the facial musculature is heavily dependent on the facial nerve (cranial nerve VII) (Fig 45–5). The orbicularis oculi, mimetic muscles, and orbicularis oris are all innervated by the ipsilateral facial nerve. It is rare for motor nerves to originate from the contralat-

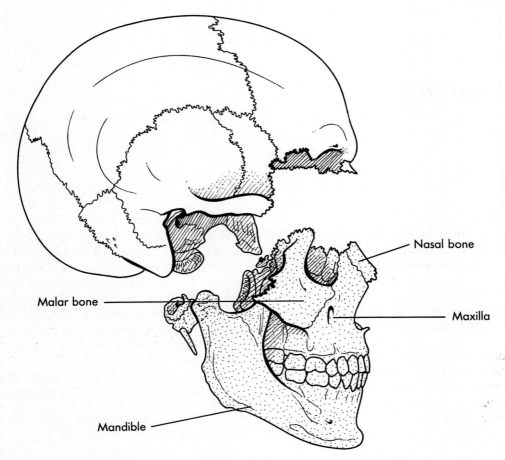

**FIG 45–1**.
The facial bones are suspended from the calvaria. (Redrawn after Pernkopf E: *Head and neck,* vol 1. In Helmut F, ed. *Atlas of topographic and applied human anatomy,* ed 2, Baltimore-Munich, 1980, Urban & Schwarzenberg. Used by permission.)

eral side. The muscles of mastication are innervated by the third division (portio minor nervi trigemini) of the trigeminal nerve (cranial nerve V).

The sensory innervation of the face is from the three divisions of the ipsilateral trigeminal nerve (Fig 45–6). The supraorbital, infraorbital, and mental nerves are major sensory nerves and are identifiable on the surface by connecting an imaginary line between the supraorbital notch, which can be detected by palpation, and the second premolar tooth, which corresponds to the location of the mental foramen (Fig 45–7). The infraorbital nerve exits its foramen approximately 5 to 7 mm below the infraorbital rim along that straight line. Anesthetic blocks of these main sensory nerves are not difficult and can be executed by infiltration of a bolus of local anesthetic.

The facial area also has a lymphatic system,

with numerous lymphatic vessels. However, it is important to understand that, although not as frequently seen as in the neck, lymph nodes are also present within the facial soft tissue. Some lymph nodes are present in the subcutaneous tissue adjacent to the corner of the nose, and others are on the outside of the capsule of the parotid gland. These lymph nodes can hypertrophy in response to either inflammatory or neoplastic involvement.

The major salivary glands have been discussed in Chapters 14 to 16. It is important to recognize that the preauricular area is the location of the parotid gland, and this area occupies primarily that space between the ear canal and the posterior portion of the vertical ramus of the mandible and even extends over the vertical ramus of the mandible to come into contact with the masseter muscle. The facial nerve courses through the pa-

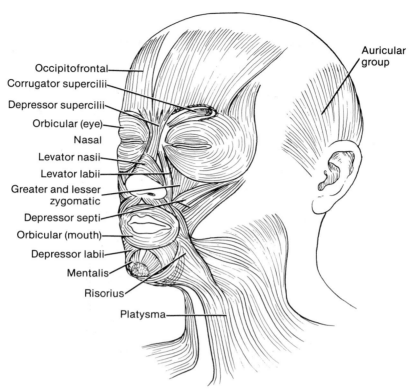

Occipitofrontal
Corrugator supercilii
Depressor supercilii
Orbicular (eye)
Nasal
Levator nasii
Levator labii
Greater and lesser zygomatic
Depressor septi
Orbicular (mouth)
Depressor labii
Mentalis
Risorius
Platysma
Auricular group

**FIG 45–2**.
The mimetic muscles are actually attached to the undersurface of the facial skin and cause movement of the skin.

rotid gland and exits anteriorly en route to the facial muscles. Any penetrating injuries to the preauricular soft tissue should alert the clinician to recall this important anatomy and therefore to test facial nerve function.

Nasal and auricular anatomy is covered in other sections of this book. It is not unusual for pathologic processes originating in adjacent structures to involve these structures.

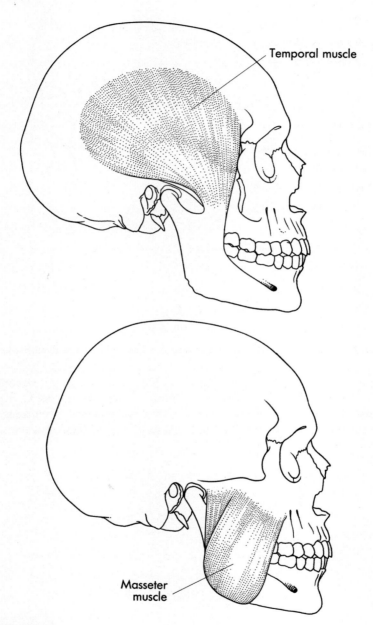

**FIG 45–3**.
The temporalis and masseter muscles are involved with closing the mandible.

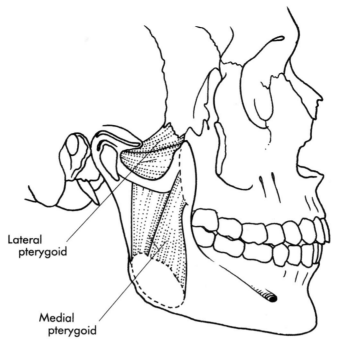

**FIG 45–4**.
The medial pterygoid muscle closes the mandible, but contraction of the lateral pterygoid displaces the mandible forward.

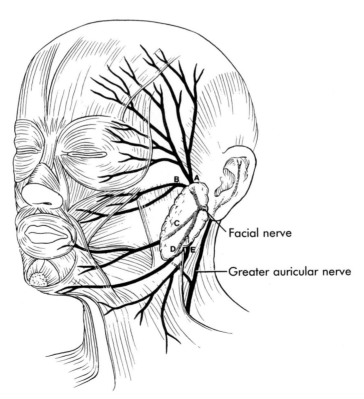

**FIG 45–5**.
The facial nerve is the main motor nerve to the facial muscles.

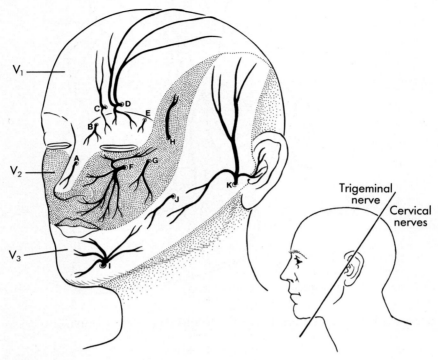

**FIG 45–6**.
Primary sensory innervation of the face is from the three divisions of the trigeminal nerve.

**FIG 45–7.**
The supraorbital notch, infraorbital foramen, and mental foramen form a straight line connecting the three.

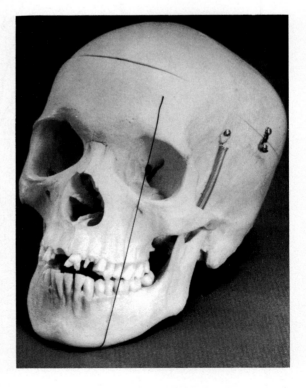

# 46

# Embryology and Congenital Disorders

The face develops below the overhanging forebrain. It originates primarily from mesoderm. The outside ectoderm covering the face actually continues to provide the lining of the embryonic mouth. It does not join the endoderm that is lining the gut until the buccopharyngeal membrane. One of the earliest events in facial embryogenesis is the development of nasal pits (Fig 46–1). The frontal nasal swelling is located between the nasal pits. It is important to understand that there is no time in normal embryogenesis that a cleft is present between this frontonasal and the maxillary swellings (Fig 46–2). The primitive auricle is also developing at the same time.

Facial embryology has special importance with reference to the cleft deformity. Clefts were previously considered to be a fusion failure problem involving the embryonic processes just mentioned. The child born with an isolated cleft palate actually undergoes an embryologic defect different from that of one born with a cleft lip with or without a cleft palate. The normal embryologic course of events regarding palate development includes a force that changes the direction of the palatal shells from a vertical to a horizontal plane. While this is occurring, the embryonic tongue is migrating in an anterior-inferior direction.

This movement provides room for the horizontal realignment of the palatal shelves. The palatal components ultimately fuse. Anything that interferes with this normal course of events, such as the proportions of the skull base or the size and/or migration of the tongue or mandible, can have an adverse effect and be associated with the development of an isolated palatal cleft.

In contrast, the cleft lip is not a fusion failure problem. It arises from the inability to maintain an epithelial bridge in an area that is deficient in underlying mesoderm, which is normally contributed by the maxillary and nasal processes. Ultimately a breakdown of the epithelium occurs, and a cleft lip is present (Fig 46–3). The presence of this cleft lip increases the possibility of a cleft palate because it alters the usual facial relationships, which can interfere with palatal fusion by obstructing tongue migration. It is easy to understand that the most common cleft deformity encountered involves clefts of the lip, palate, and alveolar processes of the maxilla.

The facial congenital disorders primarily involve the cleft deformity. The maxillofacial cleft is one of the most common congenital problems, occurring second in frequency only to the clubfoot deformity. It is more commonly seen in whites than in blacks. The incidence of the cleft deformity in the United States is approximately 1 per 700 to 850 births.

One of the most important matters requiring discussion with parents of a child with a cleft deformity is the possibility of producing another offspring with a cleft. Parents are interested not only in the affected child, but also in the chances of having other offspring with a similar deformity. This question has been extensively studied in Denmark, and those results continue to be the basis for medical advice to families who have had a child born with a cleft. Table 46–1 describes the recurrent risk rates for future offspring. The possibility of parents having another child with a cleft, even when both a parent and a sibling have a cleft deformity, is not disturbingly high. The general recommendation is for parents to proceed with their original family plans.

Another important matter involves advice to the parents about feeding the child with this deformity (Fig 46–4). This pertains primarily to

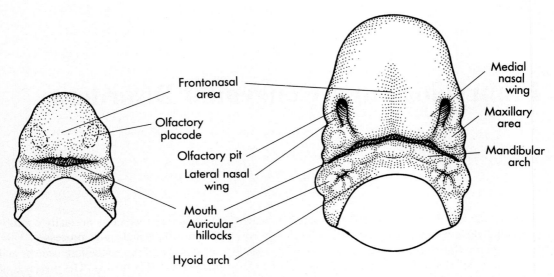

**FIG 46–1.**
Nasal pits appear early in the embryonic development of the face. (Redrawn after Davies J: *Embryology of the face, palate, nose and paranasal sinuses*. In Paparella M, Shumrick D, eds: *Otolaryngology*, vol 1, Philadelphia, 1980, WB Saunders. After Streeter: *Developmental horizons and human embryos*, 1948. Used by permission.)

children with a cleft palate with or without clefts of other structures. With a palatal cleft, the child swallows much less efficiently. This inefficiency results in an inability to generate the normal amount of negative pressure during sucking and the swallowing of an increased amount of air. There is no single feeding technique that works for all infants with a cleft. However, if the parents come to understand the basic problem, their individual creativity usually allows them to solve the problem for their particular child. A variety of cleft palate nipples are available that allow for more posterior placement of the milk and decrease the need for generating high negative pressures. In addition, the parents should be instructed to burp the child frequently to evacuate air from the stomach. With these basic concepts in mind, most parents can successfully feed the child.

Surgical repair of a cleft deformity must be

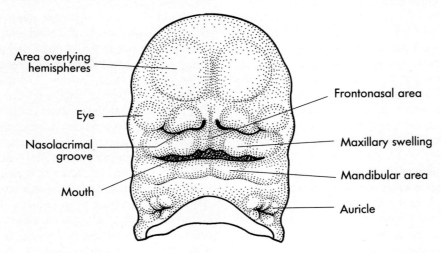

**FIG 46–2.**
A midfacial cleft is not present during normal embryonic development. (Redrawn after Davies J: *Embryology of the face, palate, nose and paranasal sinuses*. In Paparella M, Shumrick D, eds: *Otolaryngology*, vol 1, Philadelphia, 1980, WB Saunders. After Streeter: *Developmental horizons and human embryos*, 1948. Used by permission.)

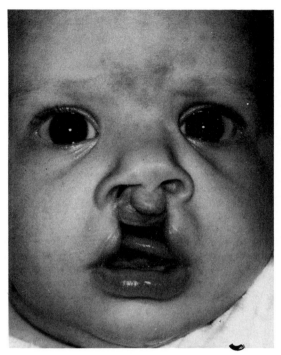

**FIG 46–3.**
Breakdown of the epithelium as a result of insufficient mesoderm produces the cleft lip deformity.

considered with respect to its impact on the child's subsequent facial growth. For this reason, the primary surgery is usually done at certain times of the child's life. The cleft lip is usually not repaired until the child is 3 to 4 months of age. It is important to allow the child some opportunity for maturation in order to evaluate for other congenital anomalies that may not have been appreciated at birth.

**TABLE 46–1.**

Recurrent Risk Rates for Future Offspring*

| | |
|---|---|
| I. Cleft lip, with or without cleft palate | |
| Chances for a child to have cleft: | |
| A. One sibling has cleft; no parent has cleft | 6% |
| B. One sibling has cleft; one parent has cleft | 14% |
| C. No sibling has cleft; one parent has cleft | 2% |
| II. Cleft palate, without cleft lip Chances for child to have cleft: | |
| A. One sibling has cleft; no parent has cleft | 2% |
| B. One sibling has cleft; one parent has cleft | 17% |
| C. No sibling has cleft; one parent has cleft | 7% |

*From Fogh-Anderson, P: *Inheritance of harelip and cleft palate,* Copenhagen, 1972, Nyt Nordisk Forlag-Arnold Busck. Used by permission.

The timing of the cleft palate repair is a different matter. Early repair of the palatal cleft will improve the child's speech development, but it may have an adverse effect on midfacial growth. The converse is true if a later repair is undertaken. It is generally agreed that delaying the palatal repair until the child is about 18 months old is a reasonable compromise to minimize the adverse effect on both of these considerations.

The primary surgery of a cleft lip involves the development of flaps, which permit elongation of the lip and closure of the cleft (Fig 46–5). This technique usually produces an improvement in both function and cosmesis (Fig 46–6). The cleft palate repair involves developing flaps that permit both medial and posterior displacement of the palate (Fig 46–7). Such technique minimizes the chance of developing velopharyngeal incompetence.

After the primary surgery is completed, the child must be followed by a group of professionals. Children born with clefts have an increased incidence of otologic, dental, and speech problems. The optimal care is usually best provided

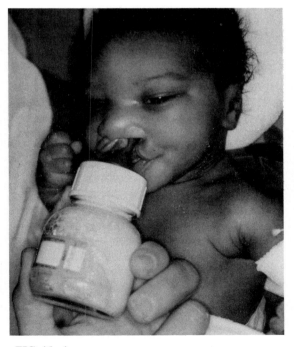

**FIG 46–4.**
The child with the cleft lip and palate has compromised feeding capabilities because of decreased ability to develop a negative pressure in the pharynx and the excessive swallowing of air.

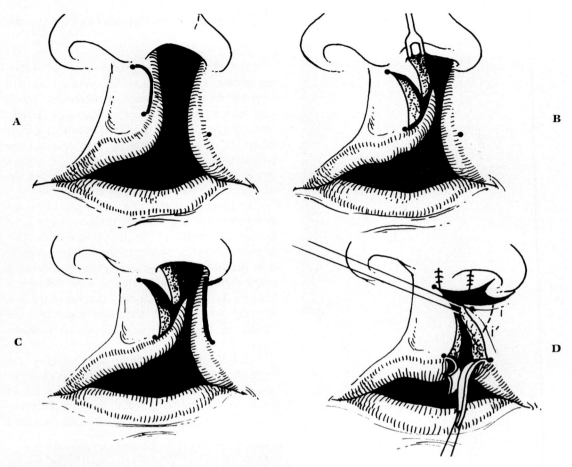

**FIG 46–5.**
The surgical repair of a cleft lip involves developing a rotation flap on the medial side of the cleft, **A** and **B,** and then filling the defect created by the rotation flap with an advancement flap from the lateral segment, **C** and **D.**

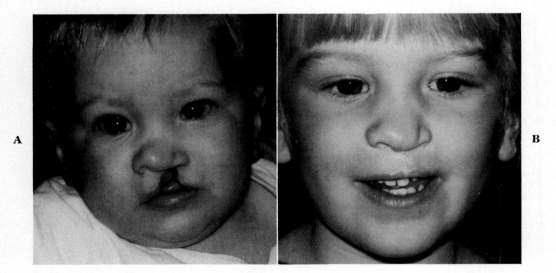

**FIG 46–6.**
**A,** a child born with a unilateral cleft lip, who then underwent rotation-advancement cleft lip repair. **B,** the postoperative results.

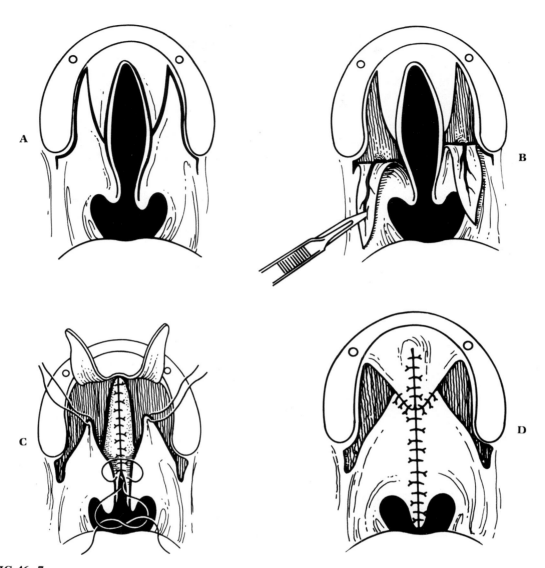

**FIG 46–7.**
Cleft palate repair involves the development of oral and nasal mucoperiosteal flaps, **A** and **B**, the approximation of the nasal mucoperiosteum, **C**, and then the medial and posterior displacement of the oral mucoperiosteum, **D**. (From Schuller D, Krause C: *Cleft lip and palate,* Washington DC, 1979, American Academy of Otolaryngology—Head and Neck Surgery, SiPac #79400. Used by permission.)

by some type of a multidisciplinary approach in a cleft palate setting that follows the child until facial growth is complete. This provides the opportunity for secondary surgery both to be done on the nasal deformity that is usually present and to improve the function and cosmesis of the lip re-

pair. When children are followed in such a multidisciplinary environment over the course of their facial growth, the results are usually dramatic and permit the child to have reasonably normal facial features and excellent facial function.

# 47

# Clinical Problems

## INFECTIONS AND INFLAMMATIONS

Primary infections of the facial skin and soft tissue are uncommon. Impetiginous lesions are sometimes transmitted from infectious sites in the skin to the facial area. This occurs almost exclusively in children. Local and systemic therapy results in prompt resolution. Acne is another facial skin problem affecting adolescents and young adults. Other, less common facial skin infections have a fungal origin. Blastomycosis is an example of a fungal infection that can affect facial skin and cause extensive scarring and destruction of normal anatomy.

Any skin infection involving the triangular area bounded by the glabella and the corners of the mouth is potentially serious. The venous drainage of the skin within this triangle has no valves and provides a direct route of flow to the cavernous sinus (Fig 47–1). Infections must be treated aggressively to reduce the chances of intravascular extension, which could result in the life-threatening complication of cavernous sinus thrombosis. Systemic antibiotics that have antistaphylococcal properties are usually prescribed after cultures are obtained when possible. Some also advocate trying to place this area at rest by minimizing talking and eating a soft diet as a means of decreasing nasal movement, which might act to promote drainage of infected fluid into the vascular system.

It is not unusual for some portions of the facial skin to become involved secondarily with infectious and inflammatory processes. Acute external otitis can cause a periauricular cellulitis, which even can progress to cause parotid adenopathy.

The periauricular facial skin is erythematous, edematous, and tender to touch. Systemic antibiotics are usually added to the treatment program for external otitis when it is accompanied by facial cellulitis. Some forms of chronic external otitis, such as eczematoid or seborrheic external otitis, can also extend beyond the confines of the external auditory canal and involve the periauricular facial skin (Fig 47–2). Antiinflammatory ointments and creams containing steroid preparations can usually decrease and sometimes totally resolve these problems.

The facial soft tissue can become secondarily infected after sinus infections. One of the most common complications of ethmoid sinusitis in children is the development of periorbital cellulitis. Systemic antibiotics are usually effective treatment. However, visual acuity and extraocular movement must be assessed on a regular basis while the eyelid edema and erythema are present. There is a potential for orbital and extraorbital abscess formation, which might limit the effectiveness of medical treatment and necessitate surgical intervention for drainage and decompression (Fig 47–3). Maxillary sinusitis in either adults or children can sometimes cause a facial cellulitis involving the soft tissue of the cheek. This usually represents an extension of the infection through a preformed pathway in the anterior or posterolateral wall of the maxillary sinus. When this complication exists, systemic antibiotics are advisable.

The greater numbers of immunocompromised patients may be responsible for an increasingly frequent presentation of atypical infectious processes. The facial soft tissue will be no exception. The clinician will encounter infectious processes

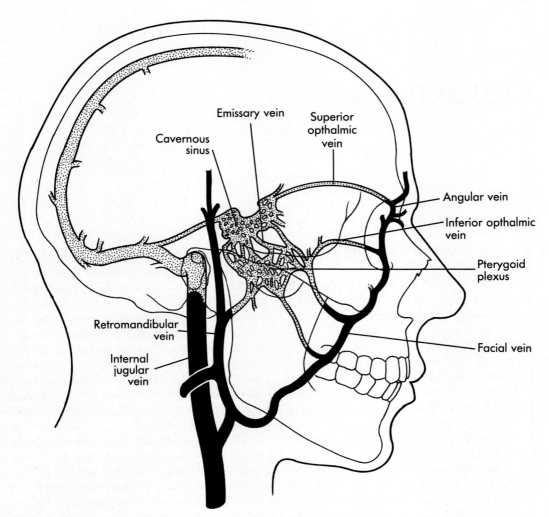

**FIG 47–1.**
The veins in the perinasal area have no valves, which facilitates extension of infection in this area into the cavernous sinus.

in patients with acquired immune deficiency syndrome, patients on immunosuppressive therapy after receiving transplants, and cancer patients receiving chemotherapy. These patient populations represent some of the people at risk for manifesting unusual physical findings associated with infections.

## TUMORS

Cutaneous cancers frequently involve the face. The most common cell type is basal cell carcinoma, followed by squamous cell carcinoma. Melanomas are encountered but less frequently

than the other two types. Although no definite cause-and-effect relationship has been established, there appears to be a strong relationship between the amount of sun exposure and the incidence of basal cell and squamous cell cancers of the skin. The face, being a relatively unprotected area, has a high incidence of these cancers, especially in the sunbelt portions of the world. Most cutaneous cancers have a propensity for local recurrence, but they rarely undergo distant metastases, especially basal cell cancers. Most previously untreated skin cancers have an excellent chance for cure and are treated with a variety of techniques, such as surgical excision, cryotherapy, laser excision, curettage, or radiation therapy.

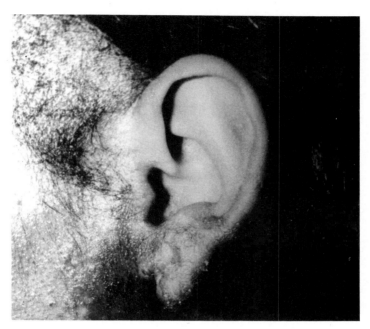

**FIG 47–2.**
Eczematoid external otitis in this patient has involved the periauricular skin.

However, conventional treatment may leave the patient vulnerable to undetected microscopic residual disease and predispose to recurrence (Fig 47–4).

Recurrent cutaneous cancers present a more formidable challenge. There is no question that involvement with underlying cartilage or bone makes treatment much more difficult. The pioneering work of Mohs has provided a technique for treating troublesome cutaneous cancers, and it

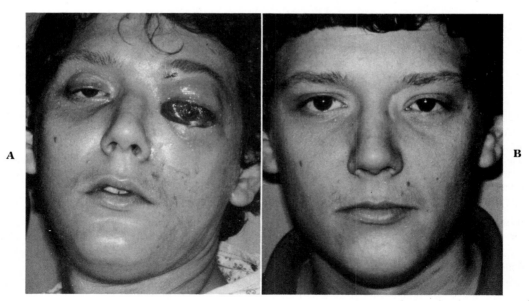

**FIG 47–3.**
This patient, **A,** developed orbital and periorbital abcesses as a complication of sinusitis with decreased visual acuity, which was preserved, **B,** by rapid surgical drainage of the abscesses and decompression of the orbital soft tissues into the sinuses.

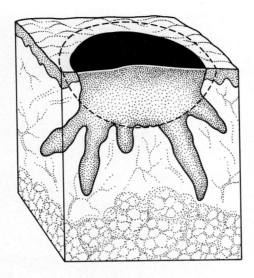

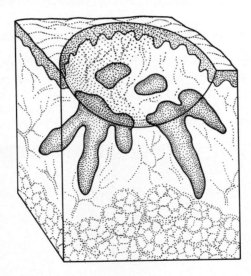

**FIG 47–4**.
Conventional treatment cannot identify microscopic cutaneous cancer cells and therefore increases the chances for a recurrence. (Redrawn after Levine H: Cutaneous carcinoma of the head and neck, *Laryngoscope* 93(suppl):1, 1983. Used by permission.)

results in dramatic improvement in the cure rates for these recurrent and certain primary skin cancers.

Mohs' surgical technique involves the horizontal sectioning of the depths of an excised skin cancer. A map of the excised tissue is drawn and histologically studied (Fig 47–5). It provides the maximal specificity of identifying the location of microscopic extensions of tumor and results in the

most accurate means of determining the amount of tissue to be removed. It minimizes the chance of undetected residual disease and of unnecessarily aggressive excisions of tissue. This exciting work with cutaneous cancers has had other positive spin-offs that are useful to all clinicians in evaluation of patients with these facial tumors.

It is now appreciated that certain areas of the face are at risk for extension of cutaneous cancer

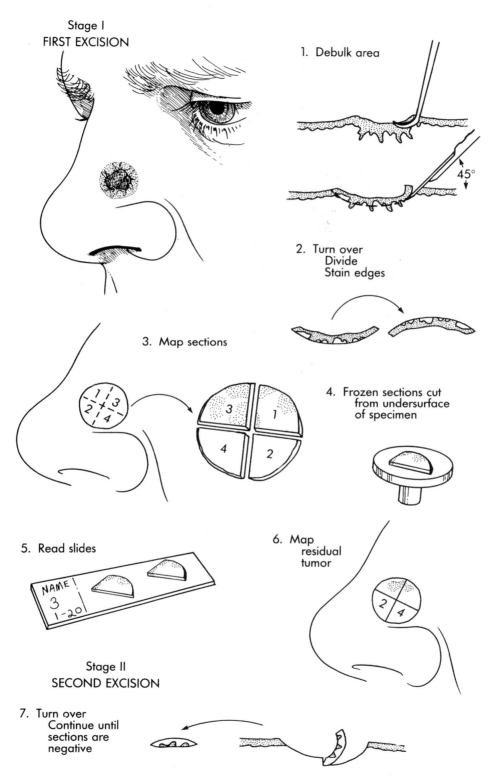

Stage I
FIRST EXCISION

1. Debulk area

45°

2. Turn over
   Divide
   Stain edges

3. Map sections

4. Frozen sections cut
   from undersurface
   of specimen

5. Read slides

NAME
3
1-20

6. Map
   residual
   tumor

Stage II
SECOND EXCISION

7. Turn over
   Continue until
   sections are
   negative

**FIG 47–5.**
Mohs' surgery involves mapping the excised tissue and histologically studying all margins. (Redrawn after Swanson N: Mohs' surgery, *Arch Dermatol* vol 119, September 1983. Used by permission.)

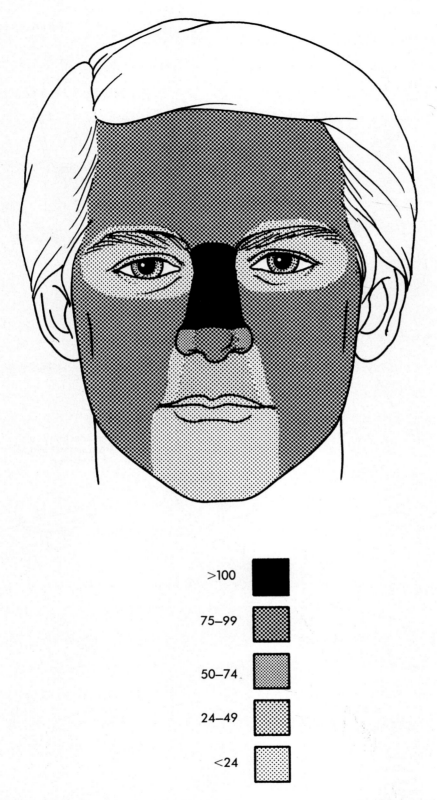

>100

75–99

50–74

24–49

<24

**FIG 47–6.**
These high-risk areas for recurrence of cutaneous cancers correspond with the embryonic fusion planes in the face. (Redrawn after Levine H, Bailin P: Basal cell carcinoma of the head and neck: Identification of the high risk patient, *Laryngoscope* 90:6, 1980. Used by permission.)

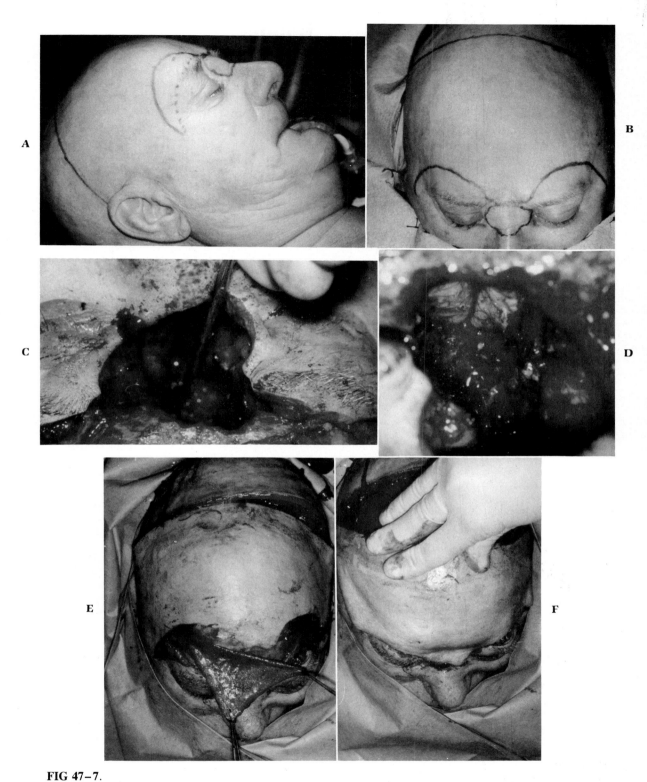

**FIG 47–7.**
**A–C,** this patient has recurrent medial canthal cutaneous cancer that eroded the skull base and required excision of the entire upper half of the nose and the inner canthal tissues, including the anterior skull base, with reconstruction using an advancement scalp flap. **D,** the frontal lobe is seen through the inner canthal defect following resection of the skull base. The bipedicle scalp advancement flap has been developed to provide the outer reconstruction, and a scalp peracranial flap, **E,** is used to seal the dural defect. A scalp rotation flap, **F,** is used to reconstruct the skin defect over hip grafts used for the nasal reconstruction.

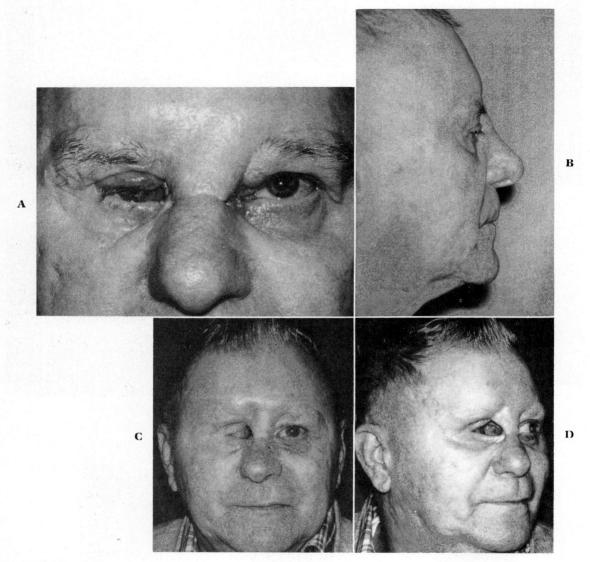

**FIG 47–8.**
Frontal, **A,** and lateral, **B,** views of the patient shown in Figure 47–7 1 year following surgery. The 5-year postoperative photographs (**C** and **D**) show this patient, following enucleation for ocular problems, free of disease.

into the deep planes. These correspond to the embryonic fusion planes in the face. Fig 47–6 identifies those areas in which control of cutaneous cancers is especially difficult.

It is also possible to approach tumors involving the skull base through the facial structures. Cooperative efforts between otolaryngologist–head and neck surgeons and neurosurgeons have increased capabilities for resecting tumors that have

eroded the skull base and were previously believed to be untreatable (Fig 47–7). An intimate knowledge of facial anatomy is necessary to maximize the surgical exposure and minimize the cosmetic impact on the patient. Transnasal skull base surgery that even involves reconstruction of the skull base is now a viable option that has the potential for long-term control of disease (Fig 47–8).

# Facial Plastic and Reconstructive Surgery

# PART X

# Facial Plastic and Reconstructive Surgery

# 48

# General Considerations

Facial plastic and reconstructive surgery is performed on patients who have deformities that are congenital, inflammatory, neoplastic, or traumatic in origin. It also includes aesthetic surgery. The goals of facial plastic surgery are to restore not only the form of the deformed part but also its function. Sometimes it is not possible to achieve both, and in that case restoration of function usually takes precedence over appearance.

The public and the media have considerable interest in this type of surgery. Sometimes information that appears in a nonmedical publication or media presentation is not accurate because it disproportionately emphasizes the dramatic and exceptional results. This information can create unrealistic expectations among some who seek facial plastic surgery. For this reason the importance of communication between patient and surgeon is emphasized. It is also useful for all health professionals to have some understanding of not only the potential for restoration but also the limitations so that they can more accurately advise their patients. A person who comes to the physician with a particular problem must be thoroughly advised about the options for reconstruction and the reasonable expectations. Health professionals must be knowledgeable about the time commitment to complete a particular reconstructive task and the potential complications and risks. When the patient is fully informed, facial reconstruction becomes a pleasant and stimulating experience for both the patient and the physician.

Some generalizations can be made about factors affecting facial plastic and reconstructive surgery. It is important to consider the patient's age. There is no question that the better blood supply of the younger patient allows the surgeon to be more aggressive with the transposition of tissue.

Sometimes liberties can be taken with certain surgical techniques in children and young adults because of this rich blood supply.

Not all of the advantages are with youth in this type of surgery. Two factors can work against them. First, between infancy and young adulthood children are vigorous scar formers. The finest surgical technique does not guarantee against hypertrophic scar formation in this age group. In contrast, it is rare for hypertrophic scarring to occur in middle-aged and older adults. Second, one of the goals of the reconstructive surgeon is to conceal any incisions in the natural skin creases present on a patient's face and neck. However, with the young there is a paucity of skin creases (Fig. 48–1). Senior citizens are blessed with a multitude of skin creases that permit concealment of skin incisions (Fig. 48–2).

It is more important to consider the physiologic rather than the chronologic age of an individual. Any disease that affects the body's vascularity will present a challenge to reconstructive procedures that require transferring of tissue. Therefore, atherosclerotic vascular disease, diabetes mellitus, and any other conditions that affect the patency of blood vessels represent a challenge, and they need to be considered when reconstruction is being planned (Fig. 48–3).

There is nothing magical about facial plastic and reconstructive surgery. It often involves techniques that permit the transfer of tissue from one part of the body to another. The success of the surgery depends on the adequacy of the blood supply of the tissue being transferred. It is necessary to be knowledgeable of and sensitive to the stress placed on the blood supply of tissue that is being transferred. Means of assessing and enhancing the blood supply are continuing to be investi-

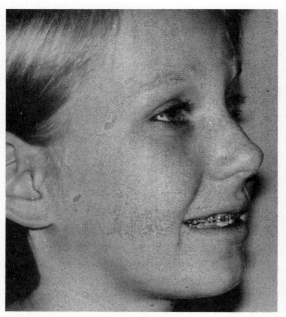

**FIG 48–1.**
The lack of relaxed skin tension lines in children minimizes the places to conceal surgical incisions in this age group.

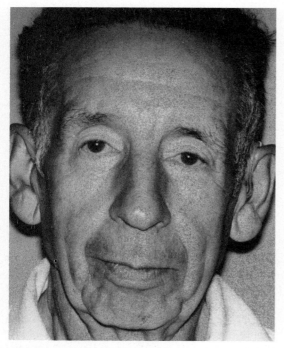

**FIG 48–2.**
Relaxed skin tension lines provide a multitude of opportunities for the placement of incisions that will provide excellent camouflage.

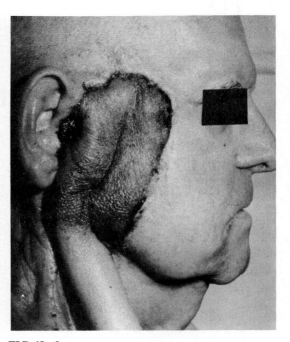

**FIG 48–3.**
This patient, who had a long-standing history of diabetes and artherosclerotic vascular disease, experienced necrosis of the distal portion of a regional skin flap used to resurface a facial defect.

gated and should provide useful information for the reconstructive surgeon.

A basic understanding of the differences in blood supply of two techniques used to transfer tissue helps to explain the rationale for this type of surgery. A considerable amount of reconstructive surgery involves the transfer of tissue into areas of epithelial defects. Skin grafts and flaps are the two common techniques to achieve this transfer. But there is a difference in the blood supply of grafts and flaps.

A *skin graft* is a thin piece of tissue that is totally detached from its donor site and transferred into a defect. It does not have its own blood supply. It is dependent totally on the blood supply of the recipient site. A recipient site will support a skin graft if it can develop granulation tissue (Fig. 48–4). Granulation tissue is a combination of capillaries and fibroblasts. If the tissue cannot form granulation tissue—such as bone devoid of periosteum, cartilage devoid of perichondrium, or tendon—a skin graft will not survive. In contrast, a *skin flap* is a piece of tissue that carries its own blood supply and is not dependent on the recipient site (Fig. 48–5). Considerations of the blood

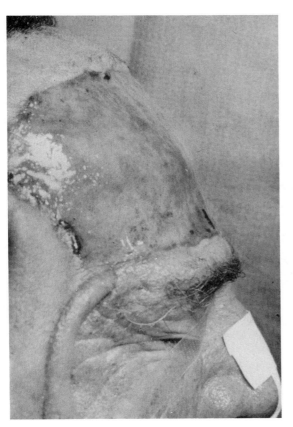

**FIG 48–4.**
Granulation tissue was permitted to develop on this man's forehead, which provided the blood supply for maintaining viability of the skin graft.

supply are paramount to the quality of the result.

Reconstruction is based on the cause of the defect, its size and location, the patient's age, the patient's desires, and the skills of the reconstructive surgeon. The algorithm in Figure 48–6 illustrates the variety of techniques used during facial reconstruction. It emphasizes the importance of the reconstructive surgeon's familiarity with numerous surgical approaches.

Current techniques in facial reconstructive surgery have improved considerably. It is necessary to be continually critical of results in an effort to stimulate thought that might provoke modifications and lead to further improvement. As mentioned, the goals of this surgery are to restore form and function. It is true that some of the techniques that will be subsequently described provide the ability to transfer tissue and restore a defect. However, critical analysis suggests that it is still not an ideal solution because in many cases it results only in resurfacing of rather than complete restoration of the form and function. The achievements in this field have been numerous, but the challenge to develop better techniques remains.

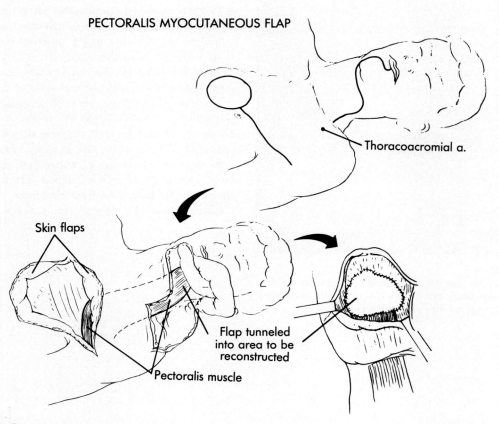

**FIG 48–5.**
**A,** the skin on a musculoutaneous flap derives its blood supply from the vasculature of the underlying musculature and can be, **B,** transposed onto another site on a nondelayed basis because of that strong blood supply.

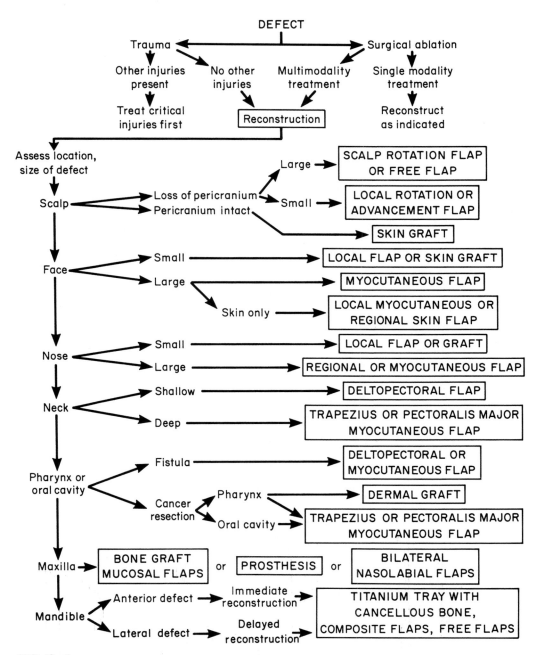

**FIG 48–6.**
Algorithm describing a variety of reconstruction options for facial deformity.

# 49

# Cutaneous and Mucosal Defects

The solution to a reconstructive problem is seldom obvious. It requires considerable thought and requires that the surgeon have a variety of alternative techniques available. To find a solution and plan a particular approach, the surgeon must first define the problem. This is especially true when encountering patients with cutaneous and mucosal defects. One must have not only a clear understanding of the size of a defect, but also an appreciation for its depth and relationship to normal anatomic landmarks. For the individual who has a loss of only skin or mucosa, a skin graft is often the technique of choice (Fig. 49–1). The postauricular, supraclavicular areas, upper eyelid, and even nasolabial folds represent good skin graft donor sites because of their suitable color match to the face. However, if a defect does not have a tissue bed that is capable of producing granulation tissue and supporting a skin graft (Fig. 49–2), or if there is a marked disparity between the thickness of a skin graft and the thickness of the defect, some type of skin flap transposition is advisable. A flap is a thicker piece of tissue because it contains not only skin but also subcutaneous fat. It may even contain muscle (Fig. 49–3).

Once again, the matter of selecting a flap depends on the surgeon's understanding of the surgical anatomy concerning the strength of the blood supply to a particular flap. Flaps can be classified according to the type of blood supply to the tissues. An axial pattern flap is based on a named artery running parallel to the long axis of the flap and has a strong blood supply. A random pattern flap has no named artery but receives its blood supply from the multiple small perforating vessels (Fig. 49–4). This blood supply is not as good as that of the axial pattern flaps.

Flaps can also be classified according to their position from the defect. Sometimes a flap that is immediately adjacent to a defect, referred to as a *local skin flap,* is the best choice (Fig. 49–5). Areas of tissue redundancy are preferred donor sites for such flaps. The glabellar region, nasolabial area, and neck are all areas that usually have some redundancy in the adult population.

If a tissue defect is reconstructed with skin not immediately adjacent to the defect, the flap is then referred to as a *regional skin flap*. These are usually larger than local flaps. However, a regional flap sometimes requires a skin graft to close the flap donor site as compared with primary closure for local flaps (Fig. 49–6).

The musculocutaneous flap is another technique that involves the transfer of skin in addition to the underlying subcutaneous fat and muscle. Anatomic studies have demonstrated that skin in certain areas of the body receives its dominant blood supply from perforating arteries that arise from the main blood supply to the underlying musculature. Therefore, one can be assured of transferring a piece of skin with a rich blood supply by incorporating the underlying musculature in the transfer process.

The pectoralis musculocutaneous flap is one of the more frequently used flaps. In this situation, an island of skin is transferred into the defect along with the pectoralis major muscle with its blood supply left intact running on the undersurface of the muscle. This particular flap allows the transfer of a large amount of skin to cutaneous or mucosal defects in the head and neck region (Fig. 49–7).

Another example of a musculocutaneous flap is the Karapandzic flap used for lip reconstruction. This involves the mobilization of the remaining orbicularis oris by detaching it from the surround-

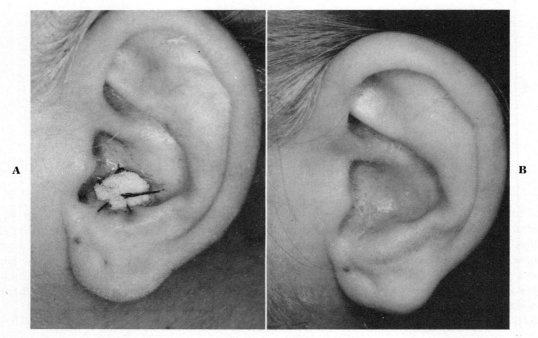

**FIG 49–1.**
**A,** this patient had an excision of skin only in the concha and underwent a full-thickness skin graft from the post-auricular area to the defect. **B,** the postoperative result was excellent because the recipient site had the blood supply for a skin graft and the thickness of the defect was comparable to that of the skin graft.

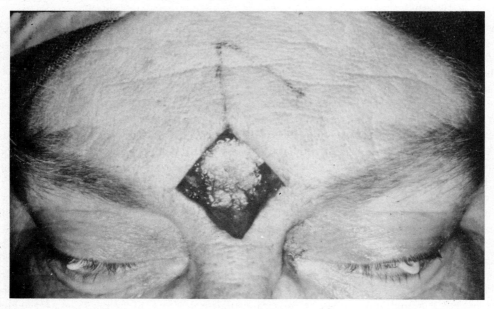

**FIG 49–2.**
This glabellar defect included a resection of the pericranium and therefore would not consistently support the skin graft because it is a nongranulating surface.

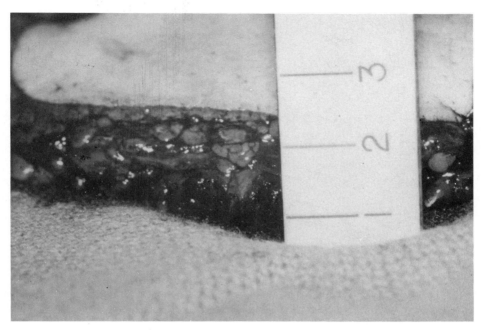

**FIG 49–3**.
Cross-section of the skin, subcutaneous tissue, and muscle of a musculocutaneous flap in which the muscle is providing the essential blood supply to the skin and therefore cannot be separated from that skin.

ing mimetic muscles but leaving the blood supply and motor nerve supply intact (Fig. 49–8). The advantage of this particular flap is that it reconstructs a defect with similar tissue, whose function is preserved even during the tissue transfer. In many respects, this flap meets the criteria of restoration of form and function better than any of the other types (Fig. 49–9).

Another exciting area of tissue transfer involves the use of microvascular surgery (Fig. 49–10) to reestablish blood flow to soft tissue that has been totally detached from its blood supply. Although technically more difficult than the other techniques, it has the potential for providing excellent results. The multiple branches of the external carotid system coupled with the numerous venous channels in the neck usually provide numerous opportunities for completing the microvascular anastomosis. Special instrumentation and suture material (Fig. 49–11) are required for this type of surgery. One of the major advantages of the musculocutaneous and free flaps is that they provide the ability to transfer tissue and complete a reconstructive task in one operation rather than multiple operations, which are required for some of the other flaps.

Mucosal defects pose another reconstructive challenge. In these defects, the existing techniques sometimes compromise the original goals of restoring form and function. If there is a small mucosal defect in the oral cavity or pharynx, it can be reconstructed by taking a mucosal graft from another area. However, as the size of the defect increases, it is no longer possible to locate a mucosal graft of suitable size, and other alternatives are necessary. These options involve the transfer of skin into the oral cavity or pharynx. The skin cannot secrete mucus and obviously does not contain taste buds. Usually for the larger defects, the underlying pharyngeal or oral cavity musculature is also included in the resection. Therefore, the reconstructive technique, whether it be a local or regional skin flap or a musculocutaneous flap, represents a compromise. It is true that the defect is resurfaced, but it does not provide a mucus-producing tissue and it is an adynamic segment of tissue because there is no muscle functioning in a coordinated fashion with the remaining pharyngeal musculature. The pectoralis musculocutaneous flap can be used for this task and usually gives satisfactory results for most patients with partial defects of the pharynx. Free flaps have also been used for this purpose.

Free flaps have also been used for the recon-

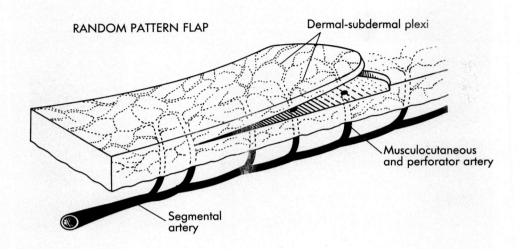

RANDOM PATTERN FLAP

Dermal-subdermal plexi

Musculocutaneous
and perforator artery

Segmental
artery

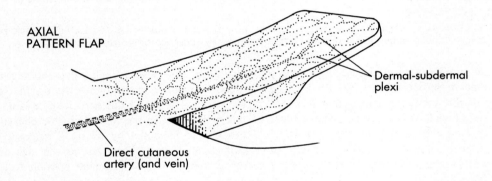

AXIAL
PATTERN FLAP

Dermal-subdermal
plexi

Direct cutaneous
artery (and vein)

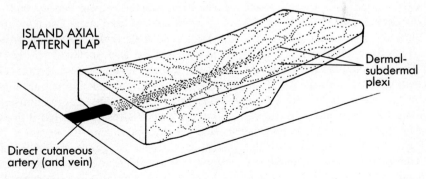

ISLAND AXIAL
PATTERN FLAP

Dermal-
subdermal
plexi

Direct cutaneous
artery (and vein)

**FIG 49–4**.
Random pattern flaps do not have the strong blood supply of axial pattern flaps.

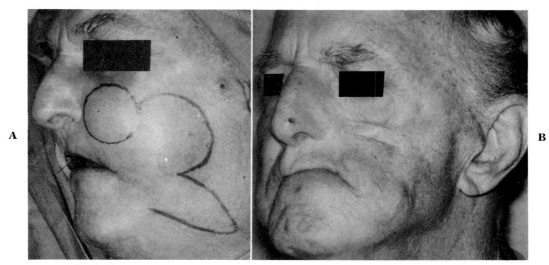

**FIG 49–5.**
This circular area, **A,** is to be resected and would include the skin and subcutaneous tissue down to the maxilla. Therefore, a local bilobed flap provides blood supply and comparable thickness for the optimal reconstruction in this patient, **B,** who also had a maxillectomy. (From Schuller, D: Cervical skin flaps in head and neck reconstruction, *Am J Otolaryngol* 2:1, 1981. Used by permission.)

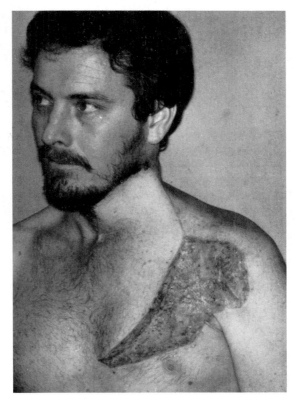

**FIG 49–6.**
The donor site of a regional skin flap sometimes has to be covered with a split-thickness skin graft, as seen in this patient who had a deltopectoral flap reconstruction of a neck defect.

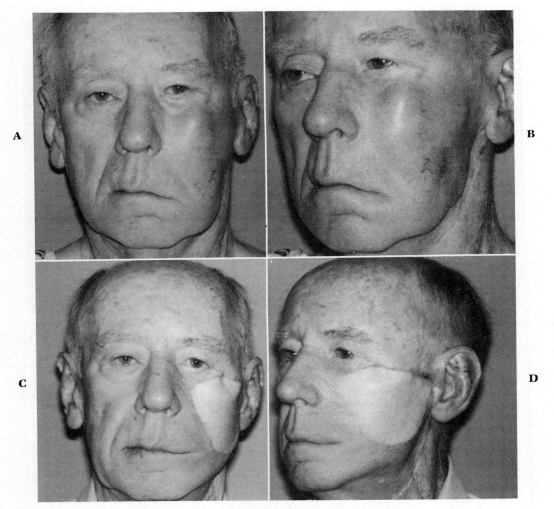

**FIG 49–7.**
This man had recurrent maxillary carcinoma involving the overlying facial tissue (**A** and **B**) and underwent one-stage resection of the maxilla and facial soft tissue with reconstruction using a pectoralis musculocutaneous flap (**C** and **D**).

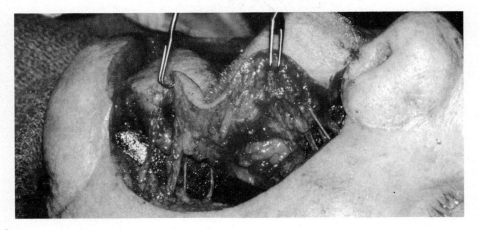

**FIG 49–8.**
This musculocutaneous flap permits the preservation of not only the blood supply, but also the multiple motor nerves to the orbicularis oris.

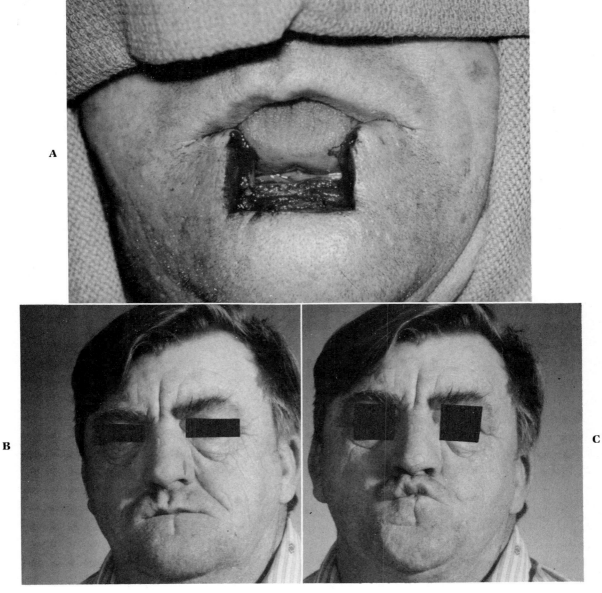

**FIG 49–9.**
The Karapandzic musculocutaneous flap was used to reconstruct this lower lip defect (**A**) and resulted in restoration of form and function, as seen in these 1-year postoperative photographs (**B** and **C**). (From Schuller D: *Myocutaneous flaps in reconstructive surgery of the head and neck*. In Wolf GT, ed: *Head and neck oncology*, Boston, 1984, Martinus Nijhoff.)

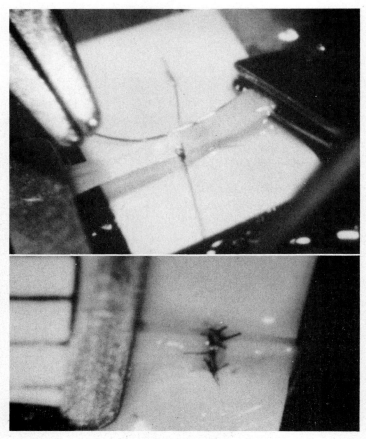

**FIG 49–10.**
Vessels as small as 1 mm in diameter can now be reanastomosed using magnification with a microscope.

struction of mucosal defects when the entire pharynx and/or cervical esophagus has been removed. This involves the transfer of a segment of jejunum with restoration of blood supply using microvascular anastomoses. Similar reconstructive tasks have been accomplished by transferring the stomach through the mediastinum and anastomosing it to whatever remains of the pharynx when the pharynx and entire esophagus are removed.

However, both of these procedures are technically difficult and potentially dangerous to the patient. Once again, the ultimate goals of the surgery are not met ideally with any of the existing reconstructive techniques. A variety of approaches exist now to transfer tissue into either cutaneous or mucosal defects, but some of these meet the goals of an ideal reconstruction better than others.

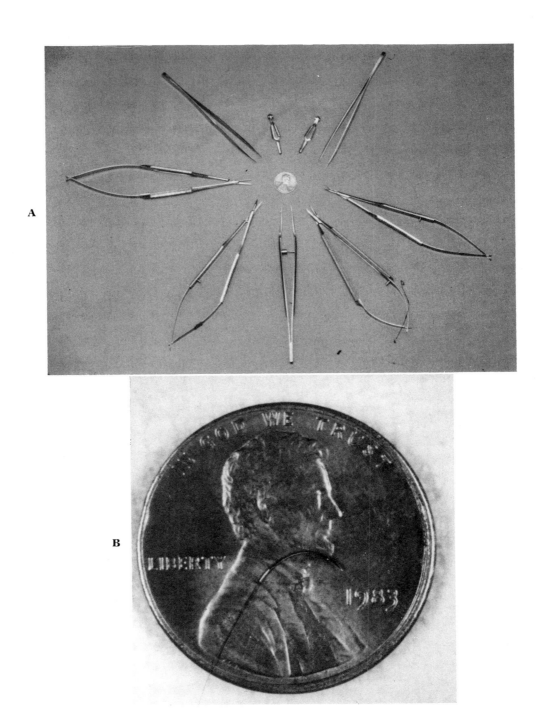

**FIG 49–11.**
**A,** special vascular surgical instruments and fine suture material, **B,** are necessary to do microvascular surgery.

# 50

# Subcutaneous Defects

Reconstruction of subcutaneous defects continues to be a major challenge. In this situation, the skin and mucosa are intact, but there is a deficiency of the underlying muscle and/or subcutaneous tissue (Fig. 50–1). It becomes necessary to augment the area of deficiency. The ideal product is one that can be easily contoured and has the same consistency as the tissue that is missing, is well tolerated by the patient's immune system, and is not prone to infection. This type of reconstruction is even a greater challenge in the head and neck because just about all areas have some degree of movement. The movement of the tissue provides a stress on the tolerance of whatever material is inserted. Currently no ideal material is available for the augmentation of subcutaneous defects.

The materials used are classified as either grafts or implants. A graft is a material inserted that ultimately becomes incorporated into the patient and is supported by the patient's blood supply. In contrast, an implant is a material that acts merely as an inert filler and is not supported by the patient's blood supply.

Living tissue donated by the patient (autologous graft) stands a greater chance of success because the immune system does not recognize it as being foreign. Rib cartilage, rib bone, and iliac bone are frequent donor materials for augmentation of facial subcutaneous defects. They have drawbacks because they sometimes cannot be easily contoured for the particular augmentation needs. Their consistency sometimes does not mimic that of the tissue they are augmenting. There is also additional morbidity resulting from harvesting the material (Fig. 50–2).

An alternative to using the patient's tissue that avoids the morbidity of a harvesting procedure is to use preserved material from another individual (homologous implant). A variety of homologous implants have been used in the past, including septal cartilage, septal bone, and rib or hip grafts. These materials appear to be well tolerated, with a low rate of acute infection. Resorption, however, can occur on a long-term basis and is a serious drawback. A modification of homologous implants involves the sterilization and preservation of homologous rib by heavily irradiating the tissue. The acute and long-term acceptance of this material is good, and the material is easily contoured. However, there are times when its consistency does not match that of the deficient tissue.

There have been multiple attempts to create a foreign material (alloplast) that would be a well-tolerated implant. A variety of materials have been advocated, some better tolerated than others. However, the possibility for infection either immediately or on a delayed basis exists. These alloplastic materials are usually easily contoured, but there are times when they also do not match the consistency of the original tissue. Expense is another limitation of these materials.

Microvascular surgery has provided a means of transferring soft tissue into large areas of subcutaneous defects. The reliable blood supply of this tissue usually decreases the amount of resorption seen when free fat grafts are placed. This type of surgery may prove to be a useful adjunct, especially for the reconstruction of large subcutaneous defects.

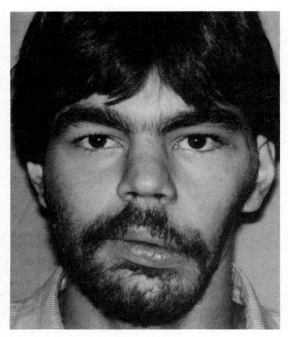

**FIG 50–1**.
This patient has a loss of the subcutaneous tissue on the left side of the face, resulting in facial asymmetry.

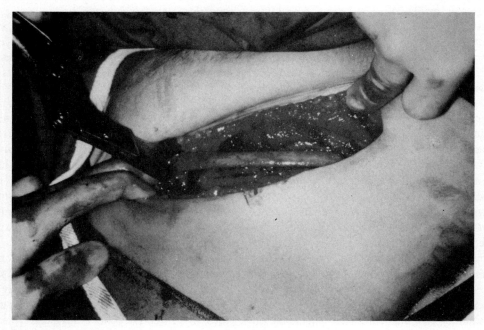

**FIG 50–2**.
Rib grafts used for augmentation of subcutaneous defects produce prolonged morbidity.

# 51

# Nasal Deformities

No other aspect of facial reconstructive surgery requires a more thorough understanding of normal anatomy and physiology than does nasal reconstruction. The surgeon performing this type of reconstruction must have a clear understanding of the impact of any surgical changes of nasal anatomy on nasal physiology. It is also imperative that the surgeon be comfortable with the use of the headlight to improve visualization of intranasal structures.

Numerous surgical techniques are available for the rhinoplastic surgeon. The proper selection of a technique is dependent on the surgeon's ability to define the nasal deformity. After the surgeon has defined the deformity and decided on a surgical solution, this must be explained in an understandable fashion to the patient.

Good rapport between surgeon and patient is essential so that each can communicate freely with the other. The surgeon must listen to the patient's definition of his or her desires regarding nasal proportions. It is advisable for the surgeon to accurately communicate the realistic potential of meeting those goals. If any difficulty in communication is encountered by either the patient or the physician, it may be advisable for the patient to seek another physician.

Both internal and external nasal reconstruction can be performed with local anesthesia. It is usually supplemented with some intravenous sedation and analgesia. Cocaine blocks of the anterior ethmoidal and sphenopalatine ganglia (Fig. 51–1), coupled with infiltration anesthesia using lidocaine (Xylocaine) preferably containing epinephrine, provide adequate anesthesia. If the patient is particularly apprehensive, however, the procedure can also be performed safely with general anes-

thesia. The decision regarding type of anesthetic is usually the patient's unless there are medical contraindications.

There is no such thing as a standard rhinoplasty. Each procedure is different and depends on the definition of the nasal deformities. The configuration of the nasal tip is dependent on the size and position of the lower lateral cartilages, the quadrilateral cartilage of the nasal septum, and the thickness of the overlying skin. The position and size of the lower lateral cartilage and its relationship to the caudal end of the nasal septum can be surgically altered (Fig. 51–2). However, little can be done regarding the thickness of the skin. There is no appreciable subcutaneous tissue that permits more tip definition by its removal.

The nasal profile can also be altered. If it is too prominent, the bone either with or without a portion of the cartilaginous septum can be removed to lower it (Fig. 51–3). The other extreme of profile alteration relates to the loss of nasal septal cartilage from either trauma or infection with a marked concavity. It is usually necessary to insert a graft to augment this concavity. If it is a relatively minor saddle deformity, often there is an adequate amount of nasal septal cartilage or bone to augment. If it is a major deformity, either rib or iliac bone autologous grafts can be used (Fig. 51–4). Alloplasts have been used in this area, as has irradiated homologous costal cartilage.

In the nose that is too wide, alterations can be made by performing osteotomies of the nose. These osteotomies not only permit movement of the bones to thin the nose, but also enable the physician to position the nose in the midline if it is crooked (Fig. 51–5).

The child with a secondary nasal deformity as-

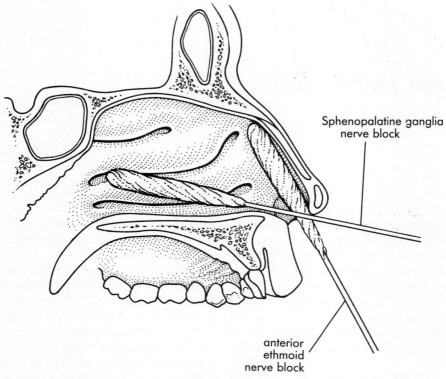

**FIG 51–1.**
The nose can be effectively anesthetized with regional blocks of the anterior ethmoidal nerves and sphenopalatine ganglia using cotton pledgets saturated with cocaine.

sociated with cleft lip and palate represents a special surgical challenge. The portion of the nasal tip on the side of the cleft lip is usually flattened so that the distance from the nasal columella to the ala is considerably greater than that on the noncleft side of the lip (Fig. 51–6). Surgical techniques used in conventional rhinoplasty are usually not adequate to make dramatic changes in the cleft nasal deformity. However, specialized techniques can elongate the nasal columella,

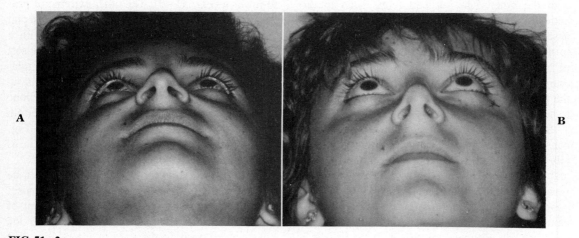

**FIG 51–2.**
It is possible to thin and reposition the lower lateral cartilages and to remove soft tissues to modify the nasal tip, as seen in **A** and the 3-year postoperative view, **B.**

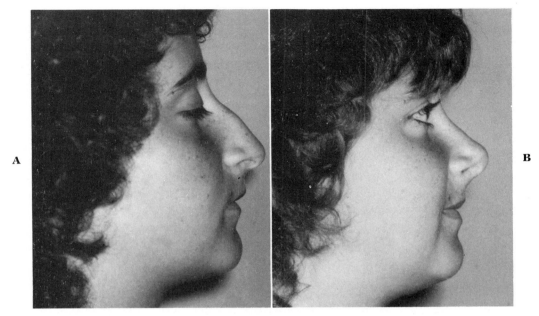

**FIG 51–3.**
The nasal profile, **A,** can also be altered by removing a portion of the bone and cartilage composing the nasal dorsum, as seen in this 3-year postoperative view, **B.**

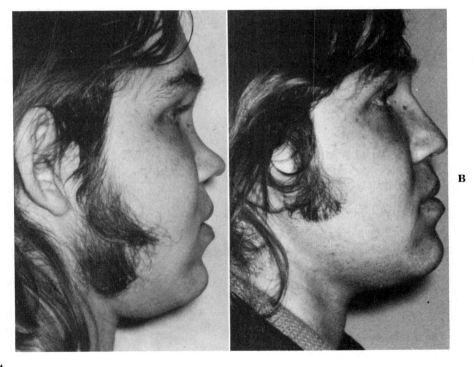

**FIG 51–4.**
This man's saddle deformity, **A,** was reconstructed with insertion of an autologous iliac bone graft, as seen in this 1-year postoperative view, **B.**

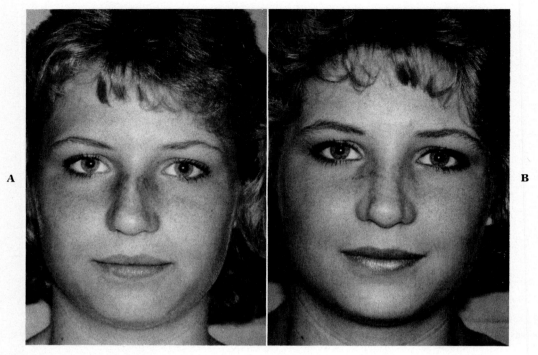

**FIG 51–5.**
The crooked nose, **A,** can be straightened and narrowed by performing osteotomies, as seen in this 3-year postoperative photograph, **B.**

move the position of the nasal ala so that it is equidistant from the columella, increase the tip projection, and thin the tip, in addition to straightening the nasal septum (Fig. 51–7). This technique can provide rather dramatic improvement in not only cosmesis but also nasal function.

The surgical approaches to nasal reconstruction are varied. Internal rhinoplasty involves placement of all incisions within the nasal cavity. The other technique involves one skin incision across the base of the nasal columella that allows for the reflection of a columellar–nasal tip flap and provides improved exposure of the underlying bony and cartilaginous structures (Fig. 51–8). This technique is called external, or "open," rhinoplasty. It is imperative that the patient who is undergoing open rhinoplasty understands the use of a skin incision across the columella and knows that a permanent scar will occur. However, criticism of this technique has been minimal because of the excellent healing of the scar (Fig. 51–9).

In those instances in which the excision of cutaneous cancers has resulted in partial or total loss of the nose, reconstruction involves a variety of techniques, such as composite ear grafts, local

flaps, and even distant flaps. As the defect enlarges, the difficulty of the reconstruction increases, as does the number of operations necessary to complete the reconstruction.

Composite auricular grafts provide excellent tissue to reconstruct full-thickness defects of the nasal ala (Fig. 51–10). However, the use of these grafts is limited by the size of the defect. Defects larger than 1.0 to 1.5 cm stand the chance of having an inadequate blood supply to support the composite graft and subsequent graft necrosis. Larger partial nasal defects can be reconstructed with local flaps (Fig. 51–11). These usually give satisfactory results with only an infrequent need for multiple operations.

Total nasal excision creates a difficult reconstructive task. The alternatives for the patient are to have a nose reconstructed with a forehead scalping flap or tubed abdominal flap or to have a nasal prosthesis created. No reconstructive technique can provide the excellent contouring that can be created with a prosthesis. The color matches are also excellent with prostheses. However, often patients have negative psychologic reactions about having to rely on a piece of plastic

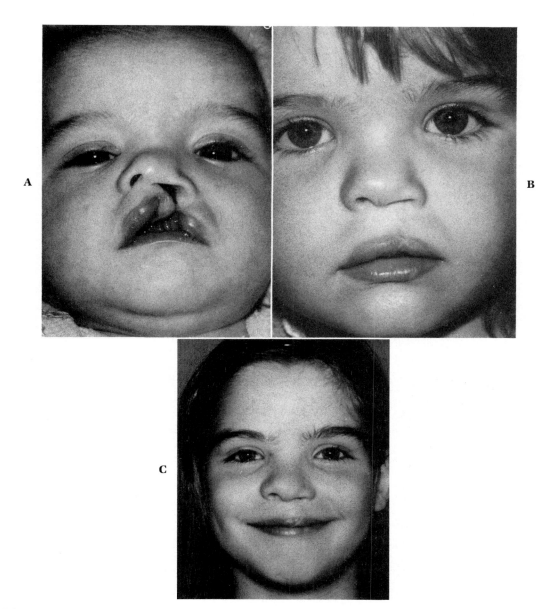

**FIG 51–6.**
This child was born with a unilateral cleft lip and had the usual nasal deformity, **A,** which was slightly improved with the cleft lip repair, **B,** but persists and will need secondary nasal reconstruction, **C,** when she is about 8 to 9 years old.

representing a significant body part. It is for this reason that most patients choose to have nasal reconstruction with autologous tissue rather than select a prosthesis, even with the knowledge that nasal contouring cannot be as good with tissue reconstruction.

The scalping flap provides a quicker means of reconstructing the nose than the tubed abdominal flap (Fig. 51–12). However, the tubed abdominal flap offers the potential for more precise contouring (Fig. 51–13). Its obvious drawback is the need for multiple stages and patient inconvenience in order to transfer the tissue to the area where it will be used.

The goals of reconstructing nasal deformities are to create a series of changes in the nasal anatomy that are well coordinated and harmonious within themselves and, as a unit, create subtle

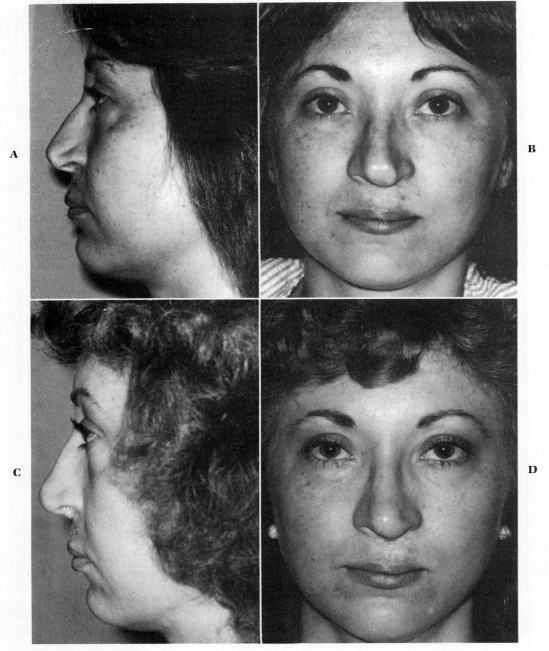

**FIG 51–7.**
The secondary nasal deformities, **A** and **B,** can usually improve nasal function and form, as seen in these 2-year postoperative views, **C** and **D.**

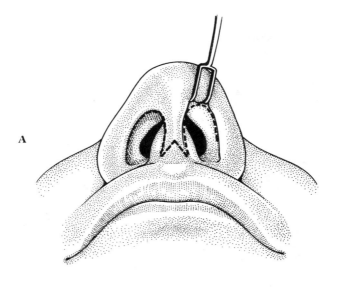

A

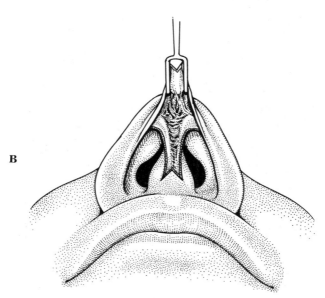

B

**FIG 51–8**.
This sketch shows the surgical technique of external rhinoplasty.

changes in the facial appearance. It is not the intent of the otolaryngologist–head and neck surgeon to create dramatic changes that drastically alter facial appearance. It is too difficult for the family and friends to adjust to dramatic changes in the patient's appearance. The surgeon must also be cognizant of ethnic and racial identity and must be sure to carefully assess the patient's desires for preservation of these features. The improvement of nasal deformities is a fascinating and challenging part of facial plastic and reconstructive surgery that often produces feelings of satisfaction in both the patient and the physician.

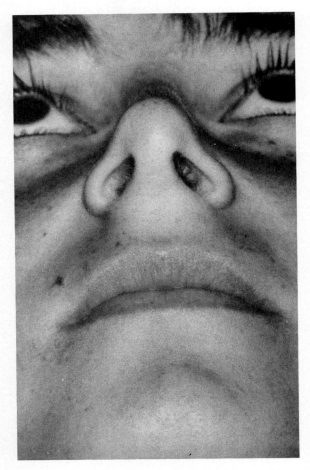

**FIG 51–9.**
A faint scar is seen across the nasal columella in this 3-year postoperative photograph, but it was not objectionable to the patient.

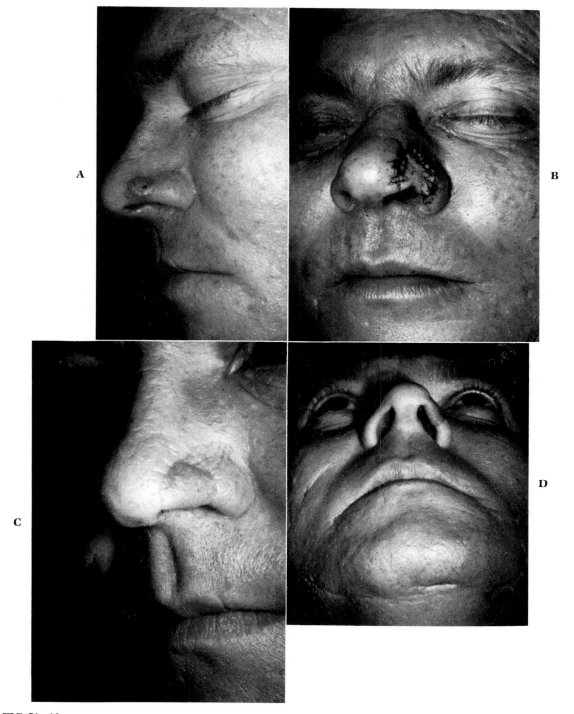

**FIG 51–10.**
This patient had a cutaneous cancer involving the nasal ala, **A,** that was small enough to permit reconstruction with a composite auricular graft, **B,** which provided excellent reconstruction as seen in the postoperative photographs, **C** and **D.**

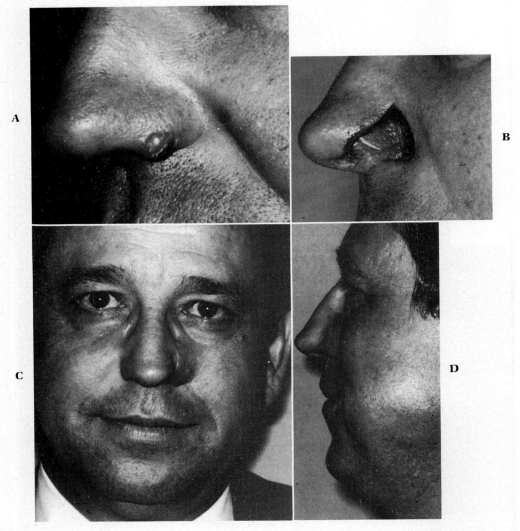

**FIG 51–11**.
Larger full-thickness nasal defects, **A** and **B,** are better reconstructed with local flaps, such as seen in these 5-year postoperative views, **C** and **D,** of a patient with a nasolabial flap one-stage reconstruction.

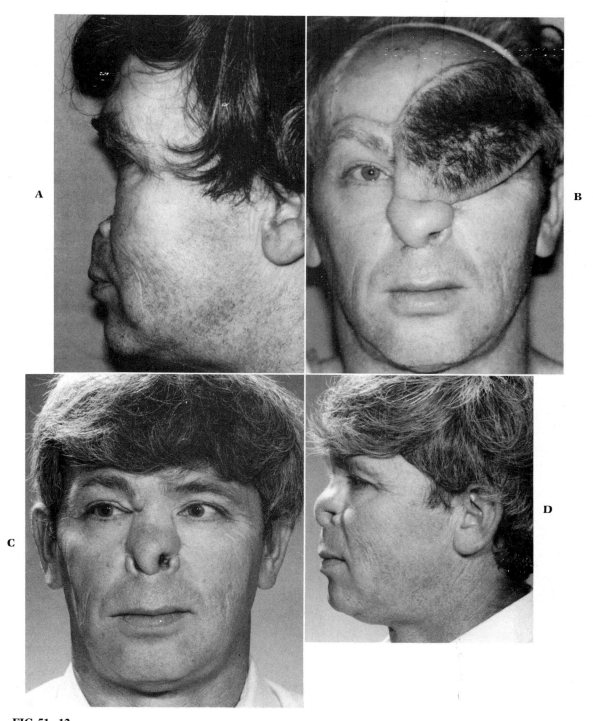

**FIG 51–12.**
This patient underwent total nasal resection, **A,** and reconstruction with a scalping flap, **B.** In the postoperative views, **C** and **D,** note the effective use of hair camouflaging of the forehead donor site.

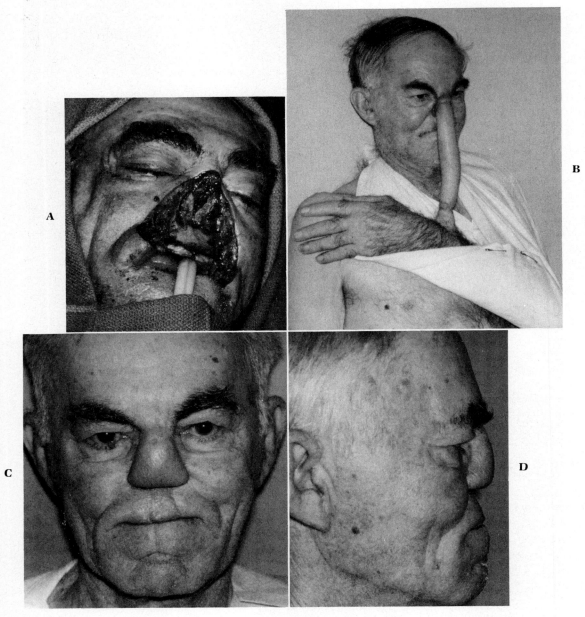

**FIG 51–13.**
This patient underwent resection of the entire nose and upper lip, **A,** and elected to have nasal reconstruction with a tubed abdominal flap following lip reconstruction, **B.** Although the technique takes longer to complete, the postoperative results, **C** and **D,** have the advantage of no additional scarring in the region that is being reconstructed.

# 52

# Mandibular Reconstruction

Mandibular reconstruction is one of the most difficult tasks facing the facial plastic surgeon. Although most of the numerous techniques developed have the potential for providing at least some components of a successful mandibular reconstruction, they also have limitations.

A full-thickness defect of *lateral* portions of the mandible results in an asymmetric pull of the muscles of mastication, with a resultant shift of the mandible toward the side of resection. This mandibular shift is more troublesome to the patient with teeth than to the edentulous patient. The malocclusion is bothersome. However, the morbidity of a lateral mandibular resection can be decreased with sliding dental guides (Fig. 52–1). This helps to maintain the proper occlusion on the nonresected side of the mandible. Most patients will adjust eventually and not have a permanent major problem with a lateral mandibular defect.

*Anterior* mandibular loss is a different matter. Whether the loss is from trauma or cancer surgery, the result is the same after healing. Whenever patients lose the anterior mandibular arch, they have lost the ability to maintain the anterior displacement of the tongue and the floor-of-mouth musculature. These soft tissue structures of the oral cavity tend to prolapse toward the pharynx, and the airway narrows. In addition, the patient loses the rigid support of the lower lip and thus can no longer control oral secretions. Persistent drooling can create a major functional, social, and psychologic problem (Fig. 52–2). It is the anterior mandibular defect that represents a critical need for reconstruction.

One method for mandibular reconstruction is the use of segments of iliac bone. This is especially useful for relatively short lengths, especially the lateral mandible. A block of iliac bone is stabilized in place with mandibular plates to increase the stability. The remaining mandible is immobilized for several weeks to permit healing. The use of autologous bone to reconstruct the short lateral segments, coupled with immobilization, is successful (Fig. 52–3). However, the success rate decreases when one tries to contour bone to the configuration of the anterior mandibular arch.

Another option for mandibular reconstruction is the transfer of bone using microvascular technique. One of the flaps used for such surgery involves transferring a portion of the iliac crest, which is supplied by the deep circumflex iliac artery. This artery is transected, and the bone flap, with or without overlying skin, is transferred to the defect. The arterial and venous blood supplies are then reestablished with microvascular anastomotic technique. This technique is excellent because it provides a bone with a strong blood supply. The iliac crest allows for a good bit of versatility regarding the configuration of the mandible. However, the drawback associated with this particular technique is the technical difficulty not only of harvesting the flap but also of performing the microvascular anastomosis.

All of the aforementioned techniques have the potential for being successful. None of them currently provides for reconstructions that will routinely permit the wearing of dentures and also permit vigorous chewing. They basically represent attempts to reestablish facial contour, protect the airway, and prevent drooling.

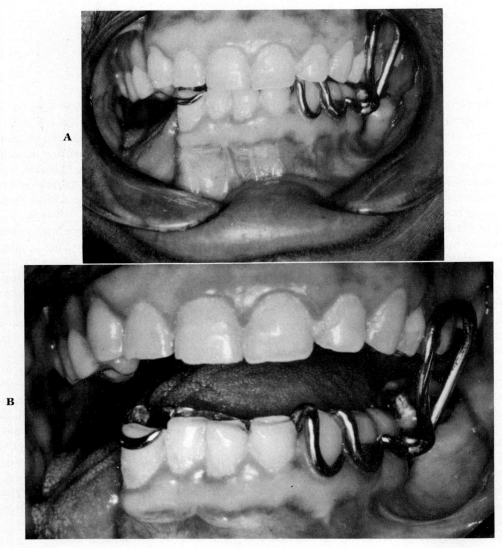

**FIG 52–1.**
A sliding dental guide, **A,** prevents drift of the mandible toward the resected side when the mouth is open, **B.**

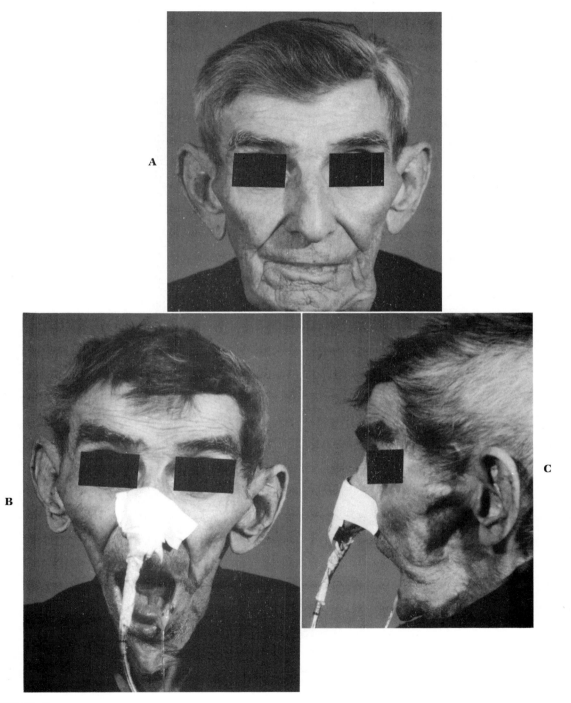

**FIG 52–2.**
**A–C,** full-thickness loss of segment of the anterior mandible creates an oral commissure that is not capable of retaining oral secretions, as seen in this man following resection of a cancer of the anterior floor of the mouth involving the mandible.

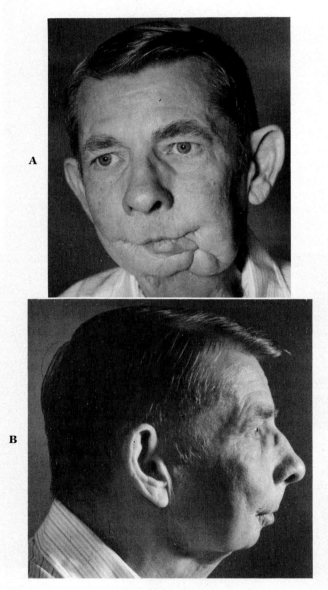

**FIG 52–3.**
**A** and **B,** postoperative appearance of a man who had a surgically created 5-cm parasymphyseal full-thickness mandibular defect that was successfully reconstructed with an autologous iliac bone graft.

# 53

# Auricular Deformities

Auricular reconstruction, like mandibular reconstruction, is a difficult task. Depending on the degree of severity, it usually requires multiple staged procedures. Auricular deformities can be the result of congenital, neoplastic, or traumatic causes. Traumatic causes are usually the result of domestic violence rather than motor vehicle injuries (Fig. 53–1). Cancer-related partial auricular deformities can often be reconstructed effectively with skin grafts. Once again, it is important to recognize that only a recipient site capable of creating granulation tissue will support a skin graft. In the event that a cancer resection includes the underlying perichondrium of auricular cartilage, it is necessary to proceed with resecting the auricular cartilage to allow exposure of the skin graft to the perichondrium of the other side. This usually gives excellent cosmetic results (Fig. 53–2).

Most auricular deformities are related to congenital causes. The auricle is the result of a fusion of the axon hillocks, which are derived from the first and second branchial arches. A partial or total lack of fusion of some or all of the axon hillocks accounts for the multiplicity of appearances of a deformed auricle (Fig. 53–3).

Congenital auricular deformities are often associated with other anatomic alterations. Once again, the clinician's understanding of basic embryology permits concentration on certain structures. The knowledge that the auricles receive contributions from the first and second branchial arches prompts a thorough inspection of other derivatives of these arches. Approximately 50% of all children born with a congenital auricular deformity will have some form of hemimandibular hypoplasia on the side of the auricular deformity (Fig. 53–4). This asymmetry is often subtle and not recognized by the parents until demonstrated by the physician. The hemimandibular hypoplasia usually improves as the child matures and does not need any specific reconstruction.

The reconstruction of an atretic auricle involves multiple procedures. Bardach has developed an approach that condenses reconstruction into four major operations. Subsequent to the four major operations, additional procedures sometimes are necessary to improve the quality of the result.

The auricle is located on the side of the head extending from a horizontal line drawn from the glabellar region to the base of the nose and usually on a plane that is somewhat parallel to the plane of the nasal dorsum. These landmarks are useful in placing the atretic ear. Reconstruction for atresia is usually not begun until the auricle has reached almost adult size. This usually occurs by the time the child is 7 to 8 years of age.

The first operation involves the repositioning of the lower portion of the vertical fold of skin, which is usually present, so that it conforms to the position and configuration of the lobule of the new auricle (Fig. 53–5). The second operation involves the insertion of a rigid framework into a subcutaneous tissue pocket corresponding to the location of the reconstructed auricle. Costal cartilage is carved into a rigid framework that mimics the contours of an auricle (Fig. 53–6). A postauricular scalp flap is then moved posteriorly to allow for the placement of a full-thickness skin graft as the third operation (Fig. 53–7). After the skin graft develops a subcutaneous sheet of fibrosis and completes its inevitable contraction, it is then ready for the final procedure.

The last operation involves the advancement of a postauricular skin graft, leaving it pedicled to the skin overlying the rigid framework into the

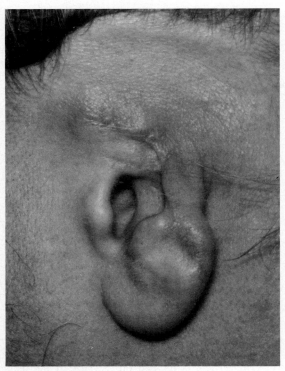

**FIG 53–1.**
This man lost a portion of his auricle when it was bitten off during a fight with his employer. He underwent excision of the conchal cartilage and a portion of the anthelix with preservation of the perichondrium on the other side, which would then support a full-thickness skin graft to reconstruct the auricle in one operation.

postauricular area to elevate the implanted costal cartilage away from the side of the head and to create an auriculocephalic crease. The previously displaced postauricular scalp flap is advanced into its normal position, which results in no abnormal position of the hairline (Fig. 53–8).

The goal of auricular atresia reconstruction is to improve facial symmetry by reconstructing an auricle that is ideally of similar dimensions and located on the same plane and at the same distance from the side of the head (Fig. 53–9). It is unrealistic to expect the creation of the fine contouring that is present in the normal auricle. The alternative to auricular reconstruction is an auricular prosthesis. Once again, most parents choose auricular reconstruction over a prosthesis for the same reasons described in Chapter 51 for patients undergoing reconstruction of the nose.

The coordination of the ear canal and middle ear reconstruction with auricular reconstruction in cases of atresia is an important matter. In children with unilateral atresia and a normal hearing ear on the other side, the ear canal and middle ear reconstructive work is usually delayed until young adulthood, when they can decide whether they want to risk injury to the facial nerve to undergo this type of surgery. When bilateral atresia is present, ear canal and middle ear reconstruction usually precedes the auricular reconstruction. However, the initial stage can be coordinated by the facial plastic surgeon and otologic surgeon so that incisions for the middle ear reconstruction do not seriously detract from the quality of the eventual auricular reconstruction.

More common than auricular atresia is the lop-ear deformity. This problem can also have familial tendencies. The deformity is the result of absence of the anthelix fold, which causes the auricle to protrude in an excessive fashion from the side of the head (Fig. 53–10). The bilateral lop-ear deformity is noticeable, and the unilateral lop-ear deformity is even more noticeable because of

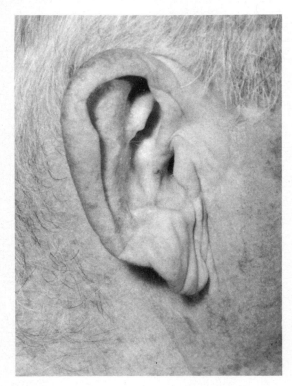

**FIG 53–2.**
This man underwent excision of an auricular basal cell cancer including the underlying cartilage so that the perichondrium provided blood supply for the skin graft.

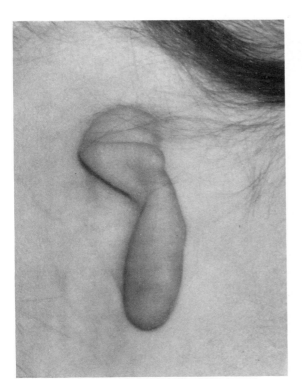

**FIG 53–3.**
The most common appearance of congenital auricular deformities is that of a vertical fold of soft tissue with underlying gnarled cartilage.

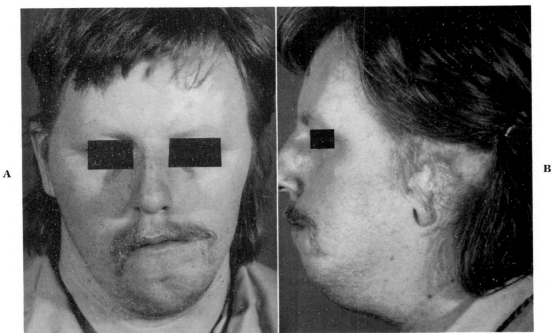

**FIG 53–4.**
**A** and **B,** this patient was born with auricular atresia and demonstrates the hemimandibular hypoplasia that is commonly seen.

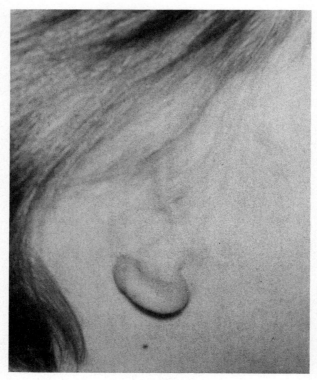

**FIG 53–5.**
The lobule is positioned into a more normal location, and the underlying cartilage is resected with the first stage of auricular reconstruction.

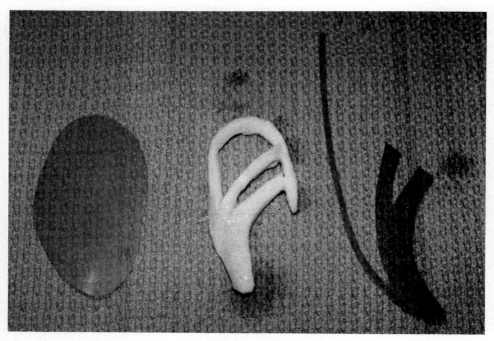

**FIG 53–6.**
Autologous costal cartilage is carved to the contour of the auricle and then implanted into the subcutaneous pocket with the second stage.

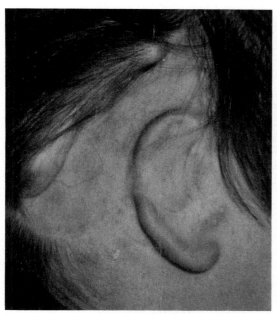

**FIG 53–7.**
A full-thickness skin graft from the groin is placed in the postauricular area during the third stage.

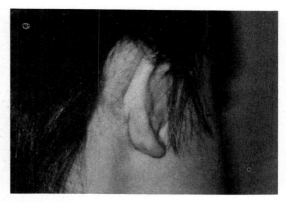

**FIG 53–8.**
The last stage involves advancement of the previously placed skin graft to create an auriculocephalic crease to displace the auricular framework of the costal cartilage away from the side of the head.

the asymmetry created. Although this does not cause any functional problems, there is no question that this deformity can be a psychologic stress to the child. Children do not like to be different from their peers. They often are subject to considerable ridicule from other children who are insensitive. To avoid psychologic stress to the child, surgical correction of the lop-ear deformity is recommended before the child enters the formal educational years. At 4 or 5 years of age a child is old enough to be cooperative and has not yet entered school.

The surgical technique to correct the lop-ear deformity is quite effective, usually involving only one operation that consistently gives good results. An incision is made on the posterior surface of the auricle, and the skin is elevated away from the auricular cartilage. Mattress sutures are placed through the auricular cartilage to create a new anthelix. This technique, which was originally described by Mustarde, is quite versatile. It is not unusual for a child with a lop-ear deformity to also have a deep auricular concha. Sometimes it is necessary to inset the concha to decrease its depth. If the lobule is protruding, an elliptical excision of skin on the posterior surface can bring it closer to the side of the head. A combination of the Mustarde suture technique with conchal setback and lobular repositioning, if needed, gives dramatic results that cause minimal discomfort to the patient (Fig. 53–11). None of the scars are noticeable because they are located on the postauricular surface. The surgical technique of reconstruction of the lop-ear deformity meets the goals of facial plastic and reconstructive surgery.

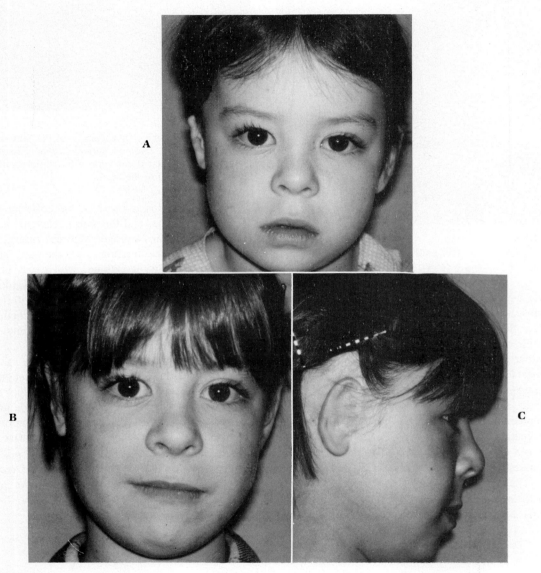

**FIG 53–9.**
This child, who was born with congenital auricular atresia on the right, **A,** underwent four-stage auricular reconstruction. **B** and **C,** postoperative result.

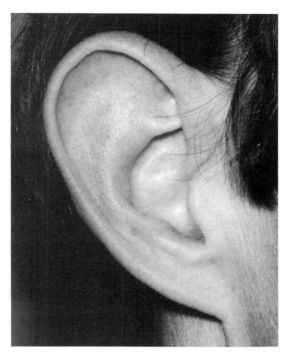

**FIG 53–10.**
Lack of the auricular anthelix causes the lop-ear deformity.

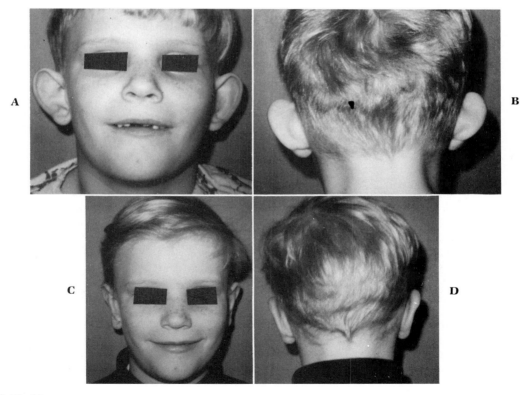

**FIG 53–11.**
Bilateral lop-ear deformity, **A** and **B,** can usually be dramatically improved with one operation, which creates scarring in the concealed postauricular area, as seen in these postoperative photographs, **C** and **D.**

# 54

# Aesthetic Surgery

Facial aesthetic surgery refers to that group of procedures intended to improve appearance when there are no identifiable functional abnormalities. Whereas this type of surgery previously was considered somewhat frivolous and performed on a relatively limited number of people, it is now socially accepted and a fully respected branch of medicine that has a sound basis. Society places so much emphasis on youth that the aging process has psychologic and even social ramifications. For some, an aged appearance that is inconsistent with the person's chronologic age can have an economic impact in terms of job promotions and even job terminations. While society's views have evolved to make aesthetic surgery a socially acceptable experience, refinements in techniques have also increased the quality of the results. Both of these factors have increased public interest and resulted in considerable focus on this field of medicine in magazines, newspapers, and television. Aesthetic surgery should be considered by both the health professions and the lay public as a means of benefiting patients both psychologically and potentially even economically. The challenge for the otolaryngologist–head and neck surgeon performing facial aesthetic surgery is to identify those patients whose desires and personalities are compatible with the surgeon's capabilities.

Patient selection is a critical component of facial aesthetic surgery. It is necessary to remember that there is no universally acceptable definition of beauty. Numerous variables such as cultural, ethnic, and racial background need to be added into the equation to define concepts of attractiveness, and it is imperative that they all be considered. The facial aesthetic surgeon must be versatile and compliant so that his or her concepts of beauty are not forced on the patient. Rather it is

important that the patient be allowed the opportunity to express and identify desires for change. The surgeon must then communicate with the patient whether or not the desires are realistic. Once again, this is an area in which thorough physician-patient communication is mandatory. If the physician has any doubts about satisfying the desires of the patient, the relationship should not be continued.

Patient selection often requires that the surgeon be able to identify what patients may not have realistic self-images and may be somewhat unstable psychologically. If the surgeon has any questions about this matter, psychiatric consultation is often helpful. If the patient has a history of previous psychiatric treatment or if there are disparities between the patient's expectations and the surgeon's ability to meet them, the situation is a potentially volatile one and may result in eventual litigation. Patient selection is a crucial aspect of aesthetic surgery for both the physician and the patient.

As mentioned, concepts of beauty are variable. They are dependent on the times, culture, ethnic and racial background, and socioeconomic level. But humans have a desire to be beautiful whatever the definition. Vanity is related to beauty. Cosmetics, jewelry, and clothing are means of self-decoration that can be used to enhance beauty.

The aging process occurs at differing rates. Generally speaking, those changes which are most noticeable relate to the skin. The gradual loss of elastic fibers creates a decreased resiliency and redundancy of the body skin. Gravity subsequently has a greater impact on the position of the skin. The loss of elastic fibers produces two general alterations in the skin: relaxation of the skin, which creates redundancy, and the development of fine wrinkles. It is important to understand that the surgical procedures developed to treat redundancy do not alter the fine wrinkles. Obviously, that point must be clearly understood by the patient seeking this type of surgery.

The multiple surgical approaches used in facial aesthetic surgery can be classified according to the definition of the problem. Those procedures which are used to correct redundant skin include rhytidoplasty (face-lift), brow lift, forehead lift, and blepharoplasty. Operations designed to alter facial profile are rhinoplasty, chin augmentation, malar augmentation, and the multiple operations for orthognathic surgery. Those used to smooth the fine wrinkles in the skin are chemical peel, dermabrasion, and cutaneous injections, such as with liquid collagen.

Rhytidoplasty is the most effective means of dealing with facial skin redundancy involving the middle and lower thirds of the face and neck region. The procedure is usually performed with the patient under local anesthesia with supplemental intravenous sedation. It involves the elevation of the redundant facial and neck skin. The fascial tissue overlying the parotid gland is often dis-

placed posteriorly to increase the support to the displaced skin (Fig. 54–1). Some techniques even use the platysma muscle to create a more dramatic change. The elevated redundant skin is then redraped, the excess is excised, and the wound is closed. The operation is usually well tolerated with a minimum of patient discomfort. Complications can occur, and they usually involve the development of hematoma under the skin flaps. Injury to branches of the facial nerve has been described but does not occur commonly. There is a variable amount of ecchymosis and edema postoperatively, but it clears relatively quickly. The results are usually gratifying to the well-informed patient (Fig. 54–2).

Brow and forehead lifts are designed to deal with the redundancy of skin that can cause some ptosis of the eyebrows and wrinkling of the forehead skin, respectively. A brow lift involves excision of a varying amount of skin directly above the eyebrows to elevate them and give the patient a more alert and youthful appearance (Fig. 54–3). Forehead lift is performed by elevating the forehead skin by means of an incision in the hairline, redraping it after transecting some of the

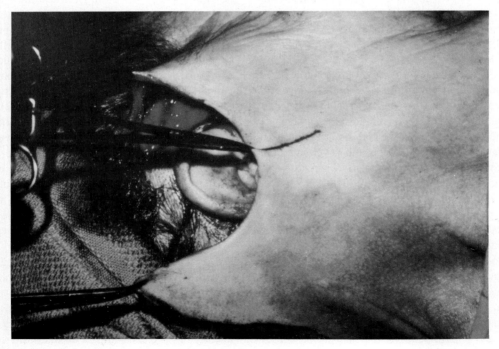

**FIG 54–1.**
The face-lift operation is performed by elevating the redundant facial and neck skin from the subcutaneous tissue, trimming the excess, advancing it and resuturing it.

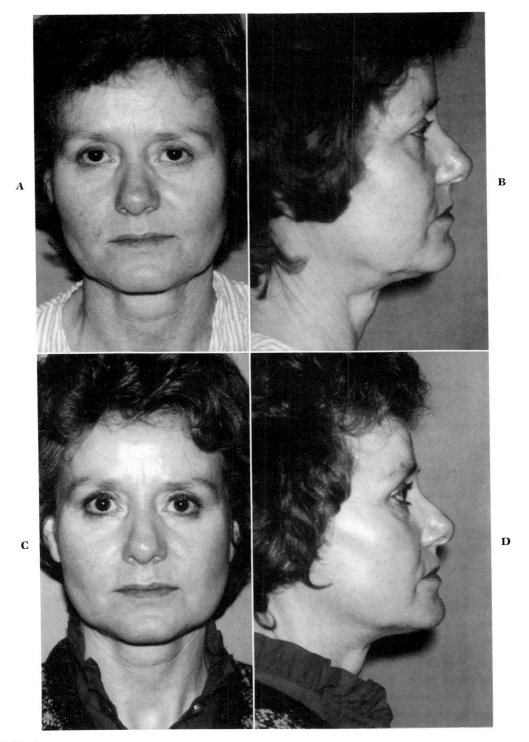

**FIG 54–2.**
Facial skin redundancy often affects the lower portion of the face and upper neck, **A** and **B,** but it can be resolved with a face-lift operation, as seen in the postoperative views, **C** and **D.**

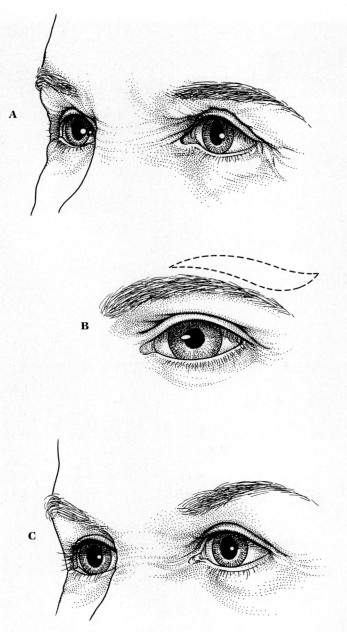

**FIG 54–3**.
The brow lift is performed by excising skin immediately superior to the eyebrows to elevate them and give a more alert and youthful appearance. (Redrawn after Tardy M, Jr.: Symposium on the aging face, *Otolaryngol Clin North Am* 13:207, 1980. Used by permission.)

forehead musculature, and excising the excess.

Blepharoplasty not only corrects the redundancy of skin that develops in both upper and lower eyelids, but also deals with the protruding periorbital fat that causes bulges in the eyelid skin. This operation requires an appreciation and understanding of eyelid anatomy. Indiscriminate removal of skin can cause excessive pressure on the eyelids, with resulting ectropion. It is important to be sensitive to the particular features of a patient's eyelid anatomy in helping to gauge how much eyelid skin should be removed (Fig. 54–4).

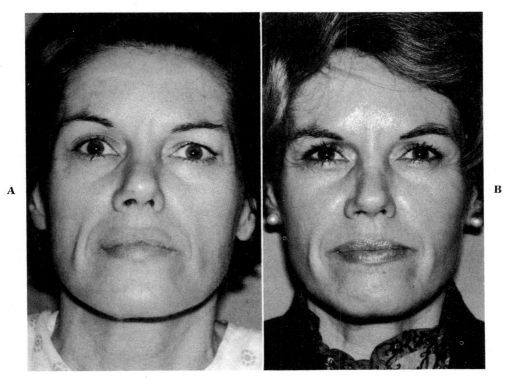

**FIG 54–4.**
A blepharoplasty coupled with a face-lift, **A,** often gives gratifying results for the patient, **B.**

It has been reported in the medical literature that blindness can occur following blepharoplasty. This is considered to be a complication of an orbital bleeding episode resulting from pressure on the optic nerve and compromise of its blood supply. Although this complication is rare, the patient must be aware of this and give consent to the surgery knowing full well that blindness may occur.

The procedures used to alter facial profile are common. Rhinoplasty is one of the most frequently performed of facial aesthetic procedures and can give dramatic results. It is a technically challenging operation that requires not only skills on the part of the surgeon, but also a certain wisdom that helps to define the problem and how it can be solved.

In the patient who has a recessed chin with normal dental occlusion, the profile can be altered with a chin implant, which is usually an alloplastic material placed either through a small skin incision below the chin or through the oral cavity (Fig. 54–5). Some surgeons prefer a small external skin incision to minimize the chance of infec-

tion that might occur with a transoral route of insertion.

Prominent malar bones are often a distinctive and attractive feature of facial beauty. In the patient who does not have prominent malar bones, alloplastic materials can be inserted either intraorally or through an extension of a lower-lid blepharoplasty incision.

The multiple procedures grouped under orthognathic surgery have the potential to dramatically alter facial profile. However, strictly speaking, these maxillofacial disproportions are associated with functional deformities and therefore are not repaired by cosmetic procedures.

The fine wrinkling of the skin can be corrected with a variety of techniques, all of which have certain limitations. The patient must understand that there are certain skin wrinkles, such as the nasolabial folds, for which there currently are no consistently reliable techniques of eradication. One approach to fine wrinkles is the so-called chemical peel operation. This involves the application of a paste that includes a concentration of phenol to the facial skin. Phenol is a caustic agent

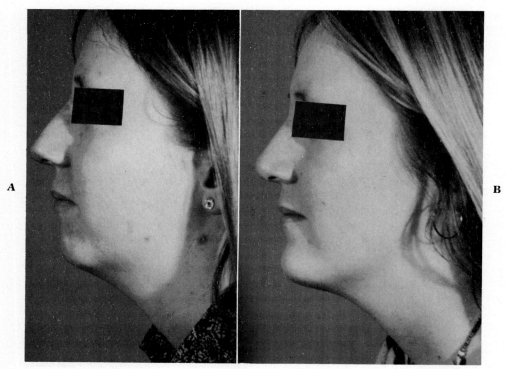

**FIG 54–5.**
A chin implant as an adjunct to rhinoplasty often provides dramatic improvement in the facial profile as seen in these preoperative, **A,** and postoperative, **B,** photographs.

that essentially produces a burn, which causes desquamation of the superficial layers of the epidermis with subsequent eradication of the facial wrinkles. However, some surgeons are hesitant to use this technique because of the apparent lack of control of the depth of the burn, depending on the patient's sensitivity to a particular phenol concentration. Arrhythmias have also been reported while the phenol-containing solution is in contact with the facial skin. In the hands of experienced users, it can give effective results.

The alternative to chemical peel is dermabrasion, which is essentially a form of sanding off the superficial layers of epidermis to remove wrinkles. This approach also requires a great deal of skill. Variable depths created by dermabrasion can create noticeable shadowing.

One of the newer approaches to dealing with fine wrinkles is the injection of liquid collagen into the skin to augment the depressed areas of the wrinkles. The liquid collagen is a bovine preparation. Patients considering this treatment must be skin-tested initially. Even with skin testing, there is no guarantee against an adverse reac-

tion. Liquid collagen can be applied in multiple settings. The results are not permanent because there is absorption after a variable period of time. The well-informed patient is often satisfied with this explanation and agrees to return for multiple injections.

There are other nonsurgical adjunctive procedures that are helpful in facial aesthetic surgery. After the surgical procedures have been performed and healing is complete, a skilled cosmetologist can add the extra touch that enhances the surgical changes. Hairstyling has an interesting psychologic effect. Studies have demonstrated that people tend to maintain the hairstyle that they were wearing during an enjoyable time of life. An example of this is a middle-aged person who is wearing a hairstyle that was popular during high school years. Often, a switch to a more contemporary hairstyle will result in a dramatic change. These nonsurgical matters should be discussed with the postoperative aesthetic surgery patient. Once informed, they can pursue the matters individually if they so desire.

Scar revision is an aspect of facial aesthetic

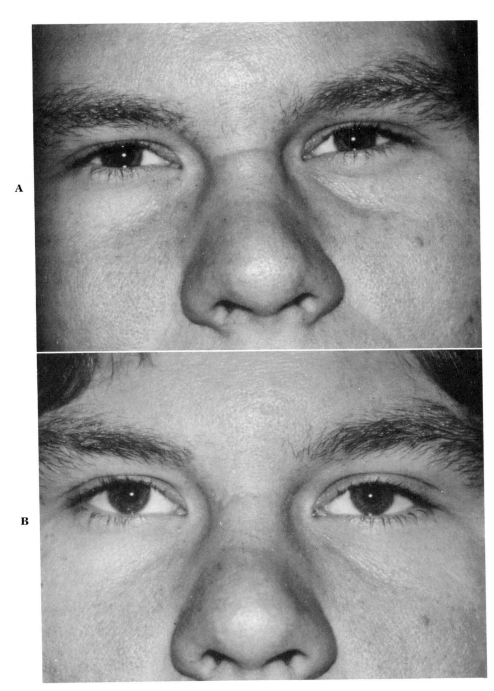

**FIG 54–6.**
Prominent nasal scar, **A,** is effectively camouflaged with scar revision, **B.**

surgery about which there is a fair amount of mis-understanding among health professionals and the public. After the skin has been injured and a scar created, nobody can make a scar disappear. The goal of scar revision is to trade the ugly scar for one that is less conspicuous. Once again, the major challenge to the surgeon is to define the problem. A scar's appearance can be improved by making it thinner and flatter and by trying to change its direction so that most or ideally all of it will lie in the usual skin creases of the face and neck.

The timing of scar revisions is important. It usually takes anywhere from 10 to 12 months for a scar to reach maturity after it is created. It is inappropriate to begin scar revisions earlier unless other factors take priority. As mentioned earlier, one must also consider the predilection for hypertrophic scar formation in the young person. It may be advisable to delay scar revision until the teenager has reached maturity.

Certain basic principles apply to how a scar revision is performed. These are based on general observations that a straight line is more noticeable than a crooked one. Sometimes a scar's direction does not need to be changed but just needs to be made thinner and converted into a crooked line to make it more difficult to see. Scar revision can be performed on an outpatient basis using local anesthesia. To the informed patient, it gives satisfying results in the overwhelming majority of instances (Fig. 54–6).

Adjunctive procedures to the initial surgical scar revision are also helpful. Sometimes, if the revised scar is slightly hypertrophic, a slight dermabrasion works to flatten it. The discreet use of cosmetics can provide the extra touch that decreases the awareness of a scar. The patient should be informed of the advisability of these adjunctive procedures, which usually results in patient satisfaction.

# Index

Tunable dye laser, 296
Tuning fork tests of hearing, 378–380
Turbinate
 anatomy of, 67, 69
 examination of, 15, 24
 hypertrophy of, 93–94
Tympanic cavity, 357–358; *see also* Middle ear
Tympanic membrane
 anatomy of, 356–357
 hearing and, 371
 infection of, 412–416
 perforation of
  chronic otitis media causing, 426–427
  traumatic, 438
 retraction of, 419
 trauma to, 437–438
Tympanography, AIDS and, 59
Tympanometry, 384
Tympanoplasty, 431, 471–475
Tympanosclerosis, 414

**U**

Ulceration, pharyngeal, drug-induced, 183
Umbo, 356
Unconscious patient, airway obstruction in, 315
Universal precautions, AIDS and, 58
Urticaria, 50
Usher's syndrome, 454
Utricle, 366–367
Uvula
 bifid, 218
 examination of, 16

**V**

Vagal body tumor, 340
Valium, for Ménière's disease, 507
Valleculae, 19
van der Hoeve's syndrome, 454
Variable nystagmus, 389
Varicosity, of tongue, 214, 216
Vascular system
 of face, 533
 neck injury and, 337
 salivary gland neoplasm and, 244
 tinnitus caused by, 490
 vertigo and, 504
Vascular tumor, of neck, 338
Vasoconstriction, 22
Vasodilator, 507
Vasomotor rhinitis, 92–93
Vehicular accident
 facial trauma from, 147–148
 laryngeal trauma from, 270
Vein, jugular, 322
Venous drainage of brain, 115
Ventricle, laryngeal, 252
 examination of, 19
Verrucous carcinoma, of buccal mucosa, 200–201
Vertebral basilar artery insufficiency, 511
Vertical mattress suture, 34, 35
Vertical nystagmus, 389
Vertical partial laryngectomy, 278
Vertigo and dizziness, 495–513; *see also* Vertigo and
  dizziness
 brainstem causes of, 512–513
 cholesteatoma and, 428
 Cogan's syndrome causing, 509
 differential diagnosis of, 499–502
 eight nerve causes of, 511–512
 examination for, 498–499
 external ear condition causing, 503
 middle ear condition causing, 503–506
 nonsystematized, 499–502
 patient history of, 496–498

perilymphatic fistula causing, 511
 positional, 511
 treatment of
  medical, 506–508
  surgical, 508–509, 510
 vertebral basilar artery and, 511
Vesicle, pemphigus causing, 183
Vestibular labyrinth, 366–369
Vestibular nerve, section of, 509, 510
Vestibular neuronitis, 504
Vestibular system
 physiology of, 376
 testing of, 388–397
Vestibule, nasal
 anatomy of, 67
 diseases of, 89–90
 examination of, 23
Videostroboscopy, 255
Vincent's angina, 183
Viral infection
 Bell's palsy and, 523
 epiglottitis as, 265–266
 hearing loss caused by, 454
 herpes zoster oticus as, 411
 laryngitis as, 266–267
 laryngotracheobronchitis as, 263–264
 pharyngeal, 181
 of salivary glands, 235
Vision
 dizziness and, 499–500
 facial trauma and, 149
Vitamin deficiency, 500
Vocal cord
 examination of, 19, 21
 inflammation of, 267–269
 laryngitis and, 267
 paralysis of
  congenital, 260
  reconstruction after, 281–282
 phonation and, 254
Vocal fold, 250, 252
Vocal restoration, 277–282
Voice disorder, 283–287
Voice testing of hearing, 378
Vomer, 15

**W**

Walkman, hearing loss caused by, 458
Wall, lateral, nasal, 24
Warthin's tumor, 240–241, 242
Wattles, 321, 323
Wax in ear, 403–404
 vertigo and, 503
Web, laryngeal, 261
Weber-Fergusson incision for maxillectomy, 132
Weber test of hearing, 378–379
Welder, ear injury to, 438
Wharton's duct; *see also* Submandibular duct
 anatomy of, 226–227
Whiplash injury, 504
Whirling, sensation of, 498; *see also* Vertigo and dizziness
Whispered voice test, 378
White lesion, oral, 219–222
Window, round, 376
Windshield accident, 148
Wound healing, 28–29
Wrinkling of skin, chemical peel for, 601–602

**X**

Xylocaine, for soft tissue surgery, 30

**Z**

Zygomatic fracture, 153–157, 158